EVIDENCE-BASEI
FOR CHILDREN WITH AUTISM
The CARD Model

EVIDENCE-BASED TREATMENT FOR CHILDREN WITH AUTISM
The CARD Model

Edited by

DOREEN GRANPEESHEH

JONATHAN TARBOX

ADEL C. NAJDOWSKI

JULIE KORNACK

Center for Autism and Related Disorders

AMSTERDAM • BOSTON • HEIDELBERG • LONDON
NEW YORK • OXFORD • PARIS • SAN DIEGO
SAN FRANCISCO • SINGAPORE • SYDNEY • TOKYO
Academic Press is an imprint of Elsevier

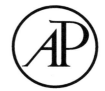

Academic Press is an imprint of Elsevier
The Boulevard, Langford Lane, Kidlington, Oxford, OX5 1GB, UK
225 Wyman Street, Waltham, MA 02451, USA

First published 2014

Notices
Knowledge and best practice in this field are constantly changing. As new research
and experience broaden our understanding, changes in research methods, professional
practices, or medical treatment may become necessary.

Practitioners and researchers must always rely on their own experience and knowledge
in evaluating and using any information, methods, compounds, or experiments described
herein. In using such information or methods they should be mindful of their own safety
and the safety of others, including parties for whom they have a professional responsibility.

To the fullest extent of the law, neither the Publisher nor the authors, contributors, or
editors, assume any liability for any injury and/or damage to persons or property as a
matter of product liability, negligence or otherwise, or from any use or operation of any
methods, products, instructions, or ideas contained in the material herein.

British Library Cataloguing in Publication Data
A catalogue record for this book is available from the British Library

Library of Congress Cataloguing in Publication Data
A catalogue record for this book is available from the Library of Congress

ISBN: 978-0-12-411603-0

For information on all Academic Press publications
visit our website at **store.elsevier.com**

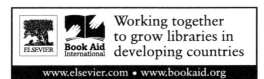

Working together
to grow libraries in
developing countries

www.elsevier.com • www.bookaid.org

Contents

II

TREATMENT PROCEDURES

8. Treatment Settings
MARY ANN CASSELL

9. Parent Involvement
EVELYN R. GOULD, VINCE REDMOND

III

PROGRAM CONTENT

10. Introduction to the Center for Autism and Related Disorders Curriculum Series
ADEL C. NAJDOWSKI

11. Language
MICHELE R. BISHOP, ADEL C. NAJDOWSKI

12. Play
JONATHAN TARBOX, ANGELA PERSICKE

13. Adaptive

JONATHAN TARBOX, ANGELA PERSICKE, RYAN BERGSTROM

14. Motor

MICHELE R. BISHOP

15. Academics

MICHELE R. BISHOP, CAROLYNN BREDEK

16. Social

JENNIFER YAKOS

17. Cognition

ADEL C. NAJDOWSKI, ANGELA PERSICKE, EVELYN KUNG

18. Executive Functions

ADEL C. NAJDOWSKI, ANGELA PERSICKE, EVELYN KUNG

IV

TREATMENT OVERSIGHT

19. Clinical Supervision

JONATHAN TARBOX, ADEL C. NAJDOWSKI

20. Data Collection and Treatment Evaluation

JONATHAN TARBOX

V

LOOKING FORWARD

Preface

Thirty-six years ago, I took a class at UCLA called Behavior Modification. It was an upper division course in psychology taught by a charismatic, funny, and very popular professor named O. Ivar Lovaas. Little did I know then that I was embarking on a journey that would shape the rest of my life. I studied with Ivar for 12 years. He taught me a great deal about autism, and he showed me how the environment can change behavior. As my mentor, Ivar gave me the foundation for what would eventually become the CARD Model. During those 12 years, Ivar introduced me to B.F. Skinner, whose work exemplified everything we now call applied behavior analysis (ABA), and to Bernie Rimland, whose foresight taught me to look beyond ABA when treating autism and to consider the value of biomedical interventions because autism is so often accompanied by comorbid conditions whose resolution optimizes the effectiveness of ABA.

When I started working with children with autism in the late 1970s, it was a very different world. Autism was rare, with a prevalence of 1 in 15,000 children. Very little research had been done on the etiology of autism, and we knew only that autism was a very debilitating, severe, and lifelong disorder. We didn't know it could be treated, we didn't think it could be overcome, and we most certainly never imagined it would one day affect 1 in 68 children.

In 1979, I started working at the Young Autism Project at UCLA. We were in the midst of experimenting with behavioral procedures to find a way to reduce the severely self-injurious behaviors of a handful of children who were living at the Autism Unit at Camarillo State Hospital, and we had just started fine-tuning the steps for teaching attention, compliance, and basic language. We called these teaching steps "Discrete Trial Training."

The Young Autism Project consisted of a handful of graduate students who were training undergraduates how to use behavior modification to teach a small number of children whom we had been treating for a few years. This "clinic" was the setting of the 1987 seminal study, *Behavioral Treatment and Normal Educational and Intellectual Functioning in Young Autistic Children* (Lovaas, 1987), which proved not only that children with autism can learn but also that they can learn to overcome the symptoms of autism as a whole. I enjoyed providing therapy to the children in that study. I learned the importance of good documentation and data collection from that study, and I realized for the first time in my life that,

xiii

with perseverance and courage, we can overcome even those things we think are impossible to change.

In 1990, I earned my doctorate from UCLA and began working with children with autism outside of UCLA. Treating children with autism was, to be honest, the only thing I knew how to do well. I had completed my training with Ivar, had worked with and supervised many children of all levels of functioning, and had conducted research on many different aspects of autism; it was time to move on. Opening my own center was really not something I had planned. A couple of Ivar's previous graduates were running autism programs at other University of California campuses, and Ivar had suggested that I consider doing the same. While the idea appealed to me, my parents had just emigrated from Iran and were living near me in Los Angeles. We had been separated by thousands of miles for years, and I was determined to stay in Los Angeles and be with them. When I left UCLA, a few children had aged out of the Young Autism Project (then called the Clinic for the Behavioral Treatment of Children). Ivar asked me to take over the treatment of these children, and so my practice began.

I was supervising a handful of children and had hired ten or so therapists to work with them. Since I had never really run a business before, I was driving from house to house, often training therapists at local coffee shops at night and paying them from my personal checkbook to make sure the children got the hours of therapy they needed. It wasn't long until I realized I needed an actual location, so I wouldn't have to waste so much time driving. Initially, I subleased an office near UCLA in Westwood, but, within a few months, I had met so many new families who needed help that I outgrew my Westwood space. I moved just north of Westwood to the San Fernando Valley, where I leased my first actual clinic space in Encino. That's where I chose the name CARD, and that's where I incorporated the business as well. CARD officially opened in June 1990.

From 1990 to 1993, the business grew from 5 children to 25. I hired therapists from the UCLA program, and I myself supervised the treatment, wrote the reports, scheduled the therapists, conducted the school observations, issued the billing, and completed the payroll. Many of those original CARD employees still work with me. One of the therapists, Niloufar Ardakani, offered to help me with some of the administrative tasks. One day, as we were filling out billing forms, with excitement over our growth, Nilou asked me, "How many children do you think we can treat?" I remember saying that I couldn't imagine we'd ever be able to handle more than 40 to 50 children since I was only able to supervise that many. It hadn't yet occurred to me that I could train supervisors as well. In 1995, when I was expecting my first child, I realized it was time to choose a supervisor to cover for me on maternity leave. That was when I suddenly realized that CARD could grow beyond the 50 children I had envisioned. With that supervisor (Evelyn Kung, who is now CARD's clinical director), we doubled our clients and began a rapid phase of expansion. (Nilou, by the way, is now in charge of one of our billing departments at CARD.)

With the realization that I could train supervisors and expand the impact of CARD, I began to establish new CARD locations. I opened a second CARD clinic in New York as a result of my relationship with Catherine Maurice, an early autism advocate and author of *Let Me Hear Your Voice* (1993), a book about the impact of ABA therapy on Catherine's two children. By this time, it was the mid-1990s, and the Internet age was just upon us. A group of families who believed in Lovaas's style of ABA had formed a group on the Internet called "ME-List," taking its name from Lovaas's first book on autism, *Teaching Developmentally Disabled Children – The Me Book* (1981). We relied on this book early in autism treatment when applying the principles of ABA to treat the symptoms of autism. The Me-List parents created a very rudimentary form of a chat room on Prodigy, one of the two existing Internet portals available at that time. Many of these families knew me from when I had supervised their children at UCLA. One of the parents, a dad who lived in the San Jose area in Northern California, had asked for my help, and I had been flying to San Jose to help his team of therapists. One day, he asked me if I could open a CARD clinic in his area, and I explained that I would need 25 families in order to make it work. He posted the following notice on the ME-list: "CARD will open a clinic anywhere there are 25 families who need help." Over the next 5 years, I opened 10 clinics, all because of that one posting on the Internet. CARD now has clinics throughout the United States, and we are opening more clinics every year. At any one time, we work with over 1,500 families and have close to 2,000 employees (therapists, senior therapists, care coordinators, case managers, supervisors, administrators, managers, and directors).

I didn't build CARD alone. The core of the company consists of people who joined me in the early years, and they have continued to grow and develop beside me. These people are called "seniors." They do almost everything, including training (Theresa Contreras, Monique Ericson, Cecilia Knight, Denise Rhine, Jennifer Yakos), quality assurance (Evelyn Kung, Sienna Greener-Wooten), family counseling and training (Vince Redmond), curriculum development (Carolynn Bredek, Kathy Thompson), administration (Hank Moore, Cathy Vizconde), daily operations (Sarah Cho), expansion (Catherine Minch, John Galle), CARD Academy (Mary Ann Cassell), training of our affiliate international sites (Soo Cho), and specialized areas of programming (Lisa Bancroft, Renat Matalon). A few non-clinical people have also made significant contributions to CARD since the early days. These include Andrea Harrington (finance), Anderson Raminelli (information technology), and Nicole

Simpson, who has managed numerous projects since 1995. These seniors have been with CARD through decades of change, and they have always welcomed new talent with humility and adjusted to change with flexibility. Their spirit and character have deeply influenced the CARD culture in which we are determined never to stop learning.

Without a doubt, CARD would not be what it is today without my colleagues Cathy Vizconde and Dennis Dixon. Cathy has literally been at my side since 1994, spending two decades helping me develop the structure that enables CARD to continue to grow. Dennis, who joined CARD in 2007, has helped take CARD into the next century. With his uncanny ability to organize our goals while always keeping our mission directly in view, we have now built educational games that will help our children learn, even when they are playing.

Together, we have learned a great deal more than we ever imagined. We have learned that autism is different from any other disorder. It affects more and more children each year, and despite substantial research, we still don't know why so many children are affected! We have learned that autism affects the whole family – the parents, the siblings, and even the extended family. We have learned that autism involves a genetic predisposition but that it is triggered by environmental factors, such as toxins and contaminants that may negatively influence a compromised immune system. We have learned that many children with autism suffer from inflammation of the gastrointestinal tract, that many have mitochondrial disorders, that numerous biochemical abnormalities interact with autism, and that viral, bacterial, and fungal infections can play a large role in the development of the symptoms we call autism. We have learned that many children have sensory sensitivities and dysregulation. We have learned that no two children with autism are the same. Most importantly, we have learned that good-quality ABA works, and children can recover! (And we have learned that it is controversial to say that children can recover, something we elaborate on in our chapter *Philosophy and Mores*.)

Together with their children, parents inspire us with their utter dedication and determination. Bryce Miler and Bonnie Yates, whose sons I treated over 20 years ago, both made careers out of securing treatment for other families. Bryce has helped hundreds of families gain insurance coverage for autism treatment, even before autism mandates took effect. Bonnie has worked tirelessly to ensure that families understood their legal rights and to secure funding for treatment. Many more parents have continued to teach me, guide me, advise me, and help me. Most of all, the parents have always given me the drive to continue to look for the answers.

People often ask me, "What's different about CARD?" I reply that CARD staff have the benefit of mentors who have treated the symptoms of autism for nearly 25 years. We have learned a lot in that time, and we are able to take that knowledge, assimilate it, and apply it with an open mind, knowing that we still have much to learn from our children and from our families. We have had many years to develop our particular type of ABA – the CARD Model – and we have been blessed by the experts who have joined us over the years. My co-editors, Jonathan Tarbox and Adel Najdowski, are not only amazing content area experts in ABA but also are courageous pioneers in the field who were not afraid to join my mentors and me in saying, "Yes, we can help recover children from the symptoms called autism. Yes, those diagnosed with autism can lead healthy, happy, and functional lives."

Autism continues to be an enigma. Each year, we learn something new that helps us understand it better. Most of all, we learn from those affected by autism themselves. Many of our children, on their way to overcoming autism, have told me how they see the world. They have told me that background noises are louder to them than voices and that they find some sounds, such as doors closing, to be funny while other sounds, such as vacuum cleaners, cause excruciating pain. Some children have shown me how brilliant they are, including a 9-year-old who finished high school academics at age 6 but couldn't make a single friend; a nonverbal 12-year-old who taught himself to play the piano and became such a virtuoso that hundreds attend his concerts; a 15-year-old who couldn't learn his basic prepositions but produced art that has been displayed in museums worldwide. The list of accomplishments goes on and on. Some children have amazing skills, and others amaze me with their patience, determination, tolerance, and kind nature.

Autism is not something to fear; it is a name that describes some "differences." Some of these differences make life harder, and some make it easier. Some of our children suffer and struggle because their symptoms and, more specifically, the underlying cause of their particular autism are painful or debilitating. Some learn ways to compensate and adapt, and others manage not only to excel but also to make extraordinary contributions to our world.

As autism prevalence has increased, CARD has grown to try to meet the demand for services. Knowing that the prevalence rates represent unique and wonderful individuals, I have always been determined not to dilute the quality of CARD treatment. Over time, it has become clear that our mission – to lead the field of autism by providing global access to the latest scientifically proven, top-quality behavioral services to our patients and their families and, in doing so, help them achieve the most they can – is more likely to be achieved by liberally sharing the CARD Model through the publication of this book and thereby enabling others to replicate the work we do. In this way, we can all work together to achieve our common goal of helping as many individuals as possible. We hope this book contributes to your understanding and your success.

Doreen Granpeesheh, Ph.D., BCBA-D

Acknowledgments

The authors would like to sincerely thank Sienna Greener-Wooten, Denise Rhine, Lisa Schrader, Soo Cho, and John Galle for their consultation on individual chapters. The authors would also like to sincerely thank Adrianna Bautista, Shirin Mostofi, Sarah Schwanz, Monica Garcia, Lena Ameripour, Tasia Wells, Carole Eden, and Kellee Chi for proofing chapters.

I would like to thank my mother, who taught me not to fear; my husband, Greg, whose love keeps me going; and my children, Nicky, Sonny, and Charly, who fill my life with joy every single day. I dedicate this book to the parents. Your courage has no bounds. I am grateful for your trust in placing your children in my care. I will do all I can to help them lead happy, healthy lives.

Doreen Granpeesheh

I would like to begin by thanking D, the first mom of a child with autism I ever met and the woman whose commitment, courage, humor, and love for her son inspired me to pursue behavior analysis and autism as a career. I would also like to thank Dr. Linda J. Parrott Hayes and the rest of the faculty at the University of Nevada, Reno Behavior Analysis Program, for the privilege of studying with them. My work on this book has built on the past 9 years of collaboration with the incredible team of clinicians and scientists that make up CARD – I am forever grateful for the opportunity to work with you. Last, I would like to acknowledge my wife, Courtney Tarbox, and my children, Johnny and Cleo, for teaching me what love is.

Jonathan Tarbox

To be able to put into writing the work that we do so passionately with individuals diagnosed with autism has been an incredible journey. It would not have been possible if it weren't for the many brilliant individuals I have learned from, beginning with Dr. Sidney Bijou and Dr. Patrick Ghezzi who taught me passion, dedication, fearlessness, and commitment in the service of autism. In addition, the knowledge and experience I have gained from working with CARD clinicians over the past 9 years is immeasurable. I also thank my husband, Adam, and my children, Conner and Kendi, for their continued support for me in all my career endeavors.

Adel C. Najdowski

No achievement of mine would be as meaningful without the loving support of my husband, Russ, and my children, Kyle, Cody, and Jake. I also want to recognize the extraordinary perseverance of parents and activists in the autism community. Unfettered access to the treatment described in this book is an ongoing challenge taken on by thousands of determined individuals who continue to fight for others long after their personal battles are won. Their stories of adversity, hope, and triumph inspire me every day.

Julie Kornack

Introduction

Doreen Granpeesheh

Welcome to *Evidence-Based Treatment for Children with Autism: The CARD Model*. Our goal in writing this book is to create the world's most practical, user-friendly, and enjoyable-to-read manual for treating children with autism spectrum disorder (ASD). Our secondary goal is to describe the way we view the world: the Center for Autism and Related Disorders (CARD) Model of treatment for children with ASD. Hundreds of different treatments are available for children with ASD, most of which have little or no research support. The CARD Model is a successful approach to providing evidence-based treatment that is based on and incorporates the principles and procedures of applied behavior analysis (ABA). There are many different specializations within ABA treatment for children with ASD, including Pivotal Response Treatment, the Early Start Denver Model, Incidental Teaching, the Picture Exchange Communication System, the Verbal Behavioral Approach, to name a few. Many approaches to ABA treatment for children with ASD are distinguished by the fact that they emphasize one particular treatment procedure or another or one particular area of functioning (e.g., language). The CARD Model is an example of a *comprehensive* approach to the behavioral treatment of children with ASD. By comprehensive, we mean that the CARD Model emphasizes the need for the use of all empirically validated treatment procedures in a customized mix that meets the individual needs of each child at any given time. In addition, comprehensive means that every area of human functioning is addressed in proportions that match the degree of need. Although the CARD Model is, in some sense, a collection of treatment procedures, at a more fundamental level it is built upon a set of basic values and philosophical beliefs that are described in more detail in Chapter 2.

We do not claim that the CARD Model is more effective than any other model of comprehensive behavioral intervention for children with ASD. In fact, virtually no research has directly compared the effectiveness of

1

different models of comprehensive ABA, so it is impossible to address this question with data at this time. However, great pains have been taken to modify and hone the CARD Model over the past 24 years, and the model continues to evolve and improve. Thus, we believe that the approach to comprehensive intervention described in this treatment manual is the best, and we sincerely hope that this book will assist clinicians who are treating individuals with ASD. Furthermore, in writing this book, we invite scientists to join us in defining other treatment modalities and detailing other unique blends of evidence-based treatment and clinical decision-making guidelines. Further articulation and manualization of the various approaches to intervention for children with ASD can only help decrease confusion, increase clarity, spur comparative research, and, ultimately, improve intervention for children on the spectrum.

Thorough program descriptions increase accessibility through replication. As more professionals are able to determine the needs and resources required to implement this model, providing CARD treatment becomes increasingly feasible. This, in turn, may increase accessibility to this effective treatment. Program descriptions remediate the limitations faced within the scientific literature regarding treatment research and efficacy. That is, treatment descriptions in research articles are limited by the space restrictions of scientific journals, and the articles focus, therefore, more on scientific methodology and treatment effects than on describing how to do treatment. It is one thing to know the results of treatment and another to understand how to implement it. Without practical expertise, there is a greater risk of poor implementation, lower quality, and inaccessibility due to lack of resources.

INTRODUCTION TO EARLY INTENSIVE BEHAVIORAL INTERVENTION

The type of autism treatment that this manual describes is commonly referred to as Early Intensive Behavioral Intervention (EIBI). Other common acronyms from the research literature that mean the same thing are Early Intensive Behavioral Treatment (EIBT) and Intensive Behavioral Treatment (IBT). EIBI consists of intervention delivered in a one-to-one format, starting as young as possible (before the age of 3), done for 30 or more hours per week, and continued for 2 or more years (Granpeesheh, Tarbox, & Dixon, 2009). The general goal of EIBI is to remediate all skill deficits that a child with ASD presents, so she can be caught up to typical development, at least to the greatest degree possible. Behavioral intervention can also be delivered at lower intensities and for older children and produce substantial treatment effects. However, EIBI is the treatment approach for ASD that is supported by the largest amount of scientific research (see Chapter 27).

FORMAT OF THIS BOOK

This book is first and foremost a treatment manual. The primary purpose of this book is to help practitioners work with children with ASD. This book is not a review of published research, although the content of the book is derived from research. Thus, in order to save space and make the book more readable, we have intentionally included only the minimum of scholarly references. For a comprehensive scholarly handbook on treatment for young children with ASD, we recommend *Handbook of Early Intervention for Autism Spectrum Disorders: Research, Policy, and Practice* (Tarbox, Dixon, Sturmey, & Matson, 2014). The primary purpose of that handbook is to provide a scholarly review of research, and it consists of 29 chapters authored by the world's leading autism researchers from prestigious universities and research institutes. The chapters in that book consist of reviews and critical analyses of research, not how-to instructions for helping children with ASD, the latter being the subject matter and purpose of this manual.

This manual is divided into five sections. Section I, Background, opens the book with a basic description of the book, describes the philosophical perspectives and mores upon which the CARD Model is built, and gives a description of the ASD diagnosis. Section II, Treatment Procedures, contains six chapters describing the procedural aspects of the CARD Model of treatment for children with ASD. In Section II, we focus on *how* to teach. Section III, Program Content, addresses *what* to teach. Nine chapters comprise this section. The first introduces the rationale and approach that CARD has taken to building the most comprehensive curriculum in the world for teaching skills to children with ASD. The next eight chapters address each major area of human functioning, giving practical advice on how to teach the myriad skills one may need to teach when implementing comprehensive intervention with children with ASD. Section IV, Treatment Oversight, is dedicated to describing practical and logistical details that are often omitted from treatment manuals. Useful tips are given regarding job descriptions, treatment settings, the clinical supervision process, and interdisciplinary collaboration. Section V, Looking Forward, concludes the book. This section includes chapters that address the burgeoning role of technology in autism treatment, global dissemination, how to maintain close contact with emerging research, and how to ensure that your treatment model revolves around research to ensure that children with ASD benefit from scientific findings that help improve the outcome of interventions.

HISTORY OF THE CARD MODEL

The Center for Autism and Related Disorders was founded by Dr. Doreen Granpeesheh after she completed her doctorate in psychology under the mentorship of Dr. O. Ivar Lovaas at the University of California, Los Angeles. After working as a researcher and clinician in Lovaas's clinic, providing treatment to the children who were participants in the seminal 1987 paper by Lovaas, Dr. Granpeesheh founded CARD in 1990 with the goal of disseminating top-quality behavioral treatment to as many children as possible. From the beginning, Dr. Granpeesheh's goals have always been to maintain the highest quality of treatment and to provide global accessibility to that treatment. Today at CARD, we continue to believe that sacrificing either of these two values is unacceptable. Children will not have the opportunity to fulfill their potential if treatment is not top quality, and millions of children will go without any treatment if more is not done to increase access to effective treatment throughout the United States and around the world. Across the 24 years that CARD has been in existence, we have always maintained a perspective that our treatment model is continuously evolving as we incorporate new research findings, update technology, and increase accessibility. Therefore, every aspect of the CARD Model has been analyzed, adjusted, and reworked countless times. The origins and foundations of the CARD Model came from Lovaas's UCLA Young Autism Project, but the CARD Model has not been recognizable as "Lovaas therapy" for many years. The version of the CARD Model presented in this manual is, therefore, the most current version, and further refinements will surely continue to be made. Nevertheless, the overall combination of treatment procedures and the scope and detail of the curriculum have reached a level of comprehensiveness such that the CARD Model is more than ready for public consumption.

TONE OF THIS BOOK

We intentionally wrote this manual using a commonsense, almost conversational tone. This approach is still somewhat uncommon in scientific writing because many fear that using everyday language may dilute the precision of what they are trying to say. While this can be true, we also believe that scientists often hide behind dry and boring language because it makes it easier to speak without having to actually say anything useful. The purpose of this book is to provide you with useful information, so we are going to "tell it like it is" – we can't think of any reason not to talk to you in the way we would if we were standing right in front of you. Writing a treatment manual that is, on the one hand, intended for everyday use by a wide variety of practitioners and, on the other hand, based on scientific principles, procedures, and research, is always going to be a balancing act. Therefore, we often explain the same idea twice: once in commonsense terms and once in technical behavioral jargon. Perhaps teachers and clinicians will prefer the former, and scientists will prefer the latter. Our one goal throughout writing this manual, however, is to provide you with information that will be useful and interesting to read, and we sincerely hope that we have done that! We hope that you will enjoy reading this manual and that you will become part of the increasing voices that speak of the benefits of the CARD Model.

Philosophy and Mores

Doreen Granpeesheh, Jonathan Tarbox

All professionals working with individuals with autism spectrum disorder (ASD) possess their own values and philosophical perspectives, and each organization consists of a unique culture, inevitably built both from an implicit blend of the individual values of the employees who work there and the values of the organization that are explicitly stated and promoted. At Center for Autism and Related Disorders (CARD), we believe that values guide action and that it is therefore crucial to clarify one's values and make them explicit, all the while being reasonable and open-minded about differing perspectives. In this chapter, we briefly describe the core values and philosophical perspectives that form the foundation for the CARD Model of behavioral intervention for children with ASD. Although values and philosophy sound like highly conceptual topics, we take a practical approach by giving concrete examples of everyday clinical and organizational decision making as examples of actions guided by CARD values.

ALL HUMANS ARE CAPABLE OF LEARNING

We believe that all human beings are capable of learning. The history of developmental disabilities, in general, and of ASD, in particular, is comprised of a long, sad series of popular misconceptions about why people with developmental disabilities cannot learn. Terms such as "untrainable" are thankfully no longer considered acceptable, but the underlying bias to blame teaching failures on children with ASD remains the same. Dozens of excuses have been offered by those who fail to produce successful learning, but they all boil down to one false notion: There is something inside people with ASD that prevents them from learning. This is just plain wrong. All human beings are capable of learning a little bit more tomorrow than they know today, and children with ASD are no exception.

Because all humans are unique, each individual child's rate of progress in learning is different. Each person's learning is affected differently by various environments, procedures, and contexts, so individualized treatment programs must be designed to maximize strengths and remediate skill deficits based on each individual's unique characteristics. This is why it is so critical that the educational, social, and behavioral development of each child is continuously monitored by highly trained experts in evidence-based treatment.

CHILDREN WITH AUTISM ARE WHOLE PEOPLE

We believe that all children with ASD are whole people, consisting of biology, physiology, sensory profiles, a family system in which she lives, and a long and complex history of reinforcement. There is an old saying that, "If you have met one child with autism, you have met one child with autism." That is to say, each child is different, and no two children are the same. This basic assumption is extremely important because it affects everything we do. For example, if you have used one particular way of teaching a particular skill to children with ASD, and it has worked with the last 20 children, that does not necessarily mean it is going to work with the next child. Every set of parents is also unique. Each family's cultural background, language status, economic status, and individual health status are going to affect the treatment that you deliver to their child since that child is part of that family system.

FEARLESSNESS

A wise soldier once said, "The difference between a hero and a coward is not fear. Everyone has fear. The difference is what you do while you are afraid." Of course, treating ASD is not the same as being shot at in a war, but the quote has implications for what we do on a daily basis. Life is full of opportunities to make mistakes and fail. It is tempting in all areas of daily life, including in the course of providing services to people with ASD, to focus on the negative, to always identify ways in which something can go wrong. This is a natural tendency, and it is probably healthy and adaptive, at least to some degree. After all, if all dangers are ignored, one is bound to do something careless that will have negative consequences. However, we have found that great things are rarely accomplished when we do what feels safe. We believe it is our duty, and it is the duty of autism treatment providers, to make a real difference in the world. Millions of individuals with ASD go without treatment day after day because treatment providers aren't available or because funding for treatment is denied. All of those individuals deserve the opportunity to fulfill their potential. We have found, almost without exception, that you simply have to step outside your comfort zone if you want to make a real difference in the world. The universe has a natural tendency to change slowly if left to its own devices, and human culture is no different. Real change requires practitioners to change their own behavior in large and often uncomfortable ways.

Many of the most important steps we have taken in making evidence-based treatment available to more children with ASD seemed reckless at the time. For example, decisions regarding how many new staff to train and hire, where and when to open new clinics, and whether to work with a new funding source that introduces bureaucratic challenges are very likely to be influenced by your fears of failure, particularly from a business perspective. We have found, time and again, that if we make top-quality treatment for children with ASD available to the community, families need it and will work with us to make treatment available for their children. Of course, expansion and growth need to be tempered by real-life financial contingencies, but if you wait until every single detail has been planned out or if you wait until you have a virtual guarantee that everything you do will work, your organization, and the entire discipline of applied behavior analysis (ABA), will never catch up with the desperate needs of the autism community.

Running an organization is full of decisions to be made and tasks to be carried out that engender fear, even in the most seasoned clinicians. To lead effectively, these fears cannot influence decision making. Dealing with problematic staff is a classic example. If leaders allow fear of disapproval or fear that their staff will not like them to stand in the way of doing what needs to be done, then negative consequences for the organization and, ultimately, for the children are unavoidable. If you avoid giving corrective feedback to an employee or colleague who desperately needs it, you do not make the problem go away; you just demonstrate to the rest of the organization that you are not willing to face the problem. Initiating any major organizational change is another classic example. In order to get better, one needs to admit that one is not "good enough" as one currently is. To admit that one needs to design and implement a better clinical staff training procedure, one must admit that one's current procedures need improvement. To admit that one needs to hire more clinical supervisors is to admit that one's current supervisors are overworked and, therefore, probably not performing at their best. All of these scenarios are real decision points that providers of autism treatment face on a daily basis, and all of them make a real-life difference in the quality of services one can offer one's clients. Being fearless means behaving how you know you should, even when it is dreadfully uncomfortable.

INNOVATION

At CARD, we believe it is important to be in front of the wave of innovation, within the fields of autism and ABA specifically, and within the economy and technology in general. In a very real sense, change is the nature of the universe, and organizations that resist change will never succeed in preventing it; they will simply be left behind. To this end, the CARD approach to innovation includes innovating the ways in which ABA treatment, training, and supervision can be done remotely through global workshop and consultation services (practical details to be provided in Chapter 28 on global dissemination). The most obvious source of change and innovation in the world today is the information technology revolution. Many in ABA have been leery of the intrusion of technology into ABA – an approach to treatment that is so fundamentally human and social. Caution is warranted, but the information technology revolution cannot be held back, and technology holds tremendous promise for bringing down the cost of ABA treatment and increasing accessibility to more people living with ASD around the world. Chapter 26 on technology will discuss this potential further.

OPEN-MINDEDNESS

We all want to be right. Unfortunately, this desire can get in the way of being as effective as we can be. The world of autism treatment is a complex one, and many players are at the table, all of whom think they are experts and that they have the right perspective. The resulting situation is incredibly complex and often contradictory. This complexity is, of course, tremendously frustrating for parents and families living with ASD, but it can be difficult for professionals as well. In the face of so much chaos, it can be tempting to "circle the wagons" and take a stand for your personal view and fight against others' influence. The reality of the situation, however, is much more complex. At CARD, we believe that we will never know everything and that we can only be our best if we are constantly open to the ideas of others. Conflicts among professionals of differing disciplines are often a source of consternation in autism treatment. There is a stereotype of the arrogant behavior analyst who believes that a hardcore ABA perspective on the world is the only thing worth talking about and that anyone who doesn't get it is stupid. Thankfully, the reality of the field is that less than 1 percent of behavior analysts fall into that stereotype. The truth of the matter is that many thousands of professionals are genuinely dedicated to helping individuals with ASD lead better lives. It is also possible that the majority of the treatment procedures that are being implemented out there do not actually work, and entire disciplines may be based on theories and procedures that are not actually effective in treating ASD. This possibility has led some behavior analysts to become frustrated with professionals who propound the myriad unproven treatments, and this frustration is understandable. However, behavior analysts are not the only professionals who treat ASD, nor will we ever be. Nor do we want to be. It is critical to the continued health and vitality of the science of behavior analysis that we remain open to the contributions of other professionals, as well as those who are not treatment professionals, such as family members and advocates. Section III, the section on the CARD curriculum, will describe in great detail how information from cognitive and developmental psychology has been used to create a more comprehensive curriculum than had been developed from a purely behavioral approach in the past. Purely behavioral procedures are still used to teach the content, but a productive, vibrant cross-pollination among the various disciplines has helped to create our curriculum and has the promise to continue to help to optimize the development of the discipline of behavior analysis.

Frequently in autism treatment, professionals from particular disciplines appear to fail to understand (or perhaps intentionally disregard) the contributions of other disciplines. For example, consider a child with ASD who suffers from diarrhea several times per day for an extended period of time and who also engages in frequent tantrums. A particularly close-minded behavior analyst might insist that the tantrums are purely behavioral and simply need to be placed on extinction. Worse yet, the behavior analyst might make medical recommendations regarding how to treat the diarrhea without referring the learner to a medical doctor. Consider another awful, and yet sadly common, example. A child with ASD sees a medical doctor who is a practitioner of unproven or off-label medical treatments for ASD. After a brief initial interview with the child's mother, the doctor prescribes methyl B-12 shots and explains that they are likely going to result in the child's increasing his language from one-word utterances to three-word sentences. In this case, the medical doctor is failing to realize that his scope of practice is to treat his patient's medical problem, not to increase language, especially by way of a treatment that has no significant research support. To be open-minded is to be willing to consider other perspectives and not sacrifice your foundational professional beliefs.

INSISTENCE ON HIGHEST QUALITY

At CARD, we believe that autism service provision must be conducted with the highest possible level of quality. The unfortunate state of affairs today in the autism community, both within the ABA field and outside it, is that the integrity and quality of treatment procedures have been se-riously compromised. Today, if one were to choose a service provider at random, one's chances of selecting a service provider who implements high-quality treatment would be unacceptably low. No research yet exists that has attempted to quantify the problem, but it is highly common to receive reports from parents of ghastly treatment quality from a myriad of treatment providers. A number of factors likely lead to the provision of low-quality services, and Chapter 22 on training and quality control pro-vides practical details on how to maintain high quality. Below, we briefly discuss some community factors that may contribute to the problem.

Financial influences. Service provision agencies are businesses that ex-ist in capitalist, consumer-based economies, so it is impossible to avoid the influence of financial matters. Billing more hours, spending less money on training and quality control, and increasing clinician caseload will all improve a company's bottom line. These facts are unavoidable. However, we believe that the moral obligation to provide the highest quality ser-vice must take precedence over the opportunity to make large amounts of money. Thankfully, the amount of funding for ABA services that is cur-rently available in many regions is such that achieving financial success and providing the highest quality services are not mutually exclusive; one can provide the highest quality service and still have a financially success-ful company.

Inadequate training. The quality of ABA services that one can pro-vide will always be limited by the quality of training one has received in the past. It is, unfortunately, very common for a professional who has only a small amount of entry-level experience at a good-quality agency to start her own agency and then act as the clinical director. It is inevitable that the quality of the service that the agency will provide will be inade-quate. Indeed, it may even approach *impossible* for the agency to provide a top-quality service because the skill sets that qualified case managers, su-pervisors, and clinical directors possess are simply not the same as those of entry-level staff, and they cannot simply be learned through books or seminars. If that agency then hires only entry-level staff and promotes only from within, as is often the case, then years or even decades can elapse without the quality of the organization ever improving. Perhaps most frightening, it may even be common in such cases for the staff at the agency *not even to be aware* that they are providing a sub-par service because they have never had experience with a top-quality level of ser-vice. The problem is compounded for society when staff at agencies such as those described above then leave and start their own agencies, further multiplying the dissemination of poor-quality practices.

Lack of an expert ABA leader. Currently, not enough expert ABA cli-nicians are available to serve all of the individuals with ASD who need their help. The desperate need for services has created a demand for the creation of new agencies. It is not surprising, then, that people from all walks of life have stepped in to fill the void. For many, such as parents or professionals from other disciplines, this is done out of benevolent motivation – they want to help people who are not being helped. This void also represents a tremendous business opportunity, and a small but significant number of agencies have been started by people who have no knowledge of ASD but simply realize the business potential of starting an ABA agency. Regardless of motivation, it has become commonplace for someone other than an expert ABA supervisor to start an ABA agency. There is no reason that a businessperson, a parent, or a professional from another discipline cannot found and run a quality ABA agency, *as long as someone is present who is qualified to make the tough clinical decisions*. In order for an agency to provide a top-quality service, the clinical services must be directed by someone who possesses at least a master's degree, is preferably a Board-Certified Behavior Analyst (BCBA), and, most importantly, has years of experience in implementing and supervising top-quality services for individuals with ASD. There is no substitute for this person in an ABA agency. If you currently own, run, or are working in an ABA agency, it is critical that you ask yourself whether you have such a person. If you do not, you must get one or arrange for one of your current leaders to obtain the training and mentorship required.

Lack of experience with ASD and skill acquisition. Another factor contributing to low-quality service provision in autism treatment is the fact that many agencies are directed by ABA clinicians who only have good-quality experience in an area of ABA other than skill acquisition for individuals with ASD. There are many other critically important areas of work in ABA, including organizational behavior management, regular education, functional analysis, and treatment of challenging behavior, among others. Supervisor-level expertise in these other areas makes one a more well-rounded behavior analyst, but it does not qualify one to supervise skill acquisition programs for children with ASD. Just as a BCBA who has only taught preschoolers with ASD would not be qualified to step into a boardroom and sell a performance-management consulting contract to the CEO of a Fortune 500 company, a BCBA who has only assessed and treated challenging behavior is not qualified to direct an entire agency that focuses primarily on skill acquisition for children with ASD. It is true that the principles of behavior analysis are applicable across behaviors, settings, and populations, but a brain surgeon nonetheless needs experience doing surgery on brains, and an oncologist needs specialized experience to become an expert in treating cancer. Just as the fundamentals of anatomy and physiology are not sufficient for a medical doctor to be an expert in any specialty, knowing the principles of behavior and passing a behavior analyst certification exam are not sufficient to ensure expertise in all specialties of ABA, particularly that of skill acquisition for children with ASD.

At CARD, we are faced with choices that gravely affect quality on a daily basis. As we fulfill our mission to expand access to ABA treatment to the maximum possible number of families affected by ASD around the world, the possibility of expansion potentially threatens the level of top-quality treatment that we maintain. Providing ABA services is a constant tightrope walk between quality and quantity. Many great university clinics, where the elite in behavior analysis receive graduate education, serve fewer than a dozen children at a given time. These clinics should be praised for an almost absurd level of quality. On the other end of the continuum are enormous agencies that serve hundreds, perhaps even thousands, of individuals with developmental disabilities but do so at such a poor level of quality that one wonders whether the services are much better than babysitting. The CARD philosophy on this balance has always been the same: Never sacrifice quality, and never give up on increasing quantity. Both can be done simultaneously; the key is to face the tough decisions that must be made at every turn and never to allow financial variables to have an undue influence.

THE RIGHT TO EVIDENCE-BASED, EFFECTIVE TREATMENT

At CARD, we believe it is self-evident that every person with ASD has a right to treatment that actually works. Just as every human has a fundamental right to dignified education and medical care, every child on the spectrum has a right to effective treatment. We believe that this right is inalienable and that it transcends cultural, ethnic, religious, and economic backgrounds. We believe that the right to effective treatment is as fundamental as any other human right and that those who are denied this right should be nothing less than outraged. Tragically, due to lack of funding or lack of trained professionals, the majority of children with ASD in the United States, and the *vast* majority of children with ASD around the world, are denied this right on a daily basis. The desperate need to spread effective, evidence-based treatment around the country and around the world is the primary catalyst for writing this treatment manual, and we sincerely hope that reading this will inspire parents, teachers, and practitioners everywhere to take a stand and do what it takes to ensure that the children with ASD in their communities have access to top-quality treatment.

GLOBAL REACH

At CARD, we believe it is the responsibility of the ABA profession to reach out and extend top-quality services to every child with ASD around the world. As will be further discussed in Chapter 28 on global dissemination, millions of children with ASD around the world are currently languishing without effective treatment, and we believe the status quo is unacceptable. As discussed earlier, we are not willing to compromise quality for the sake of dissemination, but we are equally unwilling to sacrifice dissemination for the purposes of quality. We believe we – and all ABA service providers – have a moral obligation to help to extend access to top-quality treatment to the maximum number of children with ASD around the world.

RECOVERY FROM ASD IS POSSIBLE

Recovery from ASD exists, and the willingness to acknowledge it is a fundamental part of the CARD approach to autism treatment. However, recovery is a controversial topic, so some further explanation is warranted. At CARD, we define recovery from ASD as follows: A person can be said to have recovered from ASD if that person once had a confirmed ASD diagnosis and then, after receiving treatment, no longer demonstrates clinically significant impairment. In plain English, a child has recovered from ASD when there is nothing left to treat. For the purposes of research and documentation, we use the following method of measuring recovery. A person can be said to have recovered from ASD if he demonstrates all of the following:

1. Scores in the average range (no more than one standard deviation below the mean) on standardized assessments of intelligence, language, adaptive skills, and social skills;
2. Receives passing grades in regular education without any supports or modifications (unmodified curriculum in a regular education classroom with no aide); and
3. Is evaluated by a medical doctor or licensed psychologist, who is an expert in diagnosing ASD, and does not meet diagnostic criteria for any ASD based on current level of functioning.

Most of the mainstream medical community still do not acknowledge that recovery from ASD exists, even though top-quality ABA programs have been producing it in some percentage of the children they have treated for at least a couple of decades. However, recent research has further raised awareness of the reality of recovery from ASD (Fein et al., 2013; Granpeesheh, Tarbox, Dixon, Carr, & Herbert, 2009), and the idea seems to be gaining at least a small amount of acceptance in the mainstream community.

At the current time, it is not known precisely what percentage of children with ASD who receive top-quality Early Intensive Behavioral Intervention (EIBI) will recover, but the research seems to suggest that it is somewhere between 20% and 50%. It is also impossible, at this time, to predict whether any particular child will recover from ASD. At the current time, the majority of children with ASD will not recover, even when given the best quality EIBI. The one question that all parents ask when they hear that recovery exists is whether their child will recover. It is critical to give parents an honest depiction of the facts and make it clear that recovery exists and may be a possibility but that it should not be expected or relied upon. This uncertainty naturally makes parents feel enormous anxiety and stress, and some believe that parents should not be told of the possibility of recovery in order to avoid making them feel upset if their child does not recover. Of course, it is critical to take every reasonable step to avoid making parents of children with ASD feel any unnecessary stress, but we do not believe that the possibility of recovery should be withheld from parents. It's plainly obvious that medical doctors give their patients an honest appraisal of the various possible outcomes of whatever treatment they are providing – to do otherwise would be to mislead the patient. We believe the same is true of ASD. (For a more extensive discussion of recovery, as well as the potential for prevention, see Granpeesheh, Tarbox, & Persicke, 2014).

When discussing recovery from ASD, it is critical to point out that recovery is not the only legitimate goal of EIBI treatment. The goal of any quality ABA program is to help each individual child reach his or her maximum learning potential. For some, that maximum is recovery. For the others, the maximum learning potential varies greatly, ranging from a child who makes tremendous gains across domains to another child who will remain significantly impaired across all areas of functioning but has made very real progress in core skill areas that improve quality of life. For example, even the most challenged child with ASD can learn to communicate basic needs and desires (if not through speech, then through sign language, pictures, or other means); decrease destructive behavior; become toilet trained; become more independent with daily living activities, such as dressing, eating, and food preparation; develop leisure skills; and learn to coexist with others peacefully and without strife. Although recovery is not currently possible for all children, gains such as learning to tolerate having a haircut, learning to eat at a restaurant in peace, and learning to administer one's own personal hygiene can be victories that make a very real difference in the quality of life of families living with ASD.

PERSONAL DIGNITY AND SELF-DETERMINATION

CARD believes in the personal dignity, individuality, and self-determination of every person with ASD. The right of people with developmental disabilities to determine their own fate has been denied for centuries, but the past several decades in American culture have seen a move toward acknowledging that the lives of people with ASD should not merely consist of doing what they are told and remaining calm and quiet. At CARD, children with ASD are given opportunities to express their personal beliefs, feelings, interests, and preferences. Fortunately, when done well, ABA provides the tools for maximizing independence and self-determination. By building choice into every aspect of treatment whenever possible, we automatically ensure that the child has some say over the course and format of her education and treatment. By focusing on teaching spontaneous functional communication (i.e., mands in verbal behavioral jargon), we ensure that the child with ASD has the right and ability to tell others what she wants, not merely to respond to the commands and comments of others.

SUMMARY

The field of autism treatment is comparatively young, and new funding streams attract both highly qualified service providers and grossly unqualified charlatans. Individuals who have ASD have a right to top-quality, evidence-based treatment, although many are deprived of this right due to economic, geographic, cultural, and economic barriers that must be overcome. While recovery from ASD exists, it is not the only measure of successful treatment. Behavior analysts have a responsibility to disseminate top-quality autism treatment and increase access to evidence-based treatment without sacrificing quality to ensure that individuals with ASD around the globe have the opportunity to fulfill their potential and live lives that are self-directed and as independent as possible.

The Diagnosis of Autism Spectrum Disorder

Doreen Granpeesheh, Megan Maixner, Cecilia Knight, Monique Erickson

Autism spectrum disorder (ASD) is a neurodevelopmental disorder. Neurodevelopmental disorders are characterized by onset in the developmental period and the presence of deficits that produce impairment in personal, social, academic, or occupational functioning. The *Diagnostic and Statistical Manual of Mental Disorders* (DSM), published by the American Psychiatric Association, is the standard reference that is used for medical classification and diagnosis of ASD, among other disorders. The DSM has been revised several times over the past 60 years and is currently in its fifth edition (DSM-5; APA), released in May, 2013. The diagnostic criteria for ASD changed significantly from DSM-IV to DSM-5, and this chapter will describe these changes and what they mean for you as a treatment provider. We will also review who can give a diagnosis, as well as some of the standardized assessments used to diagnose ASD.

PROFESSIONALS WHO CAN DIAGNOSE ASD

The authority to give an official diagnosis of ASD is reserved for licensed medical doctors and psychologists. Most parents bring their child to a pediatrician when they first become alarmed that something may be awry with the child's development. Pediatricians are allowed to give the ASD diagnosis, but, unless they have specialized training and experience in ASD, they should almost always refer the child to a specialist for a more thorough assessment. School psychologists are permitted to give the ASD diagnosis for use in school, but a diagnosis by a licensed medical doctor or psychologist is required for the diagnosis to be recognized outside of the school setting. Regardless of who provides the diagnosis, no formal test-ing is required, but it is highly recommended. We provide descriptions of some of the more useful diagnostic assessments included in the Center for Autism and Related Disorders (CARD) Model at the end of the chapter.

DIAGNOSTIC CRITERIA

The diagnostic criteria for ASD 299.00, according to the DSM-5, consist of two sets of symptoms: 1) social communication and social interaction deficits, and 2) the presence of restrictive, repetitive patterns of behavior, interests, or activities. These symptoms must present in the early develop-ment period, although they may not fully manifest until social demands exceed capabilities, or they may be masked by learned strategies later in life. The symptoms together must cause significant impairment in other areas of everyday functioning and must not be better described by another DSM-5 diagnosis. These criteria are discussed in greater depth below.

Criterion 1: Social Communication and Social Interaction Deficits

The first criterion is persistent deficits in social communication and so-cial interaction across multiple contexts. To qualify for an ASD diagnosis, the child must meet the criteria for all three social communication and social interaction deficits described below:

1. **Deficits in social-emotional reciprocity.** These deficits may include abnormal social approach and failure of normal back-and-forth conversation; reduced sharing of interests, emotions, or affect; and failure to initiate or respond to social interactions. These deficits often become apparent when an individual 1) does not reciprocate social exchanges (e.g., greetings), 2) does not understand the emotions of others (e.g., keeps playing and shows no reaction when peer falls down and cries), and 3) lacks empathy for others (e.g., does not appear to feel sad when a peer or family member is sad).
2. **Deficits in nonverbal communicative behaviors used for social interaction.** These deficits include poorly integrated verbal and nonverbal communication, abnormalities in eye contact and body language (e.g., avoids eye contact with others), difficulty understanding and using gestures, and lacking understanding and use of appropriate facial expressions (e.g., does not react to peer's angry facial expression).
3. **Deficits in developing, maintaining, and understanding relationships.** Deficits in this area include difficulties adjusting behavior to suit

various social contexts, difficulties in sharing imaginative play or making friends, and an absence of interest in peers. Deficits of this nature may be exhibited when an individual does not develop friendships appropriate to a developmental level beyond those with caregivers (e.g., spends no time with peers outside of times prescribed by teachers). Children may also have great difficulty maintaining any existing peer relationships. This type of deficit may also be displayed by an individual who only plays with much younger children and does not have relationships with children of the same age.

Criterion 2: Restricted, Repetitive Patterns of Behavior, Interests, or Activities

In addition to Criterion 1, an individual must meet criteria for at least two of the following four symptom areas related to restricted and repetitive behaviors and interests to qualify for an ASD diagnosis:

1. **Stereotyped or repetitive motor movements, use of objects, or speech**. Examples of these behaviors include repeating sounds, words, or phrases out of context (ranging from single words or sounds to entire scripts of movies) and repeated movements, such as hand flapping, flipping a light switch on and off, twirling objects, lining up toys, and so on.
2. **Insistence on sameness, inflexible adherence to routines, or ritualized patterns of verbal or nonverbal behavior**. Children with these symptoms may display extreme distress at small changes in schedules or routines (e.g., becoming upset when classroom schedule changes), inflexibility with changes to the organization or placement of objects, difficulty with transitions, or rigid thinking patterns.
3. **Highly restricted, fixated interests that are abnormal in intensity or focus**. Children may display unreasonably strong attachment to or preoccupation with unusual objects, carry or hoard particular objects, or have excessively circumscribed or perseverative interests. Some children perseverate on specific topics (e.g., a child may turn every conversation into a discussion about mathematics).
4. **Hyper- or hyporeactivity to sensory input or unusual interest in sensory aspects of the environment**. Children with these symptoms may display apparent indifference to pain or extreme temperatures or may overreact to differences in temperature. They may have unreasonably adverse responses to specific sounds or textures, such as tantrumming whenever the family uses the kitchen blender or crying in terror upon handling sand or uncooked rice.

Symptoms Must Appear During Early Development

In addition to meeting the criteria described above, symptoms must be present in the early developmental period. In other words, if a child develops typically and then starts to show the symptoms described above during adolescence, she would not qualify for an ASD diagnosis. However, it is important to note that some symptoms are less likely to fully manifest until the child has greater social demands placed on her. For example, if a toddler has no siblings, does not attend daycare, and has very little interaction with neighbors or peers, then her parents may not notice many of the signs of social deficits because the child has had little in the way of social demands placed on her. As she begins to interact with other children more, the seriousness of her social deficits may become clearer.

Symptoms Must Cause Clinically Significant Impairment

In order to qualify for an ASD diagnosis, symptoms must cause clinically significant impairment in social, occupational, or other important areas of current functioning. Put simply, ASD does not simply mean that the child is different from other children but, rather, that his deficits are severe enough to affect his quality of life on a daily basis. For example, social deficits that result in the child making few or no meaningful peer relationships would qualify as clinically significant. Similarly, communicative deficits that are severe enough that the child cannot tell his parents what he wants, thereby leading to tantrums, would cause clinically significant distress for him and his family. Finally, if a child's obsession with engaging in repetitive behavior takes up so much of his time that he never develops any other leisure skills, his quality of life is likely to suffer to a clinically significant degree.

As awareness of ASD has risen in recent decades, it has become a somewhat popular topic in the general media. As a result, some people may casually declare themselves to have ASD or Asperger's disorder if they are particularly good at using computers or are particularly socially awkward. It is important to keep in mind, however, that ASD is not the same as having a unique and quirky personality. If a person is highly socially awkward and would rather spend all of her time memorizing statistics, but she still engages in the social behaviors needed to make friends and function at work and at home, she likely does not qualify for an ASD diagnosis. There are likely thousands of people who find social interaction annoying and/or terrifying and who would rather spend all of their time engaging in one or two particular hobbies, but this does not mean they have ASD. For diagnostic purposes, such traits must be so severe that they prevent people from succeeding independently in their social, family, or academic lives.

Intellectual Disability and Global Developmental Delay

To receive an ASD diagnosis, the DSM requires that an individual's symptoms cannot be better explained by intellectual disability (intellectual developmental disorder) or global developmental delay. Intellectual disability and ASD frequently co-occur. However, the symptoms of each disorder are distinct, and all must be present in order for both diagnoses to be made.

Specifiers

If an individual meets the full criteria for ASD described above, the diagnosis should also include specifiers. A specifier provides the etiology and/or other important features of the presenting symptoms that are relevant to the treatment of the diagnosed condition. Specifiers are not intended to be mutually exclusive or jointly exhaustive, and therefore, more than one specifier may be given for a particular diagnosis.

Comorbidity. The DSM-5 indicates that the diagnosis of ASD is to specify the following **comorbid** (co-occurring) conditions:

- With or without accompanying intellectual impairment
- With or without accompanying language impairment
- Associated with a known medical or genetic condition or environmental factor (e.g., sleep disorder or epilepsy)
- Associated with another neurodevelopmental, mental, or behavioral disorder
- With catatonia

Age and pattern of onset. Although the symptoms of ASD are typically identified during the second year of life (12–24 months of age), these symptoms may have been observed earlier than 12 months or later than 24 months, depending on the individual and the severity or subtleness of symptoms in day-to-day life. Additionally, some children with ASD demonstrate developmental plateaus or regression, with a gradual or rapid deterioration in social or language skills. This information is important because these types of losses are rare in other disorders and can serve as a red flag for ASD, helping distinguish symptoms of ASD from other developmental delays and/or disorders (Table 3.1).

Severity. One of the most beneficial applications of the DSM-5 is that it allows the diagnostician to assign severity specifiers to the two main symptom areas. Severity specifiers rate the intensity, frequency, duration, symptom count, or other severity indicators of the social communication deficits and restricted, repetitive behaviors seen in ASD. Both symptom areas are assigned a severity, ranging from 1 (least severe) to 3 (most severe). Levels of severity are defined by how much support the symptoms

TABLE 3.1   Levels of Severity for ASD Symptoms in Social Communication and Repetitive Behaviors

Severity Level for ASD	Social Communication	Restricted Interests and Repetitive Behaviors
Level 1: Requires support	Without support, some significant deficits in social communication	Significant interference in at least one context
Level 2: Requires substantial support	Marked deficits with limited initiations and reduced or atypical responses	Obvious to the casual observer and occurs across contexts
Level 3: Requires very substantial support	Minimal social communication	Marked interference in daily life

require for that individual. Level 1 is defined as "requiring support," meaning relatively little support. Level 2 is defined as "requiring substantial support." Level 3 is defined as "requiring very substantial support." Table 3.1 gives further guidance on how levels of severity are generally defined for both symptom areas. Table 3.2 gives specific examples from the DSM-5 of symptoms of each level across both symptom areas.

CHANGES FROM DSM-IV

The largest change from DSM-IV to DSM-5 is that the various diagnostic subtypes (Autistic Disorder, Asperger's Disorder, and Pervasive Developmental Disorder Not Otherwise Specified) have been collapsed into the single diagnosis of ASD. Whereas DSM-IV delineated several separate and distinct disorders that shared characteristics of delay, the DSM-5 places these disorders under one umbrella and distinguishes subtypes not by different names but, rather, by differing levels of severity and other specifiers, as described above. The other major change is that DSM-IV included three main diagnostic domains: social interaction, communication, and restricted repetitive and stereotypic behavior patterns. DSM-5 reduces the domains from three to two: 1) social communication and social interaction and 2) restricted, repetitive behaviors. Within these two domains, the number of specific required symptoms has changed. Most notably, three types of social communication delays and two types of restricted, repetitive behaviors must be present for a diagnosis of ASD to be made.

The consolidation of separate diagnoses into one single diagnosis, the collapse of the three domains into two, the increase in the criteria for repetitive behaviors, and the inclusion of specifiers of severity level collectively

TABLE 3.2   Examples of Symptoms of ASD Across Both Symptom Areas and All Three Levels of Severity, from the *Diagnostic and Statistical Manual of Mental Disorders*, 5th Edition (APA, 2013)

Symptom Area	Severity Level	Examples
Social Communication and Social Interaction	1	Difficulty initiating and responding to social interactions. Decreased interest in others. Speaks in full sentences but difficulty with conversation. Attempts to make friends are often odd and unsuccessful.
	2	Marked impairments noticeable even with supports in place. Limited response and initiations to social interactions. Speaks in simple limited sentences. Limited and odd nonverbal communication. Interactions are limited to narrow special interests.
	3	Limited social initiations and minimal responding to others. Few words of intelligible speech. Rarely initiates and when does uses unusual approaches. Responds only to very direct social initiations.
Restricted and Repetitive Behavior and Interests	1	Marked inflexibility. Difficulty switching activities. Poor planning and organization skills that impact independent functioning.
	2	Inflexibility in behavior. Difficulty coping with change.
	3	Extreme inflexibility and difficulty coping with changes. Marked distress when needing to change focus or action. Repetitive/restricted behaviors markedly interfere with all other areas of functioning.

reflect changes that were made as part of the shift from a categorical approach to a dimensional one. DSM-5 acknowledges the need to evolve in the context of other clinical research initiatives (e.g., cognitive neuroscience, brain imaging, epidemiology, genetics, and so forth) in the field. An important aspect of that transition is recognizing that the previous rigid categorical classification system did not reflect clinical experience or scientific observations. The boundaries between the various symptoms associated with ASD are more fluid over the lifespan than the DSM-IV acknowledged, and many symptoms assigned to a single disorder may occur at varying levels of severity in many other disorders. Therefore, the DSM-5 attempts to accommodate these findings by adopting dimensional approaches to mental disorders that include dimensions that cut across categories. This approach is intended to produce more accurate descriptions of patient presentations and increase the validity of the diagnosis by presenting a thorough range of the symptoms present.

It is also interesting to note that the DSM-5 specifically acknowledges the presence of abnormal responses to sensory experiences in individuals with ASD through the inclusion of hyper- or hyporeactivity to sensory input as one of the symptoms in the restricted, repetitive behavior domain. Clinicians have widely acknowledged for years that many individuals with ASD have divergent reactions to sensory input, but the DSM-IV diagnostic criteria did not include this. We have observed repeatedly that some children with ASD are particularly challenged by sensory input of particular sorts (e.g., particular sounds or textures). On the other hand, some children have outstanding strengths in particular sensory areas, such as visual stimuli. Individual child sensory profiles must be considered in order for treatment to be optimally effective (see Chapter 6 on visual and other sensory modifications). We hope that the inclusion of sensory abnormalities in the DSM-5 criteria will help bring greater attention to the topic and, therefore, more research on how to customize treatment for sensory issues.

The inclusion of medical or genetic factors as a specifier in the DSM-5 criteria is new and interesting. To date, relatively few medical conditions have been associated with ASD. Fragile X and tuberous sclerosis are among the most well-known disorders that lead to autistic-like symptoms. For the first time, DSM-5 acknowledges the existence of associations between ASD and medical conditions. We are hopeful that this acknowledgment will lead to further research that will enhance our understanding of the etiology of ASD.

It may be important to note that a new diagnosis in the DSM-5, Social Communication Disorder (SCD), may cause confusion for the inexperienced diagnostician, as it shares some characteristics with ASD. The SCD diagnosis is given to children who have difficulty in the social use of verbal or nonverbal communication to such an extent that it affects the development of their relationships, comprehension, academic achievement, or occupational performance. While SCD touches upon a very distinct commonality with ASD (the lack of social communication), it does not account for the restricted, repetitive behaviors present in ASD. As such, it must be understood as a clearly distinct disorder.

Implications of Changes in DSM-5

The gold standard method for diagnosing ASD includes the use of standardized diagnostic assessments. The vast majority of these were developed using DSM-IV criteria, so they will need to be revised. At the time this manual goes to press, we have not yet seen the full effect of the changes in the DSM-5 on access to services and availability of third-party funding for treatment. Many are concerned that some children, who formerly would have been diagnosed with Asperger's disorder and who suffer from clinically significant impairment in their daily lives, will no longer qualify for an ASD diagnosis according to the DSM-5. Still others are concerned that funding sources will intentionally influence diagnosticians to lean toward SCD, rather than ASD with low severity, because they will be less likely to have to provide funding for treatment, given that SCD has no treatment guidelines and insurance carriers are not mandated to pay for its treatment. Research addressing these topics is still under way, and the future will provide the answers to these questions.

DIAGNOSTIC ASSESSMENTS

Autism Diagnostic Observation Scale, Second Edition

The Autism Diagnostic Observation Scale (ADOS; Lord et al., 1989) is a widely regarded semi-structured assessment for diagnosing ASD. While direct clinical observation remains paramount in any assessment, some clinicians in the field now consider the ADOS to be the "gold standard" of autism observation measures. The ADOS consists of a standardized set of scenarios that a trained clinician presents to the individual being assessed. These scenarios are designed to produce situations in which the clinician can evaluate communication, social interaction, play, and imagination skills, as well as examine any potential symptomology of ASD. That is, the contrived scenarios give the child being evaluated the opportunity to behave or react as a typically developing child generally would. In this way, if the child being evaluated reacts to the situation by performing differently or demonstrating atypical behavior, differences are apparent to the clinician.

The ADOS is now in its second edition and includes revised algorithms. The ADOS-2 (Gotham, Risi, Pickles, and Lord, 2007) can be used to evaluate almost anyone who is suspected to have ASD, from infants with no speech to adults who are verbally fluent. The ADOS-2 consists of five modules. An individual being assessed is only administered one module based on age and language abilities. Module 1 is designed for children 31 months and over who do not consistently use phrase speech; Module 2 is for children of any age who use phrase speech but are not verbally fluent; Module 3 is for verbally fluent children and young adolescents; and Module 4 is for verbally fluent older adolescents and adults. New to the ADOS is the Toddler Module, intended for use with children aged 12 to 30 months who do not consistently use phrase speech. The Toddler Module involves interacting with the child in minimally structured activities with reinforcing items. The goal is the same: to flag any behaviors consistent with an ASD diagnosis.

The time required to administer the ADOS-2 ranges from 40 to 60 minutes. Examiners need to have thorough knowledge of the exact administration and scoring procedures. A higher degree of training and experience with ASD is required for competent interpretation of test results. The clinician administering the ADOS-2 requires extensive training and supervision. To score the ADOS-2 throughout the observation period, the examiner rates the child's performance in each scenario. Items are rated on a three-point scale (0 = within normal limits, 1 = infrequent or possible abnormality, and 2 = definite abnormality). The scores on the ADOS are put into a diagnostic algorithm based on criteria for ASD. The revised scoring algorithms of the ADOS-2 reflect social and communication items as one social communication factor, and scores on the repetitive and restricted item scores are no longer included in the total score. The original algorithm cutoffs were 10 for autism and 7 for autism spectrum; the revised algorithm is 9 for autism and 7 for autism spectrum.

Autism Diagnostic Interview, Revised

The Autism Diagnostic Interview (ADI; Le Couteur et al., 1989) is a standardized, semi-structured caregiver interview that was designed to aid in the assessment of a range of behaviors consistent with diagnoses of pervasive developmental disorders. The Autism Diagnostic Interview – Revised (ADI-R; Lord, Rutter, and Le Couteur, 1994) was published in 1994. Compared to the ADI, the ADI-R is shorter, has modified items, and is intended for use with a younger population. The ADI-R can be used to assess children with a mental age of at least 18 months as opposed to the ADI, for which individuals had to be at least 5 years old to be assessed. The ADI-R consists of five sections. The sections include questions that evaluate concerns, communication skills, social development and play, repetitive and restricted behaviors, and general behavior problems. These topics address both current and previous functioning. There are three separate diagnostic algorithms that can be used to attain a diagnosis: lifetime, current behavior, and children under the age of 4 years. The ADI-R requires between 1.5 and 2.5 hours to administer. Examiners need to have thorough knowledge of the exact administration and scoring procedures. A higher degree of training and experience with ASD is required for competent interpretation of test results. DVD training in the ADI-R is recommended.

SUMMARY

In conclusion, the process of diagnosing ASD is complex and changed significantly with the publication of the DSM-5. The new criteria require that an individual has impairment across three symptom areas in social communication and the presence of restricted, repetitive behavior, as evidenced by two or more symptom characteristics. The symptoms must have emerged during the early developmental period and, taken together, must represent a clinically significant challenge to the individual's ability to function in daily life. DSM-5 criteria include specifiers that rate the severity of symptoms on a scale from level 1 to level 3, with 3 being most severe. It is also worth noting that challenging behaviors, such as tantrums, aggression, and property destruction, are still *not* part of the ASD diagnosis, despite the fact that they are common in the ASD population. This fact reflects the position that the vast majority of these challenging behaviors in individuals with ASD are learned behaviors that result from deficits in communication, not core ASD symptoms in and of themselves. Finally, the diagnostic process is something with which most applied behavior analytic service providers are unfamiliar. A greater familiarity with the process will likely give treatment providers a richer source of information about their learner's history and functioning level, thereby providing opportunities for customizing treatment programs to a greater degree.

4

Principles and Procedures
of Acquisition

Jonathan Tarbox, Doreen Granpeesheh

Comprehensive behavioral intervention for learners with autism spectrum disorder (ASD) is extraordinarily complex. Applied behavior analysis (ABA) is not a cookie-cutter "recipe" approach to treating ASD and, instead, produces highly individualized treatment. It is no exaggeration to say that a top-quality ABA program consists of arranging every conceivable detail of a learner's environment in order to teach the learner every skill that is not already developing naturally. This requires many thousands, perhaps hundreds of thousands, of decisions over the course of several years. Among the most complex and important clinical decisions is that of which combination of treatment procedures to implement at any given time, with any given learner, to teach any given skill. The "analysis" in applied behavior analysis refers to the process of making these decisions, which is an inherently complex process. The purpose of this chapter is to describe this process sufficiently to facilitate your own efforts to implement it. This chapter will describe the primary evidence-based treatment approaches used within the Center for Autism and Related Disorders (CARD) Model of treatment for learners with ASD, including discrete trial training (DTT), natural environment training (NET), and fluency-based instruction, as well as the many evidence-based treatment components used within them, including reinforcement, preference assessment, discrimination training, errorless learning, prompting and prompt fading, error correction, shaping, and chaining. In addition, practical guidance will be provided on how best to combine each component for each individual learner. Data collection and treatment evaluation are described later in Chapter 20.

BACKGROUND

We will not bore you with an elaborate history lesson on ABA's origins, but some background and basic philosophy are worth mentioning. Building upon the earlier work of Edward Thorndike and John Watson, B. F. Skinner had a remarkably simple and yet powerful idea: If we want to change a person's behavior, then we should change that person's environment. While it would be ideal if we could change people's genetics and brain structure to enable them to function better in life, for now, if we want to help people behave in a way that will improve their quality of life, all we can do is change their environment. In the behavioral way of viewing the world, a person's environment is divided into things that happen before behavior, called **antecedents**, and things that happen after behavior, called **consequences**. Behavioral intervention consists of modifying the antecedents and consequences in people's environments, such that their learning and motivation are maximized. The rest of this chapter describes the many principles and procedures that do this.

POSITIVE REINFORCEMENT

Positive reinforcement is the foundation of the entire science of behavior analysis and must form the core of any good treatment program for individuals with ASD. Behavior analysis is a science of learning, consisting of basic principles and procedures that are derived from those principles. For this reason, the same term is used to mean different things at different times, and it is therefore important to be very clear about what these terms mean. Reinforcement is a principle of learning and motivation, and it simply means that **some consequences of behavior make that behavior happen more in the future or maintain the behavior at its current rate**. A classic example of reinforcement is receiving money for working at a job. All other things being equal, as long as doing your job results in a paycheck, you will continue to carry out that behavior. Receiving money when you work reinforces the behavior of working. That is, the consequence of receiving money is *the reason* you continue to work. Of course, many other reasons may affect *where* you work, but if the paychecks stopped coming (assuming you are not independently wealthy), you would eventually stop going to work at that job. Money might seem like a crass example of reinforcement, and other reinforcement is certainly far loftier. For instance, let's say you volunteer at a homeless shelter, and one of the main reinforcers for doing that is being able to feed people who are hungry. If you were no longer able to feed people at that shelter, you would eventually stop volunteering there. Perhaps you would try a different behavior (work at a different shelter) that would likely result in the reinforcer that the original behavior no longer provides (being able to feed hungry people). The basic point is that the consequences of all of our behaviors matter and that preferred consequences reinforce and maintain our behavior. Decades of research have shown that this basic fact is equally true for learners with ASD, typically developing adults, dogs, cats, pigeons, dolphins, and so on. Reinforcement is a basic principle of learning and motivation that is amazingly effective and generally applicable.

Principles Versus Procedures

Principles and procedures are not the same. Reinforcement *as a principle* refers to any consequence that increases the future occurrence of a behavior or maintains that behavior at its current rate. The word "reinforcement," *when used as the name of a procedure,* refers to the practice of delivering a consequence with the goal of increasing the future rate of a behavior. You may implement reinforcement *as a procedure* and find that it did not work. That is, the learner's behavior did not increase in rate in the future. However, it is not possible for reinforcement *as a principle* not to work. The principle of reinforcement is defined functionally – that is, by what the consequence actually did to the behavior. If the behavior did not increase after contacting a particular consequence, then that consequence was not a reinforcer for that behavior at that time. This is not merely an academic point; it is an important distinction. We often hear someone say, "I tried that reinforcement stuff, and it didn't work." By definition, it is impossible for reinforcement "not to work." You may try a particular reinforcement *procedure,* and it may well fail, but that simply means the wrong type, amount, or frequency of reinforcement was used, not that reinforcement *as a process* did not work for that behavior or that learner. This same distinction – between principles and procedures – is critical for many other behavioral terms, as you will see below.

Negative Versus Positive Reinforcement

In everyday language, positive usually implies good, and negative usually implies bad. In technical ABA terminology, this is incorrect. The words *positive* and *negative* merely refer to whether the therapist is adding something to the learner's environment (i.e., positive) or whether the therapist is removing something from the learner's environment (i.e., negative). All forms of reinforcement have the effect of strengthening a behavior or skill. **Positive reinforcement** occurs when a therapist *adds* something to the learner's environment as a consequence of a behavior, and that behavior increases or maintains in the future. **Negative reinforcement** occurs when a therapist *removes* something from a learner's environment as a consequence of a behavior, and that behavior increases or maintains in the future. For example, if a learner with ASD says "break please" and she receives a break from work (work is removed from her environment), she will be more likely to say "break please" the next time she wants a break. Similarly, moving away from a loud noise is negatively reinforced by the sound becoming quieter (the removal of excessive volume). Negative reinforcement not only works by removing something that is present; it can also work by avoiding something that has not yet occurred. Nagging (if it works at all) usually works through negative reinforcement. If one spouse nags another spouse constantly about doing the dishes, the second spouse may be more likely to do the dishes to avoid the nagging in the future. Table 4.1 lists some common negative and positive reinforcers used in behavioral intervention.

Reinforcers are unique to each individual. As we mentioned earlier, there is a saying, "If you have met one child with autism, then you have met one child with autism." This saying emphasizes that no two learners with ASD are alike. This is true in general and is particularly true when it comes to reinforcement. Remember, reinforcers are defined 100% in terms of what they actually do to behavior, not by how we think they *should* affect behavior. What may be a powerful reinforcer for one learner may be neutral or even punishment for another learner. For example, Jimmy may work very hard to earn train toys and may avoid animal toys, whereas Sally may work very hard for her stuffed animals and may have no interest in trains whatsoever. Think about music preferences, and you will get the idea. Some people love country music, some rap, some opera, and some alternative rock. Everyone has different preferences, and reinforcement, therefore, is different for everyone.

Generally speaking, expect reinforcers to be very different for learners with ASD compared to what you might normally expect for typically developing learners. For example, social approval may not be a reinforcer for many learners with ASD when they first begin treatment, whereas it is a very powerful reinforcer for most typically developing learners. Physical

TABLE 4.1 Commonly Used Positive and Negative Reinforcers

Positive Reinforcers	Negative Reinforcers
Popcorn	Break from Work
Crackers	Playing Alone
High Fives	Being Excused from Dinner Table
Tickles	Reduced Chores
Puzzles	Dimming Bright Lights or Loud Noises
Stuffed Animals	Removing Shoes or Uncomfortable Clothing
Games	

touch, such as high fives and hugs, may be non-preferred by some learners with ASD. Some learners may have seemingly extreme preferences for reinforcers – one learner comes to mind who was only motivated by single-serving ketchup packets from one particular fast-food restaurant.

Reinforcers are not what you think they SHOULD be. Forget your preconceptions about the reinforcers that *should* be effective for an individual with ASD; using reinforcement effectively means using the reinforcers that *actually work* for each individual. Focus more on what is going to work and less on what you personally value. Of course, each learner's unique cultural and religious identities must be incorporated into this thought process, but just remember that you wouldn't want to be told what you like, and the same is true for individuals with ASD – perhaps even more so. Use what works.

Rewards versus reinforcers. Rewards and reinforcers are not the same thing. Rewards are typically items or events that are viewed as having broad appeal, and they are often applied the same across a large group of people. For example, if 100 people enter a raffle at a fair, and one person wins the reward, that reward is not personalized for that particular person. Consequently, there is no guarantee that it will reinforce that person's behavior, nor was it intended to *reinforce* that particular person's behavior. It's fine to use the term *reward* as a general non-technical term, especially when talking to people who are not as well versed on technical ABA terminology. Be careful to distinguish for yourself, though, when you are talking about a consequence that is individualized for a particular learner with ASD that is likely to be a reinforcer for that learner's behavior versus when you are talking about a general consequence that most children like (a reward).

Reinforcers are not the same for every behavior. Would you dig a ditch in the hot sun for 8 hours straight? Would you do it for one dollar? Probably not. Would you press a button once for a dollar? Probably so. So the same reinforcer, one dollar, may be extremely effective or completely ineffective, depending on which behavior it is being used to reinforce. For the exact same behavior, no matter how difficult or easy, the amount of reinforcement matters. Would you dig that same ditch for one million dollars? Keep these points in mind when using reinforcement with learners with ASD, and adjust the type and amount of reinforcement you are using to ensure that it fits the behavior and effort. It is not uncommon for ABA providers to use a lot of reinforcement initially during DTT but then to thin it out too rapidly and expect a 3-year-old learner with moderate to severe ASD to work for 20 minutes to gain access to a very small amount of reinforcement (e.g., 30 seconds of play with a puzzle). Naturally, you will want to get as much teaching done as possible so the learner can learn as much as possible, but the simple fact of the matter is that you will often need to use more frequent and larger reinforcement (e.g., 30 seconds of play with a puzzle after every 3–5 correct responses during DTT) if you want teaching to be as effective as it can be. This is especially true with younger and more severely affected learners.

Edible reinforcers. A common misconception about ABA is that providers primarily use candy to teach skills to learners with ASD. As described above, top-quality ABA programs use whatever reinforcement is going to be *effective*. Effectiveness is the first concern. Some learners have extremely limited selections of consequences that can be used as reinforcers. For example, when first entering treatment, some young learners with ASD possess no meaningful play skills, do not find any toys or tangible items reinforcing, do not find approval or attention from others reinforcing, and have no highly preferred consequences other than food. For these learners, using edible reinforcers is likely an important place to start. There is no reason that it has to be candy; it just has to be highly preferred, and *it has to work.* The vast majority of reinforcers used in top-quality ABA programs are not junk food. For a small minority of learners with ASD, though, candy really is the only effective source of reinforcement for the first few months of treatment. The objective for these (and all) learners with ASD is to build effective conditioned reinforcement (described below). If candy is to be used on a regular basis, it is critical that the learner's teeth be brushed thoroughly and at least daily (see the personal domain section in Chapter 13). If the treatment team is concerned that the learner's overall caloric intake is going to become excessive, then consider reducing the amount of calories that come from sugar and fat during regular meals. Ideally, unhealthy foods, such as candy, should be used as a last resort when selecting reinforcers. Table 4.2 lists some commonly used edible and tangible reinforcers in ASD treatment programs.

Special diets and reinforcement. A large percentage of families of learners with ASD attempt to put the learner on a special diet at some point in the learner's life. At the time this manual was written, there was little to no scientific evidence suggesting that any diets can reduce the

TABLE 4.2   Commonly Used Edible and Tangible Reinforcers

Edible	Tangible
Popcorn	Puzzles
Crackers	Stuffed Animals
Nuts	Action Figures
Chips	Pinwheels
Pretzels	Tablet or Computer Time
Crackers	Blocks
Cereal	Toy Cars
Fruit Snacks	Light-up/Musical Toys
Candy	Coloring Books

symptoms of ASD. Most special diets, however, have not been researched at all, so no real evidence exists for or against most of the diets. Clearly, if a learner has a legitimate food allergy of any kind, the learner (with or without ASD) should not eat that food. Regardless of the diet choices that families make, they will have implications for which edible reinforcers can be used. In extreme cases, some families have placed their children on such restricted diets that they genuinely do not have any foods in their life that taste good. If this is the case, effective edible reinforcement will not be possible. If the learner is one who could really benefit from edible reinforcement, then the simple fact is that an overly restrictive diet may impede the learner's treatment. In these instances, families need to weigh the pros and cons of each choice carefully. Dozens of research studies have proven that edible reinforcement works when teaching skills to learners with ASD. If edible reinforcement is ruled out by family values or is made impossible by restricted diets, families would do well to weigh the almost guaranteed learning that their child will receive from edible reinforcement against the unproven possibility of what they *might* gain from restricted diets. A good compromise might be to postpone the highly restricted diet and give edible reinforcement a month or two to work, which should be sufficient time for family members to observe the effects of the reinforcement and make an informed decision. It is worth noting that one or two months may be enough time for conditioned reinforcement to begin to work, so other reinforcers can be effectively used as well.

Lest there be any confusion, let us reemphasize one more time: We are not advocating junk food diets for the sake of ABA. It is possible for learners to have simultaneously well-balanced, healthy diets AND frequent and powerful edible reinforcement in their ABA programs. We do not believe that eliminating either is the most reasonable option for most learners.

Tangible reinforcers. From the very beginning of treatment, tangible reinforcers, such as toys, activities, puzzles, games, and so on should be used as reinforcers. These, of course, will vary for each learner. A good point to keep in mind is that most reinforcers will need to be easy to deliver and remove frequently and quickly. An excessive amount of setup or takedown time will rob the learner of precious therapy time. Prolonged activities, such as walking to the park, are better left for the end of the day or week as an overall reinforcer for a good day or week and/or as a setting for Natural Environment Training (NET) (described later). A better reinforcer to use throughout therapy might be access to a puzzle, figurines, music, or activities that can be quickly delivered for 30–60 seconds at a time.

Motivating Operations

Reinforcement produces learning, and there can be no successful comprehensive treatment of ASD (or any meaningful learning for anyone anywhere) without it. However, reinforcers do not act in a vacuum; they depend on a number of contextual variables for their effectiveness, the most important of which are referred to as motivating operations (MOs). Motivating operations are antecedent events that change the effectiveness of a future consequence as a reinforcer and temporarily affect the probability of behaviors that have produced that reinforcer in the past. Motivating operations are generally divided into establishing operations and abolishing operations. Establishing operations increase the effectiveness of a consequence as a reinforcer, and abolishing operations do the opposite. The simplest examples are satiation and deprivation. Simply put, if you have just had a lot of something, then you are less likely to want more of it than if you have been deprived of it. For example, if you have not eaten for 24 hours, food is likely to be an extremely powerful reinforcer. On the other end of the extreme, if you have just finished a 5,000-calorie meal, food is very unlikely to be an effective reinforcer, despite how much you normally like it. As a principle, the term *deprivation* refers to the fact that having less of something, as an antecedent, is likely to make that something a more powerful reinforcer and is likely to evoke behaviors that have produced that reinforcer in the past. Satiation is the opposite: Having more of a particular reinforcer as an antecedent is likely to make that reinforcer less powerful and is likely to decrease the probability of behaviors that have produced that reinforcer in the past.

Effective behavioral intervention programs depend on continuously evaluating the state of MOs for all reinforcers at any given moment. Obviously, this needs to be done within ethical limits; no one is suggesting starving a learner in order to use food as reinforcement, and individuals should never be deprived of basic needs, their senses, food, shelter, and bathroom facilities. It is not unethical, however, to deprive children with ASD of *particular reinforcers* to ensure that those reinforcers will be powerful when they are used in therapy. For example, if a learner has 6–8 hours of ABA treatment per day on the weekdays, then it is completely reasonable to isolate 5–10 of his favorite toys or items, so they are only used during therapy. This does not mean that he will not get to have these items; indeed, he will have them *frequently*, but only during therapy. In addition, out of a pool of 10 highly preferred items, it is completely reasonable to reserve particular items for particular days, such that the learner will always have access to an item on one day that he did not have a day or two earlier. Thus, the learner always has access to something he genuinely loves during therapy, but reinforcers remain "fresh" because deprivation is implemented for each item individually on different days.

Contriving motivating operations. Motivating operations can also be contrived at particular times to make normally neutral items function as reinforcers for the purpose of the particular educational task at hand. For example, when teaching a learner to request items, you want to teach her to request a large variety of different items in her everyday life, even if every item isn't necessarily her biggest reinforcer. (We all need to be able to ask for a fork when we want one, even though forks, per se, aren't powerful reinforcers.) To contrive MOs, you can create situations where the learner needs a particular item (something neutral) in order to achieve something that is highly reinforcing. For example, if a learner loves peanut butter sandwiches, and you tell him he can make one and eat it, you might contrive an MO for a knife by making all of the materials to make the sandwich available to the learner except for the knife, leaving the knife out of reach but in sight, thus creating an opportunity to teach the learner to ask for a knife when he wants one. (See more on this in Chapter 11 on verbal behavior.)

Preference Assessment

Successfully understanding, predicting, and manipulating MOs are critical to making reinforcement work, but how do you know if all of this planning has actually been effective and that a particular item is actually going to work as a reinforcer at any given moment in time? Fortunately, procedures have been developed that will help you confirm this. **Preference assessments are procedures that identify which items are likely to be effective as reinforcers by identifying a particular learner's preference for them**. Preference assessments can be classified as either 1) indirect or 2) systematic. Indirect preference assessments are procedures where you interview someone who knows the learner well (or interview the learner herself) and you ask that person what the learner likes. These procedures are helpful, but they must be supplemented with systematic preference assessments. Systematic preference assessments are procedures in which potential reinforcers are systematically presented to a learner, and the learner's response to each individual item is recorded. Several types exist, and we briefly describe how to implement each below. Before implementing any of the procedures described below, make sure that the learner has brief exposure (at least 2–5 minutes) with each item, so new items are not completely unknown.

Single-item preference assessment. The simplest form of preference assessment involves giving the learner one item at a time and allowing her to consume it for 30 seconds (Pace, Ivancic, Edwards, Iwata, & Page, 1985). This procedure is sometimes referred to as the "single-item preference assessment" or the "Pace preference assessment." Items should be presented in random sequence, and each item should be presented at least three times. Each time an item is presented, you record whether the learner consumed/interacted with it, whether the learner had no response to the item, or whether the learner actively avoided it. Data are summarized as the percentage of trials that each item was presented when the learner consumed/interacted with it. It is often helpful to make a bar graph. The items with the highest percentage are likely to be the most effective reinforcers.

Paired-choice preference assessment. One possible limitation of the single-item procedure is that the learner may interact with all of the items, and therefore all items would appear to be "100% preferred." This may be a legitimate outcome, or it could be that any real difference in preference among items is not revealed in the results. The paired-choice preference assessment procedure was developed to address this possibility (Fisher et al., 1992). In the paired-choice procedure, items are presented two at a time. The learner is asked to choose one, and attempts at taking both are blocked. When the learner has selected one item, he is given a small bite of that to consume (in the case of an edible) or given access to interact with the item for 30 seconds. Each item is presented with each other item an equal number of times (one to three times, depending on how much time you have). Data are collected in the same manner as the single-item procedure and graphed and analyzed in the same way: i.e., the percentage of opportunities each item was consumed/interacted with during the assessment. The paired-choice procedure is an excellent assessment, but it can take a long time to implement – up to several hours if many items are included. This fact makes it difficult to conduct paired-choice assessments often.

Multiple stimulus preference assessment. The multiple stimulus preference assessment involves presenting three or more items at the same time and asking the learner to choose one. The learner is then given a small bite or 30 seconds' access to the item chosen. After that, you may either replace that same item in the array for the next trial (referred to as a *multiple stimulus with replacement: MSW*) or remove it the next trial (referred to as a *multiple stimulus without replacement: MSWO*). The MSWO does not allow the learner to choose the same item repeatedly and is likely the more common procedure used. Trials are continued until all items have been chosen; thus, the total number of trials is equal to the number of items being included (unless you repeat the process once or twice and average the data, which will produce a more reliable result). The data are collected in the sequence in which the items were chosen and graphed.

Brief MSWO. If you want your reinforcers to be as effective as they can possibly be, then you need to assess preference often. Top-quality ABA programs assess preference many times during each therapy session – up to 5, 10, or more times per hour. In order to achieve this level of frequency without taking up too much teaching time, the brief MSWO is a great option. In the brief MSWO, three items are presented at once, and the learner is asked to choose the item he wants to earn. Whichever item the learner chooses is used during the particular teaching activity that immediately follows. Each time a new activity begins, the brief MSWO is repeated, often including other items each time. It is good practice to conduct a brief MSWO before each block of trials during DTT and before each major lesson within a therapy session. Since the brief MSWO is repeated so frequently and is only intended to tell the therapist which reinforcer to use in the moment, data are often not collected during it, as they are not needed in the moment. However, therapists can collect data during brief MSWOs, and the data can be summarized across the entire day, giving an overall average ranking of preference between items for that day.

Do not rely solely on judgment and opinion. Research has demonstrated repeatedly that systematic preference assessments predict the effectiveness of items as reinforcers to a *much greater degree than relying on caregiver report alone.* It does not matter how well the caregiver knows the learner, and it does not matter whether the caregiver is a parent, teacher, ABA therapist, or anyone else. A third person's opinion about what is going to work as a reinforcer is never going to be as good as giving the learner the opportunity to specify the reinforcer that she wants in the moment.

Conditioned Reinforcers

Reinforcement is the foundation of all top-quality autism treatment programs, but the numbers and types of consequences that are reinforcers for many learners with ASD are not sufficient to sustain them throughout their treatment program and later in life. For this reason, most learners with ASD will need help expanding the scope of items that they find reinforcing. This is where conditioned reinforcement is introduced. *As a principle,* **a conditioned reinforcer is any consequence that is a reinforcer because it was paired with some other reinforcer in the past**. Other than food, water, escape from extreme temperatures, escape from pain, access to sleep, and escape from fatigue, most reinforcers in our lives are conditioned reinforcers. In other words, you weren't born liking country music instead of opera; that preference was learned, and much of the learning process that accounts for conditioned reinforcement is simple pairing of a neutral stimulus with something that is already a reinforcer. A classic example of conditioned reinforcement is money. There is nothing inherently reinforcing about money, but it is a powerful reinforcer because of the other reinforcers with which it is paired and that it allows us to access. Table 4.3 lists some commonly used primary and conditioned reinforcers in behavioral intervention programs.

The most important sources of conditioned reinforcement for humans as social animals are social attention and social approval. Social attention and approval feel so natural to most of us in the typically developing population that we hardly even notice that some must learn to like attention from others, but this is the case with many learners with ASD. Many learners at the outset of treatment have no interest in attention from others,

TABLE 4.3 Commonly Used Primary and Conditioned Reinforcers

Primary	Conditioned
Popcorn	Tokens
Crackers	Money
Nuts	Toys
Chips	Games
Water	Points
Juice	Stickers
Fruit Snacks	High Fives
Candy	Praise
	Tickles
	"Rough Housing"

and therefore approval or praise from teachers, parents, or ABA therapists does not function as reinforcement for them. For these learners, making social praise a source of conditioned reinforcement is the first priority. This is why you will notice that all top-quality ABA programs pair already known reinforcers with praise hundreds of times per day from the very first day of treatment. This process is called *classical conditioning* and is well known to most people from Pavlov's experiments with dogs, wherein a previously neutral stimulus (a buzzer) was paired with an already known reinforcer (food), and the buzzer came to elicit the same response (salivation) as the food. In working with learners with ASD, this same powerful learning process is harnessed when we deliver praise immediately prior to delivering reinforcers. For example, we say, "Wow, you did fantastic!" and then give a favorite toy to the learner. This needs to be repeated many thousands of times, with a wide variety of reinforcers and with a wide variety of praise and social interactions, delivered by a wide variety of people – and with half of one second or less separating the praise and the reinforcer. Over time, the vast majority of learners with ASD who receive top-quality Early Intensive Behavioral Intervention (EIBI) will come to find that they genuinely like social attention, and interacting with other humans becomes a powerful source of reinforcement by itself.

Conditioned reinforcers may be particularly important because they do not depend on motivating operations that may affect the power of any one particular reinforcer. For example, it may take much longer for a learner to satiate on praise or tokens (see below) than it would take her to satiate on salty snacks. This is likely because conditioned reinforcers have been paired with a variety of reinforcers in the past and because they can be exchanged for a variety of reinforcers at any given time.

Tokens, points, and other conditioned reinforcers. Later in a learner's treatment program, you might find it useful to establish other, more tangible forms of conditioned reinforcement. **Tokens are previously neutral tangible stimuli that have been paired with reinforcement often enough**

in the past to function now as conditioned reinforcers. Any item that is easy to give and remove can be used as a token. Commonly used items include poker chips, pennies, stickers, and play money. Consider using stickers that depict the learner's favorite characters to make it more fun. Points can also be tallied for learners who are ready for it. Whatever item is used for the tokens, they are only effective when they can be exchanged for something else that is a powerful reinforcer, known as the **backup reinforcer**. A backup reinforcer can be any item known to be an effective reinforcer for that learner. Different backup reinforcers can be given different prices, so a learner may choose to save the tokens to earn a larger reinforcer, or a learner may spend tokens more frequently if she wants more frequent, smaller reinforcers. The classic example of token reinforcement from your daily life is money. Money has no value in and of itself; it is only a powerful reinforcer because it can be exchanged for other powerful reinforcers (e.g., food, housing, clothing, etc.).

When beginning a token system, it is critical to customize it to the verbal level of the learner. If you are working with a minimally verbal learner who has no history of using token systems, you will need to directly condition the tokens to be reinforcers. To do this, begin by giving the learner the token and immediately prompting her to give it back to you, at which point you immediately give her a highly preferred reinforcer. Repeat this process in blocks of 5 or 10 repetitions, several times per day. This process takes advantage of classical conditioning because you are pairing a previously neutral stimulus with a known reinforcer, resulting in the neutral stimulus becoming a conditioned reinforcer. You might notice the learner respond emotionally, as well. She might appear happy to get the tokens and/or might smile when she receives them.

After the learner reliably relinquishes the token to receive the backup reinforcer (perhaps following 1 or 2 days of repeated conditioning), you may be ready to start using the tokens during teaching sessions. Begin with requiring compliance with only a single task, immediately give the learner the token, and then immediately prompt her to hand it back to you, if she does not do so independently. After many repetitions of this process with little or no challenging behavior and without the need for prompting, consider increasing the work requirement to two task demands. That is, the learner now will need to earn two tokens before she can trade them in for the backup reinforcer. Many clinicians find it useful to create a "token board," a piece of paper or cardboard affixed with Velcro® to hold the tokens. When the board is "full," it serves as a visual discriminative stimulus for the learner to hand the board to you and receive the backup reinforcer.

When constructing the token board and deciding how many tokens the learner must earn before she can trade them in for the backup reinforcer, be careful to consider the value of the backup reinforcer compared to how much work the learner needs to do to earn it. The backup reinforcer has to be "worth it" to the learner. If you want the token reinforcers to be maximally effective, consider using large backup reinforcers and/or a relatively low number of tokens on the token board. Use the following steps, customizing as needed, when setting up a learner's first token system:

Steps for Implementing a Young Learner's First Token System

1. Choose an item that is easily given and removed for use as tokens (pennies, poker chips, stickers, etc.).
2. Identify a pool of highly effective backup reinforcers via a preference assessment.
3. Pair a single token with backup reinforcement repeatedly until the learner independently hands the token to the clinician as soon as he receives it.
4. Require compliance with one task (e.g., one discrete trial) before the learner receives a token and exchanges it for reinforcement.
5. Gradually increase the work requirement, only when the learner is working with little or no challenging behavior (i.e., specify a criterion and stick to it).
6. Consider using a token board to help the clinician stay organized and to serve as a visual cue for the learner.

Unfortunately, at some point you will likely have the experience of working with a learner who has already been receiving behavioral intervention services from a poor-quality treatment provider who implemented a poor-quality token system with her. Fixing this situation may be as simple as reviewing the steps here and identifying where the other treatment provider went wrong (e.g., backup reinforcer too small, work requirement too high, preference assessments not implemented, etc.). Frequently, you may need to start over with new tokens and build up an effective token system from the very beginning.

PROMPTING AND PROMPT FADING

Reinforcement is the foundation of teaching and learning in ABA programs. However, if you only used reinforcement, you might have to wait a very long time for the desired behavior to occur, or when teaching complex skills, the behavior may never occur if you just wait. This is often apparent when you observe particularly low-quality attempts at ABA therapy. It is frequently necessary to use prompting in combination with reinforcement. Prompting involves giving extra help to enable the learner to perform the response you are trying to teach, so you can reinforce it. In technical terms, a prompt is an antecedent stimulus that controls the response you are trying to establish. The antecedent stimulus – the prompt – is different from and additional to the discriminative stimulus that will eventually control the behavior. By definition, then, a prompt is something you use to get the correct behavior to occur, but it's also something that you need to discontinue in order for the behavior change to be meaningful. There are many different types of prompts, and they have been well described elsewhere (Cooper, Heron, & Heward, 2007), but brief descriptions and examples of the most commonly used prompts for teaching learners with ASD are provided below.

Types of Prompts

Physical. Physical prompts are exactly what they sound like: You use physical touch to help the learner perform the behavior. Typically, the clinician uses his hands to help guide the learner to make the desired response. For that reason, physical prompts are often also referred to as "manual" prompts. For example, if you are trying to teach the learner to touch a particular picture of an item when that item's name is spoken, you might physically prompt this by holding the learner's hand in your hand and gently placing it on top of the picture on the desk. If you are teaching a learner to wash her hands, you might hold her hands in yours and guide her hands through the handwashing process. Physical prompts range from full physical guidance to a light physical touch and everything in between. It is important to note that physical prompting is not manual restraint; it is merely the provision of gentle physical help to guide the learner.

Model. To use a model prompt, the clinician demonstrates the desired response to the learner. For example, when teaching a learner to follow simple instructions, the clinician might deliver the instruction, "stand up," while also modeling the behavior by standing up. When teaching basic functional pretend play skills, the clinician might deliver the instruction, "let's play with the trains," and then model the desired response of making a train drive back and forth while making the sound, "choo-choo." When teaching language, vocal model prompts are frequently used. For example, the clinician might deliver the instruction, "what is your name?," and immediately follow it by saying the learner's name.

Gestural. Gestural prompts involve pointing or gesturing in some way to help the learner perform the desired response. For example, when teaching receptive language, the clinician might deliver the instruction, "touch the car," and then point to the picture of the car and not the other pictures that are present. The therapist can also use her own eye gaze as a subtle prompt. For example, when working on social skills, if a learner does not greet a person who walks into the room, the therapist might prompt this behavior by looking at the learner and then making an exaggerated sideways eye gaze and eyebrow raise in the direction of the third person.

Proximity. Proximity prompts consist of placing the correct stimulus to which a learner is to respond closer to him than other stimuli. For example, when teaching a learner to receptively identify items by the function, a clinician might place a fork, a ball, and a car on the table, with the fork 2 inches closer to the learner than the other items. The instruction, "show me the one you eat with," is then delivered, and the closer proximity of the fork serves as the prompt that makes selecting the fork more likely, relative to the other items. Figure 4.1 depicts the use of a proximity prompt while teaching receptive identification of letters.

Textual. Textual prompts are written cues. Occasionally, some learners with ASD respond better to written stimuli than to vocal models or other prompts (see Chapter 6 on visual supports). For example, when teaching expressive pronouns, the clinician might place a card with the printed word *your* on his own shirt and a card with the printed word *my* on the learner's shirt. The clinician might then touch the learner's shirt and ask, "whose shirt is this?" in response to which the learner might look down, see the card with the word *my*, and respond, "my shirt." When teaching a learner to answer personal identification questions (e.g., "What is your mom's phone number?"), written cue cards are sometimes useful. Textual flashcards are a well-known prompt for teaching vocal mathematics, such as times tables.

Intra-stimulus. Intra-stimulus prompts are any type of prompt where the prompt feature is built into the instruction itself. For example, when teaching receptive identification of colors, three color cards may be placed

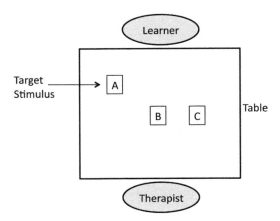

FIGURE 4.1   Use of a proximity prompt while teaching the learner to receptively identify letters. The letter that is targeted on any given trial is placed closer to the learner than the other letters.

on the table. An intra-stimulus prompt can be used by making the correct color card slightly larger than the others. A significant potential advantage of intra-stimulus prompts is that they do not require the learner to attend to some other, irrelevant stimulus (e.g., gesturing, modeling) in the environment to make the correct response. Since the prompt is *in* the stimulus, the learner only attends to the correct stimulus and nothing else, even when prompted. As with all prompts though, intra-stimulus prompts must still be faded.

Prompt Fading

The most important thing about prompting is that it has to work: It must help the learner make the correct response. The second most important thing about prompting is that you have to get rid of it! So, as soon as a prompt starts to work, you should start removing it. The process by which prompts are removed is called *prompt fading*. The importance of prompt fading cannot be overemphasized. By definition, a prompt is an extra stimulus that should not be there when teaching is done. One of the most common causes of undesirable outcomes of poor-quality attempts at ABA is "prompt dependence." Prompt dependence simply means that prompting has not been successfully faded after a response has been reinforced. And it is no exaggeration to say that teaching and learning *have not successfully occurred* if the prompting is still needed. Prompts can be faded in many ways – by duration, frequency, intensity, intrusiveness, and so on. It is useful to categorize most fading procedures as either most-to-least or least-to-most. These names refer to whether you begin with a lot of prompting and fade it out or whether you begin with minimal prompting and fade it in, as necessary.

Most-to-least prompt fading. Most-to-least (MTL) prompt fading involves starting with the largest amount of help (also referred to as the most intrusive or largest amount of prompting) in order to ensure a correct response right away. MTL prompt hierarchies that effectively prevent most errors are often referred to as "errorless learning" procedures. As the learner demonstrates the correct response at the current level of prompting, prompting is gradually faded out by transitioning to progressively less intrusive prompts. This can be done either within or across teaching sessions. For example, consider the following MTL prompting sequence: 1) full physical, 2) partial physical, 3) light touch, 4) no prompt. To implement MTL *within session*, you might deliver the first instructional trial with a full physical prompt. If the learner makes a correct response, you might deliver a partial physical prompt on the next trial, and so on. To implement the same prompting sequence *across* sessions, you might implement one block of 10 teaching trials with a full physical prompt and progress to one block of 10 trials using the next less intrusive level of prompting, as long as the learner is responding at least 80% correct at each level. No conclusive research of which we are aware has shown that within or across-session MTL works better. Both procedures work well, and it is probably best to be conscious of both options and be open to trying either or both with any given skill you are trying to teach any given learner.

Examples of most-to-least prompt sequences.

- 1) Full physical, 2) partial physical, 3) light touch, 4) no prompt
- 1) Full physical, 2) partial physical, 3) 2-second delay to partial physical, 4) no prompt
- 1) Physical, 2) model, 3) vocal
- 1) Point with finger touching correct stimulus, 2) point 2 inches from correct stimulus, 3) point 4 inches from correct stimulus, 4) point 8 inches from correct stimulus

Least-to-most prompt fading. Least-to-most (LTM) prompt fading involves gradually increasing your level of prompting when the learner is not responding successfully across successive trials. "Three-step" prompting is a commonly used LTM procedure that involves moving progressively from a vocal instruction, to a model prompt, to a physical prompt. When using three-step, the first trial of a task does not contain a prompt; you merely deliver the vocal instruction. If the learner does not respond correctly within 3–5 seconds, you then repeat the instruction while also modeling the correct response. If the learner still does not respond correctly, you repeat the instruction while simultaneously providing a physical prompt. Note that any of the prompt sequences described above for MTL prompting can also be implemented in an LTM format by simply reversing the order and progressing through the hierarchy contingent on incorrect responding, rather than correct responding.

No-no prompt. One particular type of LTM prompting strategy is often referred to as the no-no prompt procedure. To implement a no-no prompt, the therapist presents an instruction with no prompt in order to give the learner the opportunity to respond independently. If the learner responds correctly, reinforcement is delivered as always. If the learner responds incorrectly, the therapist says "no" in a neutral tone of voice and repeats the instruction once more. If the learner responds incorrectly again, the therapist again says "no" and then immediately repeats the instruction a third time, but this time accompanies the instruction with a prompt that is likely to help the learner respond correctly. The term *no-no prompt* refers to the consequences that the therapist implements across a series of three trials if the learner responds incorrectly. Originally (i.e., a few decades ago), the no-no prompt was created to ensure that the learner would be able to respond correctly at a minimum of 33% of the time. In more recent times, most agree that ensuring a higher success rate through the use of MTL prompting, particularly

TABLE 4.4 Differences Between Most-to-Least and Least-to-Most Prompting

Most-to-Least	Least-to-Most
Fewer learner errors	More opportunity to learn from errors
Maybe less challenging behavior evoked by errors	Maybe less challenging behavior evoked by prompting
More reinforcement	Less reinforcement
May take longer to fade out prompts	May encourage independence
More skill required of staff	Less skill required of staff
Maybe slower acquisition for very fast learners	Maybe faster acquisition for very fast learners

during initial acquisition, is probably more desirable. We discuss how to choose between prompting strategies in more detail below.

Choosing between MTL and LTM. Little research has compared MTL and LTM prompting, but plenty of research has shown that both are effective. Table 4.4 lists some inherent differences between MTL and LTM approaches. In general, MTL ensures fewer errors and more reinforcement and requires more skill and attention on the part of staff. In general, LTM entails more errors and less reinforcement, requires less skill and attention from staff, and may allow for faster acquisition in learners who acquire skills particularly quickly (because the learner has more opportunities to respond independently and prompts may therefore be faded more quickly). Also, note that LTM procedures fade themselves out automatically because, as the learner begins to respond independently to the instruction itself, the staff do not implement prompts, since prompts are contingent on incorrect responses.

In practice, it appears that particular clinicians and/or particular organizations often have strongly held beliefs about whether MTL or LTM is better. In reality, the best hierarchy to use will probably vary across learners, across lessons within the same learner, and across time with the same learner. For example, a very early learner may be more successful and have less challenging behavior when she does not make errors, so MTL may be better, especially for initial acquisition of skills. As that learner acquires skills, it may be better to switch to an LTM procedure for mastered skills. In addition, as the learner gets older and acquires a more advanced repertoire, she learns more complex skills and may actually learn something important from errors. In such an instance, an LTM approach may be more appropriate. This general pattern – MTL for young learners and initial skill acquisition, and LTM for mastered skills and more complex skills in older learners – is the approach used in the CARD Model. The most important thing to remember, however, is that you will need to be highly sensitive to what works and what does not work for each individual lesson and for each individual learner.

Time delay. Prompting can also be faded by using delays before the prompt is delivered. For example, when teaching manding (see Chapter 11 on language), you might hold up a preferred item and wait for the learner to say the name of the item. During initial acquisition, you will likely need to prompt the learner to say the name of the item, perhaps with a vocal model. Zero time delay would involve giving an immediate vocal model as soon as the learner makes any kind of initiation toward the item (e.g., pointing, reaching, looking). The vocal model can be faded out by gradually increasing the delay between the learner's initiation to the preferred item and your delivery of the prompt. Alternatively, you can use what is called a "constant time delay" procedure, wherein a delay of a particular duration is always used, regardless of the stage of the training. For example, you can always wait 7 seconds to present the vocal model. By doing this, you are essentially providing the learner with a choice: She can wait 7 seconds, respond to the prompt, and then get the reinforcer, or she can respond immediately and get the reinforcer sooner.

DISCRETE TRIAL TRAINING

DTT is probably the best known and yet the most often misunderstood aspect of ABA-based treatment for learners with ASD. Many in the general community still mistakenly believe that DTT is the same thing as ABA and/or that ABA consists only of DTT. This characterization of DTT has always been false; if it were true, this entire manual would consist of only a single chapter labeled DTT. It's true that DTT is an important part of EIBI, and it has formed the foundation for the EIBI programs that have been proven to work in the outcome research literature (see Chapter 27 on research). Rather than being the same as ABA, though, DTT is merely one major teaching paradigm *within* ABA.

DTT is a teaching paradigm that breaks down the teaching and learning interactions of the therapist and learner into discrete antecedent-behavior-consequence units. Each trial has a clear beginning, consisting of an instruction, then an opportunity for the learner to respond, followed by a clear consequence based on the learner's response. We discuss each component of DTT in further detail below.

The Antecedent

The antecedent portion of the discrete trial contains both the motivating operation that establishes your reinforcers as powerful and the instruction, commonly referred to as the "S^D" (which stands for discriminative stimulus). Generally speaking, instructions should be presented clearly and unambiguously. Particularly when a young learner with ASD first begins DTT, it may be important to limit the amount of additional language you present and to speak very clearly with the fewest words possible. For example, when asking Jimmy to hand you a fork, you might not want to say something like, "Hey, Jimmy boy, can you please hand me that fork over there? Yeah, go ahead and hand it to me. Thanks!" Instead, you might simply say, "Give me the fork." If it is the first time the learner is learning the meaning of the word fork, and he has no prior history with or understanding of the words "give me," and you are not trying to teach those words right now, you may want to just say "fork" and prompt the learner to hand it to you.

Guidelines for Effectively Presenting Instructions During DTT

- **Speak clearly and concisely.** In the beginning, the instruction should be stated clearly and unambiguously. You do not need to sound like a robot or a drill instructor, but your speech should be clear and should not include unnecessary words. After the learner begins to acquire the instruction, you can begin to build in extra words to make the instruction sound more natural and to help with generalization to everyday language interactions.
- **Do not state the learner's name before every instruction.** This is a common mistake. If you state the learner's name to get her attention, that is fine, but if you do this excessively, the learner may start to depend on that and only listen to instructions when she hears her name.
- **Do not repeat the instruction without providing a consequence to the learner's last response (or lack thereof).** All discrete trials must have a consequence, so close out an unsuccessful trial with error correction before you present the instruction again.
- **Make sure you have the learner's attention before giving the instruction.** If the learner is not looking at you and listening to you when you give the instruction, he will not hear it and cannot possibly learn from it.
- **The learner should respond only after the entire instruction has been presented.** Some learners will begin to "anticipate" the instruction and will begin to respond before the whole instruction is stated. While it's great that they want to respond quickly, it will lead to errors because many different instructions have the same beginning (e.g., "What's your name?" versus "What's your address?"). If the learner begins to respond early, stop her, give error correction, and move on to the next trial.

The Response

In the context of DTT, there are generally three ways that a learner can respond to the instruction: 1) correctly, 2) incorrectly, or 3) no response.

Guidelines for Responses During DTT

- **All members of the treatment team must be consistent about what counts as a correct response.** If one member reinforces a particular attempt at a response and another one does not, it will confuse the learner, produce frustration, and impede learning. Later, when the learner begins to acquire the response, encouraging varied responding is great, but you will still need to be consistent about the different variations that should be reinforced.
- **Correct response must not be accompanied by extraneous behaviors.** Early learners will often try several different behaviors that have been reinforced in the past, in addition to the correct response to an instruction. If you reinforce correct responses that are accompanied by extraneous behavior, many learners will continue to do those extraneous behaviors in the future, often resulting in long chains of strange behaviors that are not related to the instruction. Therefore, it is important to block these extraneous responses, close the trial with error correction, and move on to the next trial.
- **The learner should be given a maximum of 3–5 seconds to begin to respond to the instruction.** Many people naturally want to give learners with ASD longer to respond to an instruction because the instruction is difficult, and they perceive the learner as potentially having underlying processing difficulties. However, in top-quality ABA programs, we are teaching the learner to pay close attention to the instructor and to respond fluently. Once 3–5 seconds have passed since the instruction, it is highly likely that the learner is no longer paying attention and may begin engaging in stereotypy or some other unrelated response. If we require fast responding and we reinforce it, we will get it, and this will serve the learner much better in the future when he does not have more than 3–5 seconds to respond in real-life situations, such as classroom and social situations.

The Consequence

The consequence portion of DTT is comprised of what the clinician does immediately after the learner engages in a response. Essentially, there are only two consequences in DTT: 1) reinforcement or 2) error correction. All correct responses should be reinforced immediately, according to whatever reinforcement system you have in place for that lesson and for that particular learner.

Guidelines for Effective Reinforcement During DTT

- **Reinforce immediately (less than 2-second delay).** The research is very clear: The longer the delay to reinforcement, the less the reinforcement works. Reinforce quickly.
- **Give enthusiastic verbal praise while delivering the reinforcer.** We always want the learner to know when he is right, and we always want to focus on conditioning praise as a reinforcer (as discussed earlier). Eventually, when the learner is older and working much more independently, you will not need to praise every single good thing he does (as discussed in Chapter 7 on maintenance).
- **Make the praise genuine and varied.** Even learners with ASD who have severe social deficits can recognize insincerity. If you want your praise to work, it has to be genuine and varied; i.e., do not just say "good job" every time the learner makes a correct response.
- **Limit free access to the reinforcer.** As discussed in the section on motivating operations, free access to reinforcement decreases its potency. During DTT, the reinforcer should be delivered only for correct responses.
- **Conduct frequent brief preference assessments.** As already discussed, you will need to conduct very frequent MSWO preference assessments (at least before each block of discrete trials) to ensure that the reinforcer you are using is the most effective one available.

Incorrect responses and no response should be treated the same: They should result in an error correction procedure. There are two primary choices for error correction procedures, both of which are popular and both of which work well: 1) informational-no procedure or 2) head-down procedure. The informational-no procedure involves telling the learner that she made an incorrect response. This can consist of saying "no," "not quite," "nope," "uh-uh," and so on. The procedure is called an "informational" no because you are merely trying to make it clear to the learner that she made an incorrect response. It is for feedback, not punishment, so a neutral tone should be used, not a negative or harsh one.

The head-down procedure consists of the clinician responding to the learner's error by briefly looking away in a clear and noticeable way. This can be done by the clinician looking at his lap, turning his head to the side, or looking down onto a table. Often, the need for the clinician to collect data necessitates something of this sort at the end of every trial anyway. Very little research has compared the informational-no correction procedure to the head-down procedure. Different individuals and organizations have strongly held beliefs about which is better. The head-down procedure may make it more difficult for the learners to discriminate when they have made an error. However, the informational-no procedure may evoke more challenging behavior, especially for learners who find the word "no" aversive. Many clinicians have noted that omitting the informational-no procedure from lessons that are particularly frustrating for a learner, such as vocal imitation, works well. The important point is to be flexible and customize your error correction procedure to what works best for each individual learner and each individual lesson.

Discrimination

Discrimination means that a behavior occurs in the presence of one stimulus and not in the presence of another stimulus because that behavior has a history of reinforcement in the presence of that specific stimulus that has not occurred in the presence of other stimuli. For example, with naming behavior, a learner calls apples "apple," and he does not call other stimuli "apple." The learner comes to do this because he has received praise in the past from parents when he called apples "apple," and he did not receive praise when he called other stimuli "apple." The stimulus that controls the behavior is called the **discriminative stimulus** (S^D). In non-technical terms, the S^D "signals" to the learner that a particular behavior will get reinforced if it occurs in the presence of that stimulus. The telephone is a classic example of discrimination in everyone's daily life. The sound of the phone ringing is the S^D that signals that the behavior of answering the phone will result in the reinforcer of being able to speak to someone. If the same behavior (picking up the phone) occurs when the phone is not ringing, it will not get that reinforcer.

Teaching discriminations is fundamental to intervention for learners with ASD, as virtually all complex behavior involves discriminations of some sort. Accordingly, many types of discriminations must be taught, and many ways exist to teach them. Below, we describe how to implement the procedures that form the core of the CARD approach to discrimination training.

Mass trials and random rotation. Two key terms to know regarding discrimination training are **mass trial** and **random rotation**. Mass trial refers to presenting the same instruction repeatedly. For example, on the first trial, you might ask a learner to touch his head. Then, on the second trial, you would present the same instruction, and again on the third trial, and so on, until some criterion has been met. The purpose of mass trialing is to give repeated practice on a very simple but challenging skill. Some believe that mass trialing is crucial to early discrimination learning, whereas others believe that it is rarely, if ever, helpful. The rationale for why mass trials may not be helpful is that, by definition, they do not require a discrimination; they merely require the learner to repeat what she just did a second earlier. The rationale for why they are helpful is that they make the task as easy as possible and, therefore, provide maximum opportunity for reinforcement and maximum practice on new targets. Little research has directly evaluated the question of when and with whom mass trials should be used. It is worth noting that the major outcome studies demonstrating the most robust learning outcomes for learners with ASD have either used or not used mass trials, depending on the background of the researchers involved, so it is clear that DTT can be effective with or without mass trials. The CARD approach to teaching discriminations is to use mass trials early on, especially if a learner has learned few or no discriminations in the past, and especially when first introducing new targets. As a learner builds a history of learning discriminations, you can fade out or eliminate the use of mass trials.

Use of mass trials is sometimes done with distractors. Mass trialing with distractors is a procedure in which the same target instruction is repeatedly presented, but other stimuli are present. For example, with red, blue, and yellow objects present on the table, the teacher asks the learner to touch the red one. On each trial, the teacher always asks for red, but the positions of the stimuli change and stimuli of other colors are always present. This procedure is slightly more difficult than pure mass trials but still only requires the learner to repeat the same behavior she did a few seconds ago.

Random rotation is a procedure during which trials of the same target are **not** repeated in succession. For example, you might ask a learner to touch his head on the first trial, to touch his nose on the second trial, and to touch his ears on the third trial, and subsequent trials would randomly select from the three targets. In other words, random rotation requires the learner to choose between a stimulus that is currently being taught and one or more other stimuli.

Successive discriminations. One basic distinction to be aware of is the difference between a **simultaneous** and a **successive** discrimination. In plain English, successive discriminations require the learner to tell the difference between two or more stimuli that are not present at the same time. For example, consider the following situation: The clinician asks the learner to wave her hand, and the learner waves. Then, the clinician asks her to put her arms up, and she does so. When the clinician presents the first instruction, there is only one instruction present at the time, and there are no other stimuli from which the learner can choose; she merely responds directly to the instruction. A moment later, when the instruction is different, the learner does something different. But the learner is not choosing in any given moment between putting her arms up and touching her belly; she merely does what is asked in the moment.

Common Lessons Requiring Successive Discriminations

- **Following instructions** (one step, two step, etc.). Lessons where the therapist states a simple instruction (e.g., "stand up," "sit down," "close the door"), and the learner responds by performing the requested action

- **Receptive actions** (where the learner acts out the action). Lessons where the therapist presents an instruction that requests the learner to pretend to engage in an action (e.g., "show me sleeping," "show me running," "show me eating")
- **Expressive object labeling** (tacting). Lessons where the therapist holds up an object and asks the learner "what is it?" and the learner responds with a vocal label
- **Intraverbals** (e.g., social ID questions, categories). Lessons where the therapist asks a vocal question and the learner gives a vocal response (e.g., "what is your name?" or "can you tell me three kinds of animals?")

Three-step method for teaching successive discriminations. Most basic successive discriminations can be taught using this three-step procedure: 1) mass trial Target 1; 2) mass trial Target 2; and 3) random rotation Targets 1 and 2. For example, if you want to teach a learner to act out actions ("receptive actions"), you might start with "show me eating" and "show me running," where eating is Target 1 and running is Target 2. For step 1, you present trials of "show me eating" over and over, using prompting, reinforcement, and prompt fading, until the learner demonstrates the correct response independently, according to whatever mastery criterion you use with that learner. You then implement Step 2 by repeating the same process, but with "show me running." After meeting the mastery criterion for running, you then implement Step 3 by presenting blocks of trials where the instruction randomly switches between the two instructions. Again, prompting, reinforcement, and prompt fading continue to be used until the learner meets the mastery criterion with the two targets in random rotation. Future targets would be introduced by first mass trialing them and then placing them in random rotation with previously mastered targets. You can also drop back a step if a learner has a particularly difficult time learning a specific target. Figure 4.2 depicts hypothetical data from a learner who was taught three successive discriminations using this process.

Simultaneous discriminations. In plain English, a simultaneous discrimination requires you to tell the difference between two or more stimuli that are present at the same time. An easy way to think of this is that simultaneous discriminations are like multiple choice tests. For example, when asked "where's the cup?" in the presence of a cup and a fork, the learner responds by pointing to the cup and not the fork.

Common Lessons Requiring a Simultaneous Discrimination

- **Matching identical stimuli.** Lessons where two or more stimuli (e.g., pictures or objects) are placed on the table in front of the learner and the therapist hands the learner a stimulus that is identical to one of those on the table and instructs the learner to "match" or "put with same"

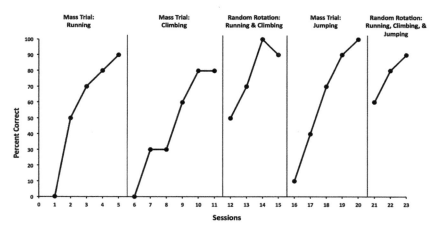

FIGURE 4.2 Sample graph of discrete trial data for a lesson teaching a learner three successive discriminations (acting out receptive actions). Note that the teaching progresses through phases of mass trials and random rotation, when the mastery criterion of two consecutive sessions at 80% correct or higher is met, across multiple targets, ending with three total targets mastered in random rotation.

- **Receptive identification of objects, categories, emotions, etc.** Lessons where two or more stimuli are placed on the table in front of the learner and the therapist asks the learner to indicate one (e.g., "touch the fork," "touch the animal," "touch happy")
- **Receptive academics (letters, numbers, shapes, etc.).** Lessons where two or more stimuli (e.g., flashcards) are placed on the table in front of the learner and the therapist asks the learner to indicate one (e.g., "touch the Q," "touch 8," "touch the triangle")

Discrimination training methods can be customized in countless ways for teaching simultaneous discriminations. We have found that the three-step method and the seven-step method work in the vast majority of cases, so we describe these two in detail here.

Three-step method. For learners who acquire discriminations rapidly, the following three-step method may be sufficient: 1) mass trial (MT) Target 1; 2) MT Target 2; and 3) random rotation Target 1 and 2. For example, when teaching a learner to recognize facial expressions indicating anger and happiness, you begin by placing a picture on the table in front of the learner of a person smiling. Step 1 involves asking the learner to "touch happy," "give me happy," or "point to happy." The learner is then prompted to respond to the picture of the person smiling (the only picture on the table). After several successful trials, prompting is faded out and the learner continues to respond correctly. To implement Step 2, repeat the process with a lone picture of a person making an angry face. To implement Step 3, place both pictures on the table at the same time. For each trial, randomly move the position of the two pictures and randomly choose whether to ask for the happy picture or the angry picture. As always, prompting is used to facilitate correct responding, correct responding is reinforced, and prompts are faded. Step 3 continues until the learner meets the mastery criterion (e.g., 80% correct on both stimuli for two consecutive blocks of trials, across two days and two therapists).

Seven-step method. For learners who are more challenged by learning discriminations, we have found this seven-step method to be effective: 1) MT Target 1 alone; 2) MT Target 1 with unknown distractor; 3) MT Target 2 alone; 4) MT Target 2 with unknown distractor; 5) MT Target 1 with Target 2 as distractor; 6) MT Target 2 with Target 1 as distractor; and 7) random rotation Target 1 and Target 2.

Let's again consider the example of teaching recognition of emotional facial expressions, this time with the seven-step method. Step 1 is identical to Step 1 of the three-step method described above: You merely mass trial a picture of someone smiling until the learner responds correctly and independently. To implement Step 2, you present the happy picture on the table next to another picture that is unknown to the learner (e.g., a picture of a piece of farm equipment). Every trial in Step 2 still only asks for the learner to touch the happy picture, but this time the learner must *avoid* touching the unknown picture, a discrimination that is, perhaps, just a small step up in difficulty from Step 1. This step is continued until the learner can consistently respond correctly and without prompting. Step 3 is identical to Step 2 of the three-step procedure; you merely mass trial the angry face alone until responding is consistently independent and correct. Step 4 is identical to Step 2 of the seven-step method, but you use the angry picture instead of the happy picture. To implement Step 5, you place both happy and angry pictures on the table in front of the learner, but you only ask for happy. So Step 5 *almost* requires the learner to discriminate between happy and angry but not fully because he can merely repeat what he did on the last prompted trial, since every trial is the same in that they all ask for the happy picture. Step 6 is the same, but now you only ask for the angry picture. As always, repeat until responding is independent and accurate. Finally, Step 7 is identical to Step 3 of the three-step method. The positions of the stimuli are randomly rotated in each trial, and the stimulus that you request is randomly determined in each trial. Accurate and unprompted performance at this step comprises the "true" discrimination you are trying to teach.

Expanded trials. For some learners, the jump from mass trials to random rotation seems too large. That is, for some learners, mass trials may seem too easy, and random rotation may seem too challenging. Yet another option for discrimination training is referred to as **expanded trials,** a procedure for gradually fading from MT to random rotation. For example, with Targets 1 and 2, you may conduct one block of trials where Target 1 is repeated for the first five trials and then Target 2 is presented for trials 6–10. During the next block of trials, Target 1 would be conducted during trials 1–4, and Target 2 would occupy trials 5–8. During the third block of trials, Target 1 would only be repeated three times before switching to Target 2. In other words, the number of consecutive trials in which a particular target is repeated before switching to the other target is gradually reduced over successive blocks of trials, contingent on continued accurate responding, until only one trial of each target is conducted before switching to the other target, thereby becoming random rotation. Table 4.5 depicts a sample progression through expanded trials while teaching discrimination between pictures of a cat and dog. Each block of trials represents 10 discrete trials and the particular stimulus that is targeted on each trial of each block. The process begins with targeting the same stimulus five trials in a row (mass trialing) and gradually progresses to randomly rotating between targeting the two stimuli (random rotation), across blocks of 10 trials. Note that the fifth block of trials (random rotation) does not simply alternate between the two stimuli, as this would be predictable and not random. Instead, the sequence is determined randomly, with the rule that the same target should never be presented three times in a row.

Random rotation only. For learners who already have extensive discrimination repertoires and/or learners who find mass trialing particularly frustrating (for whom mass trialing may evoke challenging behavior), you may consider introducing new targets directly into random rotation. If this works, then you have eliminated some unnecessary steps. If an upward trend in accuracy is not apparent fairly soon, then you may want to consider the three-step method.

Choosing among procedures. Most clinicians feel that one procedure is generally better than others, but very little research has been done that can tell you which procedure to choose for which particular learner at any given time. In general, it is critical that you think about which level each particular learner is at and how much assistance she will need to learn the discrimination, since the various procedures differ in the amount of assistance they give. The more assistance they give, the longer they will take for learners who do not need that much assistance. That being said, the procedures that provide more assistance may actually be completed more quickly overall, even though they have more steps, if they help the learner to be more successful. Table 4.6 lists the various procedures for teaching simultaneous discriminations in descending order from most assistance to least assistance.

Mastery Criteria

It is important to have a clearly defined criterion with which to determine when a particular skill is mastered and/or when a particular lesson

TABLE 4.5 Sample Progression Through Expanded Trials

Trial	Target	Trial	Target	Trial	Target	Trial	Target	Trial	Target
1	Cat	1	Cat	1	Cat	1	Cat	1	Cat
2	Cat	2	Cat	2	Cat	2	Cat	2	Dog
3	Cat	3	Cat	3	Cat	3	Dog	3	Cat
4	Cat	4	Cat	4	Dog	4	Dog	4	Dog
5	Cat	5	Dog	5	Dog	5	Cat	5	Dog
6	Dog	6	Dog	6	Dog	6	Cat	6	Cat
7	Dog	7	Dog	7	Cat	7	Dog	7	Dog
8	Dog	8	Dog	8	Cat	8	Dog	8	Cat
9	Dog	9	Cat	9	Cat	9	Cat	9	Cat
10	Dog	10	Cat	10	Dog	10	Cat	10	Dog

TABLE 4.6 Procedure for Simultaneous Discriminations

Teaching Procedure	
Seven-Step Procedure with Expanded Trials	**Most Assistance for Learner, Can**
Seven-Step Procedure without Expanded Trials	**Be Slower**
Three-Step Procedure with Expanded Trials	$\updownarrow$
Three-Step Procedure without Expanded Trials	
Straight to Random Rotation	**Least Assistance for Learner, Can**
	Be Faster

should move from one phase to the next. During DTT, it is common to require 80% correct across two or more blocks of trials, across two or more days, and across two or more clinicians. Some individuals and organizations require 90% or higher, instead of 80%. Little research has directly compared these two mastery criteria. It is logical to infer that the 80% criterion may result in faster acquisition but may allow some skills to "slip through" that were not sufficiently mastered, whereas the 90% criterion might prevent some learners from progressing as fast as they may otherwise but is more likely to ensure that the skills are truly mastered. Our clinical supervisors have anecdotally observed that some learners seem to get "bored" when a 90% mastery criterion is used. That is, they are readily able to learn new skills and something about the process of learning new material helps maintain motivation. In those circumstances, continuing to present the same material seems to serve as an establishing operation (EO) that decreases motivation. If this is true, it could lead to decreases in attending during instruction and increases in escape-motivated behaviors.

Generalization as a criterion for mastery. Another option that is rarely used and probably should be used more is requiring a demonstration of generalization across stimuli, people, and/or settings as part of the mastery criteria (see Chapter 7 on generalization). For some skills, there is no meaningful mastery without generalization because the skill is defined by generalization. For example, in teaching motor imitation, whether a learner with ASD can imitate any particular motor movement that the clinician demonstrates is irrelevant; the point of the lesson is to establish the generalized ability to imitate virtually any movement done by the clinician, so that model prompts can be used in the future. Therefore, mastery of this lesson is not achieved until generalization to untrained motor movements has been demonstrated. Although less obviously critical, the same can be true of many other lessons. For example, a learner has not really mastered the skill of labeling blue things as "blue" until he shows that he can do it with blue objects that were never present during training. Therefore, it would be wise to consider building at least some minimal demonstration of generalization into all of your mastery criteria. It's worth noting, too, that simply requiring that a trained response is demonstrated across two different clinicians does not require generalization. If both clinicians helped train the skill and the learner now does the skill in the presence of both, generalization has not been tested. To demonstrate generalization, you now need to test the skill in the presence of a clinician who was never present when that skill was trained.

NATURAL ENVIRONMENT TRAINING

DTT is the primary teaching paradigm used in comprehensive ABA to ensure that sufficient learning opportunities occur during the learner's day. However, all top-quality ABA programs these days also include some degree of naturalistic behavioral instruction, which we refer to as Natural Environment Training (NET). NET is important for a number of reasons. Although no outcome study has compared comprehensive ABA programs with and without strong NET components, a large amount of small-scale, short-term research has shown that NET has a number of benefits, including decreasing challenging behaviors and enhancing generalization, among others (Delprato, 2001). Several instructional methods can be classified as naturalistic teaching, including, but not limited to, incidental teaching, milieu teaching, and pivotal response training (see Allen & Cowan, 2008, for a review of naturalistic teaching procedures). Of course, individual features of these different models distinguish them from one another, but they have more in common than not. We use the term NET to refer to them all, and we describe the features that can be reasonably used to define the NET paradigm more generally.

Defining Features of Natural Environment Training

Table 4.7 depicts the general defining features of NET and contrasts them with their counterparts in DTT. It is important to note that this table represents an oversimplification for ease of discussion. The two teaching

TABLE 4.7 Natural Environment Training (NET) Contrasted with Discrete Trial Training (DTT)

Variables	Natural Environment Training	Discrete Trial Training
Setting	Natural	Contrived
Degree of Structure	Less Structured	More Structured
Who Initiates the Interaction?	Learner	Therapist
Prompting	Any Effective ABA Prompt	Any Effective ABA Prompt
Reinforcement	Natural Consequence of Behavior	Any Effective Reinforcer

paradigms are flexible, and actual therapy at any given moment often blends elements of both. Nevertheless, it is useful to make the DTT–NET distinction to discuss several important aspects of teaching, as we do below.

Natural environment. The most obvious defining feature of NET is that it occurs in the learner's natural environment, at least as much as possible. For example, whereas you might teach a learner to label colors in DTT while sitting at a desk, you might teach the same skill in NET while playing with the learner with toys of various colors on the floor of her living room. Similarly, you could use a DTT approach to teach a learner to button a button by using a "button board" while seated at a desk, or you could teach the same skill using an NET approach by teaching the learner in the context of putting on a shirt that has buttons while she gets dressed in her bedroom. Likewise, you could teach a learner to receptively identify prepositions in DTT by placing objects on/under/next to one another on a table and asking him to point to the corresponding items. The same skill could be taught using an NET approach by surreptitiously placing a learner's favorite toy on/under/next to his bed and then telling him where to find it when he asks for it.

In reality, it is often hard to find enough learning opportunities in a learner's truly natural environment to teach everything you need to teach without making the environment "unnatural" in some way. Therefore, NET is rarely "purely" natural. By the same token, it is rarely necessary or desirable to conduct DTT in a completely unnatural setting. DTT can be very effectively done while sitting on the living room floor with a learner. Clear instructions and consequences can be "snuck in" to natural daily interactions on a regular basis, thereby resulting in learning opportunities that look very much like DTT but occur in completely natural settings.

Less structured. NET teaching interactions are generally less structured than DTT teaching interactions. For example, in DTT, rapid trials are presented repeatedly, and there is a clear "dance" back and forth between therapist and learner. That is, the same basic structure occurs repeatedly: S^D – prompt (if needed) – response – consequence – next trial. This basic structure is highly recognizable. In NET teaching interactions, it is harder to identify the basic structure of the interaction. If the learner does not initiate an interaction (see below), several minutes may pass in between teaching opportunities, during which time the learner may be playing freely by herself. In these cases, an outside observer may not even know that teaching or "treatment" is taking place; it may merely look like an adult playing with a child in an unstructured manner. Alternatively, the learner may initiate at a high rate, thereby causing interactions to occur at a high rate. Regardless, the structure is far less visible in NET than it is in DTT. However, as you will see as you read through this section, good NET does not lack structure; the structure is merely "looser" and less repetitive.

Learner initiated. The learner, rather than the therapist, initiates NET teaching interactions. Consider the example of teaching a learner to label preferred objects. To do so in DTT, the therapist and learner are seated together, and the therapist initiates the teaching interactions by gaining the learner's attention, holding up an object, and presenting the instruction, "What is it?" To teach the same skill in NET, a preferred object could be placed on a shelf where it is out of reach but visible. When the learner reaches for the object or initiates to the therapist for the therapist to give him the object, that moment is the beginning of the teaching interaction. The therapist then responds by waiting for the learner to state the name of the object or by prompting him to do so. In NET, then, the frequency of teaching interactions is controlled purely by how often the learner initiates toward something in the environment that represents an opportunity for the therapist to teach the skills she is trying to teach.

In NET, the reason for waiting for a learner initiation before trying to teach is to ensure learner motivation. In DTT, the therapist presents as many learning trials as possible. Motivation is ensured through using powerful reinforcers and making sure that relevant establishing operations are in place for them. In NET, teaching does not occur until a learner initiates toward something. The rationale is that there must be a reason that the learner is initiating, i.e., it is not random but occurs because the learner wants something. In technical terminology, the learner initiates because there is a relevant establishing operation that evokes the initiation and ensures that the corresponding reinforcer (the thing the learner "wants") is going to be strong at that moment. In most cases, this establishing operation is deprivation of some kind. That is, the learner does not have something that she wants, and the only way she can get it is by initiating to the therapist in some way. Advocates of NET point out that this ensures that the learner is always motivated, but good-quality practitioners of DTT use frequent preference assessments to ensure that strong reinforcers are always present.

Prompting. Prompting is a crucial part of NET, just as it is in DTT. Some mistakenly believe that one just waits for correct responding to occur in NET, as though the learner will eventually figure out what to do with no help. This approach is critically flawed and will almost certainly result in the learner becoming frustrated (if the therapist really withholds instruction forever) or result in less learning (if the therapist merely "gives in" and gives the learner what she wants, even though she has not responded correctly). Instead, good NET uses effective prompting right from the beginning. For example, if a learner is learning to request (mand) for milk and currently cannot approximate the word in any way, the therapist might begin by spending time with the learner at the kitchen table. The therapist can set up the environment by pouring a glass of milk and placing it out of reach on the table. When the learner reaches for the glass, points to it, or initiates toward it in any way, the therapist looks at the learner with an "expectant look," as if to say "what do you want?" but without actually saying anything. If an MTL prompting procedure is to be used, the therapist then immediately gives a full model prompt, such as "milk." If the learner imitates the prompt, the therapist then immediately gives him a sip of milk and puts the milk back out of reach. If the learner initiates toward the milk again, the process is repeated and the model prompt is faded across successive trials.

Natural consequences as reinforcers. When teaching with DTT, the therapist uses whatever reinforcer is likely to be powerful in the moment, as determined by a brief preference assessment conducted within the past 5 minutes or so. When teaching with NET, the therapist reinforces learner responding with a natural or "functional" consequence as much as possible. For example, as a reinforcer for saying "red," the learner receives something red that she wants. Similarly, as a reinforcer for saying the action word "dance," the therapist and learner might dance to music together for 30 seconds. Finally, as a reinforcer for putting on her shoes, a learner might then get to go outside and play.

There are several aspects to the rationale behind using the natural consequence as a reinforcer during NET. First, many believe that motivation is more likely to be high. In other words, a learner would rather do something because it truly results in something good, rather than do something for some arbitrary reason. At the commonsense level, this seems logical, but an analysis in terms of behavioral principles does not necessarily support this premise. The principle of reinforcement is defined functionally: If a consequence *works* to strengthen a behavior, then it is a reinforcer. Consequences that are particularly effective at strengthening behaviors are particularly strong reinforcers for those behaviors. This is equally true whether the consequence is natural or contrived. Natural consequences, on the one hand, can be enormously powerful or, on the other hand, completely irrelevant. The same is true of contrived consequences. Consider housework. For people for whom housecleaning is not automatically reinforcing (i.e., most of us), the natural consequence of cleaning your house (having a tidy house) is sufficient to maintain the behavior at a reasonable level. But what if someone offered to pay you $500 to clean your house? Or how about $5,000 or $50,000? The basic point is that the reinforcers you use during behavioral intervention need to be enormously powerful. It's great to identify natural consequences that are powerful enough; absent such consequences, however, you will likely need to contrive them, regardless of whether you are taking primarily a DTT or NET approach at any given time.

Another important point about reinforcement during NET relates to the particular behaviors the therapist chooses to reinforce. The particular response that the therapist accepts as correct will depend on the learner and her abilities. In the example of saying "milk" above, it would depend on the learner's vocal imitation abilities. For a learner who can readily vocally imitate whole words, the therapist might only reinforce the entire word "milk." For a learner who has more difficulty, the therapist might only require an approximation, such as "muh" or "kuh." Advocates of pivotal response training (PRT; one type of NET) generally recommend reinforcing any attempt the learner makes at responding, especially at first.

Balancing Discrete Trial Training and Natural Environment Training

Many clinicians have strong opinions about the relative merits of DTT and NET, but virtually all top-quality treatment providers agree that it is not a choice *between* DTT and NET but, rather, a process of determining the best balance of the two for each individual learner and each individual skill being taught. In striking this balance, the relative strengths and limitations of both DTT and NET should be considered.

Strengths of NET. In comparison to DTT, it is likely that NET helps encourage generalization across settings and stimuli. The primary reason for this is that, when it is implemented with high quality, NET is conducted across a variety of settings and stimuli. A major goal of behavioral intervention is to establish skills that a learner will then be able to perform across all settings, including different rooms of his house, different community settings, and so on. Good NET is implemented across all of these settings, and so it is likely that the learner will be able to perform the skills across these settings. Some research has also demonstrated that some learners with ASD demonstrate less challenging behavior during NET than DTT. If the therapist is doing a better job of understanding the learner's motivation in NET than DTT, this could make sense. Or if the learner's challenging behavior is escape motivated, and he is required to do a lower rate of work in NET than in DTT, this could also make sense. Therapists, however, have successfully decreased challenging behavior during DTT and replaced it with functional alternative behaviors without having to implement NET, so a well-trained therapy team should be able to decrease challenging behaviors significantly in DTT settings. A final potential advantage of NET is that it appears to be more "normal" and often more fun than DTT. This is a significant advantage and is worth considering. However, when implemented at a high level of excellence, DTT is fun for the learner, too, because he is being challenged (but not excessively), he is earning frequent high-quality reinforcement, and he is given effective help (good prompting) when needed.

Strengths of DTT. Several relative strengths of DTT are worth considering. First and foremost, DTT causes a large number of learning opportunities to occur in the learner's environment. Simply put, NET can never produce as many learning opportunities as fast-paced DTT. The general consensus is that it is critical to maximize the number of learning opportunities for learners in EIBI programs, and DTT is a great way to do it. A second advantage of DTT is that, since it is structured and clearly defined, it is relatively easy to train staff and parents to do it and to maintain integrity. Finally, many situations in the learner's future will require her to sit still and pay attention, even when she does not want to do so. Effective DTT helps establish these "readiness-to-learn" skills, which are critical for success in mainstream educational settings. Put differently, in a regular education class, the teacher simply cannot follow the student around and wait for the student to want to learn; the teacher must teach and the learner must sit at her desk, pay attention, and do what the teacher asks.

When weighing the pros and cons of DTT and NET and deciding how best to use them both with any individual learner and for any individual skill, there are several options. We describe three general formats for balancing DTT and NET below.

NET-first option. Some clinicians believe that it is better to start teaching a particular skill with NET and then, if the learner does not progress well, use some DTT. For example, if one is teaching a young learner colors, one might do it in NET by arranging for preferred items of various colors to be just out of reach of the learner. When the learner reaches for one of the items, the clinician might prompt the learner to say the color name and then give the learner the preferred item when he makes an attempt to say the color. If the learner does not show progress across a week or two, then separate DTT time may be added to the learner's schedule, specifically to provide more practice learning colors.

DTT-first option. Others believe you should start teaching most skills with DTT and progress to NET to help generalize those skills. Using this strategy for teaching colors, you start by teaching the learner to label the color of objects in DTT until she reaches mastery criteria. Your next step resembles the first step described in the section above: Assess whether the learner will label the colors of objects in the natural environment, perhaps with preferred items at first. If she does, you give the learner the preferred items. If she does not label the colors, you might prompt the behaviors and reinforce accordingly.

Combined option. Yet a third option is to begin teaching each skill with both DTT and NET from the very start. For example, in the first 5 minutes of a session, you might conduct 10 discrete trials where you work on labeling colors. In the immediately subsequent 5 minutes, you might take the learner to a play area and play with preferred toys that are of the same color and proceed by contriving NET learning opportunities with colors.

Unfortunately, very little research has directly addressed the question of which approach to use for any particular skill with any particular learner. A small amount of research has attempted to predict which learners respond well to PRT, and some research has directly compared more structured and less structured teaching strategies for particular skills. No research of which we are aware has attempted to develop procedures to help predict whether DTT or NET (or which combination) is best when beginning to work with any particular learner or to develop any particular skill. As with everything else in ABA treatment, it is best to be flexible, open-minded, and analytic. Keep your eyes wide open and use data to try to determine which approach seems to work best for each learner. At CARD, we generally start with DTT or use the combined option. For early learners who seem to require more structure, we might start with DTT and progress to NET for each individual skill as it is acquired in DTT. For learners with more advanced repertoires, we may begin with the combined option from the start. Finally, for learners who are older and working on much more complex skills (e.g., complex perspective taking), we may go straight to a more naturalistic approach and never do anything that resembles a structured DTT approach.

CHAINING AND SHAPING

Chaining is a procedure that is used to teach behaviors that occur in sequences of two or more steps. An example of such a behavior might be making a sandwich. Many different steps are required to make a sandwich. An example of a behavior that does not occur in sequences of two or more steps is saying the word "no." There is only one step in this behavior: You simply say "no." Many of the very early skills taught to young learners with ASD are relatively simple and do not require chaining. Most basic motor responses (jumping in place, high fives, arms up, etc.), some basic words, handing over communication cards, simple toy play (basic cause-and-effect toys, etc.), and so on, do not generally need to be broken down into sequences of component steps. Many more complex skills, however, are usefully broken down into their component parts, so each part can be taught separately and more easily. Chaining is the method that is used for this process. The first step in using chaining to teach a skill is to obtain a task analysis of the skill.

Task Analysis

A task analysis is an analysis of all of the component behaviors that make up a complex chain of behaviors. An overly simplified example is making a phone call. Very discrete component behaviors make up the whole chain: First, you pick up your phone; then, you turn it on; then, you dial the first number (or choose a name from the contacts list); and then, you press the "call" button, and so on. Self-care tasks commonly require long sequences of behaviors and are, therefore, often taught using chaining. Here is a sample task analysis of washing one's hands:

Sample Hand-Washing Task Analysis
1. Turn on the water.
2. Wet right hand.
3. Wet left hand.
4. Get soap.
5. Rub fronts of hands together.
6. Rub front of left hand against back of right hand.
7. Rub front of right hand against back of left hand.
8. Rinse soap off hands.
9. Turn off water.
10. Dry hands.

Note that each step of the task analysis is somewhat arbitrarily constructed. Each step is created on the basis of how large of a chunk of behavior you think you can teach at once. For example, steps 5–7 above could be combined into one step that says "rub hands together," if you think the learner can be taught all of that behavior at the same time. For learners who are severely challenged by learning complex sequences of behaviors, you can break a task analysis down even further. For example, step 10 could be broken down into several steps, such as: Walk to towel, grasp towel with right hand, rub towel against left hand, and so on.

The most efficient way to obtain a task analysis is to get one that already exists and customize it to the needs of your learners. Commercially available curricula, such as Skills® (www.skillsforautism.com; see Chapter 26) and others, are a convenient source of task analyses. If you want or need to make your own, there are several ways you can go about it. You can ask an expert which steps are in the sequence you want to teach. This might be a useful starting point, but you are probably better off observing someone actually engaging in the behavior. For example, you could observe three different people wash their hands, videotape it, and review the videotape and write down the sequence of behaviors of each person. For very familiar behaviors, such as washing hands, this might not be necessary. For more complex behaviors, such as conversational skills, common sense alone may not be sufficient; you may need to consult a curriculum and/or conduct observations.

Forward Chaining

Chaining can be implemented in three primary ways: forward, backward, and total task chaining. The names of these procedures refer to the part of the chain that is being taught first. In forward chaining, the first step of the chain is taught first, and the remaining steps of the chain are either completed by the therapist or the therapist prompts the learner through them without expecting her to complete them independently. In the hand-washing example above, the therapist begins by telling the learner, "let's wash your hands," and then prompts her to complete the first step, that is, to turn on the water. If using an MTL approach, the therapist would implement an immediate physical prompt to ensure that the learner successfully turns on the water. The therapist then praises the correct response and either physically prompts the learner through the rest of the sequence and delivers a high-quality reinforcer or simply ends the sequence after the initial correct response and delivers the reinforcer immediately. If using an LTM approach, the therapist allows the learner to be unsuccessful at turning on the water and then responds by using increasing prompts until the learner responds correctly. Regardless of which prompting approach is used, prompts are faded across successive teaching opportunities until the learner completes the first step without prompting, according to whatever mastery criterion you have in place for that learner. When this occurs, you add the second step of the chain to the procedure. To do this using an MTL approach, the therapist responds when the learner turns on the water by immediately prompting her to wet her right hand. Correct responding is reinforced, and prompting is faded as before. As the learner masters each new step in the chain, the next step is added to the teaching procedure until the learner eventually completes the entire chain independently in response to the therapist's instruction, "let's wash your hands."

Backward Chaining

Backward chaining uses the same basic approach as forward chaining but in reverse order. That is, you start with the last step in the chain rather than the first. The therapist can either prompt the learner through the entire sequence, without opportunities for independent responding, until he gets to the final step (and then teach that step), or the therapist can initiate the teaching interaction by going straight to the last step. Either way, when the last step occurs, the therapist uses prompting to help the learner perform the step correctly, reinforces correct responding with a powerful reinforcer, and then fades prompts across subsequent trials. When the last step is mastered, then each teaching interaction begins with the second-to-last step, and so on, until the first step in the chain is mastered, at which point the whole task analysis is mastered.

Total Task Chaining

When teaching a behavioral chain with the total task method, the therapist targets all of the steps in the chain each time the task is presented.

Again, this can be done using an MTL or LTM approach. Whichever prompting method is used, every step in the chain is implemented every time the lesson is conducted, starting with the first step. In the hand-washing example, the therapist begins by saying, "let's wash your hands," and then implements either LTM or MTL, prompting for the step of turning on the water. If an MTL approach is being used, the therapist immediately prompts the learner to turn on the water at a full level of prompting. As soon as that behavior is performed correctly, the therapist then prompts the next step in the chain with a full-level prompt, and so on, for every step in the chain until the chain is complete. On subsequent occasions, the therapist would attempt to fade out the prompting slightly on each step. For example, instead of a full physical prompt, the therapist might implement a partial physical prompt. Some criterion must be set for when and how much prompts should be faded on each step of the chain. For example, each time a learner performs a step correctly on three consecutive teaching opportunities, the prompt should be faded one level on the next teaching opportunity. If an LTM approach is being used, then the therapist begins each step of the chain with no prompt. If the learner fails to perform that step correctly, then the therapist implements the smallest level prompt (e.g., a verbal instruction, such as "turn on the water"). If that prompt does not succeed in occasioning a correct response, then the therapist implements the next higher level prompt (e.g., a model prompt). If the learner still errs, the process continues on that step until a full physical prompt is used. The therapist then repeats that process, from least to most, on the next step in the chain.

Shaping

Shaping is a procedure that allows the therapist to create new forms of behavior, rather than merely reinforcing existing behaviors. Shaping consists of reinforcing successive approximations of a target response. Put simply, shaping is the use of reinforcement to make the form of a response gradually come closer and closer to the final form you are trying to teach. For example, when teaching a learner with ASD some of her first words, it is very unlikely that you will be able to prompt her to say the entire word correctly by modeling it. Instead, she will often be able to imitate some portion of the word. For example, when teaching a learner to ask for (mand) a cracker (assuming it's one of her favorite foods), you might use shaping to gradually teach the learner to pronounce the entire word correctly, even though she can only say "kuh" at first. To do this, the therapist first ensures that the learner wants the cracker by doing a brief preference assessment and then holds up the cracker and says "cracker." If the learner responds by saying "kuh" or anything closer to the actual word "cracker," then the therapist immediately gives her a cracker. On subsequent trials, the therapist would look for something closer to the actual word than "kuh," perhaps "ahkuh." When the learner says something like this, then the therapist immediately gives her a cracker and then requires this new response, or something closer, on subsequent trials in order to deliver the cracker. This general process is continued until the learner can pronounce the entire word correctly.

The particular steps in the shaping procedure must be determined by the clinical supervisor in order to make sure that the team is being consistent and that each therapist is implementing requirements that are reasonable. If the team moves forward too quickly, the process can always be stepped back one step, and earlier approximations of the response can again be reinforced for a while before moving forward. Shaping is one of the few areas of ABA that is in some ways still more of an "art" than a science. No concrete rules govern which steps to use to shape any particular behaviors, and some therapists seem to be good at it while others are not. As with any other therapist skill, the therapists' ability to use shaping can be improved with substantial amounts of training, consisting of modeling, role-play, feedback, and *in vivo* practice.

BEHAVIORAL SKILLS TRAINING

Behavioral Skills Training (BST) is a treatment package consisting of multiple treatment components that has been proven to be effective for training a wide variety of skills, simple and complex, in people in a wide variety of populations, including children and adults with and without disabilities. Several variations of BST exist, but the general model includes 1) verbal instruction, 2) modeling, 3) rehearsal or role-play, and 4) feedback. In other words, the therapist first explains the skill to the learner. Then the therapist models how to do it. Then the therapist invites the learner to rehearse the skill with the therapist. The therapist and learner can switch roles, especially if doing so makes the process more fun for the learner. During role-play, the therapist gives the learner live feedback on her performance. Role-play continues until the learner consistently demonstrates excellent performance. After role-playing is complete, the therapist should arrange for a real-life test of the skill. If the learner performs well, the skill is then placed on a maintenance schedule. If the learner does not perform well, the therapist should give *in situ* feedback and implement further rehearsal. See the safety section of Chapter 13 for examples of how BST can be used to teach safety skills. BST is also particularly useful for parent and staff training, and examples of how to use it for parent training are provided in Chapter 9.

FLUENCY-BASED INSTRUCTION

Within the CARD approach, fluency-based instruction is used to teach skills that require both speed and accuracy for proficient performance. For example, a learner may slowly count money with 100% accuracy. However, when the learner's counting speed increases, this skill can be used to buy items at a store, whereas a learner's excessively slow counting may anger or annoy the other people in line. Similarly, many social skills must be executed fluently in order to be successful. Telling jokes, friendly teasing, and even staying in a conversation require the learner with ASD not only to say something appropriate but also to do so quickly without appearing to have to think about it first.

Fluency-based instruction is founded on the idea of the free operant. A **free operant** is a behavior whose rate of occurrence is not restricted by a particular number of opportunities to respond. For example, a learner can go through a pile of flashcards by herself at whatever rate she is capable of answering them. Therefore, a learner who is particularly fluent in math facts might complete 100 math flashcards in 60 seconds, whereas a learner who is just beginning to learn the same facts and is not fluent may only be able to complete 30 flashcards in the same time period. A **restricted operant** is a behavior whose rate is restricted by the number of opportunities to engage in the behavior. In the same flashcard example, the learner's responding is a restricted operant if someone else is controlling the flashcards. That is, the learner's rate of responding is restricted by how quickly the cards are presented by the other person.

Fluency-based instruction is referred to as a free operant teaching technique because the learner is allowed to perform the target skill at his own pace. During fluency-based lessons, therapists provide the learner with several brief, timed opportunities to practice a skill, and rapid, correct responding is encouraged. Correct performance is measured by calculating the rate of correct responding per minute. Reinforcers are then presented at the end of the time period (typically 10 to 60 seconds) if the learner achieves or exceeds the goal for rate of accurate performance. As the learner becomes successful, his target rate is gradually increased across sessions until fluent responding is achieved. *Fluent performance* is defined as the rate of responding necessary for competent performance (Binder, 1996). Advocates of fluency instruction assert that the benefits of fluent responding include retention of the skill after periods of no practice, an ability to perform the skill at a constant rate for longer periods of time (i.e., endurance), stable performance in the presence of distractions, and use of the fluent skill in new ways or as a component of a more complex skill (Kubina & Wolfe, 2005). In the CARD Model, fluency-based instruction plays a small but important role in encouraging fluency and maintenance after a skill has been mastered in DTT and NET. For further reading, you are encouraged to consult *The Precision Teaching Book* (Kubina & Yurich, 2012).

SUMMARY

Evidence-based autism treatment is a complex process, requiring an intricate combination of a large variety of research-proven procedures, including DTT, NET, reinforcement, prompting, prompt fading, shaping, chaining, BST, and fluency-based instruction, among many more. Top-quality treatment programs do not base treatment decisions on dogma or tradition but, rather, design individualized combinations of procedures for each unique learner based on which procedures meet the needs of that learner and which produce the best results for that learner.

A Functional Approach to Challenging Behavior

Amy Kenzer

This chapter will describe evidence-based practices for the functional assessment and treatment of challenging behavior in children with autism spectrum disorder (ASD). The emphasis of the Center for Autism and Related Disorders (CARD) approach is on implementing the least intrusive treatment procedures possible and producing meaningful decreases in challenging behavior across all aspects of the child's life. The chapter is divided into sections on conducting functional assessments, using function-based behavioral intervention procedures, and writing behavior intervention plans.

THE NEED FOR FUNCTIONAL ASSESSMENT AND TREATMENT OF CHALLENGING BEHAVIOR

Response reduction interventions are an important component of ABA treatment programs for children with ASD. In conjunction with teaching new skills, the treatment team is concerned with reducing challenging behavior that puts an individual at risk of injury or interferes with an individual's ability to learn and/or gain access to reinforcement or less restrictive environments.

Prevalence and Type of Challenging Behavior

While challenging behavior is not a core symptom of ASD, a large percentage of children with ASD display some sort of challenging behavior. Some challenging behaviors are more common among individuals with ASD than in those with other developmental disabilities (see Matson &

Nebel-Schwalm, 2007). The primary challenging behaviors observed in ASD include self-injury, aggression, property destruction, tantrums, stereotypy, and noncompliance. This list is not exhaustive, and a child may display any number of behaviors that may not fall into one of these categories but are challenging nonetheless.

When Challenging Behavior Warrants Treatment

Many aspects of behavior can be "challenging" or "problematic" and, therefore, require treatment. Table 5.1 lists common challenging behaviors seen in children with ASD and potential negative outcomes. With some behaviors, the need for treatment is obvious, while other behaviors are only problematic under certain circumstances or when they affect the child's quality of life. Typically, treatment is warranted when the behavior:

- Poses a risk of physical harm to the child and/or others;
- Interferes with the child's ability to learn new skills;
- Limits the child's ability to access less restrictive settings;
- Increases the likelihood of intrusive interventions, such as exclusionary time-out, restraint, or management of behavior through medication;
- Reduces the child's contact with reinforcers; and/or
- Inhibits social interactions.

These problematic effects of behavior may be obvious in some cases and less obvious in others. For example, sometimes the topography of the behavior can signal the need for intervention. When behaviors such as self-injury and aggression pose risks of physical harm, the need for treatment is obvious: Self-injurious behavior poses obvious risks for the child, and aggression poses obvious risks for others. Other challenging behaviors are problematic because they interfere with treatment efforts, limit access to less intrusive settings, put individuals at risk of restrictive interventions, such as exclusionary time-out or restraint, reduce contact with reinforcers, and inhibit social interactions. Some challenging behaviors are only problematic because the frequency, duration, intensity, or context of the behavior is inappropriate. Stereotypy, for example, is often overlooked and not targeted for intervention (see Matson & Nebel-Schwalm, 2007) because its negative effects are not as readily apparent as behaviors resulting in actual or potential physical harm. Individuals who engage in aggression may be avoided out of fear. Individuals who engage in stereotypy may be avoided because they are perceived as "weird" or because people do not know how to react to their stereotypy. Given the more subtle negative effects of some problematic behaviors, aggression, self-injury, and property destruction receive more targeted and intensive treatment than stereotypy.

TABLE 5.1   Challenging Behaviors and Negative Outcomes

Negative Outcomes	Challenging Behaviors					
	Self-Injury	Aggression	Property Destruction	Tantrums	Stereotypy	Noncompliance
Increased risk of physical harm	Definite	Definite	Possible	Possible	Possible	Possible
Interference with learning	Possible	Possible	Possible	Possible	Possible	Definite
Limits access to less restrictive settings	Likely	Likely	Likely	Likely	Possible	Likely
Intrusive interventions more likely	Likely	Likely	Likely	Possible	Possible	Likely
Reduced contact with reinforcers	Possible	Possible	Possible	Possible	Possible	Possible
Inhibits social interactions	Possible	Likely	Possible	Possible	Possible	Possible

Some behaviors may only become problematic when they occur in the wrong context, happen too often, last too long, or are too intense. Even appropriate behavior may become problematic because of the frequency, duration, intensity, or context of the behavior. Examples include asking to use the bathroom too often, touching oneself inappropriately in public rather than in private, or becoming upset when a peer takes a toy and screaming "that's mine," rather than asking for the toy appropriately.

Why Challenging Behavior Occurs

At CARD, we view challenging behavior as a means of communication and/or interaction with others. Challenging behaviors, particularly aggression, property destruction, and self-injury, are very likely to evoke reactions from others. These behaviors may occur when a child is trying to communicate with someone and either does not have the skills to communicate in an appropriate way or is not motivated to communicate differently. If the appropriate communication is too difficult, effortful, or less likely to be reinforced, the challenging behavior will occur. When a child lacks the ability to communicate in a different way, challenging behavior becomes the only option. When the intervention is developed based on what the child is trying to communicate through the challenging behavior, the intervention is more likely to be effective because it directly addresses the reason that the child is misbehaving.

Traditional/Historical Interventions

Punishment is one way to decrease challenging behavior. While it may be effective, it is clearly not the ethical first choice (see Chapter 23 on ethics). Unfortunately, treatment of challenging behaviors within the autism population in the past often involved punishment procedures. Today, the general consensus is that punishment should be used very sparingly and only as a last resort. The least intrusive effective intervention is widely considered to be the most ethical and socially acceptable option. In addition, punishment procedures carry potential negative side effects, such as the child wanting to avoid the people who implement punishment and the potential of the punishment eliciting aggression and negative emotional responding. From a clinical perspective, the use of punishment fails to address the underlying cause of the challenging behavior: The child wants something, and he is using his challenging behavior to communicate that to you. If you only punish that behavior, you have not addressed what the child wants and how to help him communicate in a more productive and appropriate manner.

Function-Based Interventions

Children with ASD typically use challenging behavior as a means of communication. In order to eliminate their only or primary method of communicating, you need to teach them a more appropriate means of communicating that same information. Function-based interventions involve identifying the reason that the behavior is occurring – what the child is communicating – and developing an intervention to address the cause, rather than simply reduce the behavior. This approach to intervention is proactive because it attempts to prevent challenging behavior from occurring, rather than merely reacting to it when it occurs and attempting to stop it in the moment.

In order to develop a function-based intervention, the clinician is required to assess the behavior prior to intervention. It is important to note that behaviors that look similar may actually serve very different functions for different people. For example, one child might tantrum to escape work while another child might tantrum to get a preferred toy or food. A very common mistake is to approach treatment by thinking, "I am working with a child who hits himself. What treatment should I use?" This question skips the functional assessment portion; the first step is to ask why the child is hitting himself, that is, what function that behavior is serving.

The remainder of the chapter is dedicated to giving practical advice and instructions in a seven-step process for addressing challenging behavior: 1) identify, define, and prioritize the target behavior, 2) determine outcome goals, 3) conduct a functional assessment, 4) design a function-based behavior intervention plan, 5) write the behavior intervention plan, 6) evaluate the effectiveness of the plan, and 7) troubleshoot and follow up.

STEP 1: IDENTIFY, DEFINE, AND PRIORITIZE THE TARGET BEHAVIOR

Identify and Define

The first step of any intervention is to identify the behavior that you are going to change. In order for the intervention to be most effective, you must take care in defining the target behavior, so interventions can be consistently applied and behavior reliably measured. Target behaviors should be operationally defined, be specific, avoid reference to internal states such as being frustrated or overstimulated, and avoid inferences about a person's intentions. For example, a good definition of the target behavior of hitting might be a person's open hand or closed fist contacting another person with enough force to make a sound or leave a red mark on the skin. A poor definition of hitting might be slapping another person out of anger with the intent to harm them. The latter is vague because it refers to an emotion and intention, and these components cannot be observed by others and are therefore open to interpretation, which can cause confusion and disagreement among the members of the treatment team.

Prioritize

When a learner displays several challenging behaviors, it may be necessary to prioritize intervention targets to address the most relevant concerns first. Table 5.2 describes various challenging behaviors and factors to consider when prioritizing them for treatment. When prioritizing intervention targets, those behaviors that pose a danger to the individual or others should be addressed first. For instance, self-injurious and aggressive behaviors have the greatest potential to cause harm and should always be the highest priority for intervention. If an individual engages in several forms of self-injurious or aggressive behavior, it may be necessary to prioritize them even further. Those behaviors that have already caused damage or injury should be treated first, followed by those behaviors that have the potential to cause harm but have not yet resulted in physical damage.

The frequency of problem behavior should also be considered when prioritizing intervention targets. Problem behaviors that occur very frequently should receive priority over problem behaviors that rarely occur. For example, if a person throws food at every meal and occasionally spits milk on the floor, then food throwing should be targeted first because it happens more often than spitting. Likewise, chronic or long-standing

TABLE 5.2   Factors to Consider When Prioritizing Challenging Behavior Targets

	Challenging Behaviors			
Factors	Nose Picking	Screaming	Throwing Food	Spitting
Risk of harm	Bleeding observed	None	None	None
Severity	Infection likely	Loud and disruptive	Not severe	Not severe
Frequency	Seasonal	Daily	Daily	Occasional
Restricts access	Socialization impacted	Removed from classroom	Seated away from peers at lunch	Peers avoid briefly
Likelihood of success	Moderate – May require allergy medication	High – Teacher motivated	High – Easy access to reinforcers	Lower – Requires peer training

problem behaviors and skill deficits should be prioritized over newly emerging or sporadic problems. Oftentimes, it is necessary to balance the severity of one behavior against the frequency of another. For example, consider a child who slaps himself in the face one time per month without producing damage and tantrums every day when asked to do schoolwork and, therefore, gets no schoolwork done. In this case, it may be best to prioritize tantrums over self-slapping (a form of self-injury) because the former occurs daily and has large negative effects on daily functioning, whereas the latter occurs very infrequently and is not causing harm.

A problem behavior that is not particularly severe, frequent, or harmful may still be a priority for intervention if it prohibits an individual from accessing a less restrictive learning or living environment. For instance, consider a student who sings and hums while completing independent work assignments in the classroom. This behavior may be disruptive enough to the rest of the class that the student is often seated away from other students or in the hallway, or it could be prompting the school to consider placing the child in a special education classroom. The relocation of the student to a more restrictive environment warrants prioritizing the fairly harmless behavior of singing and humming.

The likelihood of success and/or the amount of effort required to change the behavior should also play a role in selecting intervention targets. Priority should be given to those behaviors that have a higher likelihood of successful behavior change than those behaviors that are likely to be resistant to change because the treatment team only has so many hours in the day to produce the maximum benefit possible for the learner. This does not mean that difficult-to-treat behaviors should be ignored. Rather, if you have two behaviors to change, one that you will probably be able to change quickly and easily and one that will probably prove more difficult, target the easy-to-treat behavior first and then intervene on the more difficult-to-treat behavior. For example, vocal stereotypy, such as singing, humming, or "scripting videos" to oneself, can be particularly difficult to eliminate completely. These behaviors may well produce a negative outcome for the learner, but if other behaviors that produce a similar or worse outcome (e.g., hand-flapping, excessive rigidity, tantrums, etc.) may be easier to treat, it may be wise to target them first.

STEP 2: DETERMINE OUTCOME GOALS

Once the intervention targets have been identified, the next step is to define the desired intervention outcomes or treatment goals. The behavior analyst must clearly delineate the amount of behavioral change required in order for it to be considered meaningful for the individual. Is it sufficient if the behavior occurs less frequently than before intervention, or must the behavior be occurring below a certain rate per hour or day for it to be considered a meaningful change? A note of caution: Not every challenging behavior should be decreased to zero levels. It is not reasonable to expect an individual never to engage in behavior that could be considered problematic or challenging. All children tantrum, and all adults get angry and say or do things at times that would be considered "inappropriate." Make sure that the intervention outcomes are reasonable and represent a meaningful change for the individual learner. Having a clear picture of when the desired behavior change has been met also helps to identify when the treatment service should be faded out and terminated, and/ or when the ongoing treatment should focus on other goals. Behavior analytic interventions should produce lasting changes that persist over time and generalize beyond those specific stimuli, situations, and environments used during treatment. Therefore, generalization and maintenance standards should be explicitly written into goals. It may also be useful to identify interim goals or benchmarks that can be used to monitor progress and identify intervention components that need to be modified in order to reach the terminal goal.

When selecting intervention outcomes, it is important to consider several variables, including learner preferences, current behavioral repertoire, environmental supports and constraints, and the social validity of the outcome targeted. Whenever possible, the individual whose behavior is being changed should be consulted. Caregiver input is also valuable. Parents, teachers, therapists, school districts, and other funding agencies may also have a stake in the intervention outcomes and should be considered when determining goals. However, the priority should always be placed on the individual whose behavior is being changed. Ultimately, goals should be written in a way that directly answers the question "How has this behavior change improved the quality of the learner's life?"

The learner's current behavioral repertoire will also influence the treatment outcomes identified, particularly when it comes to choosing optimal replacement behaviors. Behavior reduction is all but meaningless if it is not accompanied by increasing or sustaining a meaningful replacement behavior. Intervention outcomes will be influenced by environmental supports and constraints, as well. Many interventions require a variety of caregivers to follow specific procedures across several environments.

STEP 3: CONDUCT A FUNCTIONAL ASSESSMENT

A functional assessment serves two purposes. The first is to document the need for intervention. It allows the clinician to determine how often the target challenging behavior occurs, the severity of the behavior, and the need for intervention. The second purpose of the functional assessment is to identify the cause or reason for the challenging behavior.

Common Functions of Behavior

Functional assessments are designed to identify whether the ongoing reinforcement for the challenging behavior is delivered by someone else (referred to as "socially mediated" reinforcement) or whether it is produced automatically by the behavior (referred to as "automatic" reinforcement). The vast majority of research on the functional assessment of challenging behavior in people with developmental disabilities has identified reinforcement of challenging behaviors that falls into one or more of the following four categories:

1. Socially mediated positive reinforcement in the form of social attention: This function is usually referred to as the "attention" function. For example, a caregiver may give positive or negative attention when a child engages in challenging behavior;
2. Socially mediated positive reinforcement in the form of preferred items or activities: This function is typically referred to as the "tangible" function and occurs when a learner uses challenging behavior to get or keep access to preferred foods, toys, or other activities;
3. Socially mediated negative reinforcement in the form of escape or avoidance of a nonpreferred task or event: This function is usually referred to as the "escape" function. Escape-maintained behavior often allows the learner to avoid or escape something undesirable, such as work or self-care tasks; and
4. Automatic reinforcement: Automatic reinforcement may be positive reinforcement in that it produces a feeling or sensation that is positively reinforcing. For example, flapping one's hands in front of one's eyes may produce enjoyable visual stimulation. Automatic reinforcement may also be negative reinforcement, such as pulling on or hitting one's ears, which may produce temporary cessation of the pain of an ear infection.

Secondary Functions of Behavior

Control. In addition to these four basic functions, challenging behaviors may also have idiosyncratic functions. Functional assessment methods can be modified in a variety of ways to identify less common or unusual functions, as well. One such function that has not been evaluated by a substantial amount of research is control. The maintaining consequence of some challenging behaviors of children with ASD appears to be the opportunity to be in control of their environment in the moment. This function is distinct from the others because it is not reinforced by the opportunity to have a particular thing (i.e., tangible), nor is it reinforced by the opportunity to escape a particular demand (i.e., escape), but, rather, the child seems not to want the particular thing that someone else wants her to have or doesn't want to do the particular demand that someone else wants her to do. In these cases, you might observe that even a preferred activity becomes nonpreferred if it's someone else's idea to do it.

Access to routines, stereotypy, or "inflexibility." Another function of challenging behavior that is uncommon in research but is very commonly reported anecdotally by clinicians is challenging behavior that allows the learner to have access to preferred rituals, routines, or stereotypy. The stereotypy can be something relatively concrete, such as manipulating ripped paper in ones hands, needing to press the button on an elevator, or needing to straighten the tassels on a rug. The stereotypy can also be something relatively abstract, such as needing to walk along a particular path when walking across a room or needing to drive along a particular street when going to grandma's house. In any of these cases, the function of the challenging behavior is to allow the learner to access the event in the preferred way, that is, to allow her to have things the way they are "supposed" to be. Children with such challenging behavior are often described as highly inflexible because they want many things to be a particular way.

Conceptually speaking, it is often difficult to identify whether such functions are positive or negative reinforcement. For example, if seeing disheveled tassels on a rug evokes screaming and the reinforcer for the screaming is the opportunity to straighten the tassels, it is not clear whether disheveled tassels are aversive and straightening them represents escape from that aversive stimulus (i.e., negative reinforcement) or if the straightening behavior, itself, is a positively reinforcing event. Put simply, does the child want to make the out-of-order thing go away, or does he want to get to fix it? Practically speaking, it probably doesn't matter; what matters is being able to identify the particular idiosyncratic events that are reliable antecedents and consequences for the behavior.

Clinicians commonly discuss the potential overlap between obsessive compulsive disorder (OCD) and the challenging behaviors displayed by children with autism, although this topic has been the subject of relatively little research. Many rituals, routines, and stereotypies that children with ASD display are similar to compulsions displayed by individuals with OCD. In addition, when many children with ASD are prevented from engaging in these repetitive behaviors, they exhibit highly anxious reactions. That is, in addition to the clearly operant behaviors that serve the purpose of helping the child get access to engaging in the overt behaviors (e.g., hitting in order to get the opportunity to straighten objects), these children also display overt signs of negative affect and anxiety (e.g., overt fear responses, trembling, crying, stress, etc.). It seems likely that, in many of these cases, the function of the repetitive behaviors is similar to the function of compulsions in individuals with OCD; engaging in the overt repetitive behavior decreases the presence of aversive anxiety-related covert events. If this is the case, then two separate but related sets of contingencies may be at play: The presence of a disrupted routine functions as both 1) an establishing operation (presence of aversive anxiety) that makes "fixing" the routine a source of negative reinforcement due to escape from anxiety and 2) a discriminative stimulus that signals that engaging in challenging behavior may have the consequence of allowing the child access to the opportunity to "fix" the routine.

Social avoidance. Another less common function of challenging behavior is called "social avoidance." Social avoidance functions involve behavior that is maintained by socially mediated reinforcement in the form of escape from the attention of others. Note that this is different from escape from demands because it does not involve tasks or demands; it may be the mere presence of another person or another person interacting with the child in any way that is the thing from which the child wants to escape.

Types of Functional Assessments

All functional assessments attempt to identify antecedents and consequences associated with the challenging behavior. There are three basic formats that a functional assessment can take: 1) indirect assessment, 2) descriptive assessment, and 3) experimental functional analysis. Each format has its advantages and disadvantages. Indirect and descriptive assessments will be described in detail below. Space does not permit a thorough description of experimental functional analyses. (See Matson, 2012, for further reading.)

Indirect functional assessment. Indirect assessments are called indirect because they do not require the assessor to directly contact the child or the behavior. They are the simplest form of assessment and typically involve interviewing caregivers who are familiar with the challenging behavior. These interviews can be conducted with caregivers of all sorts, including parents and other relatives, direct interventionists, teachers, and other individuals who have observed the behavior directly. The interviews involve asking others to identify the events that typically precede and follow the challenging behavior, situations when it is more likely to occur, and situations when it is less likely to occur and may include respondents' providing their opinion regarding the function of the behavior.

The interviews can be structured, following a particular script and focused on answering a predetermined set of questions. The Questions

About Behavioral Function (QABF) (Matson & Vollmer, 1995) is a highly researched and useful tool for conducting indirect functional assessments and involves asking caregivers to answer a series of questions on a Likert-type scale. Another useful indirect assessment tool is the recently developed, web-based CARD Indirect Functional Assessment (CIFA). Appendix A displays the questions and rating system used for the CIFA.

Indirect assessments can also be unstructured, allowing for a free-flowing conversation or narrative description of the behavior by caregivers, with follow-up questions based on the information provided. Both structured and unstructured indirect assessments can provide valuable information about the function of the behavior if attention is given to identifying antecedents and consequences. Furthermore, the indirect assessment can be conducted as an in-person interview or through completion of a written or web-based form. However, conducting the interview in person allows for immediate clarification or follow-up questions to get more specific information. On the other hand, distributing a written form provides flexibility by allowing supervisors to send the forms home or get information from individuals whose schedules preclude in-person assessments (e.g., teachers at school). A web-based form promises even greater flexibility because it can be easily accessed by anyone with an Internet connection.

STEPS TO FOLLOW WHEN CONDUCTING AN INDIRECT ASSESSMENT

- Identify and define the target behavior for the caregiver to ensure that she is providing information only about the behavior you are assessing.
- Ask the caregiver to describe when the behavior is likely to occur.
- Ask clarifying questions to determine specific events, people, locations, materials, or other stimuli that typically precede the target behavior.
- Ask the caregiver to describe what typically happens after the target behavior occurs.
- Ask clarifying questions to determine specific events, people, locations, materials, or other stimuli that typically follow the target behavior.
- Ask the caregiver to describe when the behavior is not likely to occur.
- Ask the caregiver why she thinks the behavior occurs.

Use the information to compare the learner's environment prior to and following the target behavior to determine how the environment typically changes. If the information you receive is sufficiently complete, it should point to the potential function of the behavior. As the bullets illustrate below, you are looking for changes in the learner's environment from the time before the behavior to the time after the behavior. Essentially, the learner should have more of what he wants after the behavior happens. For example:

- Low or no attention before the behavior → More attention after the behavior
- Tasks/demands before the behavior → No tasks or postponement of tasks after the behavior
- No toy before the behavior → Access to toy after the behavior

PROS AND CONS OF INDIRECT ASSESSMENT

One of the greatest advantages of indirect assessments is that they are relatively easy to conduct. They can be completed in a short amount of time and do not require additional materials, multiple people to conduct them, or learner participation. Another advantage is that the assessment can be conducted without the challenging behavior occurring. This may be particularly important when the behavior poses a great risk to the learner or others or when the challenging behavior occurs infrequently.

One of the key disadvantages of indirect assessments is the secondhand nature of the information provided. Caregivers may not recognize or recall important information, may focus more on recent or annoying events than on the big picture, or may have preconceived notions about why particular behaviors occur. Results may also be inconclusive or unclear in that they may indicate that the child is attempting to communicate several things (e.g., I want a break and I want attention). This may be the case, but it is also possible that it appears to caregivers that the behavior is "happening all the time," so they may be likely to say "yes" to virtually any question about when the behavior occurs. Overall, indirect assessments often produce inconclusive or unreliable results. However, the QABF is among the most reliable indirect functional assessments, and we find it useful a high percentage of the time.

Descriptive Functional Assessment

Descriptive assessments involve observing the learner engaging in the challenging behavior and noting the naturally occurring environmental events that precede and follow it to identify patterns that point to potential functions. There are many forms of descriptive functional assessment, but the most commonly used and the most useful form is referred to as antecedent-behavior-consequence data collection (ABC data). When collecting ABC data, the learner is observed, and each time she engages in the target behavior, the observer records what occurred immediately before and immediately after the behavior. ABC data can be collected in an unstructured manner in which the observer records the antecedents and consequences of the behavior in a narrative fashion. Figure 5.1 provides a sample unstructured ABC datasheet. ABC data can also be recorded in a structured manner, in which the observer chooses the antecedent and consequence that are applicable each time the behavior occurs. Figure 5.2 provides an example of a structured ABC datasheet.

There are many factors to consider when conducting an ABC functional assessment. First and foremost, you must observe the behavior. For lower-rate behaviors, this can be challenging. You would do well to ask all

Narrative ABC Data Recording

Child: _____   Observer: _____

Setting: _____   Start time: _____   End time: _____

Date: _____

Antecedent	Behavior	Consequence

FIGURE 5.1   Sample datasheet for narrative or unstructured Antecedent-Behavior-Consequence data recording.

Structured ABC Data

Child: _____   Observer: _____

Setting: _____   Start time: _____   End time: _____

Date: _____

Each time an episode of the behavior occurs, tally ALL antecedents that were present and ALL consequences which followed.

Behavior 1_____ Definition_____

Antecedents				Behavior	Consequences			
Low Attn	Demand Given	Denied Access	None		Attn Given	Escape from Demand	Access Given	None—No Response

FIGURE 5.2   Sample datasheet for structured Antecedent-Behavior-Consequence data recording.

relevant caregivers when the behavior usually occurs, and make sure you schedule time to observe it in those settings or during those times. Second, observe a large enough sample of settings and conditions, so antecedents and consequences relevant to each function can be observed. For example, if the learner never has any demands placed on her when you are observing, you are not likely to see any escape-maintained behavior, even if it is a regular problem for her. Likewise, if the learner is constantly being given attention during your observation, she may never engage in attention-maintained behavior.

STEPS TO FOLLOW WHEN CONDUCTING A DESCRIPTIVE FUNCTIONAL ASSESSMENT

- Identify appropriate times to observe (i.e., times when the behavior is likely to occur).
- Observe the learner in the natural environment.
- Record occurrences of the target behavior.
- Record the events immediately preceding the target behavior.
- Record the events immediately following the target behavior.
- Graph and evaluate data to identify function.

PROS AND CONS OF DESCRIPTIVE FUNCTIONAL ASSESSMENTS

The clearest advantage of a descriptive assessment over an indirect assessment is the fact that you are able to directly observe the behavior in the natural environment in which it occurs, so the information you obtain is taken directly from the behavior; you do not have to rely on the recall or perceptions of others. Other advantages (compared to experimental functional analyses) are that descriptive assessments do not require the assessor to interact with the learner or his challenging behavior; one merely needs to observe. Finally, since the behavior is observed as it actually occurs, it is possible that the observer will have the opportunity to note idiosyncratic variables that might not be detected when relying on caregiver recall alone.

Perhaps the greatest disadvantage of descriptive assessments is one that is shared with indirect assessments: The information they provide is only correlational; it does not demonstrate that a behavior is actually maintained by a particular consequence. Therefore, it is often the case that descriptive assessments identify more than one function or provide inconclusive information because it appears as though many different variables are related to the behavior or that none are related consistently. Another major disadvantage of descriptive assessments is that they require the behavior to occur while the assessor is observing. An expert assessor may observe a child for hours and still not observe the child display the behavior, thereby rendering the observation useless.

Analyzing the Results of Functional Assessments

The purpose of indirect and descriptive assessments is to identify antecedents and consequences that are correlated with the challenging behavior. If you are lucky, these correlations will be relatively clear and will point directly to one or more particular functions of the behavior. For example, if the most common antecedent is that the learner is not receiving attention and the most common consequence is that the learner receives attention – and all of the other major antecedents and consequences are relatively low – then it is reasonable to hypothesize that the behavior is maintained by attention. Figure 5.3 displays sample data from indirect and descriptive assessments.

When the results are less clear, multiple factors should be considered. First, the most common reaction to a child misbehaving in most cultures is to tell the child to stop, reprimand him, or provide attention of some sort. Therefore, attention may be the most common consequence of the target behavior, regardless of whether it is actually the function. Second, escape-maintained behavior is not likely to occur if there are no demands placed, so the lack of demands as an antecedent does not necessarily rule out escape-maintained behavior. Make sure that you actually observe someone place demands on the child multiple times. Third, it is extremely rare for aggression to be automatically reinforced because there are much easier ways to get visual or tactile stimulation than hitting another person.

Multiple functions. It is extremely common for the challenging behavior displayed by children with ASD to have more than one function. For children who have significant delays in their abilities to ask for what they want, it makes sense that they would use misbehavior both to escape from activities they want to avoid and to get access to things they do want (e.g., attention and preferred items). Therefore, do not be surprised if a young child with ASD uses tantrums to tell you that he wants a break from work and to tell you he wants more of a food or toy. Indeed, this is quite common. However, it is also quite common for staff to conclude

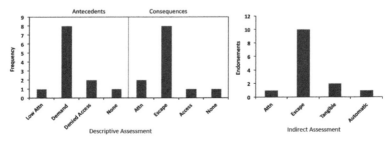

FIGURE 5.3   Sample data from indirect and descriptive assessments. Note that in this case, both forms of assessment produced clear results that agreed on the same function of escape from demand.

that a behavior is multiply maintained when they actually don't have any good evidence for any particular function. That is, the concept of multiple functions is by no means the same thing as saying that the results of a functional assessment are inconclusive. Therefore, be careful not to jump to the multiply maintained conclusion too quickly as a "dumping ground" for unclear functional assessment data.

STEP 4: DESIGN A FUNCTION-BASED BEHAVIOR INTERVENTION PLAN

After the function of the behavior has been identified, the results are then used to develop a function-based intervention to decrease the behavior and replace it with a more adaptive behavior. Many interventions can be used for each behavioral function, and space does not permit a comprehensive description of all of them. In what follows, we provide practical instructions on how to implement a selection of the most evidence-based, effective, and ethical treatment options. Each procedure is categorized as either antecedent, replacement behavior, consequence-based, or some combination of the three. Descriptions are provided on how to implement each procedure for each function.

Antecedent Interventions

Antecedent-based interventions involve changes in antecedent events to prevent challenging behavior from occurring or to evoke a replacement behavior. Therefore, antecedent-based interventions often involve the manipulation of motivating operations, discriminative stimuli, or both. Remember, motivating operations have two effects: 1) a value-altering effect that can establish or abolish stimuli as reinforcers and 2) a behavior-altering effect that can increase or decrease the current frequency of behavior. With response reduction interventions, motivating operations are manipulated primarily to prevent the problem behavior from occurring. The general goal is to abolish reinforcers that are maintaining problem behavior and reduce the current frequency of that behavior. Antecedent-based interventions can also involve the manipulation of discriminative stimuli and prompts. We commonly use four antecedent modification interventions in our behavior intervention plans: 1) noncontingent reinforcement, 2) demand fading, 3) task modification, and 4) choice.

Noncontingent reinforcement. Noncontingent reinforcement (NCR) is a procedure in which the reinforcement that previously maintained the challenging behavior is now given to the learner at predetermined times without first requiring the challenging behavior to occur. Put more technically, it is the delivery of the functional reinforcer maintaining the problem behavior on a time-based schedule of reinforcement, independent of the occurrence of the problem behavior. This means that the reinforcer is provided solely on the time-based schedule, regardless of whether the problem behavior has occurred. For example, to decrease attention-maintained behavior, one might deliver attention every 5 minutes. However, in order to avoid accidentally reinforcing the behavior, it is common to delay the reinforcer if problem behavior occurs within 5 seconds of when the reinforcer should have been delivered. Noncontingent reinforcement is most effective if the functional reinforcer is provided more frequently than the rate at which the problem behavior occurs. If the problem behavior occurs very frequently, the reinforcer may have to be provided continuously. Once the problem behavior decreases to an acceptable level, the intervals between reinforcement are gradually increased until the reinforcement schedule reflects a naturally occurring schedule. Also, note that if you are *only* delivering the reinforcer according to a time-based schedule, then you are *not* delivering the reinforcer contingent on the challenging behavior. In other words, NCR, when implemented correctly, always includes extinction, as well. NCR may be effective without extinction in some cases, but it is far more likely to be effective when implemented with extinction. (We will discuss extinction further in the consequence intervention section of this chapter.)

NCR for attention. Let's look at an example of NCR to decrease attention-maintained problem behavior. The learner engages in hitting approximately every minute, and a functional assessment indicates that this behavior is maintained by access to adult attention. To implement NCR, the clinician initially provides attention every 30 seconds, regardless of when the problem behavior occurs. Soon, the learner is no longer motivated to hit to gain attention because he already has access to the reinforcer he wants. Over the next several sessions, the learner begins to hit less frequently, so the clinician gradually increases the time between reinforcer delivery from every 30 seconds to every minute, then approximately every 2 minutes, then every 3 minutes, and so on. Eventually, the clinician is providing attention every 10 minutes, and the learner is no longer hitting.

NCR for tangible. In the example above, hitting was maintained by social positive reinforcement in the form of attention, so the clinician delivered attention noncontingently during the intervention. Had this problem behavior been maintained by access to tangible items, the clinician would have used the same process, but, instead of the attention, the clinician would have provided access to a specific object, food, or activity that the learner wanted. The specific amount of preferred item or activity that you provide according to the time-based schedule needs to be a balance between practicality and magnitude. The larger the amount of reinforcement, the more effective the procedure is likely to be, but, of course, the larger the amount of reinforcement, the more time and resources it requires.

NCR for escape. NCR procedures can also be used with problem behavior maintained by socially mediated negative reinforcement. In this case, the aversive stimulus is briefly removed according to the time-based schedule. For example, if hitting has been maintained by escape from demands, the clinician would frequently provide the learner with brief breaks from work. If a child typically hits, on average, one time every 5 minutes when being asked to do work, the clinician might start by giving a break from work noncontingently every 4 minutes.

NCR for automatic. Challenging behaviors maintained by automatic reinforcement can also be effectively treated with NCR. A substantial amount of research has shown that providing a child with an object or activity that provides preferred stimulation can replace the challenging behavior that was maintained by automatic reinforcement (often referred to as a "competing items" procedure). For example, if a child makes loud stereotypic vocalizations that are maintained by automatic reinforcement in the form of auditory stimulation (e.g., the child likes the way the vocalizations sound), then providing him with a toy that produces music when he plays with it might provide a more appropriate way for the child to get the auditory stimulation he wants. However, the most important variable is likely the preference of the competing items, so make sure to conduct a preference assessment to ensure that you are providing the child with highly preferred items to replace the target challenging behavior.

Advantages and disadvantages of NCR. A major advantage of NCR is that it is easy to do. All you need is a timer and plenty of the functional reinforcer. In addition, NCR can be effective at preventing the behavior from occurring; therefore, it is a proactive instead of reactive strategy. It probably also has the positive side effect of making the learner happy since he is getting more of what he wants. One major disadvantage is that it actually may be very challenging to implement if the rate of reinforcement is initially very high. For example, providing attention every 15 seconds may not be practical. Keep in mind, though, that if it works, then you will likely be able to reduce the reinforcement schedule to a more reasonable level. Another major disadvantage of NCR is that it *does not teach a replacement behavior*. Considering that establishing and maintaining a replacement behavior is likely the most important function of a behavior intervention plan, this is a significant limitation. Therefore, NCR by itself should almost never be considered a complete behavior intervention plan. It is also possible that, in a minority of cases, giving the learner some access to a reinforcer can actually function as an establishing operation and make challenging behavior more likely in the near future. For example, some children who are given free access to engage in stereotypy in particular locations (e.g., in the bathroom or bedroom when alone) actually engage in higher rates of stereotypy immediately afterward.

Demand fading. Demand fading is an antecedent-based intervention designed specifically to reduce challenging behavior maintained by escape. To implement demand fading, you decrease the amount of work the learner is asked to do until the he does not display the challenging behavior. For example, if a learner is normally asked to complete 20 problems on a worksheet before taking a break, demand fading might begin by asking the learner to complete only one problem before taking a break. If this works, you gradually increase the demand until the learner is able to tolerate a reasonable level without displaying the challenging behavior.

Demand fading works by eliminating the establishing operation for the problem behavior. The initial reduction in the number of demands decreases the aversiveness of the demands. If the demands are less aversive, the learner is less motivated to escape them. Advantages of demand fading include the fact that it is easy to implement and generally is preferred by the learner. A major disadvantage is that it does not necessarily help strengthen a replacement behavior. In addition, very little research has shown that it successfully decreases escape-maintained behavior when implemented by itself. Therefore, demand fading should always be considered as one possible component of a larger intervention package.

Task modification. Task modification is another antecedent-based intervention designed specifically to reduce problem behavior maintained by escape from demands. Task modification involves changing some aspect of the task, so the task is less aversive to the learner. In nontechnical terms, the point of task modification is to make work more fun. Task modification may involve changes to any aspect of the demand context, such as the materials used, order of task presentation, task difficulty, or instructional location, or any other change to the task that reduces the aversiveness of the demand context. Once the problem behavior decreases to an acceptable level, the modifications are gradually eliminated until the task no longer differs from naturally occurring tasks.

Let's look at an example of task modification to reduce property destruction. In this example, the learner crumples up her paper every time she is asked to complete her math worksheet. In order to reduce this problem behavior, the behavior analyst has copied the math worksheet onto a piece of pink paper and added fun stickers around the edge of the page. (In this case, the color pink and the particular stickers used were already determined to be highly preferred by the learner.) Once the learner no longer crumples up her worksheet, the clinician gradually removes the number of stickers and lightens the color of the paper, until he finally presents the original math worksheet on white paper with no stickers. Many task modifications are so low effort and low cost (e.g., using pencils that are a preferred color, sitting on the floor instead of at a table, and so on) that it is not critical to fade them out anytime soon.

Choice. Providing individuals with developmental disabilities and challenging behavior the opportunity to make frequent choices can help decrease challenging behavior. To address escape-maintained behavior, choice can be provided as to the sequence of work, the types of work, the way in which work is presented, and the reinforcers to be earned for work completion, to name a few. For attention-maintained behavior, choice can be offered for the type of attention the learner wants (e.g., tickles, playing a game, roughhousing, etc.). For challenging behavior maintained by access to tangibles, choice can be given between which items and activities the learner wants to earn or access. For automatically reinforced behavior, choice can be given among different competing items that the learner can access. The basic point is that choice is good and should be given to the learner as frequently as possible, not only because it works but also because we have a moral imperative to facilitate self-determination by ensuring that individuals with developmental disabilities receive what they want and engage in activities they prefer as much as possible. Recall the section on preference assessments in Chapter 4, and focus on interweaving choice as frequently as possible into your daily interactions with children with ASD.

Replacement Behavior Intervention Procedures

The single most important role of a behavioral intervention for decreasing challenging behavior is to establish and maintain a functional replacement behavior. There are both ethical and practical reasons for this. From an ethical standpoint, challenging behavior occurs because a child with ASD wants something. Generally speaking, if she had the language to ask for it appropriately, she probably would. Therefore, if your behavioral intervention successfully reduces the challenging behavior but does not replace it with a functionally equivalent replacement behavior, you may well have just eliminated the child's only means of communication – quite a serious error when working with a child who is likely grappling with communication challenges. Practically speaking, establishing a functionally equivalent replacement behavior just works better; if the child has a more appropriate, lower-effort way of getting what she wants, she is less likely to resort to challenging behavior to get it.

Differential reinforcement. *Differential reinforcement* is a general term that means reinforcing some behaviors and not reinforcing others. Generally speaking, this includes everything we do in applied behavior analysis (ABA); we never reinforce every single behavior. When applied to the treatment of challenging behavior, however, differential reinforcement usually means using extinction for the challenging behavior and using reinforcement to strengthen some other behavior. The most commonly used forms of differential reinforcement are 1) differential reinforcement of alternative behavior (DRA), 2) differential reinforcement of incompatible behavior (DRI), 3) differential reinforcement of low rate behavior (DRL), and 4) differential reinforcement of other behavior (DRO). We discuss each type of differential reinforcement in the sections most pertinent to each procedure below.

Functional communication training. Functional communication training (FCT) is one of the most well-researched interventions for challenging behavior in individuals with developmental disorders and is widely considered the gold standard treatment for challenging behavior. Therefore, in virtually every case you will ever treat, it should be the first procedure you consider when designing an intervention plan. FCT has two components: 1) extinction of the challenging behavior and 2) teaching the learner to request the functional reinforcer. Note that FCT is one form of differential reinforcement of alternative behavior (DRA), a procedure in which you place the challenging behavior on extinction and give reinforcement of a more appropriate alternative behavior. However, FCT deserves its own special name because it is by far the most useful, ethical, and desirable form of DRA, all other things being equal. We will discuss how to do extinction later in the chapter, and we elaborate on how to teach the communication response in FCT here.

Selecting a communication response for FCT. The communication response must be a request for the same reinforcer that previously maintained the challenging behavior. It does not matter whether the response is communicated vocally or using sign language, gestures, picture exchange, or a voice output communication device. (Each of these options has their strengths and limitations; see Chapter 6 on visual supports.) The communication response must be easy for the child to learn and execute; e.g., initial FCT training is not a good time to worry about a child using a full sentence spoken with correct prosody. In addition, the FCT response must be easily understood by caregivers in the child's environment, so they can immediately reinforce it.

FCT for attention. FCT for attention involves teaching the learner to ask for attention instead of displaying the challenging behavior to get it. Good vocal options include requests such as "play with me," "hug," "tickles," "hi," etc. Of course, all of these same requests can be represented in sign language, pictures, and voice output devices. Simple gestures, such as waving or tapping someone on the shoulder, may also be useful options initially. Naturally, make sure that the particular types of attention you are teaching the learner to request are ones that are actually preferred by her.

FCT for tangible. Good FCT options for tangible include requests such as "more," "please," "share," "my turn," and so on. Much better alternatives are to teach the learner to name the specific item or activity that he wants (e.g., mand for it; see Chapter 11 on language). Teaching the learner a variety of mands for different objects and activities will give him a much more powerful and flexible requesting repertoire. However, when first trying to eliminate severe tangibly maintained behavior, it may be easier and work faster to teach one of the "generalized mands" described above.

FCT for escape. Implementing FCT for escape-maintained behavior involves teaching the learner to ask for cessation of whatever it is about demands that he does not like in the moment. Good options include requests such as "break," "help," "all done," and "no thanks."

Teaching the FCT response. One of the most critical things you can do to help children with ASD who have challenging behavior is make them fluent in asking for what they want. Regardless of the particular form of request that you choose, your job is to make the learner an expert at doing it. Four steps are critical: 1) prompt and reinforce frequently, 2) ensure generalization to all relevant caregivers and environments, 3) thin out reinforcement, and 4) ensure maintenance.

Prompt and reinforce frequently. It's hard to overemphasize how important it is to prompt the communication response frequently in the beginning. If you are new to this, a general rule is that the amount that you should prompt the communication response is more than an amount that will feel natural to you. The most important thing is to prompt the communication response more frequently and more immediately than the challenging behavior occurs. For example, for escape-maintained behavior, it could be appropriate to prompt the learner to ask for a break immediately after you deliver the first task demand. In other words, you want to prompt the learner to ask for a break so quickly that he does not even have the opportunity to engage in challenging behavior. And, of course, you need to give the functional reinforcer immediately after the prompted communication behavior occurs – in this case, give an immediate 30-second break. If the function was attention, you might want to begin by telling the learner that she needs to play by herself and then immediately prompt her to ask you to play, and then immediately give her attention. Similarly, for tangible, you might begin by removing a learner's toy, immediately prompt him to ask for it back, and then immediately give it back to him.

In all of the above scenarios, you are setting up the environment in a way that would normally evoke the challenging behavior but then immediately prompting and reinforcing the communication response before the learner has a chance to engage in the challenging behavior. In technical ABA terminology, you are setting up an establishing operation that makes the functional reinforcer powerful in the moment, providing immediate prompting, and then providing the functional reinforcer immediately contingent on the communication response.

As with all skill teaching, you should start to think about how to fade out the prompting for FCT right from the beginning. (See section on prompting and prompt fading in Chapter 4.) If you choose to use a most-to-least prompt fading procedure, you can start fading the prompting on the very first day. For example, if the communication response is happening reliably after five or so prompts using full physical prompting to hand over a communication card, then try a partial physical prompt for a few trials. If the communication response is still happening reliably for 3–5 times, consider proceeding to a light-touch prompt or consider adding a 1-second delay to the partial physical, and so on, until the communication response is happening independently. If you are using a least-to-most prompting procedure, such as three-step prompting, the procedure should fade itself out; e.g., as the learner starts to respond to the model prompt, the physical prompt will no longer be implemented, and so on.

Ensure generalization to all relevant caregivers and environments. As soon as you see the prompting and reinforcement described above start to work (i.e., the communication response starts to occur more frequently and more reliably), you should start to work on generalizing it. The best way to do this is to have as many caregivers as possible practice it with the learner across as many settings as possible (see Chapter 7 on generalization). In general, the more, the better, but only include caregivers who are certain to implement the prompting and reinforcement procedure correctly.

Thin out reinforcement. Once the communication response occurs frequently and reliably, you may notice that the learner is constantly getting what he wants, and this leaves you and other caregivers very little time to do anything else. This can be challenging, but keep in mind that it is temporary and that the best results will always be obtained by reinforcing the communication response very strongly and frequently at first. However, after the behavior occurs very frequently and reliably across all relevant caregivers and settings, it's time to start thinning out the reinforcement schedule to resemble something that is more reasonable and practical. One great way to do this is to introduce a wait period. As with everything else in ABA, it's going to work best if you do it slowly and gradually. On the first day, you might ask the learner to wait 1 second after requesting what she wants before you give it to her. If challenging behavior remains low, you might proceed to 2 seconds on the second day, and so on. Some clinicians find it useful to use a visual support to represent the waiting period – e.g., a red card that says "wait." When the red card is visible, the learner must wait. As soon as the wait period is over, the clinician removes the red card and gives the learner what she requested.

For escape-maintained behavior, a great way to thin out the schedule of reinforcement is to insert a work requirement. For example, you can require the learner to complete one problem on a worksheet or fold one piece of laundry or put away one toy, etc., before his request for a break is honored. Many clinicians find it useful to include a visual support for this procedure. Token systems are frequently used to visually represent how much work a learner needs to complete before he can ask for a break (or before he gets one even if he doesn't ask). To use a token system, you might start by showing the learner a board with one small square of Velcro®. After she completes one demand, give her a token and prompt her to place it on the "empty spot" on the board. The board is then full, so prompt her to hand it to you, at which point you give her a break from work. If challenging behavior remains low, you can add another piece of Velcro® to the board every few days (each one representing one more demand that is required before a break request is honored) until a reasonable amount of work needs to be done before a break is given. The most important thing to remember when thinning reinforcement during FCT is to do it gradually and only thin further when challenging behavior remains low. If challenging behavior returns, you may need to reverse your thinning procedure slightly and progress again after you have regained low rates of challenging behavior. *The key is patience.* You may feel as though the process is taking forever, but think about how long the learner has been engaging in the challenging behavior; it is worth a few months of hard and patient work to produce a lasting change!

Ensure maintenance. As we discuss in Chapter 7 on maintenance and generalization, maintenance is very frequently overlooked. Do not assume that caregivers will automatically remember to reinforce the communication response, even though it is in their best interests to do so. It is critical that you check on the learner's communication response frequently to make sure she is still using it, even after all prompting is removed and after the reinforcement schedule has been thinned to something that resembles normal everyday life. If you find that the communication response is no longer occurring (and especially if the challenging behavior is back), do not be afraid to begin prompting and reinforcement again – and, of course, prompt fading.

Other forms of DRA. Although FCT should usually be your first consideration, other forms of DRA are often helpful as well. One very common example is when treating automatically reinforced stereotypy in children with autism. In the section on NCR for automatically reinforced behavior above, we discussed how merely providing a learner with a "competing item" may give her something else to do that provides automatic reinforcement, rather than engage in stereotypy. If this works, then great – it's quick and low effort. Often, however, a child may not have another item that competes effectively with stereotypy. In these cases, an alternative behavior may need to be directly taught and reinforced. For example, to replace hand-flapping, one might teach a child with ASD to play with "cause-and-effect" toys, i.e., toys that produce lights or sounds. If the child does not already enjoy playing with the toys, you may initially need to use prompting and contrived reinforcement. Very frequently, the child will eventually learn to like playing with the toys after he has learned how to use them. (See Chapter 12 on teaching play skills for more on this.)

Another commonly used form of DRA is differential reinforcement of incompatible behavior (DRI). DRI is identical to DRA, except that the form of the alternative behavior is physically incompatible with the challenging behavior. For example, stroking a pet dog softly cannot physically occur at the same time as hitting the dog, at least not with the same hand. Similarly, manually playing with a toy that produces visual stimulation is physically incompatible with hand-flapping in front of one's face. Very little research has compared DRA to DRI, but many clinicians find DRI useful.

Consequence-Based Interventions

As we described in Chapter 4, the term *consequence* simply means events that occur immediately after a behavior. Therefore, in behavioral terminology, *consequence* does not have negative connotations, as it does in everyday language. The consequences of behaviors, whether they are good or bad consequences, have lasting effects on the future probability of those behaviors. This is a general rule that applies to adaptive and maladaptive behavior, displayed by all humans (and virtually all other animals), with or without ASD. Consequence-based interventions for challenging behavior involve the manipulation of events that follow the behavior to make it less likely to occur in the future. The vast majority of challenging behaviors displayed by children with ASD can be effectively decreased and replaced without the use of punishment, so we do not include a significant amount of discussion of punishment procedures in this book. The consequence-based procedures we discuss include extinction, differential reinforcement of other behavior, differential reinforcement of low rate behavior, and response interruption and redirection. We also briefly discuss response cost because, even though it is technically a punishment procedure, it is commonly used and generally very nonintrusive. If you have exhausted all of the reinforcement and extinction-based procedures in this book and the learner's challenging behavior continues to present a severe problem, consider seeking help from a consultant who specializes in severe behavior.

Table 5.3 depicts positive and negative reinforcement and punishment and sample procedures for each. Note that whether a consequence is called positive or negative depends only on whether you add or remove something from the learner's environment. And, of course, a consequence is considered reinforcement or punishment based only on whether it increases or decreases behavior. Consequences that increase behavior are reinforcers, whereas consequences that decrease it are punishment. Finally, note that extinction is not included in the table because it neither gives nor removes a consequence; rather, it is, itself, the lack of a consequence.

TABLE 5.3   Positive and Negative Reinforcement and Punishment

	Adding Something	Removing Something
Increases Behavior	*Principle*: Positive Reinforcement *Example*: Giving a toy when child asks for a toy	*Principle*: Negative Reinforcement *Example*: Removing work when child asks for a break
Decreases Behavior	*Principle*: Positive Punishment *Example*: Response interruption and redirection for stereotypy	*Principle*: Negative Punishment *Example*: Taking away a toy when child hits

Extinction. Extinction is probably the most-researched and most-likely-to-work procedure for decreasing challenging behavior in children with ASD. Extinction is the process by which previously reinforced behavior no longer receives reinforcement and, therefore, decreases or stops altogether. Implementation of extinction is different for each function of challenging behavior and is, therefore, dependent on the results of a functional assessment. In what follows, we describe how to implement extinction according to each major function of behavior, and we include discussion of what to do when extinction may not be possible.

Extinction for attention. In principle, extinction for attention-maintained behavior is very simple: You must not give the child an increased amount of attention as a result of his challenging behavior. In practice, it's not always easy. Let's consider an example of attention-maintained spitting. When spitting occurs, the child's peers yell and tell him not to spit. The clinician has conducted a functional assessment and determined that the peers' attention is maintaining the problem behavior of spitting. The peers are instructed to stop providing attention of any kind when spitting occurs. The peers no longer look at the learner, say "ew," or tell him to stop when he spits. As a result, the learner's spitting gradually decreases until it no longer occurs to a significant degree. In this example, the functional reinforcer, attention, was no longer provided following the occurrence of problem behavior. Extinction for attention-maintained behavior is also called *planned ignoring* because the clinician plans to ignore the behavior when it happens. We will discuss what to do when it is impossible to ignore attention-maintained behavior shortly.

Extinction for tangible. In the previous example, the problem behavior was maintained by attention, so attention was no longer provided. In the case of problem behavior maintained by access to tangible items, the specific toy, snack, or activity that previously reinforced the behavior is withheld. A classic example of tangible extinction is the child in the candy aisle of the grocery store who cries until his parent gives him candy. Extinction for this behavior would require not giving the child candy in the store, nor even immediately after leaving the store, if crying occurred in the store. Assuming that you are in control of the preferred item or activity, this can be relatively straightforward.

Extinction for escape. Extinction for challenging behavior maintained by escape or avoidance of demands is called *escape extinction*. In these cases, escape from the nonpreferred demand or setting is the functional reinforcer, so escape extinction requires that the child not be allowed to escape from that demand or setting. For example, if a child tantrums when task demands are present, the same amount, frequency, and difficulty of task demands continue to be presented, regardless of crying.

It is critical to note that escape extinction is *not the same thing as ignoring the person*. Indeed, if you are asking a child to complete a task and he engages in challenging behavior and you then ignore him, you are likely giving him escape from the task because you are no longer requiring him to do it. For all types of extinction, it is probably more accurate to say that you *ignore the behavior,* not the person. That is, when the behavior happens, you pretend you didn't even notice and you continue to behave just as you behaved before the behavior occurred. For attention extinction, you continue to give the same amount of attention (or lack thereof) that you were already giving right before the behavior occurred. For escape extinction, you continue to place the same amount of demands as you already were. Generally speaking, extinction means that you never increase the amount of attention or decrease the amount of demands that the learner is receiving immediately following an occurrence of the behavior.

Extinction for automatic reinforcement. Preventing automatically reinforced behavior from producing the sensory stimulation that reinforces it is called *sensory extinction*. For example, an individual frequently takes chairs away from the kitchen table and pushes them around the house, scratching the tile floor. A functional assessment reveals that the reinforcer maintaining this behavior is the sound the chairs make and the vibration of the chair in the learner's hands as it scrapes across the floor. The clinician attaches runners to the bottom of the chairs, and now they glide easily and quietly, no longer making the screeching sound or vibrating the learner's hands when pushed along the floor. Sensory extinction *does not* involve depriving a child of his senses nor restraining the child in any way. It is often very challenging to prevent automatically reinforced behavior from producing its own stimulation, and for this reason, sensory extinction is rarely used.

Extinction bursts. An extinction burst is a temporary increase in frequency or intensity of a behavior when it is first placed on extinction. Figure 5.4 depicts hypothetical data for a typical extinction curve. During baseline, the challenging behavior results in the usual functional reinforcer, and it is relatively stable. When extinction begins, the behavior initially increases, followed by a gradual decline with occasional spikes.

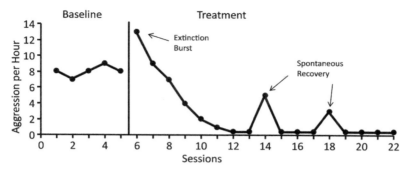

FIGURE 5.4   Hypothetical data of challenging behavior during baseline and during extinction. Note the initial extinction burst and later occurrences of spontaneous recovery. Both are common but temporary, so long as extinction continues to be implemented consistently.

Extinction bursts are very common in real-life treatment of challenging behavior in children with ASD, and they can be difficult. However, by definition, extinction bursts are temporary, and *they will go away* as long as you continue to implement extinction. In fact, extinction bursts can be interpreted as a good thing because they are a sign that the treatment is working and that you are probably implementing extinction successfully. Put nontechnically, from the learner's perspective, the reason she is doing a burst is that she is wondering why the usual behavior is no longer working, so she is trying to see what will work.

However, be aware that extinction bursts may present an opportunity to make the behavior worse if you are not consistent with extinction. If you try to implement extinction, the behavior worsens, and *then* you give in and give the child what she wants, you have just taught her that the normal amount of challenging behavior no longer works and that now she needs to engage in worse challenging behavior than ever! This is why it is critical to begin implementing extinction only when you are sure that you and all caregivers are able to follow through with it consistently.

Spontaneous recovery. Spontaneous recovery is the temporary reoccurrence of a behavior after it has decreased due to extinction. The right side of Figure 5.4 depicts hypothetical occurrences of spontaneous recovery after extinction has occurred. Research has not revealed *why* it occurs, but it is common in real-life applications of extinction. The good news is that spontaneous recovery is, by definition, temporary. The behavior will go back down if extinction continues to be implemented consistently. However, it is quite common for caregivers to become alarmed during occurrences of spontaneous recovery, and sometimes it is incorrectly interpreted as evidence that the behavior intervention plan is not working. This is yet another example of why careful data collection and graphing are so important. If the graph clearly shows a decrease in the behavior due to extinction and a single subsequent data point shows a high level of the behavior, there is no reason for alarm. The most prudent course of action is to continue with extinction. If the behavior does not decrease within a few days, then there may be a reason to reconsider the plan. If it's merely spontaneous recovery, however, then the behavior will decrease. If the increase was due to spontaneous recovery, the team changed the intervention plan immediately, and the behavior went back down, the decrease would be incorrectly interpreted as caused by the change in plan when, in fact, the increase was never real to begin with; it was only a temporary case of spontaneous recovery.

When extinction is unsafe or impossible. Conceptually, extinction is the simplest possible procedure: Just stop giving the reinforcer contingent on the behavior. When it comes to actually doing it in real life, however, it can be quite difficult and sometimes even impossible. For example, if a child hits peers to get attention from adults, then it is impossible for the adults to have no reaction whatsoever to the hitting because the peers are going to get hurt. However, just because an adult needs to react to prevent injury does not mean that the adult needs to provide a significant amount of attention. Physically blocking or redirecting the hitting, without making eye contact or talking to the aggressor in any way, may be enough to prevent injury and may be a small enough reaction that it does not reinforce the hitting behavior. In some cases, even the slightest reaction from an adult (even a change in facial expression) can be a reinforcer for a child's challenging behavior. In such cases, even the slightest reaction to prevent injury may constitute reinforcement. In all of these cases, it is critical to remember why it is so important to include frequent prompting and reinforcement of the replacement behavior. If the learner is being reminded frequently to ask for attention and he receives it immediately when he does ask, he will be far less motivated to hit for it. You would also be wise to "tip the scales in your favor" by providing a much larger amount of the reinforcer for the replacement behavior than the learner might inadvertently get for the challenging behavior. In other words, the learner may still be able to get a slight reaction out of you by hitting, but if he gets a *huge* positive reaction of out you by asking for attention, you are making it much more likely that he will make the better choice.

Differential reinforcement of other behavior. Differential reinforcement of other behavior (DRO) is a procedure whereby you provide reinforcement only if the challenging behavior has *not* occurred for a specified period of time. Thus, the procedure is sometimes called "differential reinforcement of omission" or "differential reinforcement of zero rates of behavior." Ideally, the DRO should be *functional,* meaning that the functional reinforcer for the target challenging behavior should be the one the learner earns for not engaging in the behavior. In addition, DRO is going to be much more successful if it is combined with extinction. In other words, a good DRO is one wherein the only way the learner can get the reinforcer that he used to get by engaging in the challenging behavior is if he does *not* do so anymore.

The duration of time that must pass before reinforcement is delivered is determined by the frequency of the problem behavior in baseline, so the more frequently the behavior occurs, the shorter the interval should be. This means that if the problem behavior occurs approximately every 10 minutes, the initial DRO interval should be less than 10 minutes. Once the problem behavior decreases to an acceptable level, the length of the DRO interval is gradually increased until it reaches a reasonable schedule.

Steps for Implementing a DRO
- Get a timer and datasheet ready.
- Tell the learner the rules; e.g., "If you have a nice voice for 10 minutes, you get a break with the iPad."
- Start the timer.
- If the target behavior occurs, reset the stopwatch and tell the learner that he needs to try again; e.g., "Oops, you cried. Let's try again. If you have a nice voice for 10 minutes, you get a break with the iPad."
- If the timer expires and the target behavior has not occurred, give the learner the reinforcer immediately and tell him why; e.g., "Wow, you had a great voice for 10 minutes! That's so awesome! Let's go get you the iPad!"

Strengths and limitations of DRO. One benefit of a DRO is that it makes sense to people: You reward a child for not doing the behavior that you want him to stop doing. Moreover, a significant amount of research has demonstrated that it can be effective as long as it is implemented with extinction of challenging behavior. One major limitation of DRO is that it does not help establish a replacement behavior. For this reason, DRO should virtually never be considered a complete behavior intervention plan. Another limitation is that it can be labor intensive to implement, especially if the challenging behavior occurs at a high rate. You may sometimes need to start with an interval as short as 10 seconds. However, keep in mind that the DRO interval can be gradually lengthened and that you are more likely to be successful if you start with a shorter rather than longer interval, all other things being equal.

Differential reinforcement of low rate behavior. Differential reinforcement of low rate behavior (DRL) is another form of differential reinforcement. DRL consists of giving the learner reinforcement as long as the behavior occurs at or below a specified rate. DRL can be useful for behaviors that are not maladaptive, per se, but are problematic because they occur at too high a rate. For example, a child with ASD who has learned to raise his hand to participate in class discussion may then raise his hand too frequently and attempt to respond to every single question his teacher asks the class. The teacher could use DRL by calling on that student only when he raises his hand at least 5 minutes after the last time the teacher called on him. Thus, the behavior of hand raising still gets reinforced with teacher attention but only when it occurs at or below once per 5 minutes.

Response interruption and redirection. Response interruption and redirection (RIRD) is used to treat repetitive behaviors maintained by automatic reinforcement. RIRD is particularly useful for behaviors that are persistent and occur across a variety of contexts and for long durations of time and for behaviors that have been resistant to other treatment. RIRD involves blocking or interrupting the problem behavior by providing immediate instruction to engage in a competing response until the learner stops engaging in the problem behavior and engages in a more appropriate behavior. Initially, reinforcement is provided contingent on the first occurrence of the appropriate behavior, but as progress is made, the learner must engage in more appropriate behavior for longer periods of time before reinforcement is provided, e.g., until she complies with several consecutive instructions. Brief praise and removal of demands are contingent upon compliance. The process is repeated every time the child engages in the target problem behavior.

Steps for Implementing RIRD
- Interrupt the target problem behavior by physically or vocally blocking the behavior.
- Request the child to engage in a more appropriate behavior until the specified number of appropriate behaviors have occurred (e.g., imitation of three gross motor actions).
- Cease the requests when the specified number of appropriate behaviors have occurred, and return to whatever you were doing before the challenging behavior occurred.

Technically speaking, RIRD is something that you add to the child's environment as a consequence of her behavior that results in a decrease in the behavior. This procedure may work because of punishment or because it increases the more appropriate behaviors. In any case, it should not be considered a complete behavior intervention plan because it is primarily reactive, rather than proactive, and because it does not explicitly include a plan to increase other particular alternative behaviors. Therefore, RIRD should always be combined with FCT, DRA, or similar strategies.

Response cost. Response cost is a punishment procedure wherein the clinician removes some amount of a reinforcer from a learner as a consequence of a challenging behavior. A common example of response cost from everyday life is a traffic citation. The city takes money away from you as a consequence for your speeding. Although response cost is punishment, it is also a very common part of everyday life for most people, and it is generally considered one of the least intrusive punishment procedures. In addition, it is commonly used in the treatment of children with ASD. Therefore, for all of these reasons, we include a brief discussion of it, even though punishment is not a recommended part of the CARD Model.

Perhaps the most commonly used form of response cost in treating children with ASD is the removal of a token contingent on the occurrence of challenging behavior. (See Chapter 4 for more on tokens.) For example, a learner may be earning a token for each discrete trial in which she responds correctly. A common way of incorporating response cost into such a system would be to remove a token from the token board, immediately contingent on a particular challenging behavior, such as hitting or biting. Other forms of response cost include taking a toy away from a child if she uses the toy in a way that will damage it, turning off the television if a child engages in stereotypy while watching it, and taking a toy away from a child if she refuses to share it with a peer. All of these forms of response cost can be effective augmentations to the learner's behavior intervention plan, depending on the particular child and the functions of the behaviors. But keep in mind that response cost, by itself, is never an adequate behavior intervention plan because it is based on punishment and does not help establish a functional replacement behavior. Also, clinicians too commonly resort immediately to response cost when a challenging behavior first arises, rather than considering the function of the behavior and implementing a reinforcement-based behavior intervention plan first.

STEP 5: WRITE THE BEHAVIOR INTERVENTION PLAN

A behavior intervention plan is a detailed written description of the problem behavior and the treatment designed to decrease it, as well as a description of a functionally equivalent replacement behavior intended to replace the problem behavior. Good behavior intervention plans include at least four basic sections: 1) description of the child and background information, 2) identification of the target behavior and its function, 3) description of the intervention, and 4) description of the data collection methods and reporting requirements. We provide examples of each below.

Description of the Child and Background Information

This section of the behavior intervention plan should include a brief description of all relevant background information about the child. This section generally includes the child's name, age, diagnoses, sex, living arrangement, school placement, medications, history of illness, and treatments for the challenging behavior that have been attempted in the past.

Identification of the Target Behavior and Its Function

Operational definition. A clear operational definition of the target behavior and functional replacement behaviors must be provided (see Chapter 20 for more on operational definitions). Don't forget to include examples and nonexamples, as well as descriptions of particular settings or contexts in which the challenging behavior is particularly likely to occur.

Function of behavior. This section of the behavior intervention plan should summarize the results of the functional assessment. Identify the function of the challenging behavior, including the general category (socially mediated positive or negative reinforcement or automatic reinforcement) and the specific form of that function (e.g., attention, tangible, escape from demands), as well as any specific or idiosyncratic features of the function that were identified during the functional assessment. For example, the function may be socially mediated positive for tangible but only with one specific toy or escape from demands with one type of task.

Description of the Intervention

This section of the behavior intervention plan should include a detailed description of the treatment for the target challenging behavior. Critical information that must be present includes antecedent modifications, procedures for teaching and maintaining replacement behaviors, consequence modifications, who is responsible for implementing the treatment, and the settings in which it must be implemented. Make instructions exceedingly clear, and avoid jargon and sounding "too technical." Include a clear, bold-faced heading for each of the sections in your plan. Several resources exist to help you write behavior intervention plans. One useful resource is the Skills® BIP Builder, a web-based tool for selecting behavior intervention plan components (www.skillsbipbuilder.com; see Chapter 26 for more). The tool contains a series of questions and descriptions, based on the function of the challenging behavior, that guide the clinician through the process of deciding which treatment components to include. It emphasizes the use of function-based, evidence-based, and least intrusive intervention components. Research has shown that the Skills® BIP Builder improves the quality of behavior intervention plans (Tarbox et al., 2013).

Antecedent manipulations. This section describes exactly what all caregivers should do to prevent occurrences of the challenging behavior, when they should do it, and how often they should do it. Many antecedent manipulations begin with a dense schedule and are gradually faded out. The schedule and criteria for fading out must be clearly specified. Examples:

- **Demand fading for escape-maintained tantrums.** "Implement only one discrete trial at a time with Jimmy, and give him an immediate 1-minute play break after each trial. Increase the number of trials required before the break by one for each set of two consecutive days that tantrums remain at or below an average rate of 1 per hour."
- **Noncontingent reinforcement for attention-maintained behavior.** "Give Sally 1 minute of high-quality positive attention (e.g., high fives, tickles, etc.) every 10 minutes as long as she has not hit within the last 30 seconds. If Sally has hit within the last 30 seconds of when attention was supposed to be delivered, delay the attention for an additional 30 seconds, deliver it, and then return to the normal schedule of attention."
- **Functional communication training for tangibly maintained pinching.** "Give Johnny a highly preferred toy (e.g., train, puzzles, action figures), and tell him that he's all done with the toy. Begin to remove the toy from him, and use an immediate vocal model prompt to say "my turn." If Johnny says "my turn" or any close approximation, immediately give the toy back to him for 30 seconds. Conduct 10 trials of this training every 30 minutes. If Johnny responds correctly on 8 out of 10 trials for two 10-trial blocks, fade your vocal model prompt to a partial vocal model. When he responds correctly at this level of prompting at least 8 out of 10 trials for two consecutive 10-trial blocks, insert a 1-second delay to your partial vocal model. Continue to add an additional second to the delay before the prompt according to this criterion. Discontinue prompting when Johnny responds correctly *without prompting* on at least 8 out of 10 trials for two consecutive 10-trial blocks."

Replacement Behaviors

This section of the behavior intervention plan should indicate what the replacement behavior is, the reinforcer to be delivered when it occurs, and the schedule of reinforcement to be used for the replacement behavior.

Consequence Modifications

This section of the behavior intervention plan describes exactly what to do when the challenging behavior occurs. By default, this section should include how extinction is to be implemented, at least to the greatest degree possible. In rare cases when extinction is expressly *not* to be implemented, this should be described in detail, along with a justification for it. In addition, this section of the plan should describe any emergency procedures that may need to be in place in case the child's behavior becomes out of control or excessively dangerous to himself or others. Emergency procedures vary widely based on the region and setting in which you are doing treatment, and space does not permit a description of them here.

As a general rule, the consequence modifications section of the behavior intervention plan should be shorter than the antecedent and replacement behavior sections. Good behavioral interventions focus on preventing challenging behavior and on teaching a replacement behavior, not merely on extinction or punishment of the challenging behavior. If you find that you have many treatment components in the consequence modifications section, it should be a red flag for you to examine the rest of your intervention plan more carefully to make sure that it's a balanced plan.

Description of the Data Collection Methods and Reporting Requirements

The last section of the behavioral intervention plan provides a description of the procedures for collecting data on the challenging behavior and the replacement behavior, including the measurement system, who should do it, and when it should be done (see Chapter 20 on data). Examples:

- **Rate data all day for screaming and FCT.** "Jenny's aide should collect frequency data on her tantrums and her functional communication throughout the school day. Data collection should begin when Jenny arrives at school and should end when she leaves school grounds. Data should be summarized as an average hourly rate by dividing the number of occurrences of each behavior by the number of hours Jenny is at school, and the data should be graphed at the end of each day."
- **Partial interval data for hand-flapping and toy play.** "Jimmy's therapist should collect partial interval data on Jimmy's hand-flapping and appropriate toy play during ABA therapy sessions. Since collection of these data will interfere with other ongoing teaching activities, the therapist will only collect these data during 5-minute samples of free play once every hour. During 5-minute samples, the therapist will collect partial interval data on both behaviors during continuous 10-second intervals. Data for each behavior should be summarized and graphed at the end of each day as the average percentage of intervals in which each behavior occurred."
- **Duration data for tantrums and frequency data for FCT.** "Sonny's parents will collect duration data on his tantrums during weekday evenings when ABA staff are not present. Sonny's parents will each have a stopwatch accessible at all times and will record the start and stop of each tantrum. The durations of all tantrums each day will be totaled, summarized, and graphed as the total number of minutes spent

engaging in tantrums each day. Sonny's parents will also collect data on the frequency with which he asks for preferred items or activities. They will tally each occurrence with a golf tally counter and summarize and graph the data as the total frequency of requesting each day."

Short-Format Intervention Plan for Daily Use

Quality behavioral intervention plans can be lengthy, often up to 20 pages long or more. It is critical for all caregivers and staff working with the child to read the plans thoroughly and familiarize themselves with all aspects. However, it is often useful to have a shorter version of the plan that can serve as a quick reference for daily use. If a staff member has a question about the plan and needs a quick reminder, it may not be possible to read through 20 pages to find the answer to the question. Therefore, a one- or two-page version of the plan in bulleted format can be highly useful. If the child has a logbook or a clipboard that contains all of his daily treatment information and datasheets, the short version can be kept there. Appendix B provides an example of a short-format version of a behavior intervention plan.

STEP 6: EVALUATE THE EFFECTIVENESS OF THE PLAN

The critical elements of how to evaluate the effectiveness of any behavioral intervention have been described at length in Chapter 20, so we will not elaborate them further here. However, the basics include collecting a baseline, implementing the intervention, and evaluating the effects on the challenging behavior by comparing the level of the behavior during the intervention phase to the level of the behavior during baseline. If the behavior intervention plan is not sufficiently effective, then consider trying other function-based treatment components until you find a combination that works. After you identify the plan that works, you will need to continue troubleshooting and following up on a longer-term basis.

STEP 7: TROUBLESHOOT AND FOLLOW UP

No intervention is perfect. When you run into trouble, you may need to troubleshoot to make your plan more effective. Many factors contribute to the success of a behavior intervention plan, but space only permits a brief discussion of some of the most important ones.

- **Training.** Make sure everyone knows what to do, and remember that merely telling someone is often not enough. You will often need to do role-play and give feedback to ensure excellent staff performance. (See Chapter 22 on training and quality control.)

- **Consistency.** Make sure everyone is following the plan the same way and doing the same thing every time they are supposed to do it. If the child sometimes "gets away" with the behavior and sometimes doesn't (i.e., inconsistent extinction), then you are teaching him to keep trying the challenging behavior because it occasionally works.
- **Buy-in.** Do the staff and parents believe the intervention will work, and do they value it? If not, they are much less likely to do it when they are not being observed. You may need to have a talk with them and discuss why the intervention is important or whether other options should be evaluated.
- **Difficulty.** Evaluate the ease of implementation. Is it just too difficult for staff or parents to implement consistently, and can you make it simpler or easier for staff?
- **Data.** Are the data being collected accurately? Have staff gradually become less stringent in their data collection?
- **Change in function/wrong function.** If the intervention worked for a while and is no longer working, is it possible that the behavior changed in function? In other words, did the child learn that he can use the old behavior to get new things that he wants? Or is it possible that the behavior has multiple functions and your initial functional assessment only identified one?
- **Stepping up too fast.** It is very common for treatment teams to be encouraged by the initial success of a plan and to begin thinning out reinforcement or fading out prompting too fast. It is also very common for treatment teams to become impatient with how slow a treatment really needs to be faded in order to maintain good effects. Consider stepping the treatment fading back a bit to regain low rates of the behavior.
- **Replacement behavior too difficult.** Is the replacement behavior easy for the child to do, and is he fluent in it? Consider making it easier and/or spending more time teaching it to fluency. Especially consider whether the replacement behavior is easier than the challenging behavior.
- **Inadequate reinforcement for replacement behavior.** It is common for staff and caregivers to think that the child "should" do the replacement behavior because "he knows that he is supposed to do it." The child may well know it, but he still needs lots of reinforcement for the behavior if you want the behavior to remain high. Consider upping the reinforcement for the replacement behavior.
- **Too deprived of functional reinforcer.** Remember that deprivation is a strong establishing operation and that establishing operations make behaviors more likely. It is common for a child who displays a high

rate of challenging behavior to have difficulty earning reinforcement, but this is unacceptable. It is the job of the behavior intervention team to make the child earn the functional reinforcer frequently, regardless of what it takes to do so. This will drive down the motivation for challenging behavior and help strengthen whatever replacement behavior produces the reinforcer.

Of course, all possible sources of treatment failure cannot be addressed here, but the variables above should provide you with a practical checklist to reference each time your behavior intervention plans underperform. Check each variable systematically and without bias. It is not your job to assign blame to individuals; it is your job to find out how the child's environment can be changed to help him succeed. Blame the environment, not the child, parents, or staff!

SUMMARY

Top-quality treatment of challenging behavior in children with ASD consists of the following steps: 1) identify, define, and prioritize the target behavior, 2) determine outcome goals, 3) conduct a functional assessment, 4) design a function-based behavior intervention plan, 5) write the behavior intervention plan, 6) evaluate the effectiveness of the plan, and 7) troubleshoot and follow up. Good behavior intervention plans are based on the function of behavior, they establish adaptive replacement behaviors that are based on the function of the challenging behavior, and they include intensive training of all caregivers, as well as follow-up and maintenance.

Visual and Other Sensory Modifications

*Carolynn Bredek, Doreen Granpeesheh,
Kathy Thompson, Renat Matalon*

Behavioral intervention for learners with autism spectrum disorder (ASD) generally relies very heavily on vocally delivered instructions and vocal responding on the part of the learner. That is, the child is required to learn through contacting auditory stimuli and respond by producing vocalizations. However, some learners with ASD have great difficulty learning via auditory instruction and/or vocal responding. The challenge may lie in the learner's ability to produce speech, respond to spoken language, or both. Some learners with ASD may have other sensory challenges. Indeed, the DSM-5 now includes abnormal responses to sensory stimuli in the diagnostic criteria for ASD, thereby clearly acknowledging that some portion of children with ASD suffer from these difficulties (American Psychiatric Association, 2013). As with many facets of ASD, sensory abnormalities differ greatly across children. Some children learn particularly well from visual stimuli, while others have significant comorbid vision deficits and may need to have instructions heavily modified to utilize auditory or tactile stimuli. Some children have unreasonably large avoidance responses to loud noises or other complex auditory stimuli (e.g., noisy classrooms), while others seem not to notice sudden loud noises in their environment, suggesting that auditory stimuli severely lack saliency. Still other children have severely abnormal reactions to tactile stimuli; for example, the feeling of sand or uncooked rice on the hands evokes crying, avoidance, or fear.

The key point to remember about sensory stimulation when planning treatment for children with ASD is that every child is different, and many (but not all) children's success in learning will be greatly impacted by how you do or do not adjust your treatment procedures to accommodate their existing sensory abnormalities. Although research is not conclusive yet, it appears that visual sensory input may be the most common modality that requires modification in planning treatment for children with ASD. Therefore, the majority of this chapter will be dedicated to describing how to embed visual modifications into evidence-based behavioral intervention for learners with ASD in order to maximize the child's learning and success. The chapter will also briefly touch on modifications involving other sensory modalities.

The Center for Autism and Related Disorders (CARD) approach to visual modifications aims to increase each learner's opportunity for success by including visual supports that enhance learning. This chapter will describe the CARD approach to incorporating visual modifications into the behavioral intervention process and how these modifications can be used to enhance skill acquisition across a variety of domains. *Visual modifications* refers to the use of textual stimuli (written or typed words), iconic stimuli (pictures or picture representations), or motor responses (e.g., sign language or gestures) that are used in place of or in conjunction with speech or auditory stimuli. These modifications can be used with learners who struggle to produce or learn from spoken language. Many learners who have substantial difficulty learning via traditional vocal teaching strategies can be helped significantly by using visual modifications. Communication via means other than speech is commonly referred to as Augmentative and Alternative Communication (AAC), and the use of AAC is quite common among treatment providers and educators who work with learners with ASD. However, it is rarely sufficient merely to provide visual supports to a struggling learner with ASD. As with all other successful skill acquisition efforts, effective use of visual modifications depends on the practitioner's understanding and use of evidence-based behavioral principles and procedures of learning and motivation.

Generally speaking, visual supports can be categorized as response modifications and stimulus modifications. A **response modification** replaces or supplements what would traditionally be a vocal response form on the part of the learner with a nonvocal response. Response modifications are used with learners who have difficulty producing or learning vocal speech and/or struggle with articulation. The modified response form could consist of: 1) an iconic stimulus, such as photos or icons; e.g., the learner hands his mom an icon from his communication book or touches an icon on a tablet device in order to gain access to a preferred item); 2) a textual stimulus, such as prewritten words or typing; e.g., the learner responds to the question "What is she doing?" by handing over a card with the prewritten word "running" on it; or 3) a motor response wherein the learner engages in sign language or gestures to communicate.

A **stimulus modification** consists of an additional visual stimulus that the therapist presents in conjunction with the vocal stimulus that she

TABLE 6.1 Vocal Programs Versus Visually Modified Programs and Learners Who May Benefit from Them

Traditional Vocal Program	Visually Modified Program	
Vocal Stimulus	Stimulus Modification	Learner Profile
Instruction is spoken by the therapist.	Therapist presents visual stimuli+vocal stimulus.	Difficulty learning vocal instruction Difficulty with acquisition of complex or abstract concepts
Vocal Response	Response Modification	Learner Profile
Response is spoken by the learner.	The learner touches visual stimuli or engages in motor response.	Difficulty learning to produce speech Little to no vocal imitation skills Poor articulation

would normally present. The visual stimulus could consist of: 1) an iconic stimulus, such as photos or icons; e.g., the therapist holds up a picture of an apple when instructing the learner, "Name some fruits"; 2) a textual stimulus, such as prewritten or typed words; e.g., while presenting a field of three objects and instructing the learner, "Give me shoe," the therapist holds up the written word "shoe"; or 3) a motor stimulus, such as sign language; e.g., while giving vocal instructions to the learner, the therapist also signs.

Table 6.1 summarizes differences between traditional vocal programs and visually modified programs and provides descriptions of learners who may benefit from each type of modification. Next, we will review both response modifications and stimulus modifications in more detail.

THE RESPONSE MODIFICATION

As discussed above, visually modified responses can include sign language or gestures, touching or exchanging pictures or symbols, and writing or typing to communicate. Response modifications can be used to teach anything from basic requests to commenting and conversational language. A common concern about using nonvocal means of communication is that it may hinder the acquisition of vocal speech. This is actually a misconception, as research has documented the fact that the utilization of AAC promotes the acquisition and use of speech to communicate (Charlop-Christy, Carpenter, LeBlanc, & Kellet, 2002). Further, procedures for the use of AAC should always include modeling of speech and continued efforts to teach and reinforce speech and vocal communication attempts made by the learner. A learner who possesses or develops speech, but whose speech is unclear, should never stop using speech but can use AAC to enhance her speech. A learner who has not yet developed intelligible speech might begin by using AAC to communicate all of her needs. However, as the learner's speech becomes more easily understood by others, she may only need to use response modifications in limited situations. Whenever possible, response modifications should be used to enrich, not replace, a learner's vocal communication.

CLINICAL INDICATORS FOR USE OF RESPONSE MODIFICATIONS

Clinical indicators that point to a potential need for response modifications include limited to no speech or vocal imitation skills, poor articulation, and/or difficulty initiating vocal communication. We often notice that the learner has limited-to-no functional communication skills and demonstrates slow progress or a lack of progress altogether with foundational lessons that require a vocal response. Often, we also observe problem behaviors related to the learner's inability to communicate his needs appropriately. Finally, we have also noted (although research has not yet evaluated) that learners who are particularly strong in visually based lessons, such as matching, tend to do particularly well with visual response modifications in other lessons. This may be the case because tapping into the strengths and interests of the learner helps increase motivation and therefore enhances acquisition of new skills.

Response Forms

Most visually modified response forms fall into two categories: 1) topography based and 2) selection based. **Topography-based** response forms, which are also known as unaided forms of communication, require no external devices and rely on the learner using her body to communicate. Topography-based forms of communication include sign language, as well as use of gestures, facial expression, and writing. They are called topography based because the factor that distinguishes one "word" from another is the topography or form of the behavior that the learner exhibits; e.g., the manual sign for "drink" is physically different than the manual sign for "eat."

Selection-based response forms are responses wherein the learner makes a choice between different responses that are visually available at the same time. They are not topography based because the topography is always the same, regardless of what the learner is communicating.

For example, a learner might point to a picture of a cup to ask for a drink or point to a picture of food to ask for a snack, but the topography of both responses is pointing. Examples of selection-based forms of communication include pointing to or exchanging pictures, icons, or prewritten words using a binder, voice output communication device, or tablet computer. Selection-based response forms always require external devices or materials because the learner always has to *select* from something.

Commonly Used Forms of Response Modifications

Sign language. Sign language uses specific motor responses, including movements of the fingers, hands, arms, and/or body, to communicate. A major advantage of sign language is that no devices or systems are needed for the learner to communicate. This often means that communication can occur more immediately because it does not rely on manipulation of stimuli as with other forms of AAC. The disadvantages are that sign language requires prerequisite motor skills, such as the ability to make specific fine motor movements to perform the signs. Further, sign language itself (beyond gestures and facial expression) is not a universally understood form of communication, so this limits communicative partners. In essence, the audience for a learner with ASD who relies primarily on sign language for communication is limited to people in her immediate family and/or treatment team, as well as the hearing-impaired community. In addition, sign language depends on recall, whereas picture systems allow for recognition, and all other things being equal, recognition is generally acknowledged to be easier than recall.

Picture communication systems. Selecting and/or exchanging pictures or icons as a means to communicate is a very commonly used response modification in the autism community. A major advantage of picture communication systems is that the pictures are generally understood by virtually anyone, and printed words can easily accompany the pictures in order to aid others in understanding the communication of the learner with ASD. Another major advantage is that picture systems do not require complex fine motor skills. Multiple commercially available programs exist that house vast libraries of picture communication symbols. These programs make creating the needed stimuli quite simple. Further, today's technology allows photographs of specific items that are relevant to a given learner to be taken and shared easily across different devices. The disadvantages are that the learner's vocabulary is limited to the pictures on hand, the pictures tend to be easily lost or damaged, and the need to create, organize, and maintain the pictures continually can be a chore. In addition, anytime the learner does not have access to his communication binder or communication device, he is left with no means to communicate.

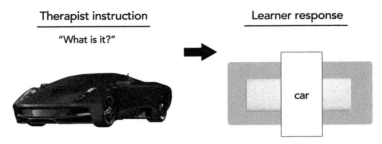

FIGURE 6.1   Example of visual response modification. In the presence of a car, the therapist asks, "What is it?" The learner responds by placing a card containing the written word "car" onto a sentence strip.

Prewritten words. The use of prewritten words is similar to the use of pictures in that the learner selects or exchanges the prewritten words as a means to communicate. Figure 6.1 depicts an example of how prewritten words can be used to modify responses during labeling (tacting) training. The advantages and disadvantages are also similar to those of pictures. Often, intervention begins with pictures or symbols and gradually transitions to written words after the learner has acquired a very large and fluent repertoire of communication pictures/symbols. This transition can be aided by printing the word on the picture and gradually increasing the size of the written word while gradually fading out the picture in order to transfer stimulus control from the picture to the written word.

Typing. Keyboards can also be used for the learner to communicate by typing out words. The advantages of typing are that there are no limits to the learner's vocabulary (outside of his capacity to learn to spell and type the words), and there are no stimuli to organize and maintain. Further, reading typewritten words is a universally understood form of communication. The disadvantages of typing are the required prerequisite skills, which include the fine motor movements of selecting letters on a keyboard and the capacity to spell. A learner's age can certainly limit typing as a possible option.

It is important to note that using typing on a keyboard as a response modification in the context of an evidence-based behavioral intervention program is *not* the same thing as "facilitated communication." Facilitated communication is a scientifically disproven procedure for facilitating people with disabilities to communicate via typing. Research has repeatedly shown that inadvertent prompting on the part of the "facilitators" was actually guiding many individuals to type what the facilitators were thinking, not what the person with the disability was trying to communicate. Beware of any typing or other selection-based response modification program where the learner never learns to communicate without the physical touch of another person. If a learner depends on someone else physically touching him to communicate, then he is not actually able to communicate independently.

System/Device Options

A variety of different systems or devices can be used across the different response forms that we just reviewed.

Communication boards or books. Communication boards or books typically employ the use of picture symbols, photos, or written words that represent items or concepts that are meaningful to the learner. The most common methods for communication include direct selection through a motor response, such as pointing, touching, or physically exchanging the stimuli with a communicative partner. The system design can be as simple as a single board with a small set of meaningful and functionally important icons, or it can be a book containing multiple pages of written words that are categorized by subject.

The advantages of communication books or boards are that they are simple and inexpensive to create. Moreover, unlike expensive devices, communication boards and books are not fragile; you do not have to be concerned that a young learner might drop her book, and you do not have to be concerned about malfunction of the device. The disadvantages are that the picture symbols or written words can be difficult to maintain, and a book or board can be cumbersome to carry. In addition, large, cumbersome boards or binders can appear socially awkward and make the learner's challenges more apparent to her peers. However, portable and less cumbersome versions can be purchased or made with a little creativity. For example, a keychain can be used to carry strips containing some of the learner's most preferred and/or relevant pictures when the learner is mobile in the community. Another disadvantage is that communication boards or books do not offer the feature of voice output, so the learner must rely on the communicative partner to model all vocal communication.

Speech-generating devices (SGDs). SGDs are machines that produce voice output. SGDs are also commonly referred to as voice output devices, voice output communication devices, and voice output communication aids. SGDs can be classified into two categories: dedicated and nondedicated devices.

Dedicated devices. Dedicated devices refer to those that are developed purely for the purpose of AAC. One advantage of dedicated devices is that you can often rent them from the manufacturer. Dedicated devices can be considered medically necessary Durable Medical Equipment (DME). As a result, funding for dedicated devices is sometimes available through both public and private funding sources, such as school districts and insurance carriers. Further, manufacturers of dedicated devices offer a great deal of training and support related to the use of the device.

Nondedicated devices. Nondedicated devices are those computers or tablets that host software or applications used to support AAC. One advantage of using nondedicated devices is that many different communication-based software programs and applications can be used that are significantly less expensive than a dedicated device. Therefore, nondedicated devices may be more affordable and offer more software choices. Further, nondedicated devices, such as laptops, tablets, and smart phones, are mainstream devices that are socially accepted and typically perceived positively by the learner's peers, so their use in different settings does not make the learner stand out in a negative way. These devices are more adaptable and offer access to the Internet and a camera, both of which can be quite useful in some cases. Finally, nondedicated devices usually tend to be lighter and smaller than dedicated devices, making their transport easier. One disadvantage of nondedicated devices is that third-party funding for their purchase is very limited, although some state legislation has mandated insurance carriers to fund tablets and several nonprofit organizations, such as iTaalk Autism Foundation and ACT Today!, fund tablets themselves or work with families to secure funding from the learner's insurance carrier. Another disadvantage of these devices is that access to the Internet, games, and applications outside of the AAC programs may serve as a distraction to the learner, although such access can often be restricted by the caregiver, if necessary.

Choosing a Response Form and Device

When determining which response form and device best meets the needs of the learner, it is important to recognize that use of AAC is dynamic, so the needs of the learner should be assessed continuously and response forms modified accordingly. Oftentimes, the most simplistic type of device is introduced first, and as the learner becomes more proficient with communication, the device can become more sophisticated to meet his needs. Ideally, the decision should be based on each learner's unique needs and which response form and device most effectively addresses those needs, although economic circumstances may be a factor. Here are some additional aspects to consider:

Communicative needs. Does the response form and device allow the learner to communicate his needs efficiently and effectively?

The learner's audience. Who needs to understand the learner? Is the response form one that will be understood by the learner's most consistent communicative partners? Will the form of communication be understood by the learner's peers? What level of instruction, if any, will be required for communicative partners to understand the learner?

Prerequisite skills. Does the response form and use of the device require specific prerequisite skills? Does the learner already possess these skills? If not, can they be easily taught and acquired? Further, if choosing symbols, the level of abstraction of the symbols themselves should be considered. Does the learner have a history of learning to respond effectively to line drawings and icons, or is she likely to require clear, high-quality photographs for all pictures in the system?

Acquisition. Do you have any evidence to believe one particular method will be more easily acquired by the particular learner in question? Does she have a history of success with learning to discriminate between pictures and/or learning sign language?

Interests of the learner. Does the learner have a particular interest in the response form or device? For example, does the learner highly prefer and show interest in letters and words? Does the learner show an interest in electronic devices? Can these interests be harnessed to increase motivation to communicate? On the other hand, are the learner's interests so strong that they may actually interfere with the therapist's ability to influence how and when the learner uses the system?

Stakeholder buy-in. Do the parents, caregivers, and teachers understand how to use the system? Do they support the use of the system and will they be willing to implement it consistently across all settings?

Introducing and Implementing the Response Modification

Space does not permit a full description of all of the steps of teaching visually modified communication systems. We recommend readers refer to *The Picture Exchange Communication System Training Manual* (Frost & Bondy, 2002) for step-by-step, practical instructions on how to teach the Picture Exchange Communication System (PECS), a popular and effective picture communication system. Below, we give general recommendations on teaching visually modified response systems that are equally applicable, regardless of which particular modifications you use.

Model vocal speech. When the learner uses a visually modified response, the communicative partner should immediately provide a vocal model for the learner. For example, if the learner hands the therapist an icon representing juice, the therapist should say "juice," modeling the vocal response for him. If the learner is just beginning to use an SGD, repeating a simple message is still advised, even though the device provides vocal output. The model can be a vocal confirmation of the intended message communicated using the device. For instance, if the learner touches the juice icon and the word "juice" is produced by the device, you could say "juice" to the learner, confirming his request or acknowledging his communication. Vocally modeling the response for the learner increases opportunities for him to imitate the spoken response.

Reinforce the modified response immediately. When first introducing response modifications, do not require the learner to attempt a vocalization in order for his response to be reinforced. Rather, always provide reinforcement for the modified response. Once the learner is fluent with the modified response form and you know the learner is able to provide a vocal approximation, you can begin to consider changing the response required for reinforcement to include an attempt at a vocal response. Frequently, the learner will make attempts to vocalize without being required to do so. Our job is to shape the learner's vocal response and reinforce successive approximations toward the target word or phrase while pairing use of the response modification.

Prompting and reinforcement. Regardless of response form or device, prompting and differential reinforcement are the most powerful tools for establishing the initial communication repertoire. Begin by presenting an opportunity to communicate by making a highly preferred item, food, or activity visually present. Immediately prompt the learner to engage in the modified response, and then immediately deliver the reinforcer. Use whatever prompting procedure is going to ensure an accurate response immediately, often a physical prompt, as long as the physical prompt is not highly nonpreferred for the learner. Fade out the prompting over successive communication opportunities (see Chapter 4 for more on prompting and prompt fading). As the learner becomes more independent, gradually fade in longer distances between the learner and the communicative partner, begin teaching other responses for other items, and make sure to practice across a variety of different settings and communicative partners.

Establishing operations. The first several communication responses you should teach when implementing a new visually modified response system are mands, that is, requests for something the learner wants in the moment (see Chapter 11 on verbal behavior). Remember that mands, by definition, have to occur when the learner actually wants something, not necessarily when the therapist wants her to communicate. Therefore, for your teaching to be successful, the learner needs to genuinely want the item/activity/food you are trying to teach her to request in that moment. See Chapter 4 on optimizing establishing operations.

Fading the Use of Response Modifications

For some, the use of AAC will be lifelong and should be viewed as an accepted and valued means of communication, as it enables appropriate functional communication, fosters independence and dignity, and facilitates learning. For others, the use of response modifications may only be necessary as a stepping stone to vocal communication, and the use of visual modifications can be faded. Often, the learner begins to make attempts to vocalize, either in response to the model given by the communicative partner or vocal output device. In some cases, the learner begins to vocalize even before these models are given, meaning that the learner begins to vocalize as he is issuing the modified response. When you notice this behavior, you can begin to reinforce the vocal response immediately as a means to fade the use of the device. However, the process of fading must be done in such a way that the learner never loses his ability to communicate effectively. It is important not to abandon a visually modified system simply because the learner has acquired some speech. You must ensure that the learner can be understood by all relevant communicative partners. In most cases, the option for using response modifications should be made available as a means to supplement and enhance the learner's communication until he is able to vocally communicate his needs effectively across relevant communicative partners and environments.

THE STIMULUS MODIFICATION

Stimulus modifications consist of the use of a visual stimulus in conjunction with the vocal instruction that is typically spoken by the therapist. The visual stimulus can be anything from a textual stimulus (e.g., prewritten words or typing) to an iconic stimulus (e.g., photos, icons, or picture representations) or motor stimulus (e.g., sign language). Stimulus modifications may also be referred to as visual supports which might include visual schedules, timers, and visual reinforcement systems. Stimulus modifications can be used across a wide population of learners with different needs. Generally speaking, stimulus modifications support the learner's understanding of language and concepts. We will address the use of stimulus modifications across two categories: 1) visual modifications to traditional vocal instruction and 2) visual supports that help organize the learner's life and environment.

When to Introduce Stimulus Modifications

As with the use of response modifications, the goal of using stimulus modifications is to provide a means of communication and to facilitate learning and overall success. Specifically, you are supporting the learner's *understanding* of vocal communication and abstract concepts and how this understanding relates to day-to-day activities in his environment. Generally speaking, stimulus modifications are less intrusive than response modifications and are easier to fade in most cases. This means you can more readily introduce a stimulus modification to support a specific need or to use only within a specific condition. Most of the time, you can use stimulus modifications as prompts to facilitate learning and quickly fade their use. However, in some cases, the stimulus modification may be necessary for the learner's success in a given environment, and fading, therefore, is not an option. This should not deter you from its use if it is facilitating success for the learner.

Several of the same considerations made for the introduction of response modifications should also be made for stimulus modifications. Specifically, you should consider the length of time the learner has been participating in an intervention program that is primarily vocally delivered and how many attempts have been made to teach a particular target skill without the learner experiencing success. If you determine that stimulus modifications should be attempted, begin by making modifications to targets within a single lesson, and compare the learner's rate of acquisition with that of the rest of the traditional vocal program. If the learner's progress with the modifications is better than his progress within the rest of his lessons, you may consider making more widespread program modifications.

The forms that stimulus modifications can take are similar to those of response modifications, except that they apply to the instruction, rather than to the learner's response. That is, with stimulus modifications, the therapist or communicative partner is using the written words, picture symbol, or signs in conjunction with her vocal instruction or communication with the learner, rather than or in addition to the learner responding visually. Consider the following example (depicted in Figure 6.2) of a stimulus modification using printed words embedded into a receptive language lesson:

- **Instruction**: The therapist presents the learner with a field of objects, including a train, ice cream cone, and a jacket. The therapist presents the written word *jacket* simultaneously with the vocal stimulus "Give me jacket."
- **Response**: The learner gives the therapist the jacket.

Here is another example of embedding visual modifications into receptive language training using sign language rather than printed words:

- **Instruction**: The therapist presents the learner with a field of objects, including a ball, a shoe, and a cup. The therapist demonstrates the sign for ball simultaneously with the vocal stimulus "Give me ball."
- **Response**: The learner gives the therapist the ball.

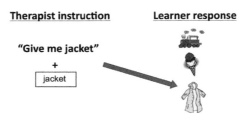

FIGURE 6.2 Example of visual stimulus modification. The therapist says, "Give me jacket," while presenting a card with the written word "jacket" (printed word stimulus modification), and the learner selects the picture of the jacket.

Fading

The purpose of providing an additional visual stimulus during instruction is to facilitate more rapid learning. However, in many cases, this additional visual stimulus is not part of the learner's real-life environment, so dependence on it essentially amounts to a type of prompt dependence. To the greatest extent possible, the goal is to fade out the use of the visual stimulus and return the learner to traditional vocal teaching strategies (i.e., being able to respond solely to vocal instructions and make auditory discriminations). As with any prompt, there are multiple ways that visual supports can be faded out (see Chapter 4), but we have found two procedures to be particularly effective: 1) fading the intensity or size of the visual stimulus and 2) time delay procedure.

Fading intensity or size. Visual stimuli can be faded out by systematically decreasing the size of the text or image on the stimulus card until the card is eventually blank. It is also possible to gradually make the text or image more and more transparent, until it is no longer visible. Whatever method you use to fade out the size or intensity of the visual stimulus, the vocal stimulus should continue to be presented in conjunction, and positive reinforcement should continue to be presented for correct responding. Thus, if successful, stimulus control will gradually be transferred from the visual stimulus to the vocal instruction.

Time delay procedure. Generally speaking, when using visually modified stimuli, the therapist presents the visual stimulus at the same time as the vocal instruction. Instead of, or in addition to, fading the intensity or size of the visual stimulus, you can fade in a time delay. This is done by gradually increasing the amount of time between the presentation of the vocal instruction and the presentation of the visual stimulus, starting with less than 1 second and gradually increasing by 1 second, as long as the learner continues to respond correctly. By gradually increasing the time delay between vocal and visual stimuli, you are essentially giving the learner a choice: She can wait for the visual stimulus and, therefore, wait longer before getting reinforcement, or she can attempt to respond to the vocal stimulus immediately and receive reinforcement sooner. As the time delay gets larger (several seconds or more), many learners will begin to respond to the vocal stimulus, rather than wait for the visual one. When they respond correctly to the vocal stimulus, you reinforce immediately with a very highly preferred reinforcer and, therefore, begin to bring the correct response under stimulus control of the vocal instruction before the visual is even presented.

It is also possible to fade out the visual stimulus by systematically decreasing the amount of time that the visual stimulus is present. You begin by presenting the stimulus modification simultaneously with the vocal instruction, keeping the visual stimulus present until the learner responds. Then, systematically decrease the amount of time the visual stimulus is present, perhaps in half-second increments, until the presentation is a brief flash that is barely visible and, eventually, a flash that is so brief that it is not functionally visible.

Difficulty with fading. If you are finding it particularly difficult to fade out visual stimulus modifications, there is no need to worry. You can continue including stimulus modifications in your teaching procedures, thereby ensuring a high rate of learning for the learner, and continue to probe for the ability to fade on a regular basis. Most learners will acquire the ability to learn from vocal stimuli at some point; however, some learners may continue to need visual supports indefinitely, and this is okay. While the goal is to return to traditional vocal programming, you must remember that some learners may have never been able to make any gains via traditional teaching strategies. Use of stimulus modifications allows the learner to acquire new skills and experience success. Some learners may only be able to learn from vocal instruction in some parts of their intervention program and not others. Some learners may continue to need visual supports during the acquisition phase of lessons but can easily be faded off them during generalization and maintenance. Some learners may be able to acquire specific skills via vocal strategies but require visual supports for others. As with all aspects of behavioral intervention for learners with ASD, the use and fading of visual modifications require a constant process of analysis and adjustment.

VISUAL SUPPORTS FOR ORGANIZING THE ENVIRONMENT

Stimulus modifications that assist the learner in organizing his environment represent another important category.

Visual Schedules

Visual schedules can be helpful in organizing tasks as simple as playing for 10 minutes or as complicated as preparing one's schedule for an entire school day, and everything in between. Visual schedules can represent tasks and activities with pictures, icons, or written words. Space does not permit a description of the many steps involved in implementing picture activity schedules, but activity schedules have been shown to increase independence and decrease stereotypy across a variety of children, tasks, and settings (see Krantz & McClannahan, 2014, for a thorough review).

Wait Cards

When teaching a learner with ASD to wait for a preferred item before engaging in an impulsive behavior (Chapter 18) or when teaching a learner to wait for attention or a break from work when teaching functional communication (Chapter 5), it can be helpful to include a visual cue for waiting. "Wait cards" help the learner discriminate that her request is going to be reinforced but that she merely needs to wait a bit. Wait cards can take a variety of forms, including the printed word *wait* on a card, a blank red card, or even a bracelet of a particular color that the learner puts on when she must wait. To maximize success, make sure to start with requiring the learner to wait for very short intervals (e.g., 1 second) when first teaching the wait card, and only increase the interval when the learner is consistently successful with the current interval.

Visual Timers

Visual timers are timers that display a visual representation of how much time is remaining before the timer sounds, usually with a red or green strip that slowly decreases in size. Visual timers can be useful in a variety of situations. For example, they can be used as "wait cards," as described above. They can also be used as a warning stimulus for learners who have particular difficulty with transition away from a preferred activity. The visual timer can provide a clear cue that indicates to the learner how much time she has left with the preferred activity. If you are consistent with its use (i.e., when the timer is up, the transition always happens, regardless of challenging behavior), then the timer will also become a cue that indicates to the learner that there is no reason to engage in challenging behavior because it will not work. (In technical jargon, the timer becomes an S-delta, signaling the absence of reinforcement available for challenging behavior.)

First-Then Contingencies

Visual supports can be used to help indicate to the learner the contingencies that are in place for completing a nonpreferred task and the positive reinforcement that will occur as a result. First-then visuals can consist of a board that has two hook-and-loop squares, the first affixed with a picture that represents a nonpreferred task and the second affixed with a picture that represents a highly preferred reinforcer. The therapist then shows the board to the learner and states the contingency, such as, "*First*, you do your math; *then*, you get your iPad." Through repeated use across multiple exemplars, the vocal stimuli "first-then," along with the visual representations of the task and reinforcer, will come to function as a discriminative stimulus that increases the likelihood of task completion.

OTHER SENSORY MODIFICATIONS

Although visual modifications are probably the most well-known sensory modifications and the ones that receive the most attention within the autism treatment community, each learner is different, of course, and a small but significant minority of learners benefit from modifications of other sensory modalities.

Visual Challenges

If you suspect that a learner suffers from some kind of visual impairment, the first step is, of course, to refer them to an ophthalmologist and/or developmental optometrist. Naturally, eyeglasses can help a great deal for visual impairment. Some visual challenges can also be addressed with practice and training, that is, by treating seeing, per se, as behavior that can be strengthened (see visual motor section in Chapter 14). If a learner has significant visual challenges, it is critical to modify her treatment program so that it relies *less heavily* on visual stimuli – the reverse of everything that was described earlier in this chapter. Consider presenting visual stimuli in much larger sizes (i.e., bigger pictures, printed words in larger font sizes), presenting them at different distances from the learner, orienting stimuli upright, and increasing the use of auditory and tactile prompts, if possible.

Auditory Challenges

The "typical" child with ASD who requires heavy visual modifications, as discussed throughout this chapter, might be described as being less sensitive to auditory stimuli than would be ideal. However, some children with ASD appear to present with the opposite sensory profile; that is, they are overly sensitive to auditory stimuli to the point that it interferes with learning. For example, sudden loud noises (e.g., a blender, a school bell, a motorcycle driving past, etc.) can evoke fear and avoidance responses. If such a child is blocked from avoiding the sound, he may resort to tantrums or aggression, and caregivers may inadvertently reinforce these challenging behaviors by allowing the child to continue to escape the noise when he displays the challenging behavior. For learners such as these, it is critical to limit the extent to which they are exposed to these loud noises, especially early in therapy. Later on, it may be necessary to implement desensitization procedures by gradually exposing the learner to louder noises in very small increments and positively reinforcing calm, coping behaviors (e.g., deep breathing, counting, etc.).

Other children with ASD are sometimes overly stimulated by ambient sounds. For example, some children find it extremely challenging to focus on instruction from a therapist when any other sounds can be heard (e.g., other therapists talking to other learners, music on the radio, someone walking down the hallway, the hum of fluorescent lightbulbs, etc.). For these learners, it is critical to decrease or eliminate the ambient noise during early stages of therapy, at least to the greatest degree possible. You can also attempt to treat selective attention as a behavioral skill, in itself, and teach it through practice and reinforcement (see attention section in Chapter 18). In very extreme cases, it may be useful to have the learner wear noise-canceling headphones and deliver vocal instruction through a microphone connected to the headphones. These accommodations should be considered temporary and need to be faded out gradually if the learner is expected to functional successfully in natural environments that contain ambient noise.

Tactile Challenges

Many children with ASD have serious challenges with tactile stimulation. Textures, such as sand, rice, grass, and the feeling of shirt tags touching the backs of their necks, can be genuinely aversive for many such children. If tactile stimulation is highly nonpreferred by a learner, care should be taken during the early stages of the therapy program to eliminate such stimulation to the greatest extent possible. For example, many daycare programs use sand or rice tables in activities for children. If sand and rice are strongly aversive for your learner, you should seriously consider whether it is worth the time and effort required to teach the learner to tolerate the activity, especially if the main point of the activity is to play with other children. You would do well to find a less aversive activity for the learner with ASD to do with peers. Some children need to have their clothing tags removed. Other children do not respond well to significant amounts of hugs, tickling, or other forms of physical praise. For these learners, especially in the early stages of therapy, it is wise to find other reinforcers that are highly preferred, so you can successfully reinforce learning during therapy. You may well want to teach the learner to tolerate hugs and high fives later in his therapy program, but it is probably not the highest clinical priority in the early stages of therapy.

SUMMARY

Effective evidence-based treatment for children with ASD should take into consideration any unique responses (or lack thereof) that each learner displays. The CARD Model incorporates the use of sensory modifications (especially visual) into treatment for learners with ASD who struggle with learning in the more "standard" applied behavior analysis (ABA) formats. This includes: 1) teaching learners to use visual supports (e.g., pictures, icons, text, sign language, etc.) to produce or in place of spoken language (response modifications) and 2) the use of such visual supports in combination with vocal instructions presented by therapists. Visual modifications can be used to support learners across a wide variety of needs. The following are a few final thoughts to consider with regard to effectively designing and using visual modifications:

- Use visual modifications as a means to support the acquisition of speech. Do not give up on speech, and always pair speech with the modification being used as a means to model vocal speech for the learner.
- Consider the learner's audience and environment when choosing a response form and type of device.
- Program for generalization. Use visual modifications across settings and people. Educate stakeholders, so they can use, understand, and support the system. Choose programs and targets that are relevant and functional for the learner.
- Use professional resources that may be available to you with regard to choosing, implementing, and funding the use of specific devices.
- Be creative and always consider the needs of the learner first, above and beyond clinical tradition or dogma.

The central point regarding sensory modifications is that every child is different. Some are particularly adept with visual stimuli, and some are particularly challenged by it. There seems to be a common belief within the ABA community that all sensory modalities have equal potential for use as avenues for instruction. For many children with ASD, this is simply not true. You would do well to approach each case with the assumptions that the learner may have unique sensory challenges, that conducting assessments to identify sensory challenges is worthwhile, and that accommodating these sensory challenges is likely to make learning happen at the highest rate possible.

Generalization and Maintenance

Angela Persicke

The primary objective of applied behavior analysis (ABA) treatment for children with autism spectrum disorder (ASD), whether teaching language, social, or other skills or reducing challenging behavior, is to ensure that the learner will demonstrate the improvements outside of the training setting in all of the real-life circumstances in which they are needed. For example, when teaching a child to mand (i.e., request), the desired outcome is for her to ask independently for what she wants across any setting, without needing to be prompted to do so. If the child only learned independent requesting when you were present and only in the classroom at lunchtime, this would represent a major deficit in manding across other aspects of her life and would clearly require further intervention. The application of a learned skill across all relevant aspects of a learner's life is referred to as **generalization**. Another critical outcome of skill acquisition is that the learner will continue using newly learned skills indefinitely. The persistence of a skill long after the teaching of that skill has ceased is referred to as **maintenance**. The skills that we teach our learners are only useful if they are applied in the real world, outside of the training environment, and they are maintained for the foreseeable future. Generalization and maintenance bridge the gap between the training experience and real-world outcomes.

Maintenance and generalization are absolutely critical to all treatment programs implemented within the Center for Autism and Related Disorders (CARD) Model. Indeed, there is virtually no point in beginning intervention if you are not planning to spend as much time and effort focusing on maintenance and generalization as you spend on initial treatment. Unfortunately, maintenance and generalization do not occur automatically. Particularly in children with ASD, it is probably reasonable for you to expect maintenance and generalization *not* to occur if you do not explicitly plan to promote it. Fortunately, decades of research in ABA provide effective procedures for doing so.

In the CARD Model, clinical supervisors develop a maintenance and generalization plan and monitor ongoing performance in order to ensure that their learners continue to display newly learned skills over time in the natural environment. This chapter provides a description of the evidence-based procedures we have found to be most useful in promoting generalization and maintenance.

GENERALIZATION

Generalization is the application of a learned skill across all relevant aspects of a learner's real everyday life. Two main categories of generalization are critical: 1) stimulus generalization and 2) response generalization. **Stimulus generalization** is when a response is trained in the presence of some stimuli and then it occurs in the presence of other stimuli which were not present during training. An example of this is if you use five different red objects to teach a learner to label red things as "red," and then she is able to label other red objects as "red," even though she was never taught to label those other objects as "red" in the past. **Response generalization** is when a particular response is trained and then a different response occurs in the future. This might happen, for instance, if you give a learner positive reinforcement for greeting others and you reinforce the particular behaviors of "hi," "hello," and "what's up?" and then, in the future, the learner says "hey" upon seeing someone, even though you never taught him to say "hey." In short, stimulus generalization involves the same behavior occurring in the presence of different stimuli, whereas response generalization involves a different behavior occurring in the presence of the same stimuli.

Generalization is imperative to the development of a robust repertoire of behavior and for success in real-life settings. Decades ago, generalization was treated as something that occurred naturally as a potential side effect of intervention, rather than something that was explicitly planned and supported. This perspective on generalization is problematic for many reasons, but the greatest concern is the central fact that generalization will *not* occur for many children with ASD unless it is explicitly planned. In their classic article, Stokes and Baer (Stokes & Baer, 1977) described common approaches used to program for generalization that have informed behavioral intervention practices in the decades that followed.

The following section describes how to implement a few of the procedures that we have found to be the most useful. Although each procedure is distinct and merits its own description, one basic principle underlies all of them: *If you want to get generalization, don't do exactly the same thing over and over.* We want newly learned skills to be flexible, applicable across all environments, and *not* rote, so *our teaching strategies must be flexible, occur across all environments, and not appear rote.*

Procedures for Promoting Generalization

Train across multiple settings. To promote generalization across all relevant settings in a learner's life, training must occur across as many different settings as possible. For example, rather than only teaching Johnny in his "therapy room," Johnny is taught expressive letter identification at a desk in his room, in other rooms in the house, outside the house, during rides in the car, and in any other setting that is feasible. Once Johnny reaches mastery criteria on particular letters, the team can then test for generalization in other untrained environments to determine if the skill has generalized across untrained settings. If the skill is not demonstrated accurately in untrained settings, then it must be trained across additional settings until it is performed accurately in *settings in which it was never trained.* In other words, you are not done with generalization training until the learner demonstrates generalization to untrained settings.

Train across multiple people. Promoting generalization across people is procedurally similar to promoting generalization across settings: Clinicians should teach each new skill across as many different people as possible. The best way to ensure that the learner will be able to apply the newly learned skill in the presence of other people who were never present during training is to include as many instructors, therapists, parents, nannies, and teachers as possible. For example, if the learner is being taught sharing and turn-taking skills, it is important to target these skills during training with siblings or peers, rather than only with adult therapists or parents. Similarly, if the target lesson is assertiveness, teach the skill across peers/siblings and adults, so the child learns not only to apply the skill across different people but also to discriminate when it is appropriate to be assertive with adults as compared to peers. Again, you are not done training for generalization across people until the skill has been accurately demonstrated with people who were not present during training.

Train across multiple materials. Perhaps you are detecting a pattern here: To promote generalization across different materials/objects/stimuli, you need to train the same skill across as many relevant materials/objects/ stimuli as possible. For example, Susie is learning the label "apple," and she is initially taught with a picture of a red apple on a white 2" × 2" laminated card. If this is the only item used to teach Susie to label an apple, it is possible that she will learn to respond to an irrelevant aspect of the card, such as the fact that it is a red circle on a white square, and not actually learn to label the critical features of apples as "apple." In order to ensure this does not occur, use multiple pictures of different types of apples and multiple examples of different kinds of real apples throughout training.

Training across multiple stimuli that are examples of a particular label (or other verbal operant) works because it results in the nonrelevant features changing frequently, therefore preventing those features from gaining stimulus control over the behavior. The only features that do not change are the ones that define the operant; they are always present, every time a new example is shown. In the apple example, the apple is always round, is always either green or red or a combination, almost always has a dip in the top, and may often have a short stem. Apart from extreme exceptions, these features define an apple, and these are the features of stimuli that we want to control the behavior of saying "apple." Irrelevant features are the size of the picture card, the background color, whether it is a two-dimensional picture or a three-dimensional object, whether the card is laminated, whether the card is new or old and tattered, etc. By using many different stimuli to teach "apple," you ensure that it is very unlikely that any of these irrelevant features will be consistently present when you are teaching, thereby ensuring that none of them will come to have stimulus control over the word *apple*. In nontechnical terms, you are making sure that the learner does not come to think that "apple" means the size of the picture card, the background color, the shape of the object, and so on.

Training across multiple exemplars of the same concept helps prevent stimulus overselectivity. **Stimulus overselectivity** is the tendency for some learners to focus too much on particular irrelevant features of a stimulus, rather than attending to a stimulus as a whole. For example, when learning to identify gender, as in labeling pictures either "boy" or "girl," a child with ASD might attend only to the color of the shoes, rather than attending to the highly complex combination of stimulus features that allow one to make the discrimination accurately. If only a few pictures are used to teach this skill, there might not be enough variation in the color of shoes between the pictures, such that the learner may therefore be able to attend only to color and respond "accurately" frequently enough to obtain intermittent reinforcement, thereby making it more difficult to learn the correct discrimination.

It is possible to predetermine all of the defining features of every single thing you are trying to teach and to create stimuli that systematically vary in every conceivable dimension, except for those features. This process is known as **general case analysis** or **general case instruction** (Cooper, Heron, & Heward, 2007). While this process is appealing, especially from a scientific standpoint, it is labor intensive. Fortunately, it is usually not necessary. Simply including many different examples of stimuli, referred to as **multiple exemplar training**, is usually sufficient.

Train loosely. In their seminal paper, Stokes & Baer (1977) identified "training loosely" as one procedure for promoting generalization.

Training loosely is one of the less well-defined and understood of the generalization procedures, but it can be useful. Basically, a therapist is training loosely when she does not do the same thing every time she teaches a particular skill. At first blush, this may sound counterproductive, especially if you understand the importance of consistency in ABA programs. However, it is based on the general principle that if you want a child to learn to behave flexibly and creatively (the essence of generalization), then you need to be flexible and creative when teaching. Finding the right proportion of consistency versus looseness is a tricky balance to strike and is going to be different for every learner and for each skill you are teaching. A good general rule of thumb is to begin teaching a new skill with a higher level of consistency and quickly start to fade in a looser approach as the learner begins to acquire the skill. This general pattern can occur across phases of teaching, within a single lesson, and it can also occur across years of intervention. When a young learner with significant global deficits first begins an ABA program, it is probably better to begin with more consistency and gradually fade in looser training as she progresses through her program.

For example, if the learner will have to use a recently learned skill in a classroom setting, procedures should be implemented to teach the behavior in a real classroom or mock classroom to promote generalization to classroom settings. The idea here is that training occurs in various environments, so the skill generalizes to all appropriate settings where the skill will be used. You can begin with a more controlled training environment and gradually transition to more natural environments, while including stimuli in the training environment from the beginning that are going to exist in the natural environment.

Generalization as Mastery Criteria

It is still common in many ABA programs to think that, once a learner has demonstrated mastery criteria on the stimuli with which he was directly trained, he has "mastered" the skill, and the skill can now be considered for generalization training or can be put on a maintenance schedule. However, the vast majority of skills that you teach learners with ASD require generalization as part of the skill itself. In other words, generalization is not something that occurs after acquisition or mastery; *generalization is mastery* of the skill. And the only way to know generalization has happened is to test the skill with untrained stimuli, in untrained environments, and with people who did not train it. For example, a learner should not be considered to have mastered the skill of labeling the letter *A* until he can do it with untrained examples of the letter *A* that are different fonts, different sizes, different colors, written on different surfaces, and present in different settings than those included in training. Similarly, he has not mastered the skill of washing his hands until he can do it independently in bathrooms in which he was never trained, with different sinks, different towels, different soap dispensers, and so on. Finally, a learner has not mastered the skill of inferring causes and effects until he can do so with new materials on which he was never directly trained.

It is very common for ABA practitioners merely to make sure to practice skills in multiple locations (which is great) but to forget that they must be tested in novel locations *without any prompting*, and the skills must be performed with high accuracy in those settings for the skills to be considered mastered. Another common mistake is for clinicians to think that their job is the initial acquisition part and that it is the job of others, perhaps the parents, to worry about generalization. This perspective is unrealistic and harmful. If you want the skills you are teaching to be meaningful and durable, then you should not consider them mastered until you have demonstrated that they have generalized across untrained exemplars, settings, and people.

Figure 7.1 displays hypothetical data on a multiple exemplar training procedure to teach the learner to tact balls. Figure 7.2 displays four sets of three exemplars that were used to train the skill and test for generalization to untrained exemplars. Note that, after the first set of exemplars were trained, the learner was tested on set 2 and did not perform accurately. Set 2 was then trained and, after acquisition, sets 3 and 4 were tested. At this point, the learner responded with 100% accuracy, thereby demonstrating generalization to untrained exemplars of balls. Note that this learner required two sets of three exemplars to be trained before she responded accurately to untrained stimuli.

Overgeneralization

It is not uncommon for children with ASD to display generalization of a learned behavior too frequently or in inappropriate situations. This is

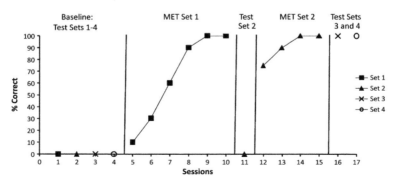

FIGURE 7.1   Sample graph of multiple exemplar training.

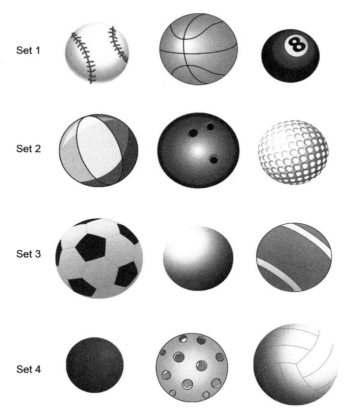

Set 1

Set 2

Set 3

Set 4

FIGURE 7.2 Sample sets of exemplars used for teaching a learner to tact (label) balls. Sets are trained one at a time, and new sets are tested for generalization after each previous set is acquired.

often referred to as **overgeneralization**. Overgeneralization may occur for various reasons. If behaviors are occurring in inappropriate situations, it is possible that irrelevant features of the generalization environment have become discriminative stimuli occasioning the behavior. In this case, the clinician should analyze the environmental variables that could be occasioning the behavior and continue training in the absence of the irrelevant variables. Here is a common example of overgeneralization:

> Susie has recently learned to expressively label genders of people in pictures, familiar people, and people in public (e.g., grocery stores). Today, while Susie and her mom were at the mall, a woman with very short hair walked by, and Susie turned to her mom and said, "Look, a boy!"

In the example above, Susie's gender-naming behavior overgeneralized, likely because it was controlled primarily by hair length, rather than a combination of the many stimulus factors characteristic of gender. Overgeneralization can occur frequently when children are learning categories, resulting in the learner erroneously assigning multiple items to a category based only on one specific feature. As stated above, it is important to include a variety of exemplars during the initial training phase to demonstrate the range of items that may be identified by a specific category, as well as nonexamples to facilitate discrimination of items that are not included in the category. If overgeneralization does occur, additional training using more novel examples and nonexamples may be necessary until the learner is able to identify novel examples of the category or concept correctly and therefore discriminate accurately between that category and others.

MAINTENANCE

As previously described, maintenance can be defined as a child's ability to continue to perform a skill or engage in a behavior with minimal errors over time after the intervention has been withdrawn (Cooper, Heron, & Heward, 2007). Maintenance is observed when, after a period of no practice, an opportunity to perform a previously learned skill arises, and the learner responds appropriately with little-to-no delay. Often, a learner masters a skill and then the clinical team focuses on new skills, with the unfortunate result of neglecting the mastered skills. When this happens, learners appear to "forget" skills or "regress," all but negating the effects of treatment, as well as disrupting the foundations upon which any new skills can be meaningfully taught. Because maintenance may not occur spontaneously, we have to include specific teaching procedures within treatment programs to ensure that the learner maintains the skills that we are teaching, especially if these skills are prerequisites for more complex skill sets.

Maintenance Procedures

Repeated practice in the same training conditions. A basic law of human learning is that repeated practice (with reinforcement) promotes both acquisition and maintenance. For example, all other things being equal, someone who practices basketball free throws 1 day per week is not going to be as good at free throws as someone who practices every day. As an extreme example, Olympic athletes and master musicians practice their critical skills for many hours every day. Maintenance of a skill for a child with ASD may actually be fairly comparable to mastery of a sport by an Olympic athlete: Both require tremendous practice and dedication. Consider the following example:

Eric has been learning receptive labels (e.g., pointing to items the therapist names) in his in-home treatment program. Eric recently met mastery criteria for the receptive targets "car" and "shirt" during daily therapy sessions. In order to ensure that he maintains these receptive labels, continued practice with car and shirt is needed. The therapist will continue to present these items by mixing them in with future items that the child is learning, thereby providing practice for maintenance while simultaneously teaching new material.

The fact that you should include repeated practice of learned skills does not mean you need to do exactly the same thing over and over. Repeated practice does not require you or the learner to be repetitive, rigid, or rote. It simply means that many practice opportunities need to be built into the learner's day. For example, if a child learns a new conversational exchange, she should be provided with at least five or ten opportunities across the day to use it in the context of different settings and different conversational partners. It is common for treatment providers to remember to provide only one or two such opportunities, perhaps when they naturally arise during recess, but this will not likely provide sufficient practice opportunities.

Repeated practice in new/advanced training conditions. It is important to extend repeated practice to various training conditions that were not included in initial training. This may include training conditions with more distractions or with various training materials not included in the original training conditions. For example, in the previous scenario, Eric learned the receptive labels for car and shirt in a structured therapy session. To promote maintenance of this skill, the therapist conducts practice trials of the receptive labels during unstructured play sessions with the same objects used in the original training condition. For example, during an unstructured play break, the therapist and learner are playing with various toys, and the therapist says, "Can you hand me that car?" while the car, a ball, and a shirt are present. The learner hands the car to the therapist, and the therapist provides specific praise, saying, "Thanks! This is a car! Let's race our cars!"

Natural practice in daily environments. Practice should also be provided in naturally occurring daily settings in which the skill will be needed. For example, when teaching colors, if Henry and the therapist are playing with toy cars, the therapist may put them out of reach and require Henry to name the color of the car he wants before the therapist hands it to him. As we described in the generalization section earlier in this chapter, practice trials of new skills across multiple natural settings has the added benefit of promoting generalization.

Intermittent reinforcement schedules. When mastered skills are placed on a maintenance schedule, it is crucial initially to continue providing reinforcement whenever the skill is performed correctly (continuous reinforcement). However, mastered skills should not continue to be reinforced every time they occur, forever. An important strategy for supporting maintenance is using intermittent schedules of reinforcement. An **intermittent schedule of reinforcement** is when the behavior is not reinforced after every single occurrence but is reinforced intermittently. The ultimate goal is for these skills to come under natural contingencies of reinforcement, and natural contingencies are usually intermittent. For example, when first teaching a learner to ask for a preferred toy (i.e., mand for it), you should give her the toy every time (i.e., continuous reinforcement). But in the real world, children do not always get what they want. They might need to share a toy or wait for it. To place manding on an effective maintenance schedule, the schedule of reinforcement should gradually be made more intermittent. This can be done by requiring the learner to wait for gradually longer periods of time after manding (from 1 second to up to 5 minutes) and by gradually increasing the frequency with which you say something like, "Sorry, it's not available right now, but you can have it later."

The frequency with which skills are practiced during maintenance must be determined by the clinical supervisor, as well as by the specified schedule of reinforcement for each maintenance skill. This information should be made clear for each lesson and target in the maintenance logbook described below. The particular intermittent schedule of reinforcement that you should use varies for each individual skill and for each individual learner, but the overall idea is to transition gradually from reinforcing every correct response to a schedule of reinforcement that mimics the natural environment. The general rule is that schedules of reinforcement should be thinned very gradually. If the skill begins to weaken, it is possible that you have thinned too rapidly.

Tracking Maintenance

Simply knowing that it is important for your team to conduct maintenance procedures is virtually never enough for maintenance procedures to be integrated into treatment. As with everything else in ABA, successful maintenance depends on accountability. It is critical for the supervisor to do something organizationally that will result in the therapists' conducting maintenance procedures frequently, so the team can be accountable for the effectiveness of the procedures. Keeping a logbook is one of the simplest and most reliable ways to keep track of whether staff have conducted maintenance procedures and whether the learner is maintaining learned skills. The maintenance logbook should include all programs that are placed on maintenance with instructions for the clinical team on how frequently the programs in the maintenance log should be targeted and how it should be done. In addition to specifying how and when the procedures for promoting maintenance should be implemented, the logbook should specify when and how to conduct "maintenance checks." Maintenance checks are quick probes of previously mastered skills. For example, if Emily has mastered counting objects up to 20, a maintenance check of this skill may be performed once per week by asking Emily to count items ranging from 1 to 20 to ensure that the skill has been maintained. If she fails to perform this skill correctly on any of these maintenance checks, the skill can be probed again the next day to ensure that the data are giving an accurate picture of the status of the skill. If Emily continues to perform at a low level, her supervisor may reintroduce the counting program into her treatment plan as a current therapy target.

SUMMARY

Promoting generalization and maintenance is essential to successful treatment of individuals with ASD, especially because maintenance and generalization can be challenging for children in this population. In summary, maintenance can be programmed in a typical treatment program by:

- Repeated practice in the same training conditions,
- Repeated practice in new/advanced training conditions,
- Natural practice in daily environments,
- Intermittent reinforcement schedules, and
- Documenting maintenance (in a maintenance logbook or similar arrangement).

Generalization can be incorporated into the learner's typical treatment lessons by teaching and testing across multiple:

- Settings,
- People, and
- Stimuli.

Generalization and maintenance do not occur naturally for many children with ASD, but using these well-established methods is sure to make the process more successful.

Treatment Settings

Mary Ann Cassell

The Center for Autism and Related Disorders (CARD) Model of autism treatment has expanded over the years from providing services in learners' homes to include school-based services, center-based services, and licensed private day schools. Top-quality autism treatment, in general, and early intensive behavioral intervention (EIBI), in particular, can be implemented across all of these settings, and each has its own advantages and disadvantages. Many factors influence how families select the most appropriate treatment setting for each individual child. Some of these factors include requirements or restrictions based upon the funding source for the treatment, the family dynamics, and the age of the child. For example, certain funding sources, such as regional centers in the state of California or Medicaid services in the state of Virginia, may specifically state that all or the majority of the treatment hours must be in the child's home. Many early intervention programs (birth to age 3 years) require that services be in the child's home with at least one parent present during treatment. Beyond the requirements of the funding source, the age of the child may also influence the appropriate setting. Once the child reaches school age, compulsory school attendance becomes a factor. For a child of school age, an applied behavior analysis (ABA) program that enables the learner to access education may be the best option for continuing to provide intensive services. In families where all parents/caregivers need to work outside of the home, center-based services may be the best option.

THE HOME SETTING

The home setting was the original setting for EIBI treatment for children with autism spectrum disorder (ASD), and it continues to be the setting most documented by research, as well as the most commonly used setting. (For a recent review of research on home-based behavioral intervention for children with ASD, see Tarbox, Persicke, & Kenzer, 2013.) In home-based EIBI programs, the vast majority of the learner's treatment occurs in her home or immediate community. In almost all cases, a parent or caregiver needs to be present in the home during these sessions. The therapist reports to the child's home on a scheduled basis to conduct treatment. Most clinics (i.e., team clinical meetings; see Chapter 19 on clinical supervision) occur at the CARD office location; however, they can also be conducted in the home when necessary. Supervisors provide parent training hours, direct observation of the therapists conducting treatment, and further clinical supervision at the child's home in between team meetings.

Designing the Therapy Environment

The "therapy room." The particular location inside the family's house that is used for teaching will vary depending upon the nature of the treatment program, the layout of the home, and the family make-up and needs. Typically, the majority of therapy takes place in a designated space in the house. This space is often in the child's bedroom but may also be a playroom. If there are other children in the home, a bedroom may be preferable to minimize distractions, except during those times when sibling interaction is integrated into treatment, particularly when practicing language, social, and play skills. For learners who are in the early stages of their treatment program, distractions may need to be eliminated from the therapy environment to the greatest degree possible. This may require the removal of extraneous toys, visual distractions such as artwork, and highly reinforcing items to which the child previously had or currently has free access. As learners progress through treatment, distractors should be added back into the environment to approximate the distractions in a typical learning environment, such as a classroom or other less controlled setting, more closely.

Materials and furniture. Standard items that are almost always needed include a child-sized table and chairs for both the learner and the therapist. Other necessary furniture items include storage for therapy materials, log books, and appropriate toys and activities that will be targeted as play items, as well as reinforcer items. A locked closet or storage cabinet is beneficial, so materials remain together and in appropriate condition between therapy sessions. Additional organizational strategies for both materials and reinforcers include some type of file system, so materials are organized and easily accessible. An example of this type of system would be an expandable file in which each section corresponds to a lesson in the child's program and items can be separated into mastered, current, and to-be-taught targets.

Perhaps the single most important set of materials are the reinforcers to be used with the learner. These, too, will need to be organized for ease of use. The number and types of reinforcers obviously vary from one child to the next and from day to day. (See Chapter 4 on reinforcers.) Therapists should ensure that there are enough items to prevent satiation from occurring. (See Chapter 4 on motivating operations.) The number of reinforcers, therefore, is dependent on how quickly the child exhibits satiation of each. A general rule of thumb for children receiving 30–40 hours of treatment per week is to identify a minimum of 30 reinforcing items through the use of preference assessments (Chapter 4), and categorize them by their level of reinforcing effect. Generally speaking, in a 2-hour session, you need to be able to offer at least 10 reinforcers that were not used in the previous session. These reinforcers need to be kept secured and separate from the toys that are accessible to the child outside of therapy to prevent learners from accessing reinforcers outside of therapy time.

In addition to reinforcers, items that are going to be used to teach play skills also need to be organized and readily available. If possible, these items can be left out to promote generalization during nontherapy times, as long as they are not likely to become lost or broken. It is also important to have items in the room that the child can access during breaks and downtime activities. These items should be mastered items or items that will hold the child's interest for several minutes at a time. Finally, the sensory needs of the child should be incorporated into the therapy room. These may include proprioceptive items, such as a mini-trampoline or swing, visual items that light up, or auditory items such as musical toys.

Other rooms in the house. It is critical for learners to spend at least some amount of time working in other areas of the house for several reasons. First, this is absolutely crucial for generalization (see Chapter 7). Second, many skills that the child needs to learn are normally executed in other rooms and might be inappropriate to practice solely in the "therapy room" (e.g., dressing, brushing teeth, snack preparation, etc.). Third, it is very important that the child learns to function with distractions, and limiting therapy to the highly controlled environment of the therapy room inhibits this. Other factors that influence where therapy takes place include the family dynamic, the individual child's progress and targets for generalization, parent involvement, and so on. It is generally advisable that all learners begin to respond and generalize skills outside of the therapy room as soon as possible, certainly within the first month of treatment.

Skills that are normally executed in other parts of the house represent ideal opportunities to move therapy outside of the therapy room. In addition to working on the particular lesson that you are intentionally targeting in a particular room, use the opportunity to work on generalization of other targets, too. For example, during feeding intervention in the kitchen, work on generalization of receptive object labeling, mands for objects, gaining attention, requesting cessation, and conversational skills. Gross motor skills are another area where conducting therapy in other locations is a natural choice. To teach outdoor skills, such as climbing or throwing, move to the backyard or a playground.

Home-Based Therapy Team

The structure of the home-based team is also an important piece of the overall program. The therapy team consists of the 1:1 therapists and senior therapists who work with the child, the supervisor of the child's program, and, in some cases, a case manager for the child's team. (See Chapter 21 for job descriptions.) The number of staff members depends on many factors. These include the number of therapy hours per week the child is receiving, the requirements of the funding source, family preferences and constraints, and scheduling factors that affect all of the providers.

The first consideration is the number of therapy hours that the child is receiving each week. The more hours of therapy per week that a child receives, the larger the number of staff required to treat the child. In all cases, there is typically one supervisor and possibly a case manager or co-supervisor per child. Most often, the largest source of variation is the number of therapists. When possible, it is advisable to place a senior therapist on the treatment team, and generally speaking, there should always be a minimum of two therapists on a learner's therapy team (Table 8.1). This ratio allows for generalization of skills across people and provides built-in checks and balances for therapy staff regarding treatment validity and integrity. In addition, conducting therapy for more than 10 hours per week with the same child can be very challenging for the therapist (as well as the child) and increases the potential for burnout for both. Even if you have a therapist who is willing and able to work with the same learner for 30–40 hours per week, and even if the logistical realities (e.g., scheduling, location, etc.) favor it, be aware that it is not the best choice for the child's learning.

On the other hand, scheduling too many therapists on one learner's therapy team can have a negative impact, as well. As a general rule, each

TABLE 8.1   General guidelines for how many therapists may be assigned to a home-based therapy team, depending on the weekly number of treatment hours the learner is receiving

Number of Therapy Hours per Week	Number of Therapists on the Team
10	2
20	2–3
30	3–5
40	3–6

therapist should work with the learner for no less than 4 hours per week. Anything less than 4 hours is likely to contribute to procedural inconsistency. Keep in mind that the more therapists there are on a team, the more potential there is for logistical and scheduling challenges (e.g., being out sick, car trouble, traffic, etc.) and the more staff that will have to be trained anytime a program change is made.

SCHOOL-BASED SERVICES

School-based services are those services where all or a significant portion of therapy hours take place in a public or private school setting that is not operated by the ABA provider. (See licensed ABA-based schools below.) There are at least two different types of ABA-based treatment that a learner can receive in the school setting: 1) school shadowing to help facilitate success in mainstream classrooms and 2) brief or full-day pull-out direct treatment services. The type and combination of services depend upon the individual child's needs, as well as the decisions of her Individualized Education Program (IEP) team.

School Shadowing

School shadowing involves a trained therapist accompanying the learner in a regular education classroom. The main goal of school shadowing is to encourage generalization of the skills that have been learned in the home or other 1:1 setting to the mainstream classroom setting. Typically, the child follows the general classroom routine, and the regular education teacher is considered the primary instructor. The role of the therapist is to provide support to the child through the use of prompting and reinforcement, so the child can successfully engage in the classroom activities in a way that is similar to his peers. That is, the primary goal of the therapist is to help the learner be successful in the classroom, not to conduct direct teaching as the therapist does in 1:1 intervention. That being said, the therapist occasionally also teaches specific skill targets, as needed.

Several factors that affect the success of the school shadowing process are worth considering. First, the number of therapists who shadow the child should be considered. In almost all cases, the ABA therapist who shadows a child will be serving as an aide in the classroom. As there are already multiple personnel (e.g., teachers, specialists, aides, etc.) who come in and out of the classroom, most schools prefer as few therapists as possible, often no more than two.

Unknown shadow. Learners who are progressing particularly well and are near the point where they no longer need any assistance to succeed in regular education classrooms may benefit from an unknown shadow. Unknown shadows are therapists whose job it is to shadow the learner in the classroom but in a manner such that the learner does not know the reason that the shadow is there. Teachers typically introduce an unknown shadow to the classroom as a "student teacher" or "classroom volunteer" or some other role. Obviously, for shadows to remain unknown, they must conduct very little or no direct intervention with the learner. Instead, they interact with many different students each day and surreptitiously collect data on the learner's success in the classroom. Essentially, as far as the learner or other students can tell, the unknown shadow is simply an aide who is especially thoughtful and attentive to everyone in the class.

In the CARD Model, the general progression of school services begins with a known one-to-one shadow who provides as much support as needed to ensure the learner's success in the classroom. As the learner becomes successful and gains more and more of the skills needed to function independently in the classroom, the goal is to fade out the shadow's support, eventually culminating in the use of an unknown shadow and, finally, no shadow at all. Of course, every learner is different, and some children with ASD will require continued support throughout their educational career to be successful in mainstream classes.

Team Meetings

Another common difference between school and home-based programs is how team meetings are conducted. If the school shadowing is being provided as one part of a larger home-based program, then the school shadow may merely attend clinics. (See section on clinics in Chapter 19.) Extra effort, however, needs to be made to include the input of the regular education teacher and other professionals at the school to ensure consistency. If the shadows for the child are unknown to the child, then those therapists obviously cannot attend clinics. If school-based services constitute a substantial portion of the learner's program, it may be more practical, or even a requirement of the funding agency, for the team meetings to occur at school.

Advantages of School-Based Services

Generalization. Generalization of skills is paramount in the successful treatment of ASD, particularly generalization to the school environment where the learner likely spends a great deal of her time. Teaching in the school setting is likely to promote generalization to that setting. The school environment provides ample opportunities to work on generalization of skills to different people, instructions, and settings since schools are such large and diverse environments.

Access to peers. In addition to the increased opportunities for generalization, consistent access to peers in a school setting offers ongoing opportunities to teach language, social, and play skills. Working in the school environment ensures access to many similar-age peers and provides opportunities for the therapist to help the learner to foster friendships with those peers and, when necessary, teach peers to be empathetic toward classmates with disabilities.

Access to general curriculum. Therapists who work in the school environment have direct exposure to the curriculum that the child is expected to know and have firsthand knowledge of the deficits and challenging behaviors that must be addressed in order to cultivate appropriate school behavior. Contriving situations to teach these behaviors in the home setting can be artificial and may create difficulties with generalization. Being in the school environment allows for natural environment teaching of skills and for those skills to come into contact with the natural contingencies of the school environment.

Parent presence. One of the major disadvantages of home-based programs is the requirement that a parent or guardian be present during 100% of the child's treatment time. This requirement may prevent both parents from working in an already economically stressed household, or it may result in insufficient treatment hours when other commitments limit parental availability. When services are provided in the school environment, it frees all potential income-earners in the household to work and ensures that the learner receives sufficient treatment hours.

Disadvantages of School-Based Services

While there are many advantages of providing services in the school environment, there are also challenges that require extra planning.

Distractions. The gradual transition to school settings represents one of the final phases of the CARD Model, which typically begins treatment in carefully controlled environments, such as the home or quiet center-based settings, and gradually fades to less controlled environments, such as mainstream classrooms. The school environment, whether classroom, playground, gym, or cafeteria, is full of distractions. Very rarely do learners have individual classrooms in the school environment; instead, shared spaces are the norm. Consequently, there are always distractions from other people, more complex environments, and all manner of unplanned sights and sounds. Therefore, the clinical supervisor should carefully assess these distractions and the child's readiness to learn in their presence. Accordingly, the learner's rate of acquisition in the school setting should be monitored to ensure that progress is occurring at an acceptable rate. Similarly, any major change in school placement should be accompanied by a careful analysis of its effects on the child's learning.

Competing activities. School days are full of preprogrammed times for academics, lunch, recess, and assemblies that can decrease the actual amount of therapy time. While some of these activities may be appropriate for the learner and may be excellent learning opportunities, many may not. Different members of the IEP team will likely have differing opinions regarding the most ideal times to conduct 1:1 therapy during the school hours, as well as which other activities may have higher priority. Often, it will take careful planning to develop a compromise to maximize exposure to the curriculum, teaching times with staff, supplemental services such as speech-language therapy, and therapeutic time that may include social goals.

Treatment integrity. Another factor to consider is the large number of people who will likely be involved with the learner in the school setting. Whenever the number of staff working with a child increases, consistency inevitably decreases. Environmental constraints may also affect the implementation of some behavioral techniques. For example, an extinction protocol may be impossible in a regular education classroom if the resulting extinction burst disrupts the other students' learning. There may also be inconsistency in procedural details, such as prompting. Careful use of data recording by all team members, as well as very clear protocol descriptions, can help maximize consistency across staff.

Staff breaks. Labor laws regarding lunch and other breaks vary greatly from state to state, so you should familiarize yourself with applicable laws in your area. The opportunity for breaks for therapists providing school-based services becomes a challenge because, in many cases, some of the most critical times for shadowing are during traditional teacher break times, such as lunch and recess. Lunch and recess are not only prime opportunities to teach social interactions and often the only times to teach social skills, but they are also unstructured times with fewer staff present. These times can be difficult for children with ASD to be successful independently. In many states, employees who work 6 hours in a day need to have a 30-minute nonpaid and nonduty lunch break. Other breaks may also be required. There are several different options for how these breaks can be given. In some cases, it may be possible to schedule a break during a time when the classroom teacher or another aide can work with the child in a group setting. There may also be times during the school day when the team agrees that school shadowing services are not needed, perhaps during library or computer periods.

Scheduling. Staff scheduling can also be a challenge in any school-based program. As discussed earlier, schools will inevitably have strong preferences regarding their scheduling needs. In addition, occasional staff absences are an unavoidable reality. If an outside ABA provider is sending the therapist shadow to work with the learner in the classroom, it is often the provider's responsibility to arrange substitutes for therapist absences.

In extreme situations, if substitute support cannot be found, then the child may not be able to go to school or will go to school with no support, which can lead to increases in maladaptive behavior. Having a specific plan, such as spare fill-in therapists, can help prevent such issues.

Confidentiality. Anytime services are provided outside of the child's home, maintaining confidentiality is a chief concern. When providing school-based services, the sheer number of people in the school provides the reason to make extra efforts to protect patient confidentiality. Obviously, several people, including the classroom and special education teachers, service providers, and administrators, will know specific protected information about the child. However, multitudes of others in the school environment, including other teachers, parents or other volunteers, and peers, do not have a right to the learner's protected information. Several procedures to protect the child's confidentiality should be put in place. First, all data and notes should be protected. In many cases, this means that the child's name should not be written on the datasheet. The names of other peers should not be listed, either. Instead, the use of initials is recommended. Materials should also not depict company logos, letterhead, or other information that might reveal the learner's diagnosis. In general, data should be maintained in a covered binder or folder that is kept in the possession of needed staff.

In addition to protecting data, staff members need to protect confidentiality when interacting with others. Staff members should receive training on how to answer questions related to their position and the child who is receiving treatment. In some situations, it may be necessary to prepare an explanation for staff, such as a student teacher or college intern, to provide to peers in the classroom. If peers ask questions about the child, age-appropriate answers should be prepared beforehand to ensure that confidentiality is maintained.

CENTER-BASED SERVICES

Center-based services refer to behavioral intervention implemented in a clinic-based or "day treatment" format. In this setting, the learner travels to the center to receive therapy for the recommended number of hours per week. These services are typically 1:1 in format or primarily 1:1 with some limited small group instruction. Center-based services differ from school-based services in that the setting generally does not fulfill the child's education requirement. The focus of instruction is generally more on developmental progression of skills rather than exposure to the general education curriculum. This setting also differs from a licensed special education school that uses special education methodology. Center-based services typically are not licensed by the department of education but, rather, are therapy centers where children receive treatment.

Physical Layout

Center-based facilities generally contain one or several "classrooms" where services take place. The option for classroom design ranges from 1:1 spaces to rooms where six or more children can receive 1:1 treatment simultaneously. The amount of space required varies depending upon a number of factors and regulations. Some states and certain funding sources may have specific guidelines for space requirements per student or per adult. For example, in Virginia, regulations require 50 square feet of space for each child. In all cases, occupancy loads need to be observed for the space.

The specific configuration of the learning space depends a great deal on personal preference. In general, larger rooms are divided into individual work areas using partitions or furniture. Cubicle-style office dividers can be fastened to walls to increase stability. If a more flexible design is needed, then portable bulletin boards and dividers can also be useful. The individual learner work spaces need to be large enough to accommodate a table and chairs for the student and therapist, as well as the container of work materials and reinforcers. In general, these spaces can be fairly small, and smaller sizes may help to eliminate distractions that may interfere with learning. When planning the number of individual learner spaces in a room, consider the amount of noise that may potentially be generated when all of the learners and therapists are in the room simultaneously. The more learners and therapists you assign to the same room, the louder the noise level will be when instructions and reinforcement are provided or when learners engage in challenging behavior. In addition to the individual work spaces for each learner, an open area to bring children together for group activities or a break/play area is recommended.

Another option for a center-based program is the utilization of more typical office-sized rooms that are approximately 10′ × 10′ and serve as individual work spaces for learners. This configuration should still include a larger room for groups of learners to come together for lunch and snack time, to work on social and play skills, and so on.

Grouping learners. Several factors need to be considered when choosing which learners to place together in particular rooms. If a learner is highly distractible or engages in high levels of tantrum and other challenging behavior, an individual space may be the best option. If that setting is not feasible, then it is important to consider many variables when grouping that learner with other children in a larger setting. For example, some learners may imitate the inappropriate behavior of others. Therefore, it may be more appropriate to use more environmental barriers or to group the more challenging child with learners who are more likely to ignore or carry on despite the tantrum behavior.

Grouping students whose treatment programs contain lessons at approximately the same level provides the most opportunities to work on similar skills in small groups with the least amount of modifications. This grouping also gives the treatment team the advantage of being able to use and share many of the same materials. However, it may not be an advantage to place many learners with maladaptive behavior in the same room. Some learners may be sensitive to noise and may begin to engage in problem behavior themselves when others do. This behavior can create a chain reaction where it is more difficult to redirect problem behavior.

Age is also a consideration when grouping children. As children will spend the majority of their day in their classrooms, it is usually better to group them with similarly aged peers. In some cases, large differences in physical size among differently aged peers can be problematic and increase the risk of injuries during normal play.

Materials

Materials management for center-based programs is similar to that of home and school-based programs. Each learner needs individual materials that are kept close to work areas and easily accessible by staff. The use of three-drawer carts often works well to organize materials and also to ensure that frequently used items, such as crayons, scissors, pens, and pencils, are easy to access. In addition to these types of materials, many learners also have flashcards and other materials for specific lessons. The use of accordion-style file systems allows these materials to be organized efficiently. Items are conveniently separated into mastered, current, and to-be-introduced materials. Well-organized systems such as these minimize downtime.

Scheduling

If children are only going to be at the center for a short period of time, such as a 2- or 3-hour shift, then these sessions will run similarly to home-based sessions with the exception of drop-offs and pick-ups, which are addressed later in this chapter. For learners who are staying for a full day of 6–8 hours, other considerations need to be made, including the scheduling of breaks for both learners and staff, the ratios of 1:1 therapy times to group play, and the provision of meals and snacks throughout the day.

If learners are attending the center-based program for the entire day, then breaks are necessary for both students and staff. The length and frequency of breaks for staff are similar to that of school-based programs and vary from state to state. In general, restroom and lunch breaks need to be planned. Typically, lunch breaks for staff can be scheduled during the children's lunchtimes. If relief staff cannot be brought in, then therapists can often work with two learners, giving another therapist the opportunity to take a break. Restroom breaks can often be managed as the need for them arises.

Of course, learners need to have breaks for meals and snacks and to use the restroom. Since we are working with children who may be in various stages of toilet training, bathroom breaks often need to occur on an as-needed basis. Scheduled restroom breaks should be provided 2–3 times per day. These may be at the arrival time, before the learners' lunch break, and then during the last 30–45 minutes of the day.

If the child is at the center for 6 hours, then a snack and lunch need to be incorporated into the child's day. If the child is at the center for 8 hours per day, then a lunch and two snack times are appropriate. These times need to be structured times for the learners and should be used as an opportunity to teach the child new skills and generalize language skills that are being taught in lessons.

Many states require meals or snacks that are served to children to be approved as nutritionally sound by a dietician. Additionally, many children with ASD may be on special diets at the request of their parents. The solution for both of these concerns is for the parents to provide all meals and snacks for their children. This arrangement only requires refrigeration and heating. All food should be well marked, and procedures should be put in place to ensure that children do not share food and are not able to access others' food. If a learner has a severe allergy to a specific food, it may be necessary to institute a center-wide policy, such as a no-nut policy, for either the specific classroom or for the entire center, depending on where food is kept and where it is eaten.

Finally, the ratio of 1:1 therapy to small group interaction must be considered. This greatly depends upon the functioning level of and goals for each individual learner. One of the advantages of the center-based setting is the access to other children to work on social and play skills. For children who are at the center for 6–8 hours per day, a reasonable amount of social interaction time may add up to 1 hour per day. This number will then increase depending upon the learner's skill development and other goals.

Communication with Parents

Good center-based programs take great pains to maintain excellent communication with learners' parents on a regular basis. While pick-up and drop-off times may provide some opportunity for interaction with parents, these tend to be chaotic periods and are not very conducive to effective communication. Daily communication sheets are, therefore, a good practice. Daily communication sheets include some representation of the learner's progress on lessons for the day, as well as information on challenging behavior that may have occurred throughout the day. Communication sheets also include narrative notes on the learner's successes throughout the day and any requests for the parents, such as the need for extra clothing or a reminder to avoid sending prohibited foods. Clinic meetings should be held for center-based learners just as they are for home-based learners. Given that parents observe less therapy when their child participates in a center-based model, clinic meetings are critical for communication and to help parents stay on the same page as the child's therapy team. Parents are also provided with access to their child's Skills® (see Chapter 26) account, so they can monitor their child's progress at any time via the Internet.

Dropping Off and Picking Up

There are several different options for dropping off learners at the beginning of the day and picking them up at the end. Some parents may feel more comfortable walking their children directly to their classrooms. However, if many children are being dropped off at the same time, this may cause a more chaotic environment. To help reduce chaos, a curbside drop-off and pick-up policy may be more feasible. With both scenarios, the most important consideration will always be the safety of the children during this time. The children should always be delivered directly to staff or to the parent. All parents/guardians should provide sufficient information to ensure that the clinicians know who is picking up the children each day, especially on those occasions when parents may make arrangements for others to pick up their child. If someone other than a parent has permission to pick up the child at the end of the day, always check that individual's picture identification to ensure the safety of the child. Any changes regarding parental permissions for picking up the learner should be given in writing.

Medication

Some learners, especially those who are at the center for most or all of the day, may require medication during the day. If this is the case, on-site staff need to be trained and certified to give medications. This requirement applies not only to prescription medication but also to nonprescription medication that is given for more than 10 consecutive days. Some learners may have life-threatening allergies that require allergy medication or an epinephrine autoinjector to be available; these medications often require additional training. Check with your state and local funding agencies for guidance on requirements.

Absences

Learner absences from treatment sessions due to illnesses, vacations, appointments, and other reasons will inevitably occur. For most center-based therapy sessions, if the learner is not present, then the session cannot be conducted and therefore should be rescheduled as soon as possible. Staff absences are another concern. One of the main reasons that parents select center-based programs is to be able to work while their child is at the center. Therefore, asking the learner to stay home if a therapist is going to be absent is not a reasonable option in many cases. Plans for coverage of absent therapists need to be made ahead of time. One solution is to have a fill-in therapist who is trained to provide services but does not have a caseload, so she is available to fill in for absent therapists. Many parents may feel hesitant about a fill-in therapist working with their child since that therapist has not necessarily been directly trained to work with their child. Certainly, consistency is an important concern in these situations. However, having novel therapists work with a learner is critical for generalization. During fill-in sessions, fill-in therapists can work on generalization and maintenance, making sure to probe all recently mastered skills. (See Chapter 7.) If done properly and not excessively, fill-in sessions like these will actually enhance learner outcomes, not hinder them.

Severe Behavior

Depending on the center's learners and on the challenging behavior they exhibit, specific accommodations may need to be made for managing severe behavior at the center. In particular, in order to prevent some learners from hurting themselves or others, a safe space may be needed for temporary use. The space may need to be free of windows or breakable objects, may need to have sharp corners of furniture and door jams padded, and may even require padding on walls or the floor, depending on the severity of behavior. Having a safe space for staff to manage severe behavior by no means necessitates a secluded timeout room or the use of punishment but, instead, requires an area where staff can keep everyone safe.

Advantages of Center-Based Services

Several advantages of center-based treatment should be considered. One major advantage is the control you have over the environment. Since all staff present are trained by and work for the center, a much greater degree of staff consistency is achievable in center-based programs relative to other settings. The challenges that arise in home-based therapy when multiple different family members are present during treatment sessions, and the challenges of working with many different professionals with a wide variety of training and competence, as is the case in school-based therapy, simply are not issues in center-based programs.

The fact that all therapists, supervisors, and learners are present in the same building at the same time presents a major advantage in terms of clinical supervision and problem solving. In home-based programs, if a clinical supervisor wants to observe four different therapists working with the learner in the normal therapy environment (rather than at a clinic meeting), she must make four separate trips to the learner's home. Hours of travel time may be required to accomplish this. In a center-based program, that same clinical supervisor can walk 20 feet down the hallway four times, for a total travel time of perhaps 3 minutes, and accomplish the same set of observations. This level of convenience in center-based programs naturally enables clinical supervisors to have more frequent contact with each learner's case, which can only be a good thing.

The substantially reduced need to travel when working in a center-based program can have a positive impact on staff as well. One of the chief complaints of therapists is the driving that is required for home-based programs. Particularly if a home-based program is located in an area with high traffic levels or when the distance to a learner's home requires a long commute regardless of traffic, therapists can spend much of their day in their cars. This can seriously impact the quality of life for therapists. Therefore, driving once to work in the morning and driving home at the end of the day can represent a significant advantage to therapists and will ultimately lead to higher morale and lower turnover.

Another advantage of center-based programs is that they automatically involve having other children present. Having other children present who are of similar ages and functioning levels provides more frequent opportunities for social interactions and social and play skills training. In a home-based program, parents may be hard pressed to schedule one playdate for their child per week. In a center-based program, social interaction sessions are scheduled every day. Since each peer will be staffed, specific prompting strategies that carry over day to day can also be implemented. These types of activities can also include mock school activities that can provide extra practice for children who are getting ready to transition to a school program.

Disadvantages of Center-Based Services

Perhaps the greatest disadvantage of conducting behavioral intervention in center-based settings is the automatic disconnection that inherently occurs with the learner's family. In a good program, this disconnection may be merely geographical and need not have a negative impact on the learner's treatment program. Center-based programs should maintain a high degree of parent involvement and parent contact. Many centers find it useful to conduct regularly scheduled sessions in the home in order to facilitate this. For example, the clinical supervisor can visit the learner's home once or twice per month to conduct parent training sessions, as well as to probe how well the learner's skills are generalizing to her home setting.

Center-based programs require a much larger degree of overhead to get started, and this may represent a significant disadvantage to some. Center-based programs require far higher rent for space compared to home-based programs and may require additional certifications and inspections from local regulatory bodies, depending on the region in which the center is located.

LICENSED PRIVATE SCHOOLS

Licensed private schools can also deliver autism treatment at a top level of quality. The advantages and disadvantages of doing so are similar to those of center-based programs. Therefore, for the sake of space, we only describe the differences below. The primary difference between a private school setting and a center-based setting is in the curriculum and the licensing, which then can result in differences in funding for the learners. As a note, not all private school settings have to be or are licensed by the department of education of the residence state. However, in almost all cases, if the school wants to receive state funding for educational purposes or through school systems as an IEP placement, then licensure is required. Once a licensed school or private school is operating, then not only are therapeutic services being provided as in a center-based program, but educational services are provided as well. As such, the licensed school must provide an educational curriculum that is aligned with state standards. Each individual state has its own requirements for the procedures and rules that private schools for children with disabilities must follow. These regulations can most often be found on the department of education website for each state.

Staff

Operating as a licensed private school also requires the inclusion of special education teachers in addition to therapists. The special education teachers must then be trained as behavioral therapists if they do not already have this training. A special education teacher who is also trained as a behavioral therapist can provide direct therapy to children, as well as supervision.

Related Services

Most learners in a school setting receive related services of some type, and these services need to be incorporated into the student's schedule. The most common related services are speech-language therapy, occupational therapy, and physical therapy. The number of hours for each service varies and is determined by each student's IEP. To maintain consistency, providers of related services should be well versed in the behavior management and teaching protocols being used with the student. Having the student's therapist accompany him to the related services helps achieve this. Related service personnel should also be included in all team meetings and IEP/Individual Program Plan (IPP) meetings for the student.

Scheduling

Efficiently scheduling staff can be a complicated task in the school environment. In CARD schools, we generally rotate staff between students on a 90-minute schedule. Each staff member, therefore, works with four different students throughout the day. Another system is to have each therapist in each classroom work with each student in that classroom every day. (Both of these options work well in center-based programs, too.) Therapist rotation serves several purposes. First, it promotes generalization across people, so students do not become dependent upon one particular staff member or way of presenting instruction. Second, staff report that they enjoy their job more when they have the opportunity to work with multiple students throughout the day. Therapists are more likely to maintain high levels of energy and enthusiasm when they work with the same student for approximately 90 minutes versus longer periods of time. Finally, rotating staff is particularly important when you have students who engage in high rates of challenging behavior, as this can be stressful and physically exhausting for staff.

One factor to consider in scheduling is that state guidelines often must be followed regarding the amount of instruction that needs to take place in the core areas of instruction of language arts, math, science, and social studies. Some states also have requirements for related curricula, such as physical education, music, and art instruction. In almost all states, there is a minimum requirement of 5½ hours of instruction per day.

Schedules should be created ahead of time for each classroom and learner. The ratio of 1:1 to group instruction will vary depending upon the needs of the students. The students' skill levels also affect the ratio of specific ABA therapeutic programming to the mandated academic curriculum. Creative programming can help with this issue, as many therapeutic tasks are the beginning levels of other curricula. For example, the language task of teaching past tense and recall can be seen as the beginning steps of learning history. Almost all of the students are at different levels academically, even if they are in the same grade. This difference means that most of the academics are also taught in a 1:1 environment for the students. Students can be grouped for some activities, such as art lessons, science experiments, or independent work times, when several students may have similar goals or where instruction can be scaffolded to meet the levels of different students. As the goal of any ABA program is to help the students to gain the skills necessary to return to a less restrictive setting, start students with higher levels of 1:1 time and then, as skills develop, increase the amount of small group work that takes place.

Other Regulations

In addition to requiring compliance with the IEP process, most states also have testing requirements. The type of testing depends upon what has been deemed appropriate for the child, as well as the plans for the child for graduation from high school. The assurance that testing is completed remains the responsibility of the school system, whereas the implementation of the testing resides with the private placement. Each private school has a designated testing coordinator who oversees the testing of its students.

For students who are privately placed in a special education school – typically by parents rather than the school entity – different documentation may be required, depending on the state. Most often, the school creates a plan to delineate progress on specific goals and objectives and reports these to the parents at specified intervals.

Advantages of the Licensed Private School Setting

Many of the advantages of the licensed private school setting, including controlling the setting, maintaining consistency, and accessing peers, are the same as those for center-based programs. However, a licensed private school environment has added advantages as well. Licensed private school programs can often serve a broader population of children than center-based programs. By far the greatest advantage of a licensed private school program is the treatment team's ample access to the learner. That is, the learner's extracurricular schedule never gets in the way of therapy because therapy is provided during school hours. Home-based and center-based programs require considerable scheduling gymnastics to provide medically necessary therapy hours, and often real gymnastics, piano lessons, or soccer practices and the like reduce the availability of the learner, whose compulsory school attendance limits his therapy to the hours between 3:00 p.m. and 7:00 p.m. The licensed private school option, then, allows for the continuation of 30–40 hours per week of ABA services for older children who still require the service.

Finally, licensed private schools also offer the advantage of having a continuum of services. While many of our learners will progress to the point that education services in less restrictive settings are beneficial, a proportion of students will continue to learn only with intensive 1:1 behavioral support. Having an intensive behavioral support setting that also meets the compulsory school attendance requirement is a great advantage to these students and their families.

Disadvantages of the Licensed Private School Setting

Among the greatest disadvantages of the licensed private school setting is the much larger number of regulations that are involved. The initial process of becoming licensed can be long and frustrating. However, in many states, once this process has been completed, it does not have to be repeated for each new site in the same state. Depending on the state, requirements of addressing particular curricula, which may or may not actually be clinically appropriate for individual learners, can also be burdensome. Added requirements in areas such as physical education, art, and music instruction may necessitate creativity to make them a high clinical priority for particular learners.

Depending on the state, additional regulations may impose guidelines regarding floor space and staffing ratios, and each facility needs someone trained to give medications or a school nurse. Finally, keep in mind that, since students are receiving public education that is free to them, the school may need to purchase additional materials, rather than asking the parents to do so.

SUMMARY

The decision to provide autism treatment services in a home, center, public school, private school, or some combination is a complicated one. Each setting has unique strengths and limitations. Parents and clinicians should take this decision seriously and weigh the pros and cons carefully and separately for each individual case. In many situations, a child will transition through more than one of these settings throughout the course of a comprehensive treatment program. Fortunately, research has shown that all of these settings can be successful in providing top-quality treatment, resulting in excellent learner outcomes.

Parent Involvement

Evelyn R. Gould, Vince Redmond

The inclusion of parents and other caregivers is widely accepted as a critical component of effective treatment programs for learners with autism spectrum disorder (ASD) (National Autism Center, 2009). Parents are essential to the process of curriculum development, as they are an ongoing source of information regarding the learner's skill deficits and behavioral challenges. In order to make appropriate initial clinical recommendations and begin formulating a treatment plan, clinicians rely on parents to develop a thorough clinical history and skill profile of the learner.

In addition, training parents to implement applied behavior analysis (ABA) interventions dramatically increases the number of learning opportunities that children with ASD can access throughout their day, helps ensure consistency of program implementation, and maximizes the likelihood that treatment gains will be maintained and generalized outside the therapy setting. In addition to enlisting the parents' support and participation in the treatment plan, training parents to understand ABA and to implement intervention procedures can positively impact the family as a whole by improving the quality of parent-child interactions, broadening family access to social and leisure activities, increasing feelings of parental competence, and decreasing parent stress. Parent involvement, therefore, plays an integral role in every treatment program at the Center for Autism and Related Disorders (CARD).

The overall goals of parent training are to teach parents strategies to address the skill deficits and challenging behaviors displayed by their children, to promote the generalization and maintenance of gains acquired through the course of therapy, and to increase the overall quality of life for the whole family. Optimally, parents acquire parenting strategies as their children begin to make gains in therapy, decreasing parent stress and expanding the family's access to social, educational, and community activities that begin to seem more manageable. Because the needs of every parent and learner are different, the individualized nature of autism treatment extends to parent training. To increase the likelihood of parents' maintaining the skills taught in parent training, clinicians must ensure that they prioritize parent training goals appropriately. In order for parents to feel comfortable with and adhere to treatment protocols, there must be a good "contextual fit." That is, targets and procedures must be responsive to the values and goals of parents and compatible with the family's typical routines and culture and must optimize the parents' experience, knowledge, and skill sets. Finally, the goal should be to create programs that maximize the extent to which parents can be successful without professional support after the training program has ended.

BUILDING A THERAPEUTIC RELATIONSHIP WITH PARENTS

Establishing Expectations

During the initial intake process, clinicians should ensure that parents are fully informed about ABA treatment and, specifically, what to expect as they move forward in the treatment process. At this initial stage, it is crucial to ensure that the family is able to make an informed decision regarding the appropriateness of evidence-based behavioral intervention services for their child. Because parent participation is so critical, clinical supervisors should communicate the importance of parent involvement in the treatment process as early as possible. At CARD, parents are asked to sign a contract stating their commitment to their child's program throughout treatment, which includes a willingness to participate in ongoing parent training. Initially, some parents may not understand or appreciate the essential role they play in determining their child's outcome. One way to emphasize the importance of parent involvement is to highlight the fact that we only work with the learner for a comparatively small portion of his waking hours and that optimizing the home as a learning environment is likely to increase the effectiveness of the program. It is essential to make parents feel empowered to change their child's life for the better.

In addition to ensuring parental participation, establishing realistic expectations is a critical part of the initial process of relationship building with parents. First and foremost, inform parents that they should expect their child to learn and make progress, regardless of the child's age or level of impairment, and that rates of progress are different for every child. To the greatest extent possible, clinicians should prepare parents for the hard work and challenges that lie ahead. Olympic athlete training is a useful analogy. While Olympic-level training requires dedication, hard work, and a great deal of time, it is the most reliable way to produce the best outcomes. In summary, parents should expect progress for their child and should expect to have to invest a great deal of effort in order to obtain it.

Of course, in addition to conveying the upcoming challenges, clinicians should underscore the benefits of the treatment program, so parents understand that they are giving their child the best possible chance to maximize her potential and improve the quality of her life and the lives of those who love her. It is also worth noting that the overall stress level for many children with ASD and many of their parents actually decreases after the first few months of intervention. Good treatment programs target basic communication skills (e.g., manding) from the very beginning, so, after a few months, many young children with ASD are able to express their basic wants and needs to their parents for the first time – an outcome that is a very real improvement in quality of life for both children and parents.

At the outset, it is important to establish realistic expectations and appropriate boundaries regarding the parent relationship with the therapy and supervision staff. Parents should expect clinicians to make their child's outcome a top priority, and they should expect constant, vigilant dedication to quality. While parents should consider clinicians an important resource, they need to recognize typical professional boundaries; e.g., it is not reasonable to contact supervisors on their personal mobile phones after normal work hours unless the child has an emergency. Establishing reasonable expectations from the beginning can prevent hurt feelings in the future, especially when emotions run high during stressful periods of the learner's treatment. A good model for the relationship between parents and clinicians is that which exists between parents and pediatricians. For everyday needs, parents are expected to make an appointment ahead of time (or wait until the next clinic), but clinicians should be accessible to parents in emergencies.

Establishing Effective and Empathetic Trainers

Clinicians are highly skilled at designing and implementing ABA techniques with learners, but that does not automatically guarantee that they will be good at training parents in how to use these techniques. Thus, it is important for clinicians to receive specific training on how to train others effectively, and they should thoroughly demonstrate competency with respect to delivering parent training prior to being assigned to a training role. Combining confident behavioral training skills with an empathetic instructional delivery style and well-developed rapport-building skills will contribute to better parent training outcomes. Clinicians benefit from specific training that targets rapport building (e.g., instruction in active listening, observing, and validating a parent's experience). All CARD supervisors receive training to cultivate those skills that facilitate a strong parent-clinician collaborative.

Building Collaborative Relationships with Parents

Collaborative relationships between parents and staff have been shown to predict the outcome of treatment services often better than any other variable (Martin, Garske, & Davis, 2000). Empathy and compassion on the part of the trainer are likely crucial for developing an effective therapeutic relationship and maximizing treatment outcomes. Developing collaborative and supportive relationships with parents is thus a key goal for supervisors in the CARD Model. However, this can be a challenge for clinicians who may not have children themselves or lack life experiences that might enable them to empathize with parents. Sometimes, supervisors do not understand what a parent is experiencing unless they have truly been in the parent's shoes; however, they can learn how to listen, make a parent feel heard, and bring empathy to their ongoing interactions.

Prior to designing and implementing a parent training program, clinicians should consult closely with caregivers in order to identify the family's specific needs and priorities, as well as the parents' willingness to participate in parent training and subsequently follow through by implementing what they learn. If parents are unwilling to participate or do not value their contribution, the clinician should spend time sensitively discussing the parents' role and the benefits of participation for them and their whole family, including their child. Sometimes, parents may require some demonstration or evidence of training benefits before they will be fully on board with the program. Rather than just talking about the benefits, the clinician may need to show the parents how particular techniques can positively influence their child's behavior.

Knowledge

It is important for clinicians to project competence to the parents they train. Parents need to know that they are in good hands and that the clinicians in charge of their training are experts. For this reason, it is important for clinicians to be well versed in relevant terms, procedures, research, and funding issues and even be able to talk about recent developments or popular trends among parents in the autism community in an intelligent, informed manner. In short, the clinicians must convey that they know what they are doing. That being said, clinicians also need to be careful to avoid using too much jargon or sounding overly technical. Clinicians who strike this balance and manage to convey extensive knowledge in professional but jargon-free language are likely to be more effective in their parent training efforts. See Chapter 24 for recommendations on translating ABA jargon into plain English.

Flexibility

Flexibility is among the most important qualities of clinicians who excel at training parents. As clinicians, we are taught about the benefits of many different treatment approaches, and each clinician has had success with various approaches in the past. At the same time, each child and family bring a unique history and set of family dynamics that must be accommodated. For this reason, when designing treatment plans, clinicians should be open to new perspectives. What works for one learner might not work for another learner. Every clinician's parent training efforts can be enhanced by an approach that avoids dichotomous thinking and embraces flexible thinking. Clinicians can easily become accustomed to doing things the same way repeatedly, but no particular procedure is going to work for every family. Many clinicians find it hard to be flexible because they perceive challenges to their ideas as challenges to themselves or to their authority or competence. A much more productive perspective is to think of holding procedures, not people, accountable for effectiveness. From that perspective, if a particular procedure doesn't work, it's time to find a new one, not blame the person whose idea it was. Flexible thinking opens clinicians to unique points of view, strategies, and interventions and ultimately results in the clinicians' learning new approaches that make them better trainers in the long term.

DESIGNING THE PARENT TRAINING PROGRAM

Format

Parent training can be effectively delivered in a number of different formats, including one-to-one, group, or self-directed. (For a recent review of research on parent training, see Najdowski & Gould, 2014.)

One-to-one versus group. At CARD, parent training is typically conducted on a one-to-one basis. One-to-one training allows a high degree of flexibility in terms of individualizing training to suit the family's particular needs. One-to-one training sessions are easier to fit around a family's schedule and enable training to be provided across different settings, which likely maximizes treatment outcomes and promotes the generalization of skills. Finally, one-to-one training allows for high levels of individualized feedback, which is helpful for facilitating learning. On the other hand, parent training has also been effectively delivered in a group format. Group training is more cost effective and offers parents an additional source of social support and opportunities to benefit from peer modeling and feedback. However, group training may decrease opportunities to provide parents with individualized feedback and recommendations.

Clearly, there are advantages and disadvantages associated with both one-to-one and group formats, and the most optimal model likely depends on the family, available resources, and targets of intervention. Another option is to provide group training combined with one-to-one. Initial topics of training can be conducted in a group, and then individual protocols can be designed for one-to-one sessions with each parent.

Self-directed. Parent training may also be delivered in a self-directed format. This modality of treatment, particularly through technology-based solutions, is gaining increasing attention due to its potential for providing cost-effective training that requires less time and effort to deliver. Self-directed programs have the potential to reach more families more quickly, particularly those in remote locations who have difficulty accessing services. Some research suggests that such programs may be effective in establishing new knowledge and skills. For example, a recent study showed that an eLearning program designed for therapists was effective in training parents in knowledge of the principles and procedures of ABA (Jang et al., 2012). For more information about this program, see the section about the Institute for Behavioral Training (IBT) in Chapter 26. However, self-directed or web-based training is likely not as effective as in-person training, so it should be considered a supplement, rather than a replacement, for in-person training, except in those cases where it is the only available method of training.

Setting

In the CARD Model, training is typically delivered both in the clinic setting during biweekly clinic meetings (see Chapter 19) and during the learner's regularly scheduled therapy hours in the home. Few studies have conclusively shown that one training setting is superior to another, thus the advantages and disadvantages of each should be considered. Conducting training sessions in the home might result in more rapid treatment gains and better generalization since the training environment more closely matches the "real world." Particular skills, such as toilet training, feeding, and other adaptive routines, may be better suited for home training. In addition, home-based training might improve attendance for families that do not own a car or otherwise have difficulty getting to the training location. There are, however, advantages to training within the clinic setting. Clinic settings allow a greater degree of control over the training environment, so fewer distractions arise during training. Additionally, generalization can be achieved from the clinic to the home setting, so the artificiality of the training setting may not be a significant factor. Still, if the majority of parent training occurs outside of the home setting, care should be taken to observe and directly assess whether generalization of parent skills occurs to the home setting.

Parents can also be trained in community settings. For example, it is often helpful to conduct parent training generalization sessions by having the supervisor accompany the parent and learner to the park, shopping mall, restaurant, hair salon, pediatrician's office, or dental office. Accompanying parents during difficult community outings can provide much-needed support, as well as the opportunity to generalize skills across additional settings and to ensure that parents are maintaining those skills. The particular community locations that you choose for your learner and parent depends, of course, on that family's unique needs, and we suggest that you be flexible and open to varying formats and settings as much as possible in order to encourage generalization and increase the likelihood of parent enthusiasm and participation.

Intensity and Duration

Effective parent training programs have varied significantly in intensity (number of hours devoted to parent training per week) and duration (length of the training program, whether that be a week or a year). Most likely, the optimal length or intensity of training depends on parent and child characteristics and the specific skills being taught. Clinicians should carefully assess how much time and energy caregivers are willing and able to devote to training. This can vary greatly, depending on whether parents work full time and have other children, family members, and/or activities outside of work that require attention. Generally speaking, parent training may be more intensive initially and will taper off over time. However, new issues will inevitably arise throughout the child's program; therefore, parent training should continue for the duration of the child's treatment program whenever possible. Often, even after the child has been discharged from treatment, it is useful for the clinician to maintain weekly phone calls or home visits for a few months in order to support the family in maintaining the gains they made during treatment.

Trainees

In some situations, it may be possible to train both parents, which promotes consistency and generalization across people. However, sometimes scheduling training sessions that include both parents can be difficult due to conflicting work schedules and/or because one parent is needed for other child or elder care responsibilities. In such cases, clinicians may need to train whichever parent has the most availability. Training other caregivers (e.g., grandparents or a nanny) with whom the learner spends a significant amount of time may also be necessary in order to promote consistency.

Prioritization of Treatment Targets

Safety first. When choosing training targets, the safety and well-being of the learner and family should be the top priorities. The clinician should assess whether particular child behaviors or parenting interactions pose a threat to the safety and well-being of the child or others. Common behaviors that may need to be prioritized are self-injurious behaviors, pica (ingesting nonedible material), and aggression toward others. Other priority behaviors are those that expose the learner to dangerous situations, such as elopement, climbing or jumping from high surfaces, or playing with hazardous objects (e.g., electrical devices and outlets, scissors, matches). Clinicians should also look for maladaptive parenting repertoires that are harmful or could potentially be harmful in the future (e.g., heavy reliance on punishment or aversive procedures, excessive use of physical restraint or physical prompting).

Choose functional targets. Next, the clinician should consider how useful or functional a particular parenting skill will be for the particular family. Clinicians should target only those skills that are likely to produce natural sources of reinforcement once treatment ends, since these are the skills that are most likely to be maintained and most likely to benefit the family in the long term. Clinicians should consider the number of opportunities parents will have to use the skills they acquire and the degree of impact those skills will have on the family's daily life and then prioritize those parenting skills that will produce immediate benefits for the family. For example, hoarding and repetitive lining up of toys are concerns because they prevent a child from using toys in a functional manner, but parents may not consider those treatment priorities. However, if this restrictive, repetitive behavior significantly disrupts the learner's ability to participate in daily activities and routines and causes a great deal of stress because the learner engages in high-pitched screaming whenever one of his siblings touches his toys, parents might view the behavior as a high priority for treatment. It is important that clinicians also consider the needs of siblings and other family members when prioritizing targets.

Choosing targets that promote the learner's integration into key educational, social, and community environments and increase his access to upcoming life events, such as a family holiday, a birthday party, or a visit to the dentist, might also be prioritized. For example, parent training might help the family cope with an upcoming vacation by working on transitioning appropriately to and from the car and training parents to increase their child's ability to wait and sit for long periods. In addition to improving the family's overall quality of life, increasing a learner's integration into new environments and targeting life events provides the learner with exposure to new learning opportunities.

Cost/benefit ratio. Clinicians should consider the amount of time involved and the likelihood of success in establishing new parent skills, particularly when trying to optimize the use of limited parent training time. Parents' individual experiences and skill sets vary tremendously, and clinicians should consider each caregiver's ability to acquire new skills when prioritizing training targets. In addition, the limited availability of caregivers or a lack of resources necessary for establishing and generalizing particular skills (e.g., access to community outings or playdates) may significantly impact the time it takes to master particular skills. If a particular skill will take a long time to establish, the teaching of other important skills could be hindered. Training parents to establish basic foundational skills in their child, such as making requests, following simple instructions, completing basic self-care skills (e.g., feeding, toileting, and dressing), and gaining the parents' attention appropriately, should be prioritized over other skills that, while important, are less functional (e.g., learning to tie shoelaces, making change, learning the alphabet).

Choose targets that set the parent up for success. Setting goals and choosing procedures that ensure that parents will quickly contact reinforcement and success are both especially important in the beginning in order to demonstrate the value of the treatment program to the parents and gain their trust. Many parents will learn new skills but can struggle to use them consistently and may give up quickly if improvements in their child's behavior are slow to emerge. It is also crucial to consider competing contingencies that offer more immediate and frequent reinforcement for parents and involve less response effort than treatment procedures. For example, it is likely much easier for a parent to allow a child to watch videos repetitively on the Internet while the parent completes household chores than to implement protocols designed to build the child's ability to play independently with toys or help with chores. In fact, a basic assumption in ABA is that, if someone continues to do something, then it works for them in some way. Unfortunately, it is virtually always easier (and more immediately rewarding) to do something other than maximize the learner's learning opportunities in the moment. In most cases, clinicians do not have control over these contingencies, and eliminating them is unlikely. However, being aware of them places the clinician in a position to design strategies that might compete with them.

First and foremost, setting goals that ensure that parents see results quickly and feel successful from the outset of training will likely increase compliance and facilitate perseverance in the face of greater challenges. Hence, initial targets for most parents will focus on more easily mastered, core skills (e.g., delivering reinforcement for desired child behavior that already occurs, at least to a small degree) that will bring them into contact with positive changes in their child quickly. Initially, the clinician might consider working on generalizing skills that the learner has already mastered in therapy. For parents who struggle to master new skills, clinicians should consider introducing fewer training targets at once. For example, the clinician might pick 1–3 skills for parents to target on a weekly basis to prevent the parents from feeling overwhelmed.

Choose targets that foster positive interactions. Skills that foster more positive interactions between the parent and child can also be prioritized, particularly for parents who are totally overwhelmed and experiencing a great deal of negative emotions during their interactions with their child. For example, the clinician might simply begin by having the parents pair themselves with reinforcement and allowing the parents to schedule "quality time" with the child every day, during which they engage in preferred activities and place no demands on the child. Clinicians might also start with simple play skills that foster positive interactions, such as having the parent practice taking turns with the child while the clinician prompts the child to respond to the parent, all in the context of an activity the child likes and which does not typically evoke challenging behavior.

Setting Parent Goals

Behavior change is closely linked to a person's goals and the specific steps he has to take in order to reach those goals. Parents are more likely to be successful when clinicians help them set goals that are specific (e.g., getting Sarah to follow specific instructions, rather than be "obedient"), proximal (e.g., getting Sarah to complete her homework daily, rather than getting her to "get good grades"), and focused on positive outcomes, as opposed to centered around avoiding negative ones (e.g., getting Sarah to ask for things she wants using her big girl voice, rather than getting her to stop whining).

Furthermore, goals are more likely reached when there is a specific action plan in place and when one can specify exactly what one will say and do in order to reach each goal. For example, parents are much more likely to be successful when they have an action plan that states a specific goal (e.g., "When Sarah screams, I will walk away and sit down on the couch and ignore her behavior until she stops screaming for 10 seconds. Ignoring means no eye contact and no reprimanding or interactions of any kind."), rather than a broad and nonspecific goal (e.g., "I will not lose my temper when Sarah screams."). Clinicians should ensure that they have clearly mapped out for parents how they will reach their goals and exactly what is expected of them at each step along the way, including the exact "who, what, where, when, and how" of each target skill. Keep in mind that a dramatic change all at once is unlikely, since most parent goals take time and perseverance to achieve. Ensuring that effective reinforcement and feedback systems are in place and identifying specific steps that the parent can take toward larger goals are both essential, particularly if there is likely to be a significant gap between parent behavior change and improvement in child behavior.

Considering Context

In order to develop an effective training package and foster the adoption of positive parenting practices, clinicians need to ensure a good "contextual fit" with respect to each individual family's needs and characteristics. Children and parents do not operate independently, as there is a reciprocal interaction between parent and child that occurs within a rich context that includes the individuals' histories, health or physiological variables, life events, physical characteristics of the environment (e.g., noise, heat, and clutter), other people, and so on. Parent training programs must thus be responsive to each family's values and goals, use parent knowledge, experience, and skills, and accommodate the family's typical routines and daily activities. Parents are unlikely to adhere to procedures if they are not comfortable with them, they do not fit with the family's lifestyle and routines, or they conflict with the family's culture.

Therefore, CARD clinicians carefully consider who the caregivers are, what their lives are like, what their needs are, what their child is like, and so on when designing parent training programs. While behavior change strategies must match the function of the target behavior, contextual variables determine whether a particular strategy is the best choice for a particular parent and child in that particular situation. By examining the context within which a parent is operating, clinicians gain a sense of the bigger picture, which might lead them to consider alternative strategies that they would not have considered if they were purely focused on the function of the learner's or parent's behavior. For example, while escape extinction might be likely to be effective for food refusal, this may not be the best strategy to give to a single parent who has three children to get through breakfast and off to school in the morning. Looking at the bigger picture might also result in simpler and less restrictive or intrusive interventions. For example, when targeting a learner's disruptive nighttime waking, you might identify that the child is eating dinner many hours before his bedtime, and simply ensuring that he eats something small and nutritious before bed might lead him to sleep more soundly, circumventing the need for a complicated behavior intervention plan.

Cultural, Educational, and Socioeconomic Variables

Clinicians should make themselves aware of cultural, educational, and socioeconomic variables that may influence the treatment program. For certain families, additional support strategies and/or accommodations may be needed to enable them to adopt positive behavior management practices in their home and community.

Culture. Cultural and ethnic differences may hinder the success of parenting interventions; thus, it is important to take a flexible, individualized approach when working with families of differing cultural backgrounds. Some potential barriers can be obvious, such as a difference in language between the family and the service provider. Other barriers can be more subtle, such as issues related to having a female or male trainer and particular home practices or family dynamics that might affect how parents view certain training protocols. Successful interactions with families depend on how well the clinician is able to acknowledge and accommodate cultural differences in training. Prior to developing a parent training program, clinicians should try to identify and be sensitive to potential cultural beliefs or parenting practices that might influence acceptance of and adherence to the treatment program.

Clinicians should make an effort to acquire knowledge about the family's culture and customs in order to ensure that the training program respects the family's perspectives. In addition to understanding the particular nuances associated with the family's culture, supervisors should ensure that families have access to a clinician or translator who speaks the same language fluently. Cultural differences are both valid and valuable, and as such, clinicians should make sure not to impose their own cultural values on the family with whom they are working. It is vital that clinicians acknowledge potential conflicts between their own cultural biases and those of the family and work to prevent such conflicts from becoming barriers to effective training. In certain contexts, if cultural or ethnic conflicts cannot be overcome, it is important to assign a different clinician to the family or refer the family to another provider who is better able to meet their needs.

Educational background. A parent's educational background should be considered during parent training. Training materials should be at an appropriate reading level, and training should be provided in a jargon-free, parent-friendly language that is easily understood. If the parents are particularly educated and prefer to learn the jargon of ABA, then you should adjust your training accordingly to avoid giving the impression that you are talking down to them or being condescending.

Socioeconomic status. Single parents, lower income parents, and parents of lower educational status may be more likely to struggle. Such families often have less time and more limited access to resources. They are also often more isolated and lacking in social support. In these cases, clinicians may need to focus first on addressing the family's broader needs before expecting the parents to participate fully in and benefit from parent training. This might include assisting caregivers in accessing additional sources of peer and social support, respite care, legal advice, Social Security benefits, and so on.

Nontraditional family unit. Trainers must acknowledge and work within alternatives to the traditional family unit. For example, in addition to an increased number of single-parent families, same-sex parents are now more common. Separated parents may have shared custody, or children might live with grandparents or other relatives or in foster care. It is also now the norm for both parents to work outside of the home. Clinicians should make sure that they are aware of the family structure and incorporate this into treatment procedures. For example, clinicians should carefully consider the amount of parent training that can be conducted with a single mother who works 8 a.m. to 7 p.m., Monday through Friday.

Values and parenting styles. The clinician should consider whether particular parent values might influence the delivery of parent training. For example, a parent who highly values promoting the child's self-esteem and autonomy will likely struggle to implement procedures perceived as punishing or restrictive. The clinician should be creative and flexible when explaining how the recommended procedures do, indeed, align with parent values. For example, some parents may view giving a child accurate corrective feedback when he responds incorrectly as overly negative and, therefore, bad for self-esteem. However, if the clinician explains that honest feedback is the fastest way to help the child learn the skill and that he will feel proud of himself when he learns it, then parents will understand that corrective feedback may actually be helpful for their child's self-esteem. In contrast, parents who highly value discipline and parental authority will likely struggle to comply with recommendations that they interpret as "being too soft" or letting the child "get away with it." For example, some parents perceive contrived rewards as bad for the learner's sense of responsibility because "he should just want to behave correctly; he shouldn't expect to get a reward for it." In order to explain how positive reinforcement can actually be in line with this value, the clinician could explain that positive reinforcement is a great way to put the responsibility back on the child because no one is forcing him to do anything; he can take the responsibility of doing the desired behavior if he wants to earn the reward, so it's up to him.

Parent Stress

Parents of children with ASD consistently experience high levels of stress. Because they are coping with constant life stressors associated with having a child with ASD, they may feel isolated, unsupported, frustrated, and as though they are living in constant crisis. Since parents who are stressed and feel unable to parent their child effectively may struggle to stay committed to their child's treatment program and adhere to treatment protocols, high levels of parental stress can negatively affect learner progress and strongly influence the success of early intervention programs. It is therefore important to help identify additional sources of support and strategies or accommodations that will decrease caregiver stress and promote the effectiveness of the training. In doing so, clinicians need to be sensitive to factors (both unrelated and related to the learner's treatment program) that may contribute to parent stress.

A factor unrelated to the learner's treatment program, for example, is the severity level of the learner's autism symptomatology. Higher stress levels have been found to be associated with higher ASD symptom severity (Hastings & Johnson, 2001). With regard to ASD symptom severity, it does not automatically follow that stress levels will decrease with effective intervention. Some parents continue to experience considerable amounts of stress even after seeing significant improvements in their child's functioning as a result of treatment. The sources of stress may change, but the experience of stress may not.

The constant stream of professionals coming in and out of the home during therapy can also contribute to parental stress for many reasons. For example, therapy sessions conducted in the home include the use of normally private areas, such as bedrooms and bathrooms, which can feel invasive and stressful for families. Other stressors have included therapists not removing their shoes when entering a home where parents have requested they do so, leaving various rooms of the house untidy, or moving items from their usual location. For these reasons, center-based treatment programs may be a better fit for some families. (See Chapter 8 for a discussion of center versus home-based treatment.)

DELIVERING PARENT TRAINING

Training Procedures

When training parents, clinicians should use the same behavioral principles and procedures that they use with learners, such as reinforcement, prompting, feedback/error correction, and multiple exemplar training. In addition, behavioral skills training (BST) is exceedingly effective, which includes a combination of didactic instruction, modeling, rehearsal, and feedback (see Chapter 4).

Didactic instruction. Initially, didactic instruction is provided to parents in person verbally (talking directly with parents and providing them with supporting written materials) or through a self-directed format (e.g., eLearning module or workbook). During didactic instruction, clinicians provide parents with a verbal description of the target skill to be acquired and a rationale for why that particular skill is important. Clinicians then provide parents with the procedures that will be used with the target skill.

To illustrate the relevance of the technique and how it might benefit them and their child, the clinician provides examples of situations in which parents might implement the procedure. Next, the clinician provides the parent with succinct, easy-to-read, written instructions outlining the procedures. The goals of these written instructions are to facilitate further comprehension and to act as a reference or reminder of procedures when the clinician is no longer present. Both verbal and written instructions should include: 1) a nontechnical definition of the skill, along with a rationale, 2) the specific steps the parent should take in order to perform the skill effectively, 3) specific prompting and fading procedures to be used, and 4) any other relevant tips for facilitating success.

Modeling. The second step in BST is modeling of the skill by the clinician. The clinician demonstrates the skill while explaining what he is doing and why and then asks the parent if she has any questions. Modeling can occur with or without the learner and can involve demonstrating the skill live, in person, via webcam, or through video modeling. Video modeling can be a particularly useful tool in situations where in-person opportunities are limited. Videos of previously recorded parent training observations can be reviewed by the clinicians and the parent together, which can allow for more in-depth discussions regarding performance than can be provided *in vivo*. This "self-evaluation" can also be useful in building parents' ability to self-monitor and correct their own behavior.

Rehearsal. The third step in BST is rehearsal (i.e., repeated practice of the new skill by the parent). Modeling alone is not enough to ensure that a person will demonstrate the correct behavior, particularly when the skill to be acquired is completely new; actual practice with feedback is crucial. Subsequent to modeling, the parent is immediately asked to imitate what she has observed. The goal is to get the parent to move from the role of observer to demonstrating the skill herself. Rehearsal typically involves the parent role-playing target skills with the clinician and/or the learner. In many cases, to build the parent's confidence and allow the trainer to hone the parent's skills more easily, role-play should initially be conducted without the learner present. It is often useful for clinician and parent to switch roles repeatedly, with one pretending to be the child and the other the parent, and vice versa. Humor can be useful at this stage – the topic of parent training is serious, but there is no reason that the process cannot be conducted lightheartedly and with fun. While the parent demonstrates each skill, the clinician provides assistance as needed with appropriate prompts, reinforces the parent's behavior, and provides constructive feedback. It is vital that the parent feels supported and successful during this stage. Clinicians repeat each step until the parent performs each target skill correctly. Clinicians should provide multiple opportunities for the parent to practice the target skill across multiple exemplar scenarios, behaviors, and settings, fading prompts to promote independence until the skill is truly established in the parent's repertoire. Clinicians should remember that, at this stage, reinforcement and shaping are vital to effectively establish and maintain newly acquired parenting skills. Skill proficiency should always be demonstrated during actual interventions with the learner, as well as during role-play with the clinician. Clinicians should encourage parents to spend time every day reviewing or practicing the skills they have learned and implementing them with their child independently as appropriate.

Feedback. Feedback has consistently been shown to be a vital component of effective training programs. Delivering feedback while training parents is a training skill that, at first blush, seems simple. However, delivering effective feedback that is motivating and not aversive to parents is actually a very complex and nuanced skill. Most expert parent trainers have acquired this skill over years of practice. The following are some guidelines to consider every time you deliver feedback to parents:

- Use four times more positive than corrective feedback;
- Feedback must be genuine; everyone can tell a "fake";
- Deliver feedback as immediately as possible;
- Deliver feedback as frequently as possible;
- Feedback should be specific, not global;
- Provide clear, specific written and verbal instructions before giving feedback on performance;
- Set goals for performance, and give feedback relative to those goals;
- Incorporate role-play, with trainer and trainee switching roles repeatedly; and
- Make feedback sessions fun – don't be overly stiff or serious.

In addition, graphic feedback (related to the parent's and learner's behavior) may be provided. The effectiveness of performance feedback depends not only on the content of the feedback but, also, on how it is delivered to parents. Feedback must be paired with positive reinforcement for desired parent behavior (partial or entire skill). Feedback alone does not change behavior; feedback only presents the opportunity for parents to improve performance. The parent's behavior will change due to the consequences directly associated with feedback or because of consequences expected in the future. If there are no consequences associated with the clinician's feedback, the parent's performance will not improve, or, at best, improvements may only be temporary. Feedback is thus most effective if it acts as a discriminative stimulus (S^D) for positive reinforcement. If clinicians pair their feedback consistently with positive consequences, their feedback might take on properties of a conditioned reinforcer and result in improved performance itself becoming a reinforcer for parents.

Positive feedback. Positive feedback involves delivering contingent, descriptive praise. When giving feedback, start with positive comments prior to offering corrective suggestions. The provision of positive comments about the parent's skills helps put both the clinician and parent at ease and focuses the conversation on what was done well, as opposed to what was not done well. Try for at least a 4:1 ratio, that is, four positive statements to every one corrective or negative statement. You want to focus on reinforcing the parent's desired behaviors in an effort to increase them. Make sure positive feedback is contingent on actual demonstration of the skill and specific to what the parent actually did. Clinicians should avoid nondescriptive, generic praise regarding the parent's behavior, such as, "You did great! You handled his tantrum really well!" In this case, the clinician could improve the effectiveness of his feedback by saying something more specific, such as, "You did really well ignoring Cormac's tantrum – you didn't give him eye contact or react to his screaming! You also did a great job prompting him to ask you appropriately for help once he calmed down." Lastly, make sure your positive feedback is genuine. Anyone can spot a fake, and artificial praise will not help establish a meaningful, collaborative relationship between you and the parent. Even if the parent is having great difficulty, it is your job to find at least one thing that the parent is genuinely doing well and praise it!

Corrective feedback. Corrective feedback should specify to parents how they can adjust their behavior to be more effective. Table 9.1 provides examples of common feedback that is given during parent training. The left column depicts information delivered in a blunt, careless manner. The right column depicts examples of how to provide the same feedback in a more positive, productive manner. For feedback to be the most helpful, it should be provided immediately following a parent's performance or as close in time as possible. This gives the parent an immediate opportunity to improve her behavior and, ideally, demonstrate the improved performance and then receive positive feedback. If the parent will not have the opportunity to try again at the moment feedback is given, it may be more effective to provide corrective feedback immediately prior to the next performance, allowing her to incorporate the feedback into her next performance. Since clinicians may not be present immediately prior to the next performance, it may be helpful to provide parents with written feedback that can be reviewed at any time. Written feedback is also an important way to ensure that the parent leaves the session with concrete goals for improvement and a sense of encouragement regarding what she did well. Of course, along with vocal and written feedback, parents should be provided with models of the desired behavior by the clinician and given ample opportunity to practice with feedback.

The manner in which clinicians deliver corrective feedback can greatly influence the likelihood that the parent will accept and implement the clinician's recommendations. Clinicians must prioritize and focus feedback on key issues and use corrective feedback sparingly. Since the training

TABLE 9.1 Examples of How to Frame Commonly Given Feedback in a Positive, Productive Manner

Negative Feedback	More Positively Framed Alternatives
"Stop giving him attention when he tantrums."	"I need you to focus on looking away and actively thinking of something else when he tantrums."
"You messed up the correction procedure again."	"Next time he makes an error, focus on presenting a full model prompt and then reinforce if he gets it right."
"You shouldn't negotiate with him after you ask him to do something."	"Next time you ask him to do something, if he tries to negotiate, physically prompt him to comply with the task."
"Just stop; I'll do it."	"Great try; let me demonstrate it one more time and then you can practice it again."
"Try not to sound rehearsed when you praise him."	"I know it's hard to seem happy 24 hours per day when situations like this are actually really frustrating. I need you to pick one aspect of your child's behavior that genuinely makes you happy and praise it, so he can tell you are proud of him. It will be a great place to start."
"Try not to use so many prompts."	"I want you to focus on asking him to do it just once and then waiting for a response. If he doesn't start to do it, then provide just one model prompt, and wait for him to respond independently."
"You have to stop giving in when he wants to escape a demand you have given him."	"This time, if he tries to escape what you ask him to do, physically block him from running away and continue to present the same request until he does it."

situation can be overwhelming for a parent, clinicians should consider not addressing every single detail of parent performance that could be improved. Instead, clinicians should focus on the most important issues at hand before getting into the small details.

Information is not feedback unless it specifies the specific behavior to be changed. For example, saying, "Johnny's hitting is still not getting any better" or merely showing a parent a graph does not address which specific behaviors the parent needs to change. Clinicians should not assume that parents automatically know what they need to do upon hearing what was done wrong or what is not working. Be sure to pinpoint exactly which skill should be performed more accurately and how to do it. For example, a clinician might say, "That was great! You were very clear with your instruction and giving Johnny the wait card. What we want now is for Johnny to listen to you the first time you give him an instruction. Next time, only tell him to 'wait' once and hand him the visual; then follow the rest of the procedures in the same way."

Clinicians should bear in mind that, for some individuals, corrective feedback can be very difficult to receive. Some parents may attempt to avoid being given feedback by engaging clinicians in lengthy discussions or finding ways to avoid having to demonstrate skills, including canceling training sessions. Other parents may react defensively or argue with clinicians. Others may perceive corrective feedback as a criticism of their general parenting and become emotionally upset. Difficulty in receiving feedback may be due to a history of feedback being paired with punishment and lack of success or positive experiences. Clinicians should remain sensitive to how different parents react to feedback and tailor their delivery style accordingly. Clinicians should work hard from the start to ensure that their presence and the feedback they give are paired with reinforcement and success. If you consistently pair feedback with reinforcement, feedback will eventually take on the properties of a conditioned reinforcer. In this situation, training might be viewed as an opportunity, rather than a stressful, demanding situation.

Prior to giving feedback, clinicians might consider asking the parent how she prefers to receive feedback and tailor their style accordingly. Clinicians should also always focus their attention on the correction of behavior, not the person, which can help take the emotions out of the situation and decrease the likelihood that parents will take feedback personally. It is often useful to tell the parents explicitly that learning new parenting behaviors and making mistakes do not reflect negatively on what kinds of parents they are – it's all just behavior. For example, you might say, "The ways that we interact with our kids when they misbehave do not make us good or bad parents. The fact that we love our children and would do anything for them makes us good parents. Learning new ways to interact with your child just means you are learning some new habits and breaking some old ones. It's all just behavior, and some behaviors work better than others. It's not personal."

Being respectful and sensitive while providing feedback is critical. Thus, before you give corrective feedback, consider each time whether it is the best time and place to do it. For example, people are not usually able to receive feedback when they are in a highly aroused emotional state. It is better to deliver feedback when parents are calm and able to attend to your instructions without distraction. It may also be inappropriate to correct a parent's behavior in front of others and more effective and appropriate to provide feedback later in private. Also, carefully consider whether you should give a parent feedback in front of the child. Especially if the child is older and more verbal, giving the parent feedback in front of her may undermine the parent's authority with the child. Even if the child is not verbal enough for this to be a problem, the parent may still perceive that you are undermining his authority, so still consider giving feedback in private.

Another way to decrease the likelihood of parents reacting defensively to feedback is to provide parents with a chance to self-evaluate what they did well and what they could do better. Teaching parents how to self-evaluate and correct their own behavior enables them to provide immediate and ongoing feedback to themselves, thus potentially facilitating a quicker adjustment of behavior. As parents build up a repertoire of self-evaluation and self-feedback, they will likely be more able to implement and maintain new protocols in the future with less training and/or maintain existing ones more successfully.

From beginning level to advanced skills training. At the beginning of training, parents most often require higher levels of support from the clinician and need to focus on more basic skills, with support gradually being faded and skills becoming more complex over time. However, the level of support needed from the clinician also depends on the parent's experience and skill set. Some parents may continue to require higher levels of support throughout their training experience. Clinicians should initially provide more concrete training examples, with structured and direct prompting procedures and more basic competency checks. For example, the clinician might review procedural techniques with parents by having them answer simple comprehension questions and instructing, "Show me how to do _____." Clinicians provide parents with concrete examples of when and where they would use target skills; e.g., "When Sasha wants milk, prompt her to mand appropriately *before* she starts to whine. If she starts to whine, ignore her until she stops whining for five seconds, and then prompt her to mand appropriately and give her milk." In order to shape the parent's behavior, clinicians should, at this stage, reinforce all attempts at proficiency.

For parents who are further along in their training, clinicians can start to focus on the development of more complex skills, such as problem solving and decision making, and prompts can become less direct. For example, clinicians might use leading questions or a scaffolding approach to help parents devise their own solutions and self-correct their behavior. Decision trees, listing pros/cons, or other strategies to facilitate a parent's ability to predict outcomes of particular courses of action might be used. Competency checks at this level might include asking the parent to analyze different scenarios and come up with potential solutions; e.g., "Why do you think Charlie's hitting is increasing? What might you do?" Having the parent start to evaluate and correct his own behavior at this stage (rather than relying on the trainer to give feedback) is also advantageous. Continuously moving parents toward independence is critical since, in the future, they will need to be able to make decisions independently regarding how to handle situations with their child once the trainer is no longer present.

Generalization and Maintenance

Even if training is successful, a newly established skill will not be useful if parents do not use it within the specific situations and settings that really matter. Skills will also not be useful if they are demonstrated inconsistently or if parents stop using the skills altogether. (Often, parents stop utilizing effective strategies once things are going well.) Generalization and maintenance are not guaranteed outcomes of parent training programs. For example, parents may demonstrate skills within the clinic but not be able to do so at home. Or, in some cases, skills might successfully be trained but not maintained during follow-up. Clinicians must therefore carefully plan for generalization and maintenance from the outset of training. (Refer to Chapter 7 for tips on generalization and maintenance.) The same basic procedures that are described in Chapter 7 for ensuring generalization of learner skills also help ensure that parents' newly learned skills will generalize. For example, make sure to train the parent across multiple settings (e.g., conduct training in different rooms of the house and across multiple community settings), across the learner's multiple challenging behaviors (e.g., practice extinction for several different learner behaviors), and across multiple learner skill acquisition targets (e.g., practice teaching parents mand training techniques across multiple different child mands).

Data Collection and Treatment Evaluation

Training parents to make data-based decisions. As part of the parent training process, clinicians should ensure that parents are provided with a rationale for recording data and should involve parents in the evaluation process on a regular basis. This helps parents understand the importance of what they are doing. Clinicians may also want to train other relevant family members to record data on the learner's behavior and/or their own and other family members' behavior. Training parents to use the data they are collecting to make good decisions regarding how to move forward with their child is also critical if parents are to be able to manage their child's behavior in the future when parent training is over. An added benefit of training parents to collect and understand data is that it will enable them to evaluate data that future treatment providers collect as well.

In order to ensure that parents are able to collect data that are consistently accurate and useful, clinicians should design individualized data collection systems that are easily integrated into the parents' daily routines and are simple and quick to administer. Clinicians should be mindful that parents are typically dealing with managing their child's behavior, running a household, going to work, and trying to meet the needs of other family members, all at the same time. Data collection (on top of implementing new parenting skills) can feel overwhelming. Accurate and consistent data collection is more likely to occur if you limit data to only a few key behaviors and require minimal information to be recorded. For example, data sheets that only require the parents to provide a simple yes/no or to circle the relevant option are a lot easier to manage than data sheets requiring parents to write out lengthy and detailed information or take running tallies on multiple different topographies of behavior.

In addition to providing good training and manageable expectations regarding data collection, clinicians should ensure that they provide reinforcement and feedback contingent on accurate and consistent data collection. Collection of inter-observer agreement (IOA) data is an important part of this process. Where clinicians are unable to collect IOA data themselves (through direct observation or video review), other family members might be trained to collect IOA. Once parents are collecting accurate and consistent data, clinicians should involve them in the analysis process and help them begin to problem solve and independently make data-based clinical decisions (see Chapter 20). It is also very common for different caregivers in the same family to disagree on the child's needs, severity of behavior, and so on. Having all caregivers collect data at the same time can facilitate a data-based discussion of the issue, rather than an emotional discussion that merely relies on memory.

Presenting graphic displays of the parents' performance and of the child's outcomes over time is an objective and direct way to provide specific feedback to parents. Once parents understand how to interpret graphic data and can see positive trends over time, feedback can become highly motivating for parents. (Graphic feedback can start to act as a conditioned reinforcer.) Graphic feedback can also be easily paired with self-monitoring systems. If self-monitoring data resulted in punishment in the past, parents might avoid taking data or report false data. In order for self-monitoring to be effective, clinicians must ensure that their feedback is established as an antecedent for reinforcement. Make sure that you reinforce accurate data collection, regardless of whether the parent is reporting positive performance changes.

Evaluating the parent training program. We strongly recommend that clinicians use data to evaluate the effectiveness of their parent training programs. Data regarding actual parent and child behavior change must be objectively collected and evaluated.

Parent skills. To assess changes in parental behavior, clinicians should compare baseline measures of performance with the parent's behavior during and following parent training. Again, direct observation, in person or via video, and analysis of self-monitoring data are both vital parts of this process.

Child outcomes. Direct measurement should also be used to assess whether the changes in parent behavior lead to changes in child behavior, including challenging behavior, skill acquisition, independence, and generalization of mastered skills. Optimally, the effects of parent training on child behavior would be evaluated by comparing child progress prior to and during parent training. Clinicians should not rely on parent report alone, since a verbal report may have little correspondence with actual behavior. For example, a parent may successfully demonstrate target skills and appear to be on board with the recommendations, but data on child behavior may show that the procedure is not effective. Changes in child behavior should be assessed through direct observation and analysis of data collected by the parent and others (e.g., therapists). In addition, permanent products (e.g., completed homework assignments) and other forms of record review (e.g., the number of days the child arrived at school on time) might be considered as further evidence of training efficacy.

Parent satisfaction. In order to assess the acceptability of training procedures and social significance of treatment, measures of parent satisfaction and social validity should be collected. Social validity might be assessed using questionnaires or informal interviews with parents and other significant people in the learner's life (e.g., grandparents, teacher, and siblings). In addition, when assessing the validity of child behavior change, actual comparisons can be made between the child with ASD and his typically developing peers. Independent observers might rate the extent to which they view the learner's behavior as similar to that of his peers by using videotapes or *in vivo* observations, for example.

Trainer evaluation. Finally, clinicians should evaluate their own practice to ensure that they are actively delivering effective parent training. This can be done through self-observation, peer observation, or mentor observation. Self-observation might involve reviewing video recordings of parent training sessions and pinpointing areas of strength and areas for professional development. Peer observation might involve having a colleague review a videotaped training session or observe training being implemented in person in order to provide feedback and aid with troubleshooting and problem solving. Similarly, mentor observation would involve a senior or more experienced clinician observing the clinician's behavior and offering feedback, help with problem solving, and so on.

TROUBLESHOOTING

Parent training does not always go smoothly. Even the most experienced clinicians encounter difficulties at times. For example, parenting skills may not result in desired changes in child behavior, or parents may struggle to participate in training or adhere to protocols. In such cases, clinicians should be careful not to blame the parent for poor outcomes. In all but the most extreme cases, clinicians should assume that parents have the ability to make the sufficient and necessary behavior changes that will lead to the best outcomes for their child and family. Poor parent training outcomes might be related to parent or child variables outside of the trainer's control; however, in most cases, improvements will be seen when something related to the training package or the clinician's behavior is altered.

Skill Deficit Versus Nonadherence

In order to identify the appropriate steps to take when desired outcomes are not achieved, clinicians must first consider the source of the difficulty. Clinicians must identify whether a lack of progress is due to a skill deficit (i.e., the parent has not acquired the necessary skills) versus an adherence issue (i.e., the parent is not applying the newly acquired skills). Skill deficits are typically due to a lack of effective training procedures (e.g., lack of rehearsal or insufficient feedback). Compliance issues can be due to a wide variety of issues, such as lack of buy-in from parents, generalization issues, competing contingencies, lack of reinforcement of target skills, programs having poor contextual fit, personal issues/life events, and so on. Clinicians might review a series of checks related to both the completeness and adequacy of their training package and parent variables, such as motivation, consistency, and skill deficits. These checks will help clinicians identify the source of the problem, so they can make appropriate changes. Each section of this chapter on designing a parent training program can serve as a "box to check" when trying to analyze the cause of failures in parent training.

Problematic Private Events

In some cases, despite the best efforts of the clinician, parents may have psychological barriers or problematic private events that interfere with their ability to benefit from parent training. For example, a parent may fail to follow through with an extinction procedure because, when her child begins to tantrum, she experiences extremely aversive feelings of guilt, anxiety, and fear, as well as thoughts such as, "I'm hurting my child," "I can't do this," and/or "I'm a terrible parent," all of which lead her to give in to her child. That is, escaping the aversiveness of these private events overrides the long-term benefits of riding out the extinction burst or other reinforcement contingencies in place to help parents follow through with the behavior plan. Parents often fail to implement newly learned procedures because their behavior is more strongly controlled by private stimuli (unhelpful thoughts or difficult emotions), rather than by environmental contingencies that would foster more adaptive parenting strategies.

It is likely that covert verbal behavior plays an important role in parent-child interactions and the outcomes of training programs. As such, it is important that behavior analytic clinicians remain aware of when parents' private events might be getting in the way of adaptive parenting behavior. Sometimes, behavior analytic clinicians fail to acknowledge or recognize interfering private events; more often, though, clinicians simply do not know how to address them effectively when they arise. Without effective strategies, clinicians tend to ignore them completely or resort to "commonsense" strategies, such as attempting to challenge a parent's thoughts, continuously reiterating how important compliance is, or repeatedly showing the parent data. In many, if not most, cases, such strategies are ineffective or may even aggravate the situation, increasing parent avoidance and nonadherence. Better outcomes will be achieved if clinicians are able to incorporate behaviorally based techniques into their practice that will reduce the influence of problematic private events on parent behavior.

Acceptance commitment therapy (ACT). ACT is a scientifically based behavioral approach to loosening the control that problematic private verbal events have on overt behavior. It is rooted in behavior analysis – specifically relational frame theory – and it offers clinicians a toolbox of behavioral techniques for helping parents address private events that are interfering with their ability or willingness to comply with treatment protocols. A great resource for parents is *The Reality Slap* (Harris, 2012), a book based on ACT that is written by a parent of a child with ASD.

At the heart of ACT is building psychological flexibility, that is, enabling individuals to respond more flexibly with respect to private stimuli, so they are more able to choose courses of action that take them in a valued direction (such as the long-term well-being of their child). ACT incorporates a variety of processes, including mindfulness and acceptance. Mindfulness training may help parents be more sensitive to environmental contingencies, so they are able to respond more effectively moment to moment. Using mindfulness to help parents be more "present" facilitates new learning and increases contact with values-oriented opportunities. For example, in a case in which a parent is experiencing extremely aversive thoughts and feelings related to her child's tantrums, the clinician might support the parent by helping her identify her values in helping her child, commit to action associated with the values, and accept and make room for difficult feelings that might arise in the process. The clinician also helps parents use mindfulness to notice when they are buying into their difficult thoughts and, instead, to get present and address what is happening in the moment with their child. Mindfulness training may inhibit the reappearance of unhelpful patterns of behavior. While increasing self-compassion, it is important for clinicians to foster acceptance in parents as well as a willingness to experience difficult circumstances, both of which are particularly important for parents of children with ASD, whose problems are typically chronic and not easily overcome by normal problem solving. In addition to helping parents cope more effectively with specific challenges, ACT-integrated parent training might also have more generalized effects, increasing the overall resilience and well-being of parents. Space does not permit a full description of ACT and its benefits for parent training, but readers are strongly encouraged to refer to the Association for Contextual Behavioral Science (www.contextualscience .org) to find out more about ACT, the basic science underlying it, current applied research, and training opportunities.

SUMMARY

Behavioral parent training has been found to be effective using various formats, procedures, intensities, and durations across multiple settings. The context of parent training, including family routines, culture, educational background, socioeconomic status, and stress level, must be considered when prioritizing treatment targets and setting parent goals that will set parents up for success. In order to obtain long-lasting effects, it is critical that you program for maintenance and generalization and teach parents how to evaluate the effectiveness of the methods they implement with their child. ACT can be a powerful tool for parents who struggle significantly with chronic stress or depression that inhibits their ability to learn or adhere to procedures presented during parent training.

Introduction to the Center for Autism and Related Disorders Curriculum Series

Adel C. Najdowski

In order to address each child's unique skill deficits and behavioral excesses effectively, it is essential to use a comprehensive, research-based curriculum that is customized to each child's individual needs. Since the goal of autism treatment is to teach the child with autism spectrum disorder (ASD) every skill she needs to learn in order to catch up to her typically developing peers, curriculum development must aim to identify all of the skills children learn in typical development. Each of the chapters contained in Section III of this manual covers one major curricular area of autism treatment (e.g., language, social, etc.). These chapters are not curricula in themselves but, rather, narratives describing the procedures to follow to teach the skills contained in comprehensive curricula for each skill area. In the Center for Autism and Related Disorders (CARD) Model, these procedures are used in combination with lessons from the CARD curriculum series, which is contained in the web-based Skills® system (www.skillsforautism.com; see Chapter 26). The remainder of this introductory chapter provides a description of the history, rationale, and framework of the CARD curriculum series.

HISTORY AND BACKGROUND

For many years, no single assessment could identify a comprehensive list of skills that should be taught during intensive behavioral intervention for young children with ASD. For some areas of human functioning (e.g., perspective taking), no assessments existed. Working with what was available, CARD clinicians conducted batteries of assessments in an effort to touch upon as many areas of child development and human functioning as possible. After an assessment battery was conducted, clinicians were faced with the many challenges involved in linking assessment results to the design of an individualized treatment program for each child. While some assessments are very useful for identifying specific skills that children need to learn, other assessments merely provide a score, quotient, or overall level of functioning in an area. These assessments are useful for identifying the extent of a child's delay or demonstrating a need for intervention in a particular area but are less useful for informing clinicians about the specific lessons or targets to teach the child. Another problem was that some of the more helpful assessments did not assess beyond early childhood years (e.g., up to 48 months of age), so they weren't useful in designing lessons for older children and adolescents. In those days, it was clear that assessments were an important tool with the potential to make treatment more effective, but no single assessment was comprehensive enough to identify delays and inform treatment for every child.

Faced with this challenge, clinicians at CARD did what all good clinicians should do: They used the results from their assessment battery as an indication of areas of child development in which the child needed curricular focus and 1) searched for lesson ideas from existing curricula, 2) read treatment research, 3) studied child development to determine milestones that typically occur within those areas, and 4) designed their own lessons to remediate deficits as best they could.

Back in the early 1990s at CARD, teaching lessons were developed on an as-needed basis, one child at a time. It was standard practice to assess the child and then develop lessons for the child that appeared relevant to the deficits identified during assessment. Then, in the course of treatment, as different issues and deficits were identified, new lessons were written. As one can imagine, this went on for about a decade, and as CARD continued to grow, the number of clinicians who could potentially be "reinventing the wheel" expanded. That is to say, clinicians within CARD could potentially be writing the same lessons that their colleagues were writing at other CARD locations, and this was likely happening over and over again.

At this point, CARD was faced with two problems. First, the absence of an age-appropriate, comprehensive, skills-based assessment made it challenging to identify which lessons and targets were needed to enable a child to catch up across all areas of human functioning. Second, resources and potential treatment hours were being wasted by duplicating lesson development on a child-by-child basis. At the same time, CARD clinicians were receiving requests for help from families all over the world who had no access to services in their region and urgently needed help to design a program for their children. These same parents were using limited information to guide their curriculum choices for their children.

Although CARD's working curriculum had already been in development for 10 years, it was not until the early 2000s that a conscious decision was made to compile every lesson ever written for every child ever at CARD and embark on a journey to further develop and eventually compose the most comprehensive curriculum series for evidence-based behavioral intervention in the world. Our mission in doing so was twofold:

1. To provide CARD clinicians and external stakeholders with the tools to implement top-quality intervention that would allow them to spend more time treating children; and
2. To provide a curriculum series to parents who were unable to obtain applied behavior analysis (ABA) services (and were essentially going without).

To optimize the CARD curriculum series it quickly became apparent that an accompanying assessment would be necessary. Regardless of the quality of the curriculum series, treatment could easily go awry without a directly linked assessment. For example, what would happen if some clinicians were to use each curriculum in the series as if it were a cookbook, introducing each lesson step-by-step like a recipe? By overlooking individualization, they could potentially waste time working on skills that the child didn't actually need. What if clinicians were to select only certain lessons from a curriculum that they wanted to teach because they were accustomed to those particular lessons? This could result in choosing activities for which prerequisite skills are not in place or that are too advanced for the child. It might also result in the clinician relying too heavily on previous clinical experience and/or preferences and creating an inappropriately lopsided or unbalanced treatment program (e.g., maybe focusing on pre-academic skills and language but nothing else). These are just a few of the potential problems that could occur without linking a comprehensive assessment directly to a curriculum.

PHILOSOPHY BEHIND THE CARD CURRICULUM SERIES

The main objective in creating the CARD series was to include lessons to teach every skill in every area of child development, from birth through elementary school age. The basic philosophy behind the development of the CARD assessment and curriculum series is that, in order to provide the most effective treatment to children with ASD, we cannot allow treatment program design to be guided by limited assessment information and our personal clinical experience alone because we may omit important skills that are not obvious to us. We must avoid only focusing on one or two curriculum areas (e.g., language and daily living skills) while ignoring other important skill sets (e.g., social and cognitive skills), and we must be committed to identifying every single skill children learn in typical development and composing lessons and targets to teach those skills. This philosophical assumption arose from our acknowledgment that no two children with ASD are the same, and all present with their own set of unique needs. In order to address those needs, no skill can be overlooked. In order to ensure that no skills would be overlooked in our curriculum series, we knew that child development had to be researched to the fullest extent to determine what children should be doing in each age range. To develop the most comprehensive curriculum series possible, standardized assessments, developmental textbooks, and journal articles associated with all areas of human functioning were consulted. A final assumption was that research and evidence should guide curriculum development first, supplemented by clinical experience where research is lacking.

DEVELOPMENT AND FRAMEWORK OF THE CARD CURRICULUM SERIES

Figure 10.1 depicts the overall structure of the CARD curriculum series. The lessons comprising the CARD curriculum series were developed across eight curricular areas: 1) Social, 2) Motor, 3) Language, 4) Adaptive, 5) Play, 6) Executive Function, 7) Cognition, and 8) Academic skills. Most of the eight curricular areas are subdivided by domains. Figure 10.2 depicts how all areas of the curriculum series are organized, starting with curriculum area (largest scope) and narrowing down to individual exemplars to be taught (smallest scope).

For example, the Motor curriculum is subdivided by the domains of fine, gross, oral, and visual motor. Each domain is composed of many lessons with a similar focus; for example, the gross motor domain includes lessons for teaching large body movements, such as Catching, Hopping, Jumping, Kicking, Riding a Tricycle/Bicycle, and Stairs and Climbing, to name a few. All of the lessons are categorized by level, from beginner lessons (level 1) to more advanced lessons (level 12). Levels are assigned based on the earliest emerging skill in the lesson. Each lesson has multiple sections which are organized according to the main concepts taught in each section; for example, the Catching lesson within the Motor curriculum has three sections: 1) catching a rolled ball, 2) catching a thrown ball, and 3) catching a bounced ball. Each lesson section is composed of various activities. For example, the lesson section on catching a rolled ball might have activities for catching a rolled ball while sitting across from someone, standing across from someone, and while standing and wearing a baseball glove. Figure 10.3 depicts sample information from the Catching

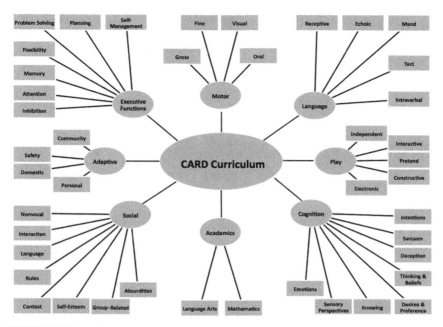

FIGURE 10.1   The eight CARD curriculum areas and their domains.

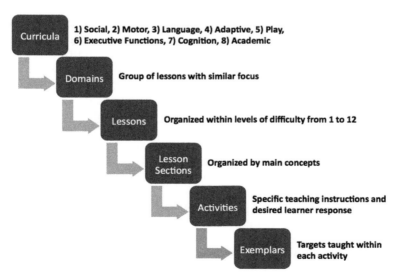

FIGURE 10.2   Structure and format of the CARD curriculum.

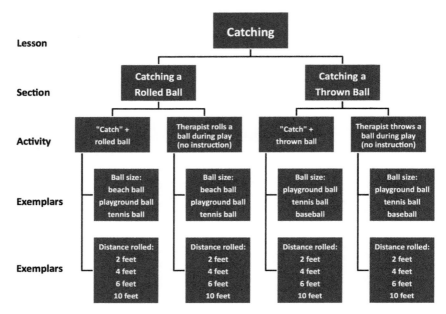

FIGURE 10.3   Example of a lesson and its sections, activities, and exemplars.

lesson in the Motor curriculum. The activities provide descriptions of the specific teaching instructions that will be delivered and the desired response from the learner that must be taught. Most activities have many different exemplars that may be targeted. For example, when teaching the learner to catch a rolled ball, various sizes of balls are targeted from various distances.

The activities in each lesson section are presented in order of emerging age in typical child development. It's not uncommon to see a lesson section start at the age of 2 or 3 and continue until the age of 7 or 8. This happens because skills evolve as a child ages. For example, from 3 to 4 years of age, a child catches a ball by scooping under it with his hands and trapping it to his chest; from 4 to 5 years of age, he extends his hands and arms to catch a thrown playground-sized ball; and from 5 to 7 years, he uses both hands to catch a ball the size of a baseball thrown from a distance of 10 or more feet. In addition to milestones categorized by age, each activity provides a wealth of information to the clinician, including the prerequisite lessons and/or lesson sections within the CARD curriculum series, examples of how to do the activity, an Individualized Education Program (IEP) goal, methods for data collection and measurement of progress toward the IEP goal, teaching points to provide helpful hints and ideas for troubleshooting, methods to program for generalization, handouts (e.g., worksheets for the learner), visual aids for prompting a correct response, and data tracking forms. See Appendix C for an abridged version of the Knowing lesson from the Cognition curriculum. In addition, Appendices D–K provide outlines for each of the eight curricula in the CARD curriculum series, listing domains, lessons, sections, and ages for all curricula.

Using the Assessment and Curriculum Series

The assessment that goes with the CARD curriculum series is intended to identify skills that the child needs to learn in order to catch up to his typically developing, same-age peers. Using answers from a series of yes/no questions, the assessment identifies the pool of activities that the child cannot do. Once the assessment is complete, clinicians choose lesson activities from the pool of identified activities the child does not know how to perform and place those activities into the child's treatment plan. The clinician starts by determining which curricular areas to address and then begins choosing specific lessons and activities to target. Usually, a couple of activities are introduced from many or all of the curricular areas in an effort to design a balanced program (although this might not be the case if working with a learner who primarily has social and executive function deficits or when working with a learner for whom funding only covers certain curricular areas), and many factors will go into which activities clinicians choose to put into the child's treatment program (see Chapter 19 on clinical supervision).

It's important to note that each lesson activity and its accompanying list of targets are considered only suggestions for clinicians to consider when designing treatment programs for children with ASD, and we fully expect clinicians to make adjustments and modifications to lessons in an effort to individualize and customize them to suit each learner's unique profile. This means that lessons, activities, and targets can be ignored if they are irrelevant to the learner's daily life and won't be maintained by natural contingencies. Clinicians are expected to use the CARD curriculum series flexibly and to be able to recognize the purpose of an activity and then modify it to suit the learner's needs.

Skills®

The CARD assessment and curriculum series are now a part of an online system called Skills® (www.skillsforautism.com; see Chapter 26) which is used both internally within CARD and also externally by other ABA service agencies, school districts, and parents all over the world. The system allows users to interact with the CARD assessment, design individualized treatment programs for learners, and track learners' progress.

SUMMARY

The CARD assessment and curriculum series are the results of decades of research and practice in evidence-based treatment for learners with ASD. By design, the CARD curriculum series will always evolve to be more comprehensive and to incorporate new information on best practices for treating children with ASD. New content is added regularly, and changes are made to activities based upon new research. In CARD's mission to extend top-quality treatment to as many individuals with ASD as possible, self-improvement and fine-tuning of the CARD curriculum series have no end in sight.

11

Language

Michele R. Bishop, Adel C. Najdowski

Language skills are an integral component of human behavior and contribute to the development of social interactions, play skills, and many academic skills. *The Diagnostic and Statistical Manual of Mental Disorders, Fifth Edition* (DSM-5) (American Psychiatric Association [APA], 2013) lists language deficits as one of the defining features of autism spectrum disorder (ASD), with delays commonly observed in the areas of speech, making requests, labeling objects, and conversation skills. Often, inappropriate behavior develops as a means of communication when appropriate language skills are lacking. Given the pervasive nature of this deficit and the central role that language skills play in most areas of human functioning, a large proportion of time must be dedicated to the development of language skills in learners diagnosed with ASD.

While many typically developing children acquire language skills without explicit intervention, language skills must be directly taught to many learners with ASD. Historically, language was taught as either "receptive," which involves understanding the language of others, or "expressive," which involves using language to communicate. To teach receptive language, the therapist would display three picture cards (e.g., chair, fork, and cookie) and instruct the learner to identify one upon instruction, as in, "Touch cookie." The learner demonstrated that she receptively understood the therapist if she touched the picture of the cookie instead of the chair or fork. Then, the therapist would teach expressive language by holding up a picture of an item, such as a cookie, and asking, "What is it?" In this case, the learner was expected to use her expressive language by communicating "cookie" through whatever form of communication was appropriate for her (e.g., speech, sign language, communication device, etc.). Once she could receptively and expressively identify an item – in this case a cookie – it was assumed that the learner had been taught the meaning of the word and that the learner should thereafter use the word whenever necessary in her daily life. The problem is that teaching language to learners with ASD is not as easy as teaching the meaning of words. Humans use and respond to words in many different ways, and most early learners with ASD will not spontaneously acquire the ability to use a word in every way after merely learning it receptively and expressively.

Verbal Behavior

According to B.F. Skinner (1957), there are seven primary functional uses of expressive language, four of which will be reviewed here: 1) echoic, 2) mand, 3) tact, and 4) intraverbal. Skinner referred to these as "verbal operants." See Table 11.1 for a representation of the defining characteristics of the four **verbal operant** categories. Each verbal operant is defined by the environmental conditions that evoke the response and the source of reinforcement for the response. The same vocal response may have a different function based on the conditions under which it is said. In other words, each verbal operant is a different way to use the same word. For example, the word *cookie* is an echoic response if it is said in response to hearing someone else say "cookie." It is a mand if the learner is hungry and says "cookie" so that someone gives her a cookie. It is a tact if she sees a cookie and says, "cookie," and it is an intraver-

TABLE 11.1 Defining Characteristics of Basic Verbal Operants

Verbal Operant	Antecedent	Verbal Response
Echoic	Verbal Stimulus *Example:* The therapist says, "Cookie."	Verbal response that has point-to-point correspondence and formal similarity with the verbal stimulus *Example:* The learner says, "Cookie."
Mand	Motivating Operation (i.e., deprivation or satiation) *Example:* A learner cannot find his favorite toy.	Verbal request that identifies a specific reinforcer *Example:* The learner says, "Mom, I want my red car." His mom gives him the red car.
Tact	Nonverbal Stimulus *Example:* A learner sees a group of people kicking a black and white ball around.	Verbal response that labels (names) the nonverbal stimulus, followed by generalized conditioned reinforcement *Example:* The learner says, "They are playing soccer," and his mom says, "That's right!"
Intraverbal	Verbal Stimulus *Example:* A parent says, "What color is the sky?"	Verbal response that does not have point-to-point correspondence and formal similarity with the verbal stimulus *Example:* The learner says, "Blue."

bal if her parent asks, "What's your favorite dessert?" and she answers, "Cookies." One cannot assume that, if a learner is taught to say "cookie" as a mand, she will also be able to say "cookie" as an echoic, tact, or intraverbal. Each verbal operant must be assessed separately to determine if explicit instruction is necessary. Especially with early language learners, single words must often be taught across all operants so as to ensure that the child can actually use those words in every way needed in her everyday life.

The first step in building functional verbal communication is to increase sound production. Unfortunately, it is impossible to manipulate the vocal cords to produce sounds, so therapists must rely on behavioral techniques to encourage sound production and then establish instructional control for sounds that are emitted. Once the learner consistently makes sounds, teaching methods can focus on developing words and eventually using those words in mands, tacts, and intraverbals. During the early stages of learning, echoics, mands, and tacts may be formally similar. For example, a learner may say "milk" under a variety of conditions: 1) when a therapist says, "Say, 'milk,'" 2) in response to the question "What do you want?" and 3) when asked "What is it?" while the therapist points to a glass of milk. The function of the verbal response in each situation is differentiated by the antecedent stimuli (e.g., an instruction or establishing operation [EO]) and the consequence following the response. (See Chapter 4 for more information on the EO.) Mands result in access to the item, while echoics and tacts result in reinforcement that is unrelated to the response. As the learner develops more sophisticated language, the function of individual verbal responses becomes more apparent. This is partially due to the use of complete sentences instead of single words when communicating with others. For instance, now a learner may say "I want some milk" as a mand and "I see milk" as a tact.

Verbal Operants Versus Concepts

In addition to teaching the learner to use the various verbal operants, language intervention consists of teaching a large repertoire of concepts. In lay terms, concepts are the content or meaning of language, and verbal operants are the ways in which the speaker uses the concepts when she speaks. The Center for Autism and Related Disorders (CARD) Language curriculum is organized into lessons that teach each individual concept, and each lesson is organized into the steps for teaching that concept across all verbal operants. For example, for the concept of actions, the learner is taught to mand for preferred actions (e.g., "swing"), respond receptively to action names (e.g., the therapist says, "Point to swinging," and the learner points to a picture of a child swinging), tact actions (e.g., "he is swinging"), and engage in intraverbals related to actions (e.g., the

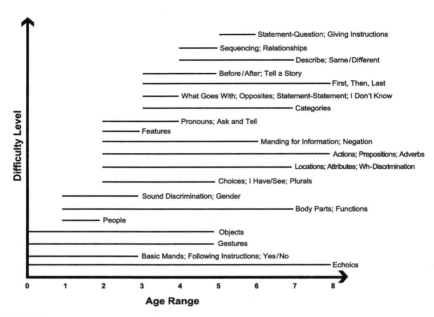

FIGURE 11.1   Language lessons by age range and difficulty level. *Reprinted from Skills®*
with permission from the Center for Autism and Related Disorders.

therapist asks, "What do you like to do at the park?" and the learner
answers, "Swing"). Figure 11.1 depicts the main lessons in the CARD
Language curriculum. The horizontal axis depicts the age range in typical
development during which children begin to learn the concepts, and the
vertical axis depicts the relative difficulty and complexity of the various
concepts. Note that many concepts begin at a young age but take years
to fully develop. Consider the Echoics lesson. Infants begin to imitate
individual sounds, and the complexity of imitation gradually increases
with age until children are able to imitate sentences containing a dozen
or more syllables by the time they are 8 years old. Appendix D provides
an outline of the entire Language curriculum.

This chapter will provide practical guidelines on how to use instructional techniques to teach echoics, mands, receptive behavior, tacts, and
intraverbals across all necessary concept areas. Space does not permit step-
by-step guidelines for every concept, so this chapter will need to be used
in combination with a comprehensive curriculum, such as Skills® (www.
skillsforautism.com). Tips for generalization, maintenance, and problem
solving are also provided. All of the teaching procedures described in this
chapter are explained in detail in Chapter 4. See Sautter & LeBlanc (2006)
for a review of the literature on verbal behavior and Shafer (1994) for a
review of interventions used to teach manding.

ECHOICS

Echoics are verbal behavior under the control of a vocal stimulus that is formally similar to the vocal response. For example, a parent says, "Ball" (vocal stimulus) and the learner says, "Ball," or a parent says, "Red" (vocal stimulus) and the learner says, "Red." These examples highlight the point-to-point correspondence between the verbal stimulus and the verbal response, which is sometimes referred to as vocal imitation.

Vocal imitation is taught to learners with ASD with the goal of eventually being able to teach them to use speech as a form of communication. Researchers have found that, for some learners with ASD, shaping vocal imitation (echoic) repertoires also results in an increase in vocalizations (Lovaas, Koegel, Simmons, & Long, 1973; Ross & Greer, 2003), which is a nice bonus. Furthermore, once learners have an established echoic repertoire, echoics can be used as prompts to establish other verbal repertoires, such as mands, tacts, and intraverbals.

Vocal Imitation

Vocal imitation is often taught using either: 1) discrete trial training (DTT), 2) DTT combined with shaping, or 3) DTT combined with chaining. As described in Chapter 4, DTT follows an instruction, response, consequence sequence. For example, the instruction "Say, 'apple'" is followed by the response "apple," and then reinforcement is delivered. While pure echoic behavior occurs in the absence of an instruction, most clinicians include an instruction (e.g., "say") when teaching vocal imitation because this is the cue that it is appropriate to imitate the sound, word, or phrase that follows the instruction (and it would be strange for children to walk around imitating everything other people say all day long).

Free Operant Reinforcement of All Vocalizations

Some learners have a particularly difficult time learning to vocally imitate and display a limited amount of vocalizations of any kind. For these learners, consider beginning by reinforcing any vocalizations that they display (except for ones that are obviously the learner's most common forms of stereotypy). To do this, the therapist should always have highly preferred reinforcers available during therapy and deliver them immediately following any vocalization that the learner makes. The rationale of this procedure is that it should increase the overall rate and variety of vocalizations that the learner makes. If this works, you can then try to bring some of these vocalizations under stimulus control with the vocal imitation procedures described above.

Embedding Echoics in Motor Sequences

Another teaching option for learners who have difficulty with vocal imitation is to embed vocal imitation trials at the end of a series of mastered motor imitation trials. For example, if a learner has already mastered raising arms, clapping, and waving, then the therapist can present one trial for each of these in rapid succession with rapid reinforcement for each correct response and then "sneak in" a vocal imitation trial at the end of the chain of motor imitations. Research has shown that this procedure can be helpful in some cases (Tsiouri & Greer, 2003).

MANDS

Mands (requests) are a unique form of verbal behavior because the verbal response specifies the reinforcer. For example, a child says, "I want juice," and his parent gives him juice. Mands occur when a person is motivated to ask for something or, in other words, the person *wants* the thing for which he is asking. For example, if a child really likes playing with cars and she is not currently playing with cars, she will presumably be motivated to mand (ask) for a car.

Along with echoics, mands are one of the first verbal operants that should be taught to learners with ASD. When learners are taught to mand, they are essentially learning that they can make good things happen by talking. Being able to mand puts the learner into a position of feeling successful and allows interactions with therapists to be positive because therapists give the learner what she wants. For sample concepts you might teach during mand training, see the example lessons and their corresponding targets for teaching mands in Table 11.2.

Naturally Occurring Establishing Operations

Manding instruction follows an EO, response, consequence sequence. The EO sets the occasion for the response, the response is a request for something, and the consequence is always directly related to the request. Natural environment training (NET) is frequently used to capture EOs relevant to the learner. EOs occur naturally in the environment during the learner's daily activities (e.g., at lunchtime, the learner is motivated to ask for food), or they can be contrived through environmental manipulations. For example, the learner is coloring, and the therapist places all of the crayons out of the learner's reach, increasing the learner's motivation to ask for a crayon. When using naturally occurring establishing operations, the therapist interacts with the learner as he moves around in the environment. When the learner expresses an interest in something (e.g., reaching for an object, pointing to an item), the therapist prompts the learner to ask

TABLE 11.2   Sample Mand Targets

Antecedent/Establishing Operation: Limited or Blocked Access to Preferred Items		
Learner's Response: A Request for a Preferred Item		
Specific Examples		
Lesson	**Antecedent/Establishing Operation**	**Learner's Response**
Objects	The learner has not had access to her bouncy ball lately.	"I want *ball*."
People	The learner sees mom in the distance and has not seen her all day.	"I want *Mommy*!"
Actions	The learner has not jumped on the trampoline for several hours.	"I want *to jump*."
Attributes	The learner is given a small piece of candy from a bowl of candy.	"I want a *big* piece."
Manding for Information	The learner has not had access to his race cars in a while, and when he goes to get them from their usual location, they are missing.	"*Where* are my race cars?"
Functions	The learner is trying to open a taped box.	"I need something *to cut with*."
Gestures	The learner sees someone open up a bag of cashews.	The learner gestures with an *open palm-up* request.
Locations	The learner has not played in the playroom for a while.	"I want *playroom*."
Gender	The learner requests a doll and is given a girl doll.	"I want a *boy* doll."
Pronouns	The learner has not had access to a highly preferred item(s)/activity.	"*I want this/that/these/those*." "*This is mine*." "*My turn*."
Prepositions	There are various items on a high shelf (multiple cars, a box, and other items).	"I want the car *next to* the box."
Negation	The learner is trying to open a container.	"Can you help me? I *can't* open this!"

for it. For example, when the learner is reaching for a cup of water, the therapist says, "Say, 'I want water.'" The learner responds, "I want water," and then the therapist gives the learner a cup of water.

Contrived Establishing Operations

When using contrived EOs, the therapist limits free access to highly preferred items by placing them in a visible location out of the learner's reach or arranging other environmental variables that increase the value of an item; e.g., smelling cookies baking or fresh popcorn increases the likelihood of asking for cookies or popcorn To confirm motivation for the item, the therapist may present the item to the learner without allowing access to it to determine if he reaches for it. For example, if the learner begins building a tower with blocks, the therapist could move all of the blocks out of the learner's reach. When the learner reaches for another block, the therapist could then prevent access and say, "Say, 'I want block.'" When the learner responds, "I want block," the therapist would then give the learner a block. See Table 11.3 for step-by-step instructions for teaching learners to exhibit mands using contrived EOs.

Reinforcing Mands

Lessons for teaching mands frequently incorporate both naturally occurring and contrived EOs to increase the number of teaching opportunities. When possible, give a small amount of the preferred item requested to encourage the learner to ask for the item again. For example, if the learner asks for a cookie, give the learner one bite of the cookie instead of the whole cookie, or if the learner asks for his favorite stuffed animal, give him brief access to the stuffed animal, and then remove it until the learner asks for it again.

TABLE 11.3   Teaching Mands Using Contrived Establishing Operations

Establishing Operation: Limited or Blocked Access to Preferred Items by Therapist Learner's Response: A Request for a Preferred Item	
Step 1	Prepare the environment by setting out preferred food, drinks, toys, and activities. Place some items in a visible location but out of the learner's reach. Set out any materials used during teaching (datasheets, etc.).
Step 2	Bring the learner to the instructional area. If the learner begins playing with something, allow brief access, and then remove the item to create an opportunity for the learner to ask for it. If the toy has multiple pieces, restrict access to the additional pieces, and have the learner ask for the pieces. You may also present items to the learner to see if she reaches for them, without allowing access to the items. Then, wait for the learner to ask for the items.
Step 3	If the learner vocally asks for something, give the learner access to the requested item. If the learner indicates nonvocally (e.g., pointing to, reaching for, or guiding your hand toward something) that he wants something, prompt the learner to request the item, and then give the learner access to the item.

Complex Mands

As the learner's mand repertoire develops, more complex requests will be taught, such as mands for objects that are out of sight, mands for information (e.g., "When are we going to the park?"or "Where are the scissors?"), and mands for someone to do something (e.g., "Mom, will you sit on the blue chair?") or stop doing something (e.g., "Please stop shaking the table."). To teach the learner to mand for information about an object that is out of sight, for example, the therapist might give the learner a piece of paper and ask him to draw a picture of his family. When the learner is not able to find the markers, he is taught to ask, "Where are the markers?" The therapist then gives the information, saying, "The markers are in the craft box in the kitchen." This information functions as the reinforcer for the learner's mand because now the learner can find the markers and complete the picture.

Spontaneous Mands

In beginning lessons for teaching mands, prompts (e.g., "What do you want?" and "Say, 'I want…'") are often used to assist the learner in engaging in a correct response. Then, over time, the use of prompts is gradually eliminated, allowing the learner's request to come under the control of the relevant establishing operations. This is done by gradually increasing the amount of time before a prompt is delivered and providing less intrusive prompts. For example, when a learner is first being taught to mand for chips, the therapist may immediately provide the prompt, "I want chips." Then, as the learner continues reaching for the chips, the therapist may begin using a partial model prompt, such as, "Say, 'I'" or asking the learner, "What do you want?" As the learner continues responding correctly, the therapist delays the prompt by a few seconds and observes whether the learner initiates the mand independently. (See Chapter 4 for a discussion about prompt fading.) The goal is for the learner to be able to use mands spontaneously on his own whenever he wants something, not only when asked what he wants.

Disguised or Softened Mands

Sometimes, it is not socially appropriate to mand directly for what one wants, so people often soften or disguise their mands by wording them in a more subtle way (Skinner, 1957). For example, if a child has cookies for dessert in his lunch, another child might say, "Wow, those cookies look yummy," rather than saying, "Can I have a cookie please?" After your learner has a strong repertoire of spontaneous mands worded in a direct way, consider teaching disguised topographies of mands. To get ideas for particular topographies of disguised mands to teach, consider observing same-age, typically developing peers and review the desires lesson in Skills® (see Chapter 17). At the same time, make sure to teach your learner to identify and reinforce the disguised mands of others, as described in Chapter 17.

MATCHING

Matching is not technically a language skill, but it can be helpful for some learners who have difficulty with receptive language (next section below). Let's say, for example, that a learner has a difficult time responding to receptive identification instructions, such as "touch shoe" when there are three items out on a table, one of which is a shoe. For some learners, a matching response with a slightly modified matching instruction that includes the name of the object can be helpful. Specifically, in this case, instead of using the traditional matching instruction "put with same" when presenting the learner with three pictures, the therapist says, "Put with *shoe*." Once the learner visually determines that the picture of the shoe in his hand goes with the picture of the shoe in the array of three pictures on the table, paired with hearing the word "shoe" across several trials, the learner might be better prepared to respond correctly when moving to the receptive instruction "touch shoe." For this reason, we include matching in the Language curriculum.

Lessons that target matching include matching identical and nonidentical objects and pictures, as well as sorting. When using DTT to teach matching, two or more picture cards or 3D objects are placed on a table, the therapist hands the learner a card or object, and then an instruction to match is presented. The learner responds, and a consequence is delivered indicating if the response was correct or incorrect. For example, a therapist places a ball, a car, and a cup in front of the learner, gives the learner a ball, and says, "Put with same" or "Match." The learner responds by placing the ball next to the ball on the table, upon which reinforcement is delivered. If it is the very first time the child is learning matching, it is likely prudent to begin with placing only one object on the table at a time and practicing several matching trials with the same object consecutively (i.e., mass trialing without distractors – see Chapter 4 on discrimination training). The number of stimuli present on the table is gradually increased and mass trialing is gradually faded out, contingent on continued accurate responding by the learner. Once basic matching skills are established, matching items with subtle differences and more complex sorting tasks are introduced.

UNDERSTANDING THE VERBAL BEHAVIOR OF OTHERS

Language interactions include two components: 1) speaker behavior and 2) listener behavior. Echoics, mands, tacts, and intraverbals focus on speaker behavior, which means that the learner is learning to communicate. All comprehensive autism intervention programs must also teach listener behavior, which means that the child is learning to interpret and understand language spoken by others. These lessons do not require the learner to say anything; instead, the learner *listens* carefully to someone else's verbal behavior and responds effectively to it.

Receptive Identification

Receptive identification involves teaching a learner to select a stimulus when she hears its name (e.g., object name, action name, color, size, etc.) in the therapist's instruction. Essentially, every lesson that is taught as a tact has a flipside wherein the learner learns to respond to that same word as a listener, thereby demonstrating comprehension of the word. Table 11.4 lists examples of lessons and receptive targets.

Discrete trial training. When using DTT to teaching receptive identification, two or more picture cards or objects are placed on a table, and an instruction is presented to select one of them based upon some named aspect of it. The learner responds, and a consequence is delivered indicating if the response was correct or incorrect. For example, a therapist places a toothbrush, comb, and spoon in front of the learner and says, "Touch comb" or "Give me comb." The learner responds by touching/giving the comb, upon which reinforcement is delivered. If the learner has not already mastered a significant number of receptive discriminations, it may be useful to begin with only one item on the table and present several trials of the same target consecutively (i.e., mass trialing without distractors – see Chapter 4).

Natural environment training. Using NET, the therapist interacts with the learner as she moves around in the environment, taking advantage of opportunities to teach receptive identification. The therapist instructs the learner to select or touch items based on an aspect of the item (object name, action name, color, size, feature, etc.). For example, while the therapist and learner are playing "tea party" with a kitchen set containing dishes and food, the therapist might say, "Give me a cup." The learner should hand the therapist a cup instead of one of the other kitchen items. Since they are playing tea party, the therapist also needs a spoon for her tea, so she says, "Give me a spoon." Again, the learner discriminates a spoon among an array of kitchen items and hands the therapist a spoon instead of some other item.

TABLE 11.4   Sample Receptive Identification Targets

Antecedent: Therapist Presents a Vocal Instruction, Consisting of the Name of an Object, Property, Feature, Concept, etc. Learner's Response: Touch, Hand Over, or Show the Correct Stimulus Specific Examples		
Lesson	**Antecedent**	**Learner's Response**
Body Parts	Therapist presents a doll and says, "Touch *arm*."	Touches *arm*
Categories	Therapist presents pictures of a cat, shoe, and car and says, "Give me an *animal*."	Gives picture of *cat*
Gender	Therapist presents pictures of a man, girl, and boy and says, "Touch *boy*."	Touches picture of *boy*
	Therapist presents felt pieces and says, "Make a *boy*."	Makes a *boy* with felt
What Goes With	Therapist presents pictures of a basketball hoop, baseball bat, and tennis racket and says, "Give me the one that goes with *a baseball*."	Gives picture of *baseball bat*
Plurals	Therapist presents pictures of one shoe, two shoes, and two balls and says, "Give me *shoes*."	Gives the picture of the two *shoes*
Sequencing	Therapist presents sequence cards, narrates them, and then says, "Give me what happened *first/last/before/after*."	Gives the correct picture in a sequence of pictures
Pronouns	"Touch *my/your/his/her* nose."	Touches correct person's nose
	"Give me *his/hers/yours/ours/theirs*."	Gives correct person's item
	"Give this to *him/her/them*."	Gives item to correct person
Adverbs	"Show me clapping *slowly*."	Claps *slowly*
Relationships	In the presence of the learner's aunt, uncle, and grandma, the therapist says, "Touch *aunt*."	Touches *aunt*

Following Instructions

Instruction-following is another critical part of the listener repertoire that must be taught to many learners with ASD. Instruction-following is different from receptive identification because it generally involves acting out behavior in some way that demonstrates comprehension, rather than discriminating between two or more stimuli (as is done in receptive identification). Instruction-following lessons often focus on teaching the learner to understand instructions to perform a variety of fine and gross motor movements.

Discrete trial training. When using DTT to teach learners to follow instructions, an instruction is presented, the learner responds, and a consequence is delivered indicating if the response was correct or incorrect. For example, a therapist says, "Stomp feet," to which the learner responds by stomping his feet, and reinforcement is delivered. One-step instructions are taught first, followed by more complex two- and three-step instructions and group instructions.

Natural environment training. When using NET, the therapist works with the learner as she explores the environment, taking advantage of opportunities to teach the learner to follow instructions. The therapist asks the learner to follow different instructions as she contacts various stimuli. For example, if a learner is getting ready to play outside, the therapist might say, "Put your shoes on," in which case the learner puts on her shoes. While outside, the therapist might say, "Climb to the top of the slide," resulting in the learner climbing up the slide. Next, when the learner walks into the kitchen for lunch, the therapist might say, "Sit down at the kitchen table," and the learner might respond by sitting at the kitchen table.

Modifying the general receptive teaching format. Receptive identification and following instructions are relatively straightforward, and it's easy to use the same general format to teach all sorts of targets across various language concepts. However, several language lessons require modification of the general format in that correct responding does not involve discriminating between two or more choice stimuli or completing an action in response to a therapist request. We describe a few examples below.

When teaching learners to understand the words "yes" and "no," one of the skills the learner must learn is to respond appropriately when the therapist says "yes" or "no" in response to something the learner does or asks. For example, when a learner climbs on furniture and the therapist says, "No," the learner's response of climbing off the furniture indicates that the learner understood the therapist's "No." Or when the learner asks whether he can have a piece of candy, and the therapist says, "Yes," then the learner gets a piece of candy, but if the therapist says, "No," the learner refrains from getting a piece of candy. This is also relevant when teaching the language concept of negation. For example, when teaching the learner to understand the words "don't" and "can't," the therapist might say, "Don't jump on the bed" when the learner is jumping on the bed, or the therapist might say, "You can't have that" when the learner is about to take something. Another example of modifying the listener behavior format involves teaching prepositions. For example, the therapist might give the learner an object and provide an instruction in which the preposition varies. The therapist might hand the learner a doll and a toy bed and provide the instruction, "put *on top*" or "put *under*."

TACTS

Tacts are verbal behavior under the control of a nonverbal stimulus. For example, a learner sees a car (nonverbal stimulus) and says, "car," or sees a group of children wearing party hats, eating cake, and playing games (nonverbal stimuli) and says, "It's a birthday party." The nonverbal stimuli evoke the verbal response. Reinforcement for a tact, unlike a mand, is not specific to the verbal response. The tact "car" is reinforced when someone says, "Yes, it is a car" or "That's right" – the listener does not *give* the speaker a car. Simply described, a tact is used to label or comment on things in one's environment.

Discrete Trial Training

Tacting should be taught using both DTT and NET. When using DTT to teach tacts, a nonverbal stimulus and instruction are presented. Then, the learner responds, and a consequence is delivered indicating if the response was correct or incorrect. For example, a therapist shows the learner a picture of a car and says, "What is it?" The learner responds, "Car," and reinforcement is delivered.

Combining receptive and tact training. Receptive trials can be effectively embedded as prompts in DTT tact training. To do this, conduct a standard receptive trial for a target that you are teaching as a tact and then immediately follow up a correct learner response to the receptive trial by conducting a quick tact trial. For example, the following teaching interaction would be conducted in rapid succession:

- **Therapist**: "Touch the car."
- **Learner**: Touches the car
- **Therapist**: "That's right!" and then immediately holds up the car and asks, "What is it?"
- **Learner**: "Car."
- **Therapist**: "Great job! It is a car!"

Just as with any prompt, the immediately preceding receptive trials need to be faded out, either within session or across successive sessions, contingent upon continued correct performance. In addition to working as an effective prompt for teaching tacts, this mixed receptive-expressive approach has been shown to be effective in teaching children the ability to generalize between tacts and receptive responses, a repertoire known as generalized naming or generalized derived symmetry (Greer, Stolfi, & Pistoljevic, 2007).

Natural Environment Training

During NET, the therapist interacts with the learner as he moves around in the environment, taking advantage of opportunities to teach him to tact. The therapist asks the learner to label things as he contacts various stimuli in the environment (e.g., playing with toys, seeing people, hearing sounds, tasting food). If the learner is playing with an animal puzzle, the therapist might point to the cow and ask, "What animal?" to which the learner would tact, "Cow." Then, when the learner's mom walks into the room, the therapist might point to her and ask, "Who is it?" to which the learner would tact, "Mom." Next, when the therapist and learner hear a dog barking, the therapist might ask, "What do you hear?" and the learner would tact, "Barking."

Spontaneous Tacts

While pure (spontaneous) tacts occur in the absence of an instruction, it is initially important to include an instruction (e.g., "What is it?") when teaching a learner to label things because this is the cue that tells the learner that it is appropriate to name things in the environment. However, the learner is not yet finished learning to tact until she is able to tact spontaneously under the control of a nonverbal stimulus instead of an instruction. It is perfectly natural for humans to tact novelty in their environments without instruction. For example, when driving on the freeway and observing someone hang gliding in the distance, most people will tact by pointing it out and saying something like, "Cool! A hang glider." Young children tact when airplanes are flying overhead or if they see a cute puppy.

To teach the learner to tact in the absence of instruction, you can bring interesting or novel things into the learner's environment and use either an echoic or gestural (point at items and look expectantly at the learner) prompt to encourage the learner to label the item. You may also label many objects per hour, throughout all activities in your therapy session, and require the learner to vocally imitate you when you do this. When the learner begins to tact spontaneously on her own, begin to fade out the tacts you are making. You might also do activities that are highly preferred by the learner and then suddenly stop until she tacts something interesting in the environment (and then restart). For example, while on a walk, you might suddenly stop walking and not restart until the learner labels something interesting that just occurred. Regardless of which prompting methods you use, you will have to fade them out over time in order to bring the learner's response under the control of the nonverbal stimuli themselves. On a side note, keep in mind that it is not normal to walk around labeling things all day long, so the goal should be for the learner only to tact things that are either new or interesting. Table 11.5 lists examples of spontaneous tacts that can be taught during tact training.

TABLE 11.5   Sample Tact Targets

Antecedent: A Novel or Preferred Stimulus Occurs in the Learner's Environment Learner's Response: Identifying/Naming/Labeling/Commenting on the Antecedent Stimulus Specific Examples		
Lesson	**Antecedent**	**Learner's Response**
Objects	An airplane flies overheard.	*"Airplane!"*
People	Mommy comes home.	*"Mommy's* here!"
Actions	During a parade, a bulldog is riding a skateboard.	"Look, the dog is *riding a skateboard!"*
Attributes	The learner sees a penny on the ground.	"The penny is *shiny."*
I Have/I See	While riding in a car, the learner is looking out the window and sees a puppy.	"I *see* a puppy."
Same/Different	The learner sees a peer wearing a bracelet.	"We have the *same* bracelet."
Sound Discrimination	A fire alarm is going off.	*"Fire alarm!"*
Features	The learner sees a fish tank full of fish.	"That fish has *spikes."*
Categories	The learner enters a petting zoo.	"Look at all the *animals!"*
Prepositions	The learner sees a lizard in a tank crawl under a log.	"He went *under* the log!"
Plurals	The learner takes three cookies; a peer only takes one.	"I have lots of *cookies."*
Negation	The learner sees Bambie fall again and again.	"Bambie *can't* walk."
Adverbs	The learner's dog is snoring.	"He snores *loudly."*
Sequences – First, Then, Last	The learner is looking at an illustration in a book.	"Mary is *first* in line, *then* comes Peter, and *last* is Suzie."
Sequences – Before/After	The learner has to wait his turn.	"I get to go *after* Brian."
Relationships	The learner sees a peer's grandma at the grocery store.	"That's Jay's *grandma."*
Opposites	The learner has an empty cup, and a peer has a full cup.	"Yours is *full*, and mine is *empty*. We have *opposites."*

INTRAVERBALS

Intraverbals are verbal behavior under the control of a verbal stimulus. However, unlike echoics, intraverbals do not have point-to-point correspondence or formal similarity to the verbal stimulus that evokes them. In other words, the response does not match the antecedent. For example, the verbal stimuli "A and B" evoke the intraverbal response "C." Similar to echoics and tacts, reinforcement for intraverbal behavior is not specific to the form of the response. Skinner (1957) discussed that much of what is traditionally referred to as conversational speech, question answering, a series of numbers, letters, or words (e.g., saying "go" after hearing "ready, set..."), word associations (e.g., saying "white" after hearing "black"), and translations (e.g., saying "gracias" in response to "thank you") is, in fact, intraverbal behavior. Table 11.6 lists examples of intraverbal targets across lessons.

TABLE 11.6   Sample Intraverbal Targets

Antecedent: Therapist Presents a Verbal Stimulus (e.g., Statement, Question, Instruction)
Learner's Response: Verbal Response (e.g., Statement, Question, Series of Words)
Specific Examples

Lesson	Antecedent	Learner's Response
Yes/No	"Do cows say 'woof woof'?"	"No."
Sound Discrimination	"What does a cat say?"	"Meow."
Choices	"What would you like to work on first?"	"Math."
Gestures	"What's the plan?"	Learner shrugs shoulders.
Features	"What has a *beak*?" / "What does a bird have?"	"A bird." / "Beak."
Functions	"What do you use a *chair* for?" / "What do you use *for sitting*?"	"To sit." / "A chair."
Categories	"What is a *bus*?" / "Name a *vehicle*."	"A *vehicle*." / "A bus."
Describe	"*Tell me about* an airplane."	"It has wings, you fly in it, and it's a vehicle."
Same / Different	"How are a pig and a dog the *same/different*?"	"They are both animals." / "One has paws, and one has hooves."

Continued

TABLE 11.6 Sample Intraverbal Targets—cont'd

Antecedent: Therapist Presents a Verbal Stimulus (e.g., Statement, Question, Instruction)
Learner's Response: Verbal Response (e.g., Statement, Question, Series of Words)
Specific Examples

Lesson	Antecedent	Learner's Response
Negation	"Do elephants fly?"	"No, they *don't*."
I Don't Know	"How old is your dad?"	"*I don't know.*"
Opposites	"What is the *opposite* of rough?"	"*Smooth.*"
Ask and Tell	"*Ask* Janie if she wants to come."	"Janie, do you want to come?"
Statement-Statement	"I like chocolate chip cookies."	"I like peanut butter cookies."
Statement-Question	"I went to the beach yesterday."	"Who did you go with?"
Tell a Story	"*Tell me a story about* the pirates finding the deserted island."	"The pirates were all sleeping on their ship when it suddenly crashed into something. They ran out on the deck and saw they had crashed into an island. It was a treasure island!"
Actions: Noun-Verb Agreement	"What *do* horses eat?" / "What *does* a horse eat?"	"Horses *eat* hay." / "A horse *eats* hay."

Discrete Trial Training

Intraverbals are often taught using DTT and NET. When using DTT to teach intraverbals, a vocal stimulus is presented, the learner responds, and a consequence is delivered indicating whether the response was correct or incorrect. For example, a therapist says, "What color is the sky?" Then, the learner says, "Blue," and reinforcement is delivered.

Natural Environment Training

When using NET, the therapist interacts with the learner as she moves around in the environment, taking advantage of opportunities to teach intraverbals. The therapist presents vocal stimuli and waits for the learner to respond, providing prompts when necessary. For example, the learner might begin building a tower with blocks and the therapist might ask, "Do you like playing with blocks?" The learner might say, "Yes." Then, the learner might request a snack, so the therapist might ask, "What is your favorite snack?" to which the learner might respond, "I like chips." Next, the learner might begin playing with ABC magnets, and the therapist might say, "Let's sing the ABC's, A, B, C, D...," to which the learner might respond, "E, F, G."

Prompting and Shaping Intraverbals

Early intraverbal lessons often focus on sentence completion and basic questions that can be answered using a single word. Echoic prompts are commonly used to establish use of an intraverbal response. Initially, an approximation of a word may be accepted as a correct response. Then, as the learner's echoic repertoire and articulation improve, the therapist begins increasing the difficulty of the target response, transitioning from an approximation of the word to the actual word and then to more complex sentences. For example, when a therapist first asks, "Where do you sleep?" the response "ba" may be accepted as correct. Next, the response "bed" is accepted, followed by "in a bed," and, then, "I sleep in a bed."

For learners who can read, textual prompts are also useful for teaching intraverbal behavior such as question answering. When teaching learners to identify categorical intraverbals (e.g., instructions such as "Name an animal"), it can be useful to use a tact response to prompt the initial behavior (by holding up a picture of an animal or by showing multiple cards, one of which is an animal). However, eventually these prompts must be faded out as the learner is successful, so the response is only under the control of the verbal stimulus "name an animal."

IMPROVING ARTICULATION AND INCREASING COMPLEXITY

Articulation

Articulation impacts the success of a learner's entire vocal verbal repertoire because verbal behavior is only useful if others can understand and reinforce it. In the early stages of language development, words may not be clear, making it difficult to understand a learner's request. Begin by requiring the learner to vocalize and reach for the object. This will confirm motivation to access the item and provide an opportunity to work on improving articulation. Initially, it may be necessary to lightly prompt the learner to reach for the object. Then, as articulation improves, reaching for the object will no longer be needed. For example, if a learner says, "waya" and reaches for a water bottle, you might give the learner a drink of water and initiate teaching trials by saying, "Say, 'water,'" in an effort to improve pronunciation of the word.

While some articulation errors may be age appropriate, it is important to emphasize correct articulation to ensure the development of functional vocal speech. Begin by assessing the conditions under which the articulation problem occurs, determining if the problem occurs when saying the single sound or when the sound is a part of a word. If the learner cannot articulate the single sound, devote time to improving oral motor skills to ensure that the learner is using the correct lip and tongue position to produce the sound (see Chapter 14 on oral motor training). Also, emphasize maintenance and continue improving articulation of the sound by frequently practicing the sounds and words that the learner is able to articulate combined with shaping.

If the learner can pronounce the sound in isolation but not when it is included in a word, divide the word into separate sounds that the learner can imitate, and then slowly blend the sounds together. For example, if a learner can say the "d" sound but pronounces the word *red* as "re," begin by instructing the learner to imitate first the beginning sounds and then the end sounds in the word. Specifically, you would say, "Say, 're,'" and when the learner responds, "re," you would say, "Say, 'd,'" followed by the learner saying, "d." Then, bring the sounds closer together by decreasing the delay between the sounds (e.g., "Say, 're...d'"), until the learner is pronouncing the word correctly. For learners who are having particular difficulty with words that contain multiple phonemes, consider starting with words that repeat the same phoneme (e.g., ma-ma) before moving on to words that consist of different phonemes (e.g., ma-mee).

Complete Sentences and Grammar

In the early stages of language development, it is common to reinforce sentences with incorrect grammar, and then as conversation skills develop, grammar becomes increasingly important. When errors occur during conversation, first ensure that the error cannot be attributed to poor articulation. If a grammar error is confirmed, begin by instructing the learner to imitate simple sentences with correct grammar, advancing to more complex sentences as grammar improves. For example, if the learner has difficulty using plural words and often says, "I see two dog" or "Can I have more cookie?" instruct the learner to say, "I see two dogs" and "Can I have more cookies?" Or, if the learner excludes articles and often says, "Give me ball" or "I want to read book," instruct the learner to say, "Give me the ball" and "I want to read a book." Initially, work on grammar in a lesson separate from other language lessons to minimize extinction of existing language skills due to poor grammar. Then, as grammar skills progress, begin requiring the learner to use correct grammar during everyday speech.

When errors in word order are observed, begin by identifying the segment of the sentence where the error happens. Then, separate that segment from the rest of the response chain, and instruct the learner to imitate that portion of the response. For example, if you were to say, "What is in the backyard?" and the learner were to answer, "I see a tree pine big backyard," the next step would be to isolate the phrase where the error occurred and say, "Say, 'big pine tree,'" at which point the learner should respond, "Big pine tree." When imitation of this phrase is consistently correct, extend the length of the phrase by saying, "Say, 'big pine tree in the backyard.'" The length of the sentence should continue to increase until the learner is able to respond using correct sentence structure when asked, "What is in the backyard?"

When using vocal imitation to extend the length of a sentence or to correct grammatical errors, a learner may have difficulty understanding whether an echoic response or intraverbal response will be reinforced if the instruction "say" is excluded. For example, if a therapist is teaching a learner to say "I want a book," the therapist may prompt by saying, "I want a...." Then, the learner may respond with an echoic response and say, "I want a book" (correct response), or the learner may respond with an intraverbal response and say, "book" (incorrect response). The inclusion of the instruction "say" assists in the discrimination between when an echoic response or an intraverbal response will be reinforced. Using the same example, the therapist may say, "Say, 'I want a,'" to which the learner might respond by saying, "I want a book." In this case, reinforcement is delivered. However, if the learner responds by saying, "book," no reinforcement is delivered. Alternatively, when targeting an intraverbal response, the therapist may say, "Let's sing the alphabet, A, B, C," and if the learner responds by saying, "D, E, F, G," reinforcement is delivered.

A textual prompt can be used as an alternative to vocal imitation if the learner is able to read. When using this prompting method, a textual stimulus is presented immediately prior to the portion of the response where the error occurs. For example, when the therapist asks, "What is in the backyard?" and the learner consistently makes an error after saying, "I see a," the therapist might show the learner the words *big pine tree in the* before the learner completes the sentence. In this case, the learner should read the words *big pine tree in the* and then complete the response by saying, "backyard." The textual prompt is only used for the segments of the response during which the error occurs and is faded out as correct responses increase.

The basic verbal operants form the foundation of language learning, but language quickly becomes more complex, with even relatively straightforward sentences consisting of multiple different operants touching on multiple different concepts. For example, the sentence "I went to the store to buy pink candy" contains pronouns, actions, tenses, locations, and colors (each of which is its own lesson, progressing through all operants). Each lesson progresses from the simplest operants (e.g., echoics, mands, and tacts) to complex operants, such as intraverbals. Intraverbals progress from relatively simple intraverbals that involve rote memorization (e.g., reciting particular songs, counting by rote, reciting the alphabet, etc.) to complex intraverbals consisting of conversations about past events and abstract topics. As more lessons progress to the more advanced levels, therapists should focus on teaching longer, more complex language in the natural environment that combines elements of many different lessons, all of which occurr in a flexible, spontaneous manner.

STRATEGIES FOR SUCCESS

Shaping

Shaping can be used across all verbal operants by reinforcing successive approximations of entire words. For example, an initial mand for a car may merely be "c," then "cah," and finally "car." It is common to use shaping when teaching echoics, whereby vocal imitation is gradually shaped, starting with the crudest approximations at imitation and progressing to precisely articulated imitation. Regardless of verbal operant, the same basic steps of shaping described in Chapter 4 can be applied.

Chaining

Chaining is another basic applied behavior analysis (ABA) procedure that can be used successfully in the context of teaching most or all verbal operants. For example, chaining can be used to increase the complexity of mands, starting with one-word mands (e.g., "cracker") and ending with mands that consist of multiple words in a chain (e.g., "Can I have a cracker please?"). Chaining can also be implemented in the context of teaching echoics, starting with echoing single words and progressing to echoing entire sentences. To use chaining to teach echoics, the therapist models the first word in the chain (e.g., "say, 'red'"); the learner imitates, and then the therapist models the second word (e.g., "car"); and then the learner imitates, and so on, until the last word in the chain is imitated, leading to reinforcement. All of the instructions in Chapter 4 on how to implement chaining can be implemented when teaching the various verbal operants.

Maximize Learning Opportunities

Every moment a learner is awake is an opportunity for her to learn something. Maximize learning opportunities throughout the day by conducting as many learning trials as possible, both structured in DTT and less structured in NET. Begin viewing everything in the learner's environment as a learning opportunity. Remember, the more teaching trials you conduct, the more rapidly the learner will learn the skill.

Focus on Establishing Useful Language

Remember that the purpose of teaching language to learners with ASD is to help them become masters of their environment. Language is the most important human repertoire because it allows us to be effective in a way that no other behavior does. Make sure that you are constantly focused on ways to make your learners' newly acquired language skills actually useful in their lives. Every mastered language item should become something that they actually want to use in their daily lives because it makes them more effective at being independent, getting what they want, and having fun with others. Avoid merely teaching the learner to memorize endless lists of language "content."

Nonvocal Options

Children who cannot vocalize words can still learn language because verbal behavior does not necessarily need to be vocal behavior. Listener behavior, such as following instructions and matching, does not require vocal speech. Also, there are nonvocal versions of mands and tacts. Nonvocal mands involve teaching a learner to touch, reach for, point to, or guide another person toward things that he wants. Similarly, nonvocal tacts and intraverbals include alternative forms of communication, such as sign language, picture communication systems, typing, and computerized talking devices. If a learner does not engage in vocal language, it may be appropriate to consider one of these alternative communication methods. An entire chapter in this book is dedicated to visual and other sensory modifications (Chapter 6), so we do not elaborate further here.

SUMMARY

This chapter reviewed several instructional procedures that are useful when teaching language skills to learners with ASD. Lessons in the Language curriculum target both speaker behavior (echoics, mands, tacts, and intraverbals) and listener behavior (matching, receptive identification, and following instructions). Initial instruction focuses on the acquisition of simple verbal responses. As the learner's verbal repertoire develops, the simple verbal responses begin interacting, and complex language emerges. Language skills are an integral part of many social skills, play, academic, cognitive, and executive functions lessons. As such, skills learned in the Language curriculum function as the foundation for more advanced lessons in these curricula.

Play

Jonathan Tarbox, Angela Persicke

Playing is central to child development in a wide variety of ways. In addition to its potential as an important source of fun, a filler of downtime, and an opportunity for imaginations to flourish, play is critical to language development and, most importantly, the first major way in which children learn to navigate the social world. Unfortunately, for many children with autism spectrum disorder (ASD), play does not develop naturally and, quite simply, may not be fun. Therefore, helping children develop rich, robust, variable, and fun play repertoires is a central component to any high-quality comprehensive applied behavior analysis (ABA) treatment program. This chapter will describe the Center for Autism and Related Disorders (CARD) approach to teaching play to children with ASD, including the different types of play repertoires that should be targeted during programming, general approaches to teaching play skills, and tips for success.

The general approach for teaching play skills begins by addressing each domain of play as it emerges in typical child development. Within each area of play, practical strategies are described for building foundational play skills, increasing independence, increasing fun, and, finally, firmly establishing play as a means for productive and enjoyable interactions with peers. It is important to note that the purpose of ABA-based approaches to teaching play skills is *never* to establish rote or memorized scripts or routines but, rather, to establish flexible, variable, and creative repertoires of play behavior. That is, the emphasis is to teach children with ASD to be good at and to love play, not to comply with play demands or simply to do what is expected of them.

WHY BOTHER TEACHING PLAY?

Parents of children with ASD sometimes wonder why their therapists spend so much time playing with their child. Some even find themselves frustrated and asking their clinical supervisor, "When are we going to get to the stuff my child really needs to learn?" There are many great reasons for teaching play. First, if you can make it fun, teaching during play helps the overall learning process become more enjoyable for the learner. Second, play helps to develop rapport between the learner and therapists and makes the learner want to participate in therapy. Third, teaching play skills facilitates varied interests and hobbies that provide the learner with activities to do independently during leisure time, allowing the learner's parents to accomplish their own daily tasks and worry less about "keeping their child busy." Fourth, being able to play is a prerequisite to making and maintaining friendships. Peers play in their free time, and if learners with ASD are to fit in and make friendships, they need to play with peers at school and be involved in playdates after school hours.

Play also serves as the perfect setting in which to develop critical skills across many other domains. Children can learn language skills, such as mands, tacts, and intraverbals, when therapists use natural environment training procedures in the context of play (as described in Chapter 11). Learners develop their gross motor skills through locomotor play, such as freeze tag and dodgeball, and fine motor skills by manipulating toys with small parts (e.g., LEGOS®, beads). Learners indirectly practice daily living skills through play, such as vacuuming with a pretend vacuum, hair brushing through brushing a doll's hair, fastening snaps and buttons when dressing dolls, and cleaning up when putting away toys. Learners practice social skills during play, such as sharing, turn taking, cooperating, negotiating (what and how to play), and conversation skills (answering/asking questions and making reciprocal statements related to the play activity). Multiple executive function skills can be addressed in play, such as flexibility when peers introduce new rules (e.g., who will play the mommy versus the daddy), play sequences (e.g., not doing an activity in the same order every time), and ways of playing with toys (e.g., using a tea set during "restaurant play" instead of a "tea party"). Furthermore, learners can practice problem solving during play when, for example, a piece is missing or broken, a structure keeps falling, batteries stop working, and so on. Likewise, learners can practice planning when they learn to follow an activity schedule for play, choose their own order of play activities (e.g., "I'll do blocks, then puzzles, and then dolls."), and figure out the order of each step of a play activity. Pretend play is also a setting in which learners can be taught basic perspective-taking skills, and learners indirectly learn and practice perspective taking during play when they take on the role of one or more dolls and create an experience for one doll that is different from another doll's experience or their own experience.

DOMAINS OF PLAY

In developing the CARD Play curriculum, we first scoured the research literature in developmental psychology to identify which types of play emerge and at what ages they emerge. The developmental psychology literature provides a rich source of information on the development of play in typically developing children. A behavioral approach to creating a curriculum for teaching play to children with ASD begins with categorizing typical play development into classes of skills or domains. In many cases, the broader classes of play skills can be taken from the developmental literature. In the CARD curriculum, play domains include **Independent, Interactive, Pretend, Constructive**, and **Electronic** play. Each domain is then broken down into smaller, more easily teachable units, each of which is taught individually or in combination with others. Lessons in the Play curriculum are organized by the age during which the skills emerge in typical child development. Figure 12.1 depicts some of the main play skills from the curriculum, in ascending order from age in typical development

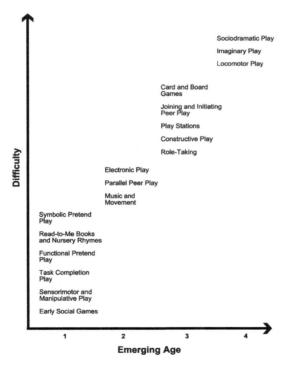

FIGURE 12.1 Types of play in the Play curriculum, organized in ascending order by age in typical development and by relative difficulty of the skills involved. *Reprinted from Skills® with permission from the Center for Autism and Related Disorders.*

and relative difficulty of the skills involved. Appendix E provides an outline of the entire CARD Play curriculum. The goal, of course, is not to teach
children with ASD to memorize particular play behaviors. Rather, the goal
is to establish generalized, flexible play repertoires that the learner can
later recombine into larger, fluid, natural play activities. Therefore, none
of the play domains – and none of the individual behaviors contained
within them – should be considered ends in themselves. Rather, they all
constitute multiple exemplars of the larger repertoire of having fun while
playing flexibly and creatively.

Helping children with ASD learn to love play is perhaps the most important goal of early play intervention, so we recommend that you read
this entire chapter with that goal in mind. Each step of teaching play skills
that you implement across the years of a learner's intervention program
should be oriented toward this goal and should be understood as one piece
of the overall strategy for achieving this goal. Of course, when working
with learners who already love playing with others and already find play
to be genuinely fun, you don't need to worry about achieving this goal.
Even in these cases, however, great care should be taken not to "ruin" the
fun of play by making the learner feel that it's something that he has to do.

Independent Play

During infancy, children use their senses and motor abilities to understand the world, beginning with reflexes and ending with complex
combinations of interactions with toys. Independent play begins with ex-
ploratory play, wherein the child is solely interested in the properties of
the object and not interested in using it in any particular way. The child
then moves on to sensorimotor play, which involves learning that specific
actions performed with the toy cause specific effects, such as pushing a
button to create a sound. Finally, the child moves on to manipulative play,
which occurs when the child has had sufficient opportunities to become
familiar with the object or toy, knows in which ways it can be used, and
performs known and increasingly complex actions to produce a pleasurable experience.

The Play curriculum includes activities in the independent play domain
to facilitate learning how to interact with items in the environment to gain
reinforcement from those interactions. Lessons include sensorimotor and
manipulative play, task completion play, and play stations. Although the
initial goal of these lessons is to imitate appropriate play actions, the ultimate goal is to teach the learner to explore his environment independently
and appropriately through these types of play activities and gain reinforcement through independent play.

Sensorimotor and manipulative play. These activities have a clear goal
and facilitate the learning of a cause-and-effect relationship (e.g., pressing a

button on a toy makes it light up and play a song). Examples of play activities included in the sensorimotor and manipulative play lesson start with simple activities, such as popping bubbles, banging on a drum, pressing hands into buckets of macaroni or beans, ringing bells, etc. These activities have a sensory component in that playing with the items allows the learner to experience different sounds, textures, sights, and motor experiences. This play then progresses into more manipulative play activities, such as jack-in-the-box toys, press-and-spin toys, ball-and-hammer sets, kaleidoscopes, and other toys that require specific play sequences in order to engage with the toy effectively.

Task completion play. These activities are another form of independent play and include play activities that require placement of a specific number of pieces until a specific task is complete, such as puzzles, Mr. Potato Head® toys, shape sorters, stacking rings, nesting cups, and other types of toys that usually have a definite end.

The independent play activities described above emerge between the ages of 1 and 3 years in typically developing populations, but children with ASD often do not demonstrate independent play skills such as these or may inappropriately engage with toys or objects during these types of play activities. Because engaging with objects through independent play activities does not result in natural forms of reinforcement for some children with ASD, it is important to contrive reinforcement for independent play activities initially and then slowly fade to more natural forms of reinforcement. For example, for task completion activities, you may need to contrive reinforcement using more primary types of reinforcement, such as edibles paired with social praise, then fade to social praise alone, and finally intermittently provide social praise, so completing the task becomes reinforcing in and of itself.

Play stations. In order to ensure that the learner is able to engage in sustained play activities and rotate between play activities such as those that are typically present in a school setting, a final lesson about play stations is also included in the independent play domain of the Play curriculum. At 3–4 years of age, children can typically stay engaged in an activity, such as playing with toys, for at least 20 minutes. Once the learner is able to play with various toys independently, you can then create various play stations, and when the learner is approximately 3 years old, you can begin to use this 20-minute marker as a goal for the time it should take for the learner to complete all the stations presented. Teaching learners to rotate between play stations offers many added benefits. For one, learners have activities that they can do independently for periods of time when an adult is unable to interact with them. Rotating between play stations teaches the learner how to start and stop an activity, clean up after the activity, and indirectly manage leisure time. Finally, it prepares learners for the "centers" that are characteristic of preschool and kindergarten classrooms.

Interactive Play

In typical child development, a child's very first introduction to the world of play is through early "games" that parents and family members play with infants, such as peek-a-boo, tickles, lifting the child up in the air, "I'm gonna get you" games, and so on. These interactions begin well before the first year and involve eye contact, physical contact, smiles, and laughing on the part of the infant and the family member. For most typically developing children, eye contact and physical touch are already sources of strong reinforcement, and these early forms of play involve frequent pairing of these reinforcers with the process of interacting with toys and objects. As a result, playing with toys becomes a conditioned source of reinforcement. In other words, typically developing children learn to enjoy playing with toys and other humans without any intentional teaching or conditioning from anyone.

Unfortunately, the whole process described above seems to have gone awry with many children with ASD. When they first enter a treatment program around the ages of 2 to 3 years, many children with ASD do not engage in any kinds of play interactions, especially those requiring early interactive play skills, and they may not show any interest in doing so. It is not yet known why this is the case, but it is possible that social attention and, specifically, eye contact and physical touch, were never strong positive reinforcers for these children. If that is the case, then it would make sense that basic play skills would not develop or become a source of positive reinforcement because they were never paired with reinforcers.

One of the first interactive play lessons is **early social games** (e.g., horsey ride, chase, peek-a-boo). These games can provide fun learning opportunities that support later development of attending skills, event anticipation, understanding sequences of behavior, and sharing humor, suspense, and excitement with another person. The activities in this lesson are also great for developing good rapport with the learner. Many early social games focus on capturing potentially reinforcing social interactions, such as games that cause laughter or surprise in a fun and playful manner. Some of these games can be used later to reinforce the occurrence of other skills. For example, the tickle game is often used to facilitate language (e.g., requests for more tickles); therefore, the tickle game itself, once learned, becomes a reinforcing interaction to use in the acquisition of other skills.

Other early play lessons in this curriculum include **music and movement** activities in which children learn to interact with others through singing and dancing. Finding reinforcement through singing and dancing with others also helps to prepare the learner to participate in unison with peers in social and classroom settings in which singing, gesturing, and dancing are frequently incorporated into the school day. Similarly, other activities, including **read-to-me books and nursery rhymes**, are targeted in the Play curriculum to create opportunities for children to find these activities pleasurable and facilitate social engagement.

The interactive play domain of the Play curriculum also aims to target peer play, including **parallel play** (i.e., playing beside a peer with similar toys but not necessarily interacting yet), **joining and initiating peer play** (now interacting), **card and board games**, **locomotor play** (e.g., follow the leader, tag, catch, keep away, etc.), treasure or scavenger hunts, and other related games and activities. In general, the goal of the interactive play domain is to create opportunities in which the child learns to enjoy interacting with others through play. When first bringing peers into interactive play teaching sessions, it is usually helpful to begin with a peer who naturally tends to lead play interactions and will thereby provide ample opportunities for the learner to imitate her. As the learner acquires the ability to play interactively with one peer, larger groups of two or more peers can be introduced.

Pretend Play

Pretend play refers to play activities that involve interactions with objects to create play scenarios, typically with peers. For instance, playing house is an example of pretend play in which a child interacts with various objects to pretend to set the table, cook a meal, or imitate some common household activity. In typical child development, pretend play begins to emerge early on and consists of several subclasses, beginning with functional and symbolic pretend play and later progressing to imaginary play and role-taking or sociodramatic play. Pretend play is among the most widely recognized deficits in children with ASD, likely because it involves nonliteral behavior (i.e., pretending something is happening that is not) and perspective taking (creating and sharing a false belief with a peer), both of which are skill areas that many children with ASD find challenging (see Chapter 17 on perspective taking). Despite the fact that pretend play does not develop automatically for many children with ASD, it is readily teachable. All of the subclasses of pretend play can be taught, one at a time and in combination, depending on the existing play skills of the learner.

Functional pretend play. Children begin demonstrating functional pretend play skills between the ages of 1 and 3 years. Functional pretend play refers to playing with an object in a manner that reflects its actual function (e.g., using a broom to pretend to sweep the kitchen or using a toy stethoscope to check a teddy bear's heartbeat). Children first begin imitating functional pretend play exhibited by others, especially caregivers or siblings. This may also include imitating housework during play. For example, a 2-year-old may pretend to use a play vacuum to imitate her father vacuuming the house. Additionally, as language develops, children pair common vocal sounds with play skills as they attempt to imitate the sound of the actual object they are using in a play activity (e.g., making a sizzling sound to represent eggs cooking in a pan).

Symbolic play. Symbolic play develops around the same age as functional pretend play and refers to the ability to attribute the properties of one object to another object for the purpose of pretend play (e.g., using a hairbrush as a microphone). Symbolic play requires behavioral flexibility by using objects in a manner different than their intended purpose in order to create play sequences that are imaginative and creative. The ability to engage in symbolic play provides learners with opportunities to obtain reinforcement from sources that are not physically present in the current environment by transforming the properties of various objects, so they can function as different objects. For example, a broom may serve its apparent function in the environment (e.g., sweeping the floor). Through symbolic play, the broom can function as a horse with which to race siblings around the house. A broom itself may not have many reinforcing properties, especially for a young child, but pretending the broom is something that does have reinforcing properties allows children to gain reinforcement by engaging with the objects.

Imaginary play. As children develop more complex forms of play sequences, they begin to engage in imaginary play. Imaginary play does not depend on toys or any other physical objects. Instead, children use language, gestures, and symbolic actions (e.g., pretending to be asleep, pretending to eat imaginary food, gesturing as though they are picking up a telephone, etc.). In typical development, imaginary play skills are observed around 4 years of age. Children begin with simple imaginary play that includes very few actions (e.g., pretending to read a book or walk a dog), and over time, they expand upon these simple forms of imaginary play to include more creative scenarios and engage in multiple action sequences without any physical objects. At this point, children should be able to describe the features of imaginary objects and the environment within the play sequence. For example, if you and the learner are pretending to ride bikes in the park, the learner should be able to describe the bike, the scenery in the park, and whether other people are in the park and what they are doing. It is not uncommon for functional pretend and symbolic play actions to be incorporated into imaginary play sequences. For example, the learner could be playing with a cat figurine (to symbolically represent a tiger) and a lion figurine (functional object) in an African jungle (imaginary location). The distinction between these types of pretend play is that both functional play and symbolic play require physical objects, albeit the physical object for symbolic play is not the actual object it represents, and imaginary pretend play involves creating a scenario in which physical objects are not necessary for the play activity.

Role-taking. Around 3 to 4 years of age, children begin engaging in play activities in which they take on roles of different people or characters during sequences of pretend play activities. For example, when rocking a pretend baby, a child may take on the "mommy" role and use language and actions that represent that character. Often, children first imitate the roles that are prevalent in their own lives, such as imitating phrases used by their caregivers or familiar TV or movie characters. Children can assign roles during play to themselves and to objects. For example, a child may take the role of a dog by crawling around on all fours and barking. A child may assign the "mommy" role to a doll by making a doll talk and act like the mommy.

Sociodramatic play. Role-taking during pretend play develops into sociodramatic play in which multiple people act out roles together. The child may assign various roles to different people as they play together. In sociodramatic play, a number of types of pretend play activities are flexibly incorporated into various pretend play sequences. The ability to engage in these types of pretend play activities demonstrates the child's ability to project multiple pretend properties onto multiple objects and people, as well as himself, to extract reinforcement from the pretend play sequences.

Constructive Play

Constructive play refers to the use of materials or objects to construct other objects or structures. The CARD approach to teaching constructive play includes five subclasses of constructive play: 1) block construction, 2) clay construction, 3) sand and water construction, 4) structure building, and 5) arts and crafts. A few of these subclasses are briefly described below.

Block construction is observed very early in typical development as a fun play activity. Children are observed to imitate the construction of simple block structures with two to five blocks during play at around 1 to 2 years of age and begin copying more complex representations of objects (e.g., a bridge or train) by the age of 3 years. The ability to imitate block structures continues to develop, and children are able to build more sophisticated block structures as they get older. As language develops, children are able to identify block representations of other objects, such as a house or boat, as well as provide narration about what they are making; e.g., "I'm making a wall around the castle." Children with ASD often are not observed to play with blocks in these manners. Including this lesson in a learner's treatment plan will help teach visual attention skills, appropriate play with blocks and representational building, and appropriate language during play. This lesson is a prerequisite to the other constructive play lessons in this category and should be targeted early in intervention. Additionally, learning to construct block structures can contribute to more advanced social play skills when building structures with others.

By the age of 3 years, typically developing children begin constructing various items using different materials, such as clay, Play-Doh®, and sand. Additionally, children begin engaging in other fun activities, including building structures out of common household materials (e.g., building a house or barn using objects, blanket forts, etc.) and undertaking various arts and crafts projects (e.g., paintings, puppets, collages, etc.). The purpose of construction and arts and crafts lessons is to teach the child to participate in, initiate, and have conversations about (e.g., answer questions about their construction, make comments in response to others' comments during play, etc.) the things they are building or creating in order to increase the learner's repertoire of possible appropriate play activities for socialization and to stimulate problem solving, planning (e.g., planning to create a fort and then building it), and creativity. Many of these activities also involve using various items in the environment to represent other items, so these lessons can incorporate the play skills discussed earlier in the section on pretend play.

Electronic Play

As technology becomes more and more prevalent in our culture, it is important to teach learners to use and engage with various electronics in appropriate and meaningful ways. The electronic play domain of the Play curriculum includes audio and video play, computer play, and video games. These lessons teach learners to identify the names and functions of different pieces of electronic equipment (e.g., power, play, pause, and stop buttons), initiate play with these devices, and use the devices independently when desired. Video game play may also facilitate learning the prosocial behaviors of sharing and turn taking, good sportsmanship, and emotional self-control when losing to an opponent. For ways that these social skills can be targeted specifically, see Chapter 16 on the Social curriculum. Additionally, video game play exposes the learner to rule-based games and fantasy role-play and potentially may develop into a hobby that will enable the learner to connect with his peers.

PROGRESSION THROUGH PLAY TRAINING

Imitation

A large proportion of early play involves learning to imitate the play behaviors of others, including parents, siblings, and so on. The goal of imitation activities in play instruction is to teach the learner the generalized ability to watch what others are doing during play and to try it herself. This generalized play imitation repertoire is established through reinforcement of multiple individual exemplars of imitating specific behaviors. For example, in functional pretend play, the therapist might take a toy train and drive it back and forth while saying, "choo choo," thereby providing an opportunity for the learner to imitate the action and the sound. At first, the therapist would deliver vocal model prompts ("do this" or "say, 'choo choo'"), reinforce when the learner imitates, and fade out prompts over time. Similarly, with symbolic play, the therapist might hold a plastic banana up to her ear as though she were talking on the phone and say, "hello," thereby providing an opportunity for the learner to do the same and receive reinforcement.

Imitation sequences. In each play lesson, once a child has learned to imitate a few basic play behaviors, you can start to chain them together and have the learner imitate sequences of known play behaviors. In doing so, make sure that you are not saying "do this" between each step of the play chain; rather, only say it once at the beginning and then add an additional action for the learner to imitate until the learner is following along with any new action you add to the sequence. Over time, you should be able to fade out the instruction "do this," as well. The point here is to increase the complexity of play behavior, not to memorize particular sequences. Therefore, present different sequences of play behaviors. For example, if the learner can already imitate pretending behaviors such as eating toy food, putting toy food on a plate, and putting pretend ketchup on toy food, you can model all possible sequences of these three behaviors at different times and prompt and reinforce imitation of the sequences.

Narration

Children often provide narration during play. For example, while pretending to cook toy food, a child might say, "I'm making a hamburger." If and when a child has sufficient vocal speech to make teaching such narration not unduly difficult, it may be time to add it to the learner's play program. Generally speaking, start small and easy with play skills that are already mastered and, ideally, ones that the learner enjoys. Provide a vocal model, reinforce, and fade out the prompting and reinforcement as the learner continues to narrate independently. As with all play skills, do not just teach one particular narration. The goal is to increase narration overall, so prompting and reinforcing a large variety of narrations are key. Ideally, you should collect data separately on new narrations that have not been directly taught, as well as directly taught narrations that occur in the presence of different play behaviors (e.g., saying, "I'm going fast" while playing with a horse, even though only motor vehicles have been included in training so far), as these will provide evidence that a generalized repertoire of narrating is emerging.

Increasing Complexity: Chains and Themes

After a child has learned a variety of basic play behaviors across a variety of different toys, she may be ready to start learning to combine them into chains that are relevant to particular play "themes." Popular play themes include cooking and eating, playing dress-up with dolls, fixing/building with toy tools, tea time, self-care routines with dolls (brushing, bathing, etc.), and so on. Some themes conventionally occur in a particular order; for example, one generally cooks food before eating it. These themes should be taught in conventional sequence, but still be cautious and make sure you are not teaching rigid sequences of play behavior. For instance, you could contrive situations in which something in the sequence is missing and the learner needs to problem solve and determine what can be used instead or determine a different way to achieve the same outcome of the conventional sequence. There should be many variations within a given sequence (e.g., cooking on a frying pan versus in an oven, putting ketchup on food versus salt and pepper, etc.). Other themes have no conventional sequence, so be extra careful not to teach the same sequences repeatedly.

Increasing Independence

The social aspect of play is by far the most important; however, as any parent will tell you, it is also important for children to have meaningful ways to fill their downtime. Generally speaking, the more fun activities that children know how to do independently, the less time they are likely to spend engaging in stereotypy or destructive behavior when they have free time. Thus, work on teaching the learner to initiate preferred play activities and to play independently for periods of time. As mentioned earlier in the independent play section, play stations are a great way to increase the length of independent play.

Teaching How to Extract Reinforcement Out of Play

Play may not be fun at first for many children with ASD. If an activity is not fun (i.e., not automatically reinforcing), then it makes sense that a child would not want to do it if given the choice. With that in mind, until play has become genuinely fun for the learner, do not be discouraged if she does not want to play on her own, nor should you expect her to do so. However, the vast majority of children with ASD do, indeed, learn to find play to be a rich source of fun in their lives if given effective training in play skills. An analogy from your own life may help to clarify the point. Imagine a new television that you do not know how to turn on and that you cannot figure out on your own. After the initial frustration of finding out that it does not work (so you think), you will not spend very much time using the television because it is not a source of reinforcement for you. Now, imagine that a teacher comes along and teaches you how to turn on your television and how to change the channels. Of course, you will use the television more in the future! In this example, the teacher teaches you how to extract reinforcement out of the television, and that is exactly what we do when teaching play skills to children with ASD.

Conditioning Play to Be a Source of Reinforcement

As discussed in Chapter 4, classical conditioning plays a major role in comprehensive Early Intensive Behavioral Intervention (EIBI) programs because many things in a child's life that were previously neutral or nonpreferred can be conditioned to become a source of enjoyment. The main example discussed in Chapter 4 was social attention and the importance of pairing social approval with other previously established reinforcers, thereby resulting in social approval becoming an effective source of reinforcement for the child. A very similar process is crucial to effective play intervention. Through positively reinforcing the behavior of playing with a previously neutral toy, the toy itself is paired with strong reinforcers repeatedly, and the toy can then become a source of conditioned positive reinforcement. As a result, we see toys that were uninteresting to the learner early in treatment become favorites later in treatment. To make this process work, you must keep in mind the basics of classical conditioning, which we will now outline.

Many pairings of the neutral toy and the established reinforcer must occur. This may be daunting, but hundreds – perhaps even thousands – of pairings may need to occur before the previously neutral toy becomes a source of conditioned positive reinforcement for the learner. Just as a learner may need to practice dozens of learning trials per day to learn a new language skill, a learner may require dozens of pairings of positive reinforcement of play behavior with a particular toy or set of toys in order for there to be a sufficient number of pairings for classical conditioning to occur. A common error is to assume that therapists will remember to implement enough learning opportunities with play targets during "downtime" or between blocks of discrete trial training without actually specifying how many of these learning opportunities therapists need to implement. A better strategy is to use a checklist or datasheet that specifies the minimum number of times the therapist is expected to reinforce particular target play behaviors with particular toys.

The neutral toy and established reinforcer must occur close in time. To ensure that a toy that is currently not pleasurable or reinforcing to the learner becomes reinforcing, the established reinforcer (e.g., food item, tickles, etc.) must be presented close in time with the presentation of the toy or activity. It is best if the established reinforcer is presented concurrently, if possible, or at least within three seconds of the presentation of the toy or activity. For example, when establishing a sensorimotor toy (e.g., a light-up musical toy) as a reinforcer, you would present the toy and then immediately present some small piece of a preferred food item that is a known reinforcer. As noted in the previous section, many pairings may have to occur before a toy or activity becomes a conditioned positive reinforcer. Therefore, consider the types of established reinforcers used during pairings, especially if food items are used, because the learner will most likely become satiated with some types of reinforcers, and these items may no longer facilitate establishing the neutral toy as a reinforcing item. For example, if a food item is paired with the toy 10 times in a short period, the learner may become full and will no longer want the food item; therefore, it will have very little reinforcing effects until the learner is hungry again.

In addition to pairing an established reinforcer immediately with the presentation of a toy, reinforcement should also be provided as the learner begins to engage in appropriate play behaviors to facilitate the likelihood that engaging with toys in appropriate ways will occur more frequently. It is likely that once the presentation of the toy becomes established as a conditioned reinforcer, the learner will show interest in the toy and will begin exploring its properties. In the beginning, it is important to provide reinforcement for any attempt to engage with the toy, including simply touching it or picking it up.

Avoid making the situation frustrating or overly demanding. Remember that the point of this activity is to make playing with the toy genuinely fun, not to work on compliance. If you are sensing that the learner wants to escape, that is a sign that you are not making it fun enough. If you have placed a clear demand, make sure you follow through (as always), but do not continue to place additional demands that make the situation frustrating or boring to the learner. Go back to the drawing board and figure out a way to make it more fun. The first thing to consider is whether you really have a powerful reinforcer to pair with the toy that you are trying to make a conditioned reinforcer.

The already-established reinforcer must be powerful. If you want a reinforcer to be effective in conditioning another stimulus to be a reinforcer, then it needs to be powerful. Pairing a weak reinforcer with a neutral stimulus is not likely to be effective, so don't bother implementing that lesson until you find a powerful reinforcer. Also, don't forget to assess preferences frequently with a brief multiple stimulus without replacement (MSWO) (see Chapter 4) in order to ensure that the reinforcer is preferred in the moment.

Requesting Play

Requesting a peer to play and/or requesting particular responses from peers during play are important parts of a child's overall play repertoire. However, it is common for clinicians to make the mistake of going straight to teaching a child with ASD to ask others to play with her before ensuring that the child actually *wants* to play with the peer. In other words, there is no reason to learn how to request something you don't actually want. Therefore, wait until there are particular play activities that are genuinely fun for the learner, and then teach her to ask other people to do it with her. When the learner is ready, you can consider teaching requests, such as "Let's play," "Play with me," "Can I play?" and so on. Keep in mind that requesting is a form of manding, so you should apply what you know about mand training in terms of contriving establishing operations, and so on (see mand training in Chapter 11).

STRATEGIES FOR SUCCESS IN TEACHING PLAY

In this section, we briefly describe a short list of strategies that are helpful in maximizing success. Each time you review your learner's play intervention, it is worth briefly considering each one of the points described below.

Be Creative, Fun, Energetic, and Positive

Play is often not reinforcing for the therapist, but she needs to appear to the learner as if she is having fun. When teaching play skills, the therapist is inevitably modeling play, even when unintended. Therefore, therapists need to model it well in all play interactions. This can be awkward for many therapists, as the honest truth is that many therapists may not know how to play with children and do not feel comfortable doing so. This is understandable but is not acceptable. Being great at playing with children is a foundational prerequisite for being able to deliver comprehensive treatment to children with ASD, and there is no way to avoid this. Fortunately, playing is a skill that can be taught to therapists through modeling, roleplay, and feedback. It may seem a bit ironic that the therapist who is going to teach the learner how to play does not already know how to play, but it is simply true in some cases, and avoiding this fact will not make it go away. Therapists may well need to be repeatedly trained and videotaped and given honest feedback with opportunities for repeated practice until mastery. Keep in mind that the same behavioral principles apply when you are training therapists in this way, and try to make it fun for the therapists. This is a perfect setting for letting loose and not taking yourself so seriously – make jokes and have fun!

Pick Compatible Play Partners

When teaching interactive play, you or the learner's parents will need to identify and recruit peers to be play partners. Recruiting play partners who are consistently available can be a challenge, and parents will often take whomever they can get. However, it is important to consider the characteristics of the play partners from the beginning. Consistent play partners may well turn into meaningful and enduring friendships for the learner, so it is important to recruit play partners whose interests overlap with the learner's. Typically developing children generally make friends with peers who like similar games, sports, music, and so on, and it makes sense for you and the learner's parents to consider the same variables when selecting potential play partners for the learner.

Include Items and Activities That Are Motivating

Children with ASD (like all children) will be more motivated to learn if the learning materials include items that are preferred. A learner may not yet know how to play with a particular toy in the way in which it is intended, but the learner is likely to have preferences between toys. Include toys that he likes, whenever possible. Accordingly, not every child with ASD needs to learn to play with every commonly used toy or engage in every commonly played game just because other children do. Just as you wouldn't force a typically developing child to play every conceivable sport, there is no reason that a child with ASD has to play everything that is common in the typically developing population.

Teach Skills in Social Context, Not Mere Mastery of Particular Behaviors

As with most skills, it is crucial that we teach play skills with flexibility, creativity, and enjoyment. Therefore, it is important when teaching play skills to avoid teaching using the exact same activities, items, or games, so play skills are not under sole control of those activities. For example, it is not necessary to focus on "mastery" of total completion of one particular puzzle; instead, focus on the learner's ability to complete various puzzles in context with a peer.

Picture Activity Schedules for Increasing Independence in Play

To promote independence during play, try using picture activity schedules that show the various toy sequences or play stations in the order that the learner is expected to engage with them. In some cases, you can also use picture activity schedules to teach or remind learners of the steps involved in a play sequence. At each play station, for instance, you could have a separate picture activity schedule that shows each step of the activity. For example, a book for teaching how to make a simple arts and crafts project might first have a picture of someone coloring a witch, then a picture of the person cutting out the witch, then a picture of someone gluing pre-cut string to the witch's head to represent hair, and so on. See Chapter 6 for more information about picture activity schedules.

Have Two Sets of Materials Available

This tip may seem obvious, but it's often forgotten: Have two sets of toys available, one for you and one for the learner. Especially when you are modeling play and teaching parallel play, having two sets of materials available will make it so that the learner and you don't have to hand toys back and forth while you model and the learner imitates.

COMMON PITFALLS IN TEACHING PLAY

In this section, we describe common mistakes in teaching play to children with ASD. When troubleshooting your learner's play intervention program, consider each of the points described below.

Being Overly Repetitive

This general tip could be included in every chapter in this book (and probably is). We want the learner to have variable play repertoires, so make sure your teaching is variable. You might be thinking to yourself, "Aren't I supposed to provide repeated practice? Isn't that how learning occurs?" The answer is yes, but repeated practice consists of repeatedly engaging in some kind of play, not literally repeating the same behavior or sequences of behaviors over and over. It's easy for therapists to fall into routines for how they teach play because it's easier to remember and it requires less planning and creativity, but it's bad for the learner's play repertoire. As a general rule, the learner should not be able to predict exactly how you are going to teach him play on any given day, and you should not be able to predict exactly which play behaviors he is going to do at any given moment. Variability in teaching procedures is key to success, and variability in child responding is the evidence that you are achieving success!

Completely Unmodified Free Play

Clinicians often do not want to upset the learner, and they want play to be fun, so they might just let the learner do whatever she wants during play. While following the learner's lead and incorporating learner preference into play lessons are both good ideas, you likely won't create enough opportunities for the child to learn something new if you only let her do whatever she wants. After all, the learner is just trying to have fun; she's not trying to teach herself new ways to play.

Waiting Too Long to Include Peers

A common mistake is to assume that a child with ASD is not ready to use her newly learned play skills with peers until she has mastered a large repertoire of play. Learners with ASD do not need to know how to do every type of play with every type of toy before beginning peer play. Once learners can imitate others when told "do this" and can follow simple instructions, they are ready to have peers included in play. Of course, a therapist needs to be present, just as he normally is during play training, in order to prompt when necessary and to make sure the interaction goes well. Particularly astute peers may even be directly involved in training efforts, if they like and if their parents permit it. A substantial amount of research has shown that peer tutoring approaches are successful in teaching a variety of skills and that involving peers typically results in improvements in relationships with them.

If the learner attends preschool, when choosing a peer, it's worthwhile to observe the learner in his preschool setting to identify another student in the class who attempts to interact with him. This shows that the peer already has an interest in the learner. Moreover, this helps to recruit outgoing and "bossy" peers who like to be the leader.

When setting up peer play sessions, have preplanned activities for the learner and peer to do together (e.g., tea party, etc.). During the session, teach the peer to instruct the learner by saying "do this" or by giving simple play instructions (e.g., "brush the doll's hair"). Make sure to provide ample praise to the peer when she helps in this way. Also, have goodies planned to give to both children at the end of the play date, so that the peer wants to come back again and the learner's participation is reinforced.

SUMMARY

Play is an integral component of behavioral intervention that is important to so many other skills that develop in childhood. CARD's approach to teaching play addresses each area of play as it occurs in typical child development with the goal of making therapy fun, increasing independent leisure activities, and helping the learner to develop skills needed for making friends, all the while further developing and practicing other skills within the CARD curricula (motor, adaptive, social, executive functions, and cognition). The particular domains of play to address include interactive, independent, pretend, constructive, and electronic play, and key strategies for teaching play skills include training imitation, instruction following, narration, and increasingly complex play themes and sequences.

Adaptive

Jonathan Tarbox, Angela Persicke, Ryan Bergstrom

This chapter will describe how to teach adaptive skills to children with autism spectrum disorder (ASD). Technically speaking, the term *adaptive* refers to any skill or behavior that will help individuals function better in their daily lives. In common usage, and in this chapter, the term *adaptive* refers to skills that promote independence and self-determination in skill domains not covered in the other chapters. The skills described in this chapter are also often referred to as "daily living skills," "independent living skills," "activities of daily living," and "self-help skills." They include skills such as dressing oneself, feeding oneself, ordering food at a restaurant, shopping, and crossing the street safely. Adaptive skills are often overlooked in behavioral intervention programs because it is common for young children, with or without ASD, to rely on their parents to assist with many activities of daily living. However, it is crucial to begin focusing on these skills at a young age because many children with ASD will not develop them without explicit treatment, and it is easy to overlook adaptive skills when focusing primarily on communication, challenging behavior, social skills, and academics. Independent daily living skills can make a great impact on the quality of life and degree of independence achieved by older children and adults with ASD, often far more of an impact than learning academic skills that individuals with ASD may have far less opportunity to use in their daily lives.

Chaining is probably the single most useful procedure for teaching many daily living skills, especially in the personal and domestic domains described below. These procedures have already been described in Chapter 4, so we will not repeat them here. However, in the personal and domestic domains below, we provide sample task analyses taken from the Skills® curriculum (www.skillsforautism.com; see Chapter 26). Keep in mind that a particular daily living skill can be analyzed in many different ways, and these examples are not exact prescriptions for what you should do with any individual learner.

ADAPTIVE SKILL DOMAINS

The Center for Autism and Related Disorders (CARD) Adaptive curriculum is divided into four domains: 1) personal, 2) domestic, 3) safety, and 4) community. Tables 13.1 and 13.2 list lessons from each domain. Appendix F provides an outline of the entire CARD Adaptive curriculum. In the following sections, we provide recommendations for how to teach sample skills in each domain.

TABLE 13.1   Personal Domain of the CARD Adaptive Curriculum

Personal Domain		
Lessons	**Activities**	
Feeding	Self-feeding Drinking from a cup/straw	Using utensils Using a napkin
Undressing and Dressing	Front-opening clothing Pull-up and pull-down clothing Socks Pull-over clothing	Shoes Coordinating clothing Dressing for weather
Unfastening and Fastening	Zippers Bows Buttons Snaps	Buckles Laces Knots
Toileting	Bladder training Bowel training	Indication training Nocturnal toileting
Preventing the Spread of Germs	Washing hands Blowing nose	Covering mouth Avoiding individuals with illness
Teeth Care	Brushing teeth Using mouthwash	Flossing
Hair Care	Brushing/Combing hair Styling hair	Using a hair dryer
Bathing	Using the faucet Washing face	Drying hair and body Washing hair and body
Health Care	Applying lotion/sunscreen Caring for minor cuts	Following special diets Taking medicine
Nail Care	Cleaning nails	Filing and clipping nails

TABLE 13.2 Domestic, Safety, and Community Domains of the CARD Adaptive Curriculum

Domestic Domain

Lessons	Skills	
Tidying and Chores	Putting items away after use Making a bed Taking the trash out Cleaning up spills	Dusting Watering plants Raking leaves
Snacks and Meals	Obtaining a snack/drink Meal preparation	Using appliances School lunch
Clothing Care	Placing dirty clothing in hamper Sorting dirty clothing	Folding and hanging clothing
Setting and Clearing the Table	Clearing the table Wiping the table	Setting the table
Pet Care	Feeding the pet Letting the pet out Brushing the pet	Walking the dog Bathing the dog Picking up feces

Safety Domain

Lessons	Skills	
Safety Awareness	Following safety rules Identifying safe versus dangerous Stranger safety Seatbelt safety	Pedestrian safety Safety signs and traffic symbols Responding to emergencies
Safety Equipment	Putting on safety equipment Removing safety equipment	

Community Domain

Lessons	Skills	
Shopping	Using a cart Finding items	Requesting information Making purchases
Restaurant Readiness	Disposing of unwanted food Ordering from a menu	Buffet lines
Telephone Skills	Answering the phone Summoning others to the phone Taking a message	Making phone calls Finding a phone number

Personal

Personal self-care skills probably represent the majority of daily living skills that you will need to teach children with ASD. Below is a sample task analysis for hand washing taken from the CARD curriculum in the Skills® system (see Chapter 26). See Skills® for a complete list of lessons to teach in the personal domain, as well as comprehensive task analyses for each. Note that the task analysis below was intentionally written to include every conceivable step that *might* need to be included in a task analysis. Many learners will not require hand washing to be broken down into such small steps, and the steps can therefore be combined into larger chunks of behavior, as you see fit. (For a simplified version of the handwashing task analysis, see Chapter 4.) If you are working with a learner who has particular difficulty learning self-care skills, you may be wise to keep all of the steps listed below in your task analysis.

Hand Washing

1. The child goes to the faucet.
2. The child turns on the faucet using his preferred hand.
3. The child tests the water temperature using his non-preferred hand.
4. The child adjusts the temperature as necessary using his preferred hand.
5. The child places both of his hands under the water to wet them.
6. The child pumps a quarter-sized dollop of soap onto his non-preferred hand using his preferred hand. (Skip this step and go to step 7 if the child is using a bar of soap.) Go to step 10.
7. The child picks up the bar of soap with his preferred hand.
8. The child rubs the bar of soap between his hands at least two times.
9. The child places the bar of soap back in its place.
10. The child rubs both of his hands together to disperse soap.
11. The child places both of his hands under the water.
12. The child rubs his palms together vigorously.
13. The child rubs his left hand over his right hand to clean the top of his right hand and fingers.
14. The child rubs his right hand over his left hand to clean the top of his left hand and fingers.
15. The child repeats steps 11–14 until all of the soap has been rinsed off.
16. The child turns off the faucet using his preferred hand.
17. The child goes to the location where the towel rack is located.
18. The child retrieves a towel from the rack.
19. The child uses the towel to dry his hands.
20. The child places the towel back on the rack.

Toilet training. Toilet training is among the most important independent living skills you can teach to an individual with developmental disabilities. It has a profound impact on independence and on the lives of the child's family and other caregivers. This lesson is categorized under the *personal* domain of the Adaptive curriculum, but because of its importance, we will devote a substantial amount of space to describing how to toilet train. Below is an example of a task analysis of a beginning toileting routine.

Toileting Routine

1. The child communicates her need to go to the bathroom (e.g., says "go potty," manually signs, or hands over a potty card, independently or when prompted).
2. The child walks to the bathroom.
3. The child pulls step tool in front of the toilet (if applicable).
4. The child pulls down her pants (if applicable).
5. The child pulls down her underwear.
6. The child sits on the toilet for a short period of time (e.g., 1 minute) or until urinating/defecating (as applicable).
7. The child gets toilet paper (if applicable).
8. The child wipes self (if applicable).
9. The child places toilet paper in the toilet (if applicable).
10. The child gets off the toilet.
11. The child pulls up her clothing.
12. The child moves step stool to sink (if applicable).
13. The child washes her hands. (Refer to the task analysis above for hand washing, if necessary.)

This task analysis represents most steps that would be included in the toileting routine, especially when the learner is just beginning to use the toilet. As you may have noticed, some of the skills in the task analysis may require additional practice outside of the toileting routine and some skills may not need to be included, depending on the individual learner. The exact procedures to teach these skills are described below.

In 1974, Azrin and Foxx published their book *Toilet Training in Less than a Day*, and the procedure they described continues to be among the most commonly used today. The Azrin and Foxx method has been successful with a variety of individuals, with and without ASD, including children and adults. The authors suggest that most children are ready for toilet training at around 20 months of age, but it is important to ensure that the learner is ready by assessing three fundamental aspects of toilet training: bladder control, physical readiness, and instructional readiness. The learner should be ready for toilet training if she is able to stay dry for a few hours, urinates completely rather than dribbling a little over a few hours, and indicates through facial expressions and/or postures when she needs to urinate or when she is urinating. Sometimes, children do not overtly indicate when they are relieving themselves or when they need to relieve themselves, so the learner may be ready if she is demonstrating just the first two components of bladder control.

Make sure the learner is physically ready for toilet training by testing a few of the fine and gross motor skills that are necessary for proper toileting behaviors. The authors suggest that necessary skills include picking up objects and the ability to walk from room to room. We would suggest that other dressing-related skills and wiping-related skills could be useful components but are not necessary prerequisite skills, and these can be taught as part of the toileting procedure.

Teaching procedures. Once you have determined that the learner is ready for toileting, you need to schedule 2 to 3 days when you can devote enough time to focus on this skill without distractions. Initially, you need to schedule frequent trips to the bathroom, so you shouldn't plan to begin toilet training on a day when you have other events planned. We also recommend that, a few days prior to beginning training, track the typical frequency of urination. This requires you to check the learner's diaper approximately every 15 minutes to determine if it is wet or dry. This allows you to determine how often the learner typically relieves himself, so you can schedule trips to the bathroom before an accident may occur. For example, if you find that urination occurs once an hour, you can schedule potty trips every 45 minutes.

Get rid of diapers. The learner has a long history of relieving himself in diapers, so he will most likely continue to urinate/defecate in the diaper if he is wearing it. This makes it very difficult for the learner to begin using the toilet instead of the diaper, especially because it requires less effort for the learner to go in the diaper. To set the occasion for toileting, remove diapers and have the learner wear "big boy" or "big girl" underpants. This will help the learner discriminate that he should not relieve himself unless on a toilet, and it will also allow the learner to experience the non-preferred feeling of being wet in case of an accident, as diapers are specifically designed to eliminate the feeling of wetness.

Increasing opportunities. As with any other skill we aim to teach, we want to increase the number of opportunities for the learner to practice the skill. With toileting, this process involves providing more access to water or juices, so urination will occur more frequently. This will potentially allow the learner to contact reinforcement more frequently, as well.

Scheduled trips. Initially, begin with frequent trips to the bathroom, and have the learner practice undressing, sitting, and waiting. We recommend that you use a timer to prompt trips to the bathroom. Because the learner is drinking more liquid, you may initially need to make trips to the bathroom every 15–30 minutes to decrease the likelihood of accidents and provide ample opportunities to go on the toilet. Take note of when the accidents occur or when the learner urinates in the toilet, so you can adjust the schedule when needed. For example, if you have toilet trips scheduled every 30 minutes and you notice that the learner is having frequent accidents, you can change the schedule to every 15 minutes. Likewise, if you are on a 15-minute schedule and you notice that the learner is only urinating in the toilet every 30 minutes, you may want to change the schedule to every 25 or 30 minutes. In addition, make sure you are teaching the learner to communicate in some manner when she needs to use the potty by pairing some form of communication with the potty trip. For example, if the learner is able to imitate words or short phrases, you can prompt her to say, "go potty," using echoic prompts right before you walk to the bathroom. You will need to fade these prompts over time until the learner can independently say the phrase "go potty" without a model. If the learner does not have the language to imitate, you can use sign language or a communication card in the same manner.

Reinforcement. Give the learner a powerful reinforcer immediately every time he eliminates on the toilet. To create motivation, make sure the reinforcer the learner receives is highly preferred and only available for appropriate toileting (see preference assessments in Chapter 4). Additionally, you can incorporate dry checks in between potty trips in order to teach the learner to discriminate between dry and wet. During dry checks, you should provide some type of reinforcing item if the learner remains dry.

Increasing independence. Once the learner is consistently urinating in the toilet during scheduled trips (and not having accidents between visits), you can begin increasing the amount of time between scheduled trips to give the learner opportunities to request to use the bathroom. When doing this, you can provide prompts in between scheduled trips, such as asking, "Do you need to go potty?" Again, differentially reinforce occurrences of urination after the learner states that he needs to go or independently requests to go. The ultimate goal is to get the learner to a point where he independently requests and uses the bathroom when needed without any adult assistance. Other skills within this curriculum, such as washing and drying hands, can be incorporated into the toileting routine once the initial skills are accomplished.

Domestic

Skills in the domestic domain include various activities that the learner will engage in at home, such as cleaning, clothing care, gardening, making a bed, pet care, setting and clearing a table, preparing snacks and meals, and tidying. As with the other daily living skills, you should first identify the skill you wish to teach and then create a task analysis that includes every single step that you want to teach in the behavior chain. See Skills® for a comprehensive list of lessons to teach in the domestic domain, as well as task analyses for each. Below is an example of a task analysis from the Snacks and Meals lesson:

Making a Peanut Butter and Jelly Sandwich

1. Prestep: The therapist puts out all materials that the child will use.
2. The child opens the bread bag.
3. The child takes out two slices of bread (or as many slices needed to make the amount desired).

4. The child may toast his bread. Skip this step, and go to step 5 if the child is not toasting his bread.
5. The child takes the bread back to the counter/table.
6. The child places the bread on the plate/napkin.
7. The child holds the peanut butter jar firmly using his non-preferred hand.
8. The child twists open the peanut butter jar using his preferred hand.
9. The child picks up the butter knife using his preferred hand.
10. The child places the butter knife inside the peanut butter jar.
11. The child scoops out a small amount of peanut butter with the butter knife.
12. The child spreads the peanut butter on one slice of bread.
13. The child repeats steps 10–11 until enough peanut butter has been spread on the slice of bread.
14. The child repeats steps 6–13 for the jelly.
15. The child puts the two slices of bread together.

Safety

Safety skills are among the most important – and yet most often ignored – skills in behavioral intervention programs for children with ASD. Of course, we hope that some safety skills will never be used (e.g., abduction prevention), but others are used on a daily basis (e.g., street crossing). In either case, safety skills are critical and if you prioritize teaching safety skills to your learners, you may literally save a life one day. Below, we briefly describe how to use Behavior Skills Training (BST) to teach three common safety skills. See Skills® for a larger collection of safety lessons and instructions for how to teach them.

Street crossing. Street-crossing skills can initially be taught in analog settings, such as a home or classroom and then generalized to real streets, or teaching can begin in the real-life setting. Some of the targets you can teach in the home/classroom setting are identifying traffic signs and lights and describing what you are supposed to do when you see them. When it comes time to teach in the natural environment (i.e., outside on a street), pick a side street with minimal traffic. Begin your BST training by teaching the learner the rules: 1) Always look for cars before going into the street; 2) stand on the curb where you can see up and down the street clearly; 3) look to the left, then to the right, and then back to the left again; and 4) if there are no cars coming, you can cross. Of course, the particular traffic laws that need to be trained depend on the country in which the learner resides.

After going over the rules, role-play each step with the learner, explaining what you are doing and asking the learner questions: for example, "I'm looking to the left. Are there any cars coming?" Then switch roles and have the learner be the one narrating what she is doing as though she is teaching you to cross the street. You can prompt the learner through this process by asking her questions, such as, "Which way do you look first?" or "I looked both ways, and it's clear, so now what do I do?" Once the learner is consistently responding correctly 100% of the time, practice on other streets that have more traffic, so she can learn that sometimes you have to wait awhile and look left, right, left several times before it is finally safe to cross. Be sure to incorporate rules about using crosswalks, heeding traffic lights, etc. It goes without saying that a therapist needs to stay next to the learner the entire time to ensure her safety.

Getting lost in public. Another important safety skill that can be taught using BST is what to do when one gets lost in public (Bergstrom, Najdowski, & Tarbox, 2012). To teach this skill in the natural environment, take the learner to various public retail stores and other locations and teach the rules: 1) If you get lost, yell for mom or dad (or whomever accompanied the learner); 2) if that doesn't work, find a worker; and 3) once you find the worker, tell him you are lost. After going over the rules, role-play the entire process, providing prompts as necessary until the learner is engaging in all of the behaviors independently. Learners who are less verbal (and won't be able to tell someone they are lost) can carry a card in their pocket that contains their name and their parents' phone numbers. For public locations that do not have workers (e.g., parks), you can train the learner to find a woman who has children with her, as this is likely the safest type of stranger to approach for help. For the final real-life test, the learner should become lost (with unobservable staff watching for safety) without the therapist or parents visually present to the learner. At least one or two people should be secretly keeping an eye on the learner to ensure his safety while practicing this skill. Obviously, at no point should the learner ever actually be lost. Make sure to train the skill in a variety of locations for generalization and to test it in untrained stores to ensure generalization occurred.

Stranger danger. Although the likelihood of a stranger attempting to abduct a child is very low, the consequences of being abducted are extremely serious, so many parents want their child with ASD to learn stranger safety skills. Stranger safety involves learning what to do when a stranger tries to lure the child to go with him (Bergstrom, Najdowski, & Tarbox, in press). Lures used by abductors include authoritative lures (e.g., "Your mom said you have to come with me right now."), incentive lures (e.g., "I have some video games in my car that you can have."), and assistance lures (e.g., "Can you come help me find my dog?"). Once again, BST is effective for teaching stranger safety skills to many children with ASD. The BST training approach begins by teaching the rules for what to do if approached by a stranger: 1) If a stranger wants you to go with him, say "No!"; 2) then run away from the stranger; and 3) tell an adult you know. After reviewing the rules, role-play different scenarios with the learner using a variety of lures, and have the learner go through all three correct steps, prompting as necessary. Once the learner is responding correctly during role-play, it is important to test this skill in real-world settings by having a person who is a stranger to the learner (but not to the parent) attempt to lure the learner away. If the learner fails to respond correctly in the real-world test, then training should begin immediately in that situation. In other words, if a therapist whom the child has never met attempts to lure the learner into his car and the learner begins to go, a known therapist should enter the situation at this point, give feedback on the error, and prompt the learner to respond correctly. This real-life setting training process should continue across different settings and different unknown therapists until the learner is responding independently to these real-world tests.

Community

The community domain includes skills that are useful for the learner in community settings, such as what to do in a restaurant (e.g., ordering, disposing of food, etc.), shopping-related skills (e.g., purchasing, using a cart, asking for assistance), and telephone skills (e.g., receiving and making phone calls from/to known and unknown callers, taking messages, finding a phone number). See Skills® for a comprehensive list of community lessons and instructions on how to teach them. The following is a task analysis from a lesson on telephone skills.

Answering the Phone and Engaging in a Brief Conversation with Known Caller

1. The child identifies that the phone is ringing (might be the home phone or cell phone).
2. The child walks to the phone (if applicable).
3. The child picks up the receiver/cell phone using her preferred hand.
4. The child opens the phone/presses the talk/send button using her non-preferred hand/finger (if applicable).
5. The child puts the home phone/cell phone on the ear of her preferred side.
6. The child says "hello" into the phone.
7. If the caller does not identify herself, the child asks the caller to do so: for example, "May I ask who's calling?"
8. The child acknowledges the caller and then listens to the message the caller called to say.
9. The child responds appropriately to the caller and continues the conversation by taking turns with the caller, waiting for a pause before speaking, and maintaining the conversation.
10. The child ends the conversation (e.g., "I have to go now") and/or responds appropriately to the caller's ending of the conversation: for example, "Okay, talk to you soon. Bye."
11. The child hangs up the phone.

Many community adaptive skills may initially be taught in the home or classroom environments, using simulated community settings and role-play. For example, the therapist can role-play a server at a restaurant to teach the learner how to use a menu and order food. As with any other skill that is taught in a simulated environment, it must be tested in the real-life setting. Many children will not automatically demonstrate the skill in the natural environment and may require additional training across multiple real-life settings.

WHEN ARE ADAPTIVE SKILLS A PRIORITY?

If you are wondering when to make adaptive skills a priority, the short answer to this question is "always." However, the heterogeneity of individuals with ASD, the challenges they face, and the various circumstances in which they live and learn necessarily make this issue somewhat complex. Generally speaking, most Early Intensive Behavioral Intervention (EIBI) programs focus heavily on increasing language, play, foundational social skills, and "readiness-to-learn" skills, as well as decreasing challenging behavior. For many young children with ASD, the reality is that it is easy enough for parents and therapists simply to do daily living tasks for the child, so these skills do not initially appear to be a priority. Indeed, most EIBI outcome research shows only modest gains in measures of daily living skills, and many authors attribute this to the fact that those skills are not prioritized in treatment. If existing outcome research is to be used as a model for treatment planning, then a relatively low focus on daily living skills may be acceptable, especially if it is specifically for the sake of increasing core language, social, and play skills.

As Children Get Older

As children begin to age out of early intervention and preschool programs, two things usually happen. First, a clearer picture of the child's developmental trajectory begins to emerge. The reality today is that there is a very large degree of variability in response to treatment across different children with ASD, and it is currently not possible to predict at intake which children will recover, which children will make substantial progress but still require minimal supports across the lifespan, and which children will still require substantial supports across the lifespan. After at least 3 or more years of EIBI, as children reach the age of perhaps 6–8 years old, the child's developmental trajectory begins to become clearer. If it appears likely that a child will still require substantial supports across the lifespan, the overall process of prioritizing domains of treatment begins to lean toward daily living skills to a much greater degree than when that child was younger.

Second, as children get older, they are expected to play a larger role in caring for themselves, so it's natural for daily living skills to become more of a priority as the child ages. For example, it is probably not overly challenging for a parent to bathe his 2- or 3-year-old child, but as the child reaches 6–9 years of age, it is probably reasonable to start to expect the child to perform some or all of the steps in the bathing task independently. The same is true for getting ready for school in the morning, preparing a bowl of cereal for breakfast, obtaining an after-school snack from the cupboard, and so on.

Limited Treatment Intensity

At the time that this manual was written, the only treatment for ASD that has been scientifically demonstrated through repeated replication to produce robust overall outcomes is EIBI, that is, behavioral intervention for more than 25 hours per week. If a child is under the age of 5 when treatment begins, the scientific evidence is clear: He should receive intensive treatment. However, the unfortunate reality is that many – perhaps even most – children with autism under the age of 5 are still denied access to this level of intensity of treatment. Many children are still only offered 10 hours per week or less. This is a significant ethical problem for the autism field and society as a whole, and it is hoped that further progress can be made toward fixing it. For now, some special considerations likely need to be made for children who receive only low-intensity behavioral intervention (defined as fewer than 25 hours per week). Probably the most important clinical priorities for children who are not able to receive intensive services are to reduce challenging behavior, replace it with functional communication, and establish non-destructive leisure skills to fill downtime. A close fourth priority is probably self-care skills. Therefore, it is probably reasonable to prioritize independent living skills higher for a child who is receiving only 10 hours per week of intervention than for one who is receiving 40 hours per week, all other things being equal.

STRATEGIES FOR SUCCESS

Reinforcement

As with virtually all learning that occurs in applied behavior analysis (ABA), daily living skills are only learned if there is effective positive reinforcement. It's easy to lose sight of how important this is to consider when teaching daily living skills because their natural consequences are usually reinforcing enough for typically developing children to learn and maintain the skills; for example, the consequence of preparing a meal is eating it; the consequence of getting dressed is getting to go outside and play, etc. It's critical to remember, however, that the natural consequences of most skills – daily living skills included – are often not sufficient to produce learning or maintenance in children with ASD. Therefore, very powerful reinforcers must be programmed frequently during initial acquisition, and it's possible that contrived reinforcers may need to be delivered for long periods of time if you want daily living skills to continue to be exhibited independently. For many children with ASD, the natural social consequences of grooming skills are not strong enough to maintain the behavior. For example, many children may not notice or care if their peers think their unbrushed hair looks bad. Hair brushing may need to be maintained through contrived reinforcement for a long time, even after the skill has been successfully taught.

Plan Sufficient Time for Teaching

Many daily living skills naturally occur (or fail to occur) during periods of the day that tend to be rushed and/or stressful. These are not the best times to teach the learner these skills. Of course, it's important to teach daily living skills (and virtually all others) in the natural environment, but it's even more important for the learner to be successful and for the teaching program not to increase stress and anxiety in the parents and challenging behavior in the children. You don't learn how to drive a car by driving a racecar on a racetrack while racing against other drivers; you learn how to drive under controlled, safe, non-stressful conditions. The same should be true for the learner who is learning to brush his teeth, take a bath, get dressed, make his lunch, and so on. In addition, if you only practice self-care skills when they are actually used in daily life, then you will likely not present enough learning opportunities to teach the learner effectively and efficiently. One learning opportunity per day is not likely going to be very effective for teaching dressing skills; you will need to plan additional learning opportunities. Remember, ABA works through *a lot of practice* and positive reinforcement.

Adapt Teaching to Customs and Contexts of Everyday Family Life

Every domain needs to be adapted, when necessary, to be relevant in each unique family culture and context, and this may be especially true for independent living skills. For example, if a family is completely satisfied with their child taking a bath, regardless of age, and never expects their child to take a shower, then taking the time to teach independent showering skills is probably not practical; teaching bath-taking skills would be far more appropriate. Similarly, with feeding issues, family food preferences and traditions need to be taken into account. In some cases, these considerations are obvious. For example, one would teach a learner in a kosher family to accept only kosher foods or a learner in a vegetarian family to eat only vegetarian foods. Many family expectations, routines, and customs are subtler but no less important. For example, it may not make sense to spend time teaching a learner to eat plain broccoli if her family always serves broccoli with some kind of seasoning or dressing or, worse yet, never serves broccoli at all. When teaching laundry skills, make sure to teach the learner to fold clothing the way his parents want the items folded. If you don't pay attention to these details, the parents may become frustrated with having to refold the clothes and may be less likely to encourage their child to help fold, thereby decreasing generalization and maintenance. Similarly, some families do not use napkins when eating a meal. Spending time teaching a learner to use a napkin is a waste of time if the family does not provide napkins during everyday meals.

Consider the Learner's Motor Abilities

Occasionally, a particular motor movement in a chain is especially challenging for a learner, much more so than the rest of the chain, such as buttoning a button or twisting a cap off the toothpaste. In these cases, there is often no point in taking the time to run through the whole chain when all you are really doing is trying to teach one challenging motor response. You may be better off using the time to target only the particular motor response, thereby producing more practice with the skill that really needs instruction and less time on already mastered steps. Once the learner can perform the difficult motor response quickly and proficiently in isolation, you can once again begin teaching the entire chain that contains it.

Include Parents

In every area of ABA intervention for children with ASD, it is critical to include parents and other caregivers. This is particularly true for many independent living skills because, after they are learned, they are *only* displayed in the presence of parents (e.g., undressing and bathing). There are multiple models for how parents can be included in teaching daily living skills. For example, it is possible to train the parents how to teach the child and for the clinician not to do any of the direct teaching herself, that is, to do a purely parent-mediated model. However, in practice, this model is far more challenging and places a large burden on the parents. Except in cases of severely limited therapy time, it is virtually always more effective if the clinician does the majority of the teaching, and the parents and other caregivers are brought in primarily to ensure generalization and maintenance. Therefore, parents are commonly included in the teaching sessions when a child begins to master some or most steps of a daily living skill. As with any parental involvement, you need to make sure that the parents are adequately trained so that when they begin to step in and conduct the teaching, they do it correctly. Common sources of error are over-prompting, under-prompting, repeating vocal directions excessively, forgetting to deliver reinforcement, and delivering it when it hasn't been earned. You would do well to watch for all of these potential sources of procedural infidelity.

As parents demonstrate that they can conduct the sessions accurately, you can begin to ask them to do so when clinicians are not present. When you do, you would be wise to ask them to document their sessions in some way. It may be possible to teach some parents to collect data on a task analysis data sheet. Other parents may prefer to videotape the sessions with a camcorder or mobile (cell) phone. If neither of these options seems feasible, you could consider merely asking the parents to write down on a calendar the days they implemented a procedure, which would provide at least a minimum degree of tracking and accountability.

Visual Supports

As discussed in Chapter 6, many children with ASD learn more rapidly when visual prompting is used. Many sequences of self-care skills involve several different tasks, each one of which contains a chain of many steps. Providing a visual prompt that depicts the steps can help many children with ASD be more independent. For example, the bathroom can be a good setting in which to use visual supports for a child who is getting ready for school. If the learner is able to read, a bulleted list of the tasks (e.g., go pee, wash hands, brush teeth, wash face, etc.) taped to the bathroom mirror may be sufficient. If the learner is not able to read words, then a sequence of pictures or line drawings may be sufficient. The presence of visual supports is, of course, a prompt. Technically, if learners continue to be dependent on the visual support, then you are building a certain level of prompt dependence into their daily lives. However, with many tasks, this level of prompt dependence is perfectly acceptable, especially in younger children. Moreover, typically developing adults are prompt dependent in many ways, relying on grocery shopping lists, work calendars, and so on. It is not entirely unreasonable for children with ASD to remain dependent on some visual supports for daily living skills while you use your therapy time to focus on teaching skills that are more crucial for everyday quality of life rather than spending additional time fading out the visual supports.

COMMON PITFALLS IN TEACHING ADAPTIVE SKILLS

Don't Start Too Early!

It is very common for clinicians to become overly excited about the effectiveness of ABA teaching procedures and, as a result, start teaching skills at an unreasonably young age. Make sure you do not start teaching an independent living skill that typically developing children of the same age are not expected to do. If you are not sure whether a particular skill is age appropriate, you can consult a comprehensive curriculum, such as Skills® (see Chapter 26), or a standardized assessment, such as the Mullen (see Chapter 25).

Targeting Too Many Skills at Once

Trying to teach too many self-care skills at once is another common source of difficulty. Little or no research has directly addressed the question of how many skills should be targeted at a time; however, given how many hours of therapy are being delivered, clinicians have often observed that decreasing the number of skills being taught can result in a smaller number of skills being mastered more quickly. It is likely that each individual skill requires at least a minimum number of learning opportunities per day or week in order for acquisition to occur, so consider teaching only one self-care skill at a time (especially if therapy time is limited), thereby ensuring many practice opportunities per day/session.

Inadvertently Prompting Already Mastered Skills

A very common mistake for parents and clinicians to make with independent living skills is to prompt the child through them, even when a skill has been mastered. This is probably because the situations in which these skills need to be displayed are often rushed and stressful. If the whole family is waiting in the car to go somewhere and the child needs to wash his hands, a parent or staff member may simply prompt the child through it because it's faster than waiting the extra 2 or 3 minutes for the child to complete it independently. Such situations are understandable, but every effort should be made to avoid them. Every opportunity that the child has to practice newly learned self-care skills should be considered an opportunity to progress toward independence, and unnecessary prompting can only impede that progress.

Ensure That Focused Learning Environments Are Relevant to Real Life

In order to create sufficient learning opportunities, it is often necessary to focus on teaching particular skills in a repetitive, non-natural way. For example, with buttoning, you may be better off teaching buttoning by having the learner repetitively button and unbutton, rather than having her do it only once when she is getting dressed in the morning. However, when contriving focused learning situations, it is critical that the task remain relevant to how and when the skill will need to be performed in real life. For example, clinicians often use "button boards" (i.e., boards covered with cloth with many buttons) to teach buttoning. If used properly, button boards can be very effective, but buttons on some button boards are oriented in the opposite manner of how the learner will be manipulating them on his clothing. Similarly, zippers can be on the opposite side of the garment, depending on whether the garment is designed for a boy or girl. Regardless of how well a learner can button a button on a button board, the skill of buttoning is not mastered, of course, until the learner can button and unbutton her own clothes, on her body, in the context of real-life dressing and undressing. This is true of all focused learning situations, which should always be undertaken with the real-life skill in mind.

Balancing Values and Efficiency

Sometimes, families and/or clinicians value certain skills that may not be the most efficient targets when planning treatment. A classic example is tying shoelaces. Every parent wants her child to learn to tie his shoes, and most clinicians probably want their learners to learn it, as well. However, especially if therapy time is limited, it might be wiser to buy the child a pair of slip-on or Velcro® shoes than to dedicate treatment hours to teaching the learner to tie shoelaces. In years past, Velcro® shoes were often viewed as stigmatizing for children with disabilities, but they are much more common in everyday fashion now, as are slip-on shoes, such as Vans®. Another classic example of inefficient treatment targets is making change or counting money. The ability to understand and use one's own money is important for maximizing independence, but many children with ASD will have few, if any, daily experiences in which they are required to count their own money while making purchases. If therapy time is limited, it may make more sense to focus on other, more critical independent living skills, such as dressing, self-feeding, bathing, snack preparation, etc.

SUMMARY

Daily living skills are crucial for helping individuals with ASD live more independent lives. Although adaptive skills are not necessarily the first thing an early learner with ASD needs to be taught, such skills quickly become necessary as the learner grows. In addition, safety skills are absolutely critical to the learner's well-being, especially for children with ASD who often lack self-preservation skills and/or lack communication skills needed to alert others when they are in danger. Overall, adaptive skills should be taught using the same basic procedures as other skills, consisting of positive reinforcement, prompting, prompt fading, chaining, and generalization training. The ultimate goal is to establish independent, spontaneous use of daily living skills, so the child with ASD can live as fully and independently as possible.

Motor

Michele R. Bishop

Motor skills play a part in almost everything a person says or does, including language, play, academic, and adaptive behavior. While deficits in motor skills are not a defining feature of autism spectrum disorder (ASD) according to the Diagnostic and Statistical Manual of Mental Disorders, fifth edition (DSM-5; APA, 2013), researchers have frequently observed delayed motor skills in children with ASD (Dewey, Cantell, & Crawford, 2007). Therefore, for many children with ASD, motor skills must be directly taught. The general process of teaching motor skills is the same as teaching any other skill. In the beginning, simple motor movements are taught with the assistance of prompts and the use of positive reinforcement. The learner may practice an approximation of the motor response as strength, flexibility, and coordination develop. Then, as motor control improves, prompts are faded, allowing for independent movements. Once a repertoire of basic motor responses is established, it can be expanded to develop more complex motor responses. Concurrently, therapists integrate teaching exercises into natural play activities to the greatest extent possible.

The Center for Autism and Related Disorders (CARD) Motor curriculum is organized into four basic categories: 1) visual, 2) gross, 3) fine, and 4) oral motor. See Table 14.1 for a list of lessons within each category. Appendix G provides an outline of the CARD Motor curriculum. This chapter will provide guidelines on how to teach motor skills. The teaching procedures described in this chapter are not intended to replace traditional therapies (e.g., physical therapy, vision therapy, occupational therapy, and speech-language therapy) used to treat visual, oral, gross, and fine motor deficits. Instead, these teaching techniques should serve as supplements to other therapies that a learner may be receiving. If a visual, oral, gross, or fine motor deficit is suspected, it is recommended that the learner be evaluated by a specialist.

MOTOR DOMAINS

Visual Motor

Research has documented deficits in visual motor skills, including ocular motility, binocular vision, and visual perception, in some children and adolescents with ASD (Kurtz, 2006). See Table 14.1 for a list of visual motor lessons.

Ocular motility. Poor ocular motility (eye movement) is associated with deficiency in fixation, tracking moving objects with the eyes (pursuits), and shifting one's eyes quickly between items (saccades). To help a learner improve her **fixation** skills, the therapist should engage the learner in activities that require the learner to shift her eyes from a near point to a

TABLE 14.1   Motor Lessons

Domain	Muscles	Lessons
Visual Motor	Eye muscles	Ocular motility Binocular vision Visual perception
Gross Motor	Arm, leg, and torso muscles	Rolling over Sitting Creeping and crawling Standing Walking Stairs and climbing Rolling/throwing/dribbling Running Balancing Riding foot-propelled vehicles Catching Jumping Kicking Hopping Riding a tricycle/bicycle Swinging a bat/racquet/paddle Physical education readiness Gross motor fluency
Fine Motor	Hand and finger muscles	Hand skills Finger skills Coloring Prehandwriting Cutting with scissors Drawing Fine motor fluency
Oral Motor	Mouth and face muscles	Oral motor

far point and from a far point to a near point (e.g., looking from the chalk-board to the paper on her desk and back again). Make the activities fun and make sure that positive reinforcement is built in for behaviors that the learner can only execute if she shifts her gaze back and forth from near to far stimuli. For example, the therapist and learner can play word games in which the learner has to tell the therapist a "secret code" that is written on either a near or far location, requiring the learner to shift her eyes back and forth between far and near locations in order to report the correct "codes" to the therapist.

To help a learner improve his **tracking** (pursuits) skills, the therapist can present activities that require the learner to fixate his eyes on a moving object (in horizontal, vertical, circular, and arc movements) and smoothly move his eyes to follow the object across the field of vision with little head movement (e.g., tracking a moving ball, flashlight on a wall, laser pointer across a wall, etc.). Tasks should progress from relatively easy to relatively difficult, and positive reinforcement should be used to reinforce accurate responding.

To help a learner improve her ability to **shift gaze** between points where her gaze has become fixed (saccades), the therapist should present activities that require the learner to shift gaze from a stationary point smoothly and efficiently with stops at the proper times and without over-shooting and/or undershooting. This can be done, for example, by having the learner name items in a line from start to finish.

To help a learner improve his **scanning** skills, which involve smooth continuous movements of the eyes in order to visually examine materials (e.g., words on a page, a list of words or letters, lines from start to finish), present activities such as having the learner trace lines with his finger (top panel of Figure 14.1) or draw lines within lines from beginning to end without pause (bottom panel of Figure 14.1).

Binocular vision. Binocular vision skills involve the ability to use both eyes simultaneously and combine what is seen by each eye into a single image. Poor binocular vision is associated with problems such as crossed eyes and double vision. Activities focusing on improving binocular vision

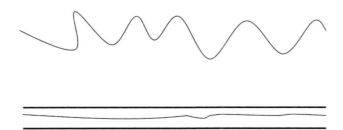

FIGURE 14.1   Sample activities for working on scanning skills.

will work on convergence, which is the simultaneous inward movement of both eyes toward each other in an effort to maintain focus on an object that is moving closer to the learner's face. For example, the therapist might place a button on a string, extend the string out horizontally from the learner's nose, and say, "Watch the button," as she moves the button toward the learner's nose. Initially, provide reinforcement when the learner watches the button move a short distance. Gradually, move the button longer distances and require the learner to keep watching it with both eyes, providing reinforcement when she is successful. This process is continued until the learner is able to watch (eyes should turn inward) the button move within 2–4 inches of her nose.

Activities in this area will also focus on improving stereopsis, which involves both eyes working together to view one image that has depth and spatial orientation. Activities that might be targeted include riding a bike, picking up toys at different distances, gauging the distance of cars when crossing the street, and standing, stopping, and starting one's body (e.g., when walking and running) without bumping into people or objects.

Gross Motor

Gross motor skills involve the development of large body movements related to balance and arm, leg, and torso movement (see Table 14.1). For example, in typical development, by the time they are 2 years old, children are able to jump 2 inches on both feet, walk up and down three stairs, and throw a small ball 3–5 feet in the direction of a target. However, researchers have reported that many children with ASD do not develop foundational gross motor skills if they are not directly taught them (e.g., Ozonoff et al., 2008).

When teaching gross motor skills, the clinician should focus on teaching the skills as they apply to functional and fun activities in daily life, such as playing with a ball, playing tag, and so on. For example, when teaching a learner with substantial gross motor delays to jump, you may need to start with prompting the learner to bend his knees and hold the position for a few seconds. Then you might move to requiring the learner to jump off of a small step or curb. This would progress to jumping up 1 inch in place. Then, you might gradually increase the number of times that the learner jumps in place and add jumping forward and backward. You might also work on increasing the height and length of jump required in small increments until the learner is able to jump over small objects. At this point, you might begin to integrate the lesson into fun games that the learner likes to play, such as tag, pretend Olympics, and so on.

Another commonly taught gross motor skill is catching. If the learner cannot catch, you can start by teaching the first form of catching that emerges in typical development: scooping under a ball and trapping it to the chest. Begin by handing the ball to the learner while standing immediately in front of him. Prompt and reinforce the correct motor movements, and gradually increase the distance between you and the learner until you are standing too far away from him to be able to hand him the ball. Then, standing a few inches from him, throw the ball. Increase the distance between the two of you as long as the learner is still able to catch the ball. Over time, begin to teach the learner to extend his arms to catch a ball in his hands (instead of his chest). Start with large balls, such as a beach ball, and decrease the size to a playground ball and, eventually, a tennis ball. As soon as possible, integrate teaching sessions into highly preferred games that involve throwing and catching. This will help to keep motivation high and will start to generalize the catching skill to the natural environment.

Fine Motor

In typical child development, a variety of fine motor skills emerge quite early. For example, children aged between 9 and 12 months are able to pick up small objects with a precise finger and thumb grasp; children aged between 18 and 24 months are able to build a tower up to four blocks high; and children aged between 2 and 3 years are able to cut with child-sized scissors. However, researchers have indicated that learners with ASD often display deficits in fine motor skills (e.g., Dyck, Piek, Hay, & Hallmayer, 2007). For example, Dyck and colleagues reported that the majority of children with ASD whom they assessed had difficulty with fine motor skills, such as putting beads in a box.

Fine motor lessons focus on the development of hand and finger strength and movement in the context of functional tasks, such as cutting, writing, and so on (see Table 14.1 for a list of fine motor lessons). Learners with severely delayed fine motor skills may need to learn to grasp small objects with a precise finger and thumb grasp. To teach this, begin with small numbers of relatively large objects and prompt and reinforce the learner to pick up objects and place them in a container (e.g., putting blocks into a bin). As the learner becomes successful with small numbers of larger objects, gradually decrease the size of the objects and increase the number of objects. Make sure to train across objects with a variety of different shapes, textures, and weights to ensure generalization. As soon as possible, integrate teaching into fun games that require fine motor skills, such as board games or crafts that are highly preferred by the learner.

When teaching a learner with substantial fine motor deficits to use scissors, you might start by teaching the learner to hold the scissors correctly by having him practice placing his preferred thumb in one hole and his first three fingers in the other hole of the scissors. Once he has the scissors in his hand, you might move on to teaching him to open and close the scissors multiple times in succession. Then you might draw thick, straight lines on small pieces of paper that the learner can manipulate and require the learner to cut as close to the line as possible until he is able to cut on the line. Give the learner positive reinforcement for successive approximations toward cutting the piece of paper in half without going outside of the line. As he becomes successful, gradually decrease the width of the line until he can cut on a line drawn with a regular pen. Then move on to shapes, such as circles and triangles, again starting with thick lines that are eventually faded to thin lines drawn with a regular pen. Finally, consider this skill to be mastered once the learner is able to move the paper in various directions in one hand in order to cut out increasingly difficult forms with the other hand.

Oral Motor

Researchers have reported that some children with ASD display deficits in oral motor skills, such as tongue movement, sucking, and lip movements (Adams, 1998). Results of a study by Adams indicate that children with ASD display significant impairments in the areas of oral movement, complex phonemic/syllabic productions, and total oral motor functioning when compared to typically developing children. Oral motor activities focus on the development of mouth, tongue, and lip movements, so they can be applied to functional skills for which they are critical, such as speech production.

We do not teach oral motor skills just for the sake of teaching. Many learners will not need oral motor activities because their oral motor skills will develop without direct training. Oral motor activities are not targeted in isolation from teaching direct sounds. Oral motor activities are targeted that are directly associated with sounds, blends, and words when they are difficult for the learner to produce. In this way, oral motor activities are used in the Echoics lesson (see Chapter 11) to supplement correct mouth movements when needed.

Mouth movements. Various mouth movements are used in the production of speech. We pucker our lips to say the sounds "ch" ("chip"), "j" ("just"), "w" ("what"), "oo" ("oops"), "ō" ("okay"), and "U" ("book"). We spread our lips wide (bilateral smile) to say the sounds "ee" ("eat"), "ĭ" ("it"), "ā" ("ape"), and "ĕ" ("empty"). We press our upper and lower lips together to say the sounds "mm" ("more"), "b" ("bat"), and "p" ("pig"). And we put our upper teeth on our lower lip to say the sounds "ff" ("four") and "v" ("very").

The therapist uses non-vocal imitation to instruct the learner to make the mouth movements associated with target sounds that the learner is finding difficult to articulate. Specifically, if the learner is having difficulty articulating the "sh" sound in the word "shoe," the therapist says, "Do this," and pushes her lips forward. As soon as the learner imitates and has his lips in the correct position, the therapist says, "Say, 'shoe.'" The learner then says "shoe" or some approximation. Successive approximations toward correct mouth movement and articulation are reinforced, and the oral motor prompt is faded out when possible.

Tongue movements are also used to produce speech. We touch our tongue to the alveolar ridge inside our mouth behind our teeth to say the sounds "nn" ("no"), "l" ("lips"), "d" ("down"), "t" ("top"), "z" ("zipper"), and "s" ("sip"). This is also the correct tongue placement when swallowing food. We place our tongue between our upper and lower teeth to say the sounds "th" ("think") and "Th" ("this"). As with teaching mouth movements, use non-vocal imitation to instruct the learner to place his tongue in the proper location. Additionally, if the learner is having difficulty imitating a particular tongue movement when instructed, you can use a variety of physical prompts to guide the learner's tongue to the correct position in or around the mouth. For example, if the learner is having difficulty lifting his tongue to the roof of his mouth when instructed to imitate touching his tongue to the alveolar ridge, you can use a tongue depressor to physically guide the learner's tongue to the roof of his mouth. This should be faded as the child learns to lift his tongue independently.

TEACHING PROCEDURES

Chapter 4 describes evidence-based teaching procedures in detail, so they are not repeated here. However, we briefly describe some of the more useful procedures below.

Discrete Trial Training (DTT)

When using DTT to teach motor skills, an instruction to perform a motor movement is presented, the learner responds, and a consequence is delivered, indicating if the response was correct or incorrect. The instruction presented by the therapist can explicitly state the action to be performed (e.g., "watch the car" [visual]; "throw the ball" [gross]; "color" [fine]; or "press your lips together" [oral]) or require the learner to imitate the therapist (e.g., saying "do this" while tracing a curvy line with your finger [visual], jumping [gross], drawing a circle [fine], or touching your tongue behind your top front teeth [oral]). Initially, responses are prompted and reinforced, but as the learner becomes successful, the prompts are faded out.

Natural Environment Training (NET)

Motor skills should be practiced as part of daily activities in the natural environment. For example, if the learner has fine and visual motor deficits, the therapist might instruct the learner to open the door of the playroom upon deciding to play in there, using this as an opportunity for the learner to practice grasping the doorknob and twisting her wrist to open the door independently (fine motor). Then, upon entering the playroom (which turns out to be messy), the therapist might instruct the learner to "find all the toy cars, so we can race" (visual motor). As with DTT, responses are prompted and reinforced initially, but prompts are faded out over time.

Prompting

Modeling and gentle physical guidance are commonly used prompts that can assist a learner in making a correct response during motor lessons. Modeling can be effective when the learner is able to see and imitate the therapist's motor movement. However, if the learner is not yet able to imitate consistently, it is likely that modeling will not be an effective prompt. Gentle physical guidance can be useful when the therapist has access to the learner's targeted muscle group (e.g., movements involving arms, legs, and fingers). However, some motor responses require muscles that therapists cannot easily manipulate, or the muscle movements are so complex that gentle physical guidance is not beneficial (e.g., running, tongue movements, ocular motility). In these situations, modeling is generally the best choice for prompting procedures, and in some cases, prompting may not be possible at all.

Chaining and Shaping

Motor skills require sufficient strength, coordination, flexibility, and balance, which are achieved through repeated practice. Chaining and shaping, combined with DTT or NET, allow these skills to develop and/or improve through the reinforcement of steps and successive approximations until the specified target response is achieved. Chaining is helpful for motor skills that involve multiple steps (e.g., bike riding and cutting with scissors). Using shaping, when a child is learning a new motor skill (e.g., hopping [gross], coloring inside lines [fine], puckering lips [oral], fixating eye gaze on distant objects [visual]), initial phases of the response are reinforced, such as hopping on one foot while holding onto a chair for support. Once the initial response is occurring consistently, the therapist discontinues reinforcement for the initial response and requires a closer approximation (i.e., hopping once on preferred foot). This shaping process continues until the learner is able to hop off the ground multiple times on both his preferred and non-preferred foot.

Increasing Independence

When beginning to teach motor skills, the therapist delivers a cue to evoke the learner's response. It is usually an instruction ("jump") and/or a model ("do this" + demonstrating the skill). Eventually, however, it will become necessary to let the natural discriminative stimuli in the environment begin to cue the motor behavior. For example, when playing catch, you shouldn't have to tell the learner "catch" every time you throw the ball. Rather, seeing a ball flying toward the learner in a game of catch should evoke the learner's response of catching. Thus, once the learner is able to exhibit a motor skill without physical prompting, begin to fade out directive and model prompts, and allow the natural discriminative stimuli to control the motor behavior.

Maintenance and Generalization

A comprehensive treatment program should include a systematic maintenance and generalization procedure for motor skills, with performance being monitored to make sure that the learner continues to display newly learned skills and abilities over time in the natural environment (see Chapter 7 on generalization and maintenance). Additionally, the acquisition of new complex skills may be expedited by continuing to practice mastered component skills. For example, practicing hand skills (e.g., squeezing objects) in maintenance may aid in the acquisition of single hand throwing.

The maintenance of skills is improved by implementing a variable reinforcement schedule, so the learner is not able to determine when a preferred item will be delivered. When preferred things are delivered less frequently, the learner experiences the naturally occurring consequences of the behavior. Over time, the learner will become more independent and efficient when engaging in personal, play, and academic activities that require strength, flexibility, coordination, and balance. Some techniques that can be used to enhance generalization include varying the teaching materials, using natural consequences, and encouraging a variety of appropriate forms of the response (e.g., teaching a learner to get dressed by sometimes putting pants on first and sometimes putting a shirt on first). It is important to note that no single technique is effective for every learner. Frequently test for generalization, and if generalization is not observed, modifications to the protocol may be necessary. (See Chapter 7 for a detailed discussion of maintenance and generalization.)

STRATEGIES FOR SUCCESS IN TEACHING MOTOR SKILLS

Build Gross and Fine Motor Strength

Sufficient strength is necessary to perform all motor responses, and strength, coordination, and flexibility gradually develop as muscles are used to perform actions. When gross and fine motor skills are in their early stages of development, it is common to reinforce less strenuous approximations of the target motor movement. It is also beneficial to target supplemental actions that boost strength. For example, if the target response is coloring and the learner has difficulty gripping a crayon, the therapist may implement a lesson that targets squeezing a ball to assist with the development of hand strength. Then, over time with repeated practice, the learner's strength improves, making it easier for her to grip the crayon and color.

Teach Fluent Motor Behavior

Some motor responses require speed for proficient performance. Speed and muscle strength are related; the stronger the muscles are, the easier it is to move quickly. At first, the learner may practice a skill slowly and focus on the correct movements, but the treatment program should not stop when the learner merely performs the movements accurately. In addition to accuracy, the speed of the response while maintaining proper form should increase if the learner is going to use the skill proficiently. Some motor skills, such as jumping, running, catching, and throwing, require sufficient speed in order for the skill to be meaningful in daily life. For instance, a learner may be able to catch a ball that is thrown at him slowly and with sufficient warning, but he may still not be able to play sports with peers because balls are rarely thrown slowly and with ample warning during play. Targeting speed should be done by instructing the learner to engage in the motor skill as many times as she can during a 30- or 60-second timing and gradually increasing how many times the learner is able to perform the skill with correct form until she demonstrates fluency. For example, when learning how to throw a ball, a child may repeatedly practice correct arm movements focusing on speed, strength, and coordination. These arm movements do not necessarily involve throwing but are components of the skill, including rotating the arm in a circle, thrusting the hand and arm forward from the shoulder, and squeezing a ball. Additionally, the learner can practice throwing the ball repeatedly, and the frequency of correct throws (including good form) is slowly increased by setting goals for the learner to gradually increase speed in order to earn positive reinforcement.

Don't Forget to Consider Fatigue

All skills that require muscle movement have the potential to cause the learner to feel fatigue when she practices them during therapy. This is especially true for repeated practice of motor skills because they tend to isolate specific muscles and use them repeatedly. When you are working on motor skills, remember that the learner's muscles may be getting sore and she may not have the language to tell you that. Make sure that you provide ample opportunities for rest during therapy in the form of breaks and switching muscle groups.

COMMON PITFALLS IN TEACHING MOTOR SKILLS

Teaching Irrelevant Skills

Avoid the trap of blindly teaching to a curriculum, as not all motor skills need to be taught to every learner with ASD. For example, visual and oral motor activities do not need to be taught to a learner unless she exhibits deficits in these areas. If the learner has been diagnosed with having poor visual motor skills by a developmental ophthalmologist or shows signs of visual motor deficiency, then visual motor teaching may be helpful for that learner. Likewise, if the learner has poor articulation due to inappropriate tongue placement or can't chew food appropriately, then oral motor lessons might be useful. For example, if a learner does not reliably pronounce the "n" sound in words, then working on the associated oral motor movement of placing the tongue behind the front teeth just prior to instructing the learner to say "n" might be helpful. Working collaboratively with a speech and language pathologist in such circumstances can often be helpful in identifying the most crucial targets to address.

Poor Communication Across Service Providers

When a learner displays a significant motor impairment, it is common for learners to receive additional intervention from other professionals who specialize in the specific motor deficit (e.g., occupational therapist, developmental ophthalmologist, physical therapist). When this occurs, there is potential for poor or even non-existent communication among providers, likely resulting in inefficiency and confusion. If a learner is participating in intervention programs with other service providers, it is important to ensure that the treatment protocols are complementary. Complementary interventions focus on similar treatment goals, reinforcing comparable skills to improve skill acquisition, maintenance, and generalization. This results in the most beneficial intervention for the learner and enhances his overall motor development. When intervention goals are not aligned, a decreased rate of skill acquisition may be observed due to the reinforcement of incompatible skills. Behavior analysts would be especially well advised to be respectful of the role of occupational therapists and physical therapists in treating motor deficits, as this is their primary area of expertise, and the same is certainly not true for behavior analysts. See Chapter 24 on interdisciplinary collaboration for more discussion on this topic.

SUMMARY

Motor skills are critical to human functioning because they impact an individual's ability to move independently and interact with people and things in her environment, and they contribute to the development of language, play, academic, and adaptive behavior. This chapter has outlined several instructional procedures that are useful when teaching motor skills to learners with ASD. Lessons in the Motor curriculum target four primary domains (visual, gross, fine, and oral motor skills). Initial instruction focuses on the acquisition of simple and less strenuous motor movements. As the learner's strength, flexibility, and coordination improve, more complex and strenuous motor movements are targeted. Similarly, as the learner masters simpler motor movements in controlled situations, it is critical to help the learner integrate those skills into functional tasks and activities in her everyday life.

Academics

Michele R. Bishop, Carolynn Bredek

Pre-academic skills are the foundational skills (e.g., knowing colors and how to hold a pencil) that prepare a learner for acquiring more advanced academic skills (reading and math) taught in kindergarten and elementary school. While deficits in academic behavior are not a defining feature of autism spectrum disorder (ASD), learning disabilities are prevalent among children with an ASD diagnosis (Mayes & Calhoun, 2006; Montes & Halterman, 2006). Mayes and Calhoun reported that 67% (n = 124) of the children with ASD whom they evaluated also displayed a learning disability. Furthermore, achievement in early academic skills is associated with continued academic success in elementary school. Given the relationship between pre-academic skills and success later in school, it is important that an adequate proportion of time is dedicated to teaching pre-academic skills to children diagnosed with ASD. A well-developed repertoire of pre-academic skills will prepare a child for successful integration into a kindergarten classroom.

A common misconception of applied behavior analytic intervention for learners with ASD is that it primarily focuses on teaching children to memorize academic content, such as shapes, letters, numbers, and counting by rote. As is described in the other chapters in Section III of this manual, the vast majority of behavioral intervention time in applied behavior analysis (ABA) programs is spent teaching communication, social, play, and other skills, not academics. Nevertheless, behavioral intervention programs can play a crucial role in providing a foundation for the academic curriculum that children with ASD may be expected to master when they go to school. In addition, some very good-quality ABA-based schools offer alternatives to public education, such as the Center for Autism and Related Disorders (CARD) Academy (see Chapter 8), and are therefore responsible for teaching all of the academics a child might need. The majority of ABA services for children with ASD, however, tend to occur before children enter school full time and/or tend to be supplementary to the academics that are taught in schools. For these reasons, and for the sake of space, this chapter will provide a brief overview of how to teach only pre-academics and the earliest foundational academic skills. We will use the term *academic skills* from here forward in the chapter to refer both to *pre-academic* and *academic* skills. This chapter will describe how to teach these skills across two broad areas: 1) language arts and 2) mathematics. Specifically, this chapter will address the core academic skills that help to build the foundation for successful learning in a classroom setting and will describe strategies and specific teaching procedures that can be used for teaching these skills. See Table 15.1 for example lessons.

Our goals in teaching pre-academic skills are to make the transition to learning in a classroom setting as smooth as possible and to facilitate long-term academic success for the learner. Learning in a classroom setting requires a host of prerequisite skills, including, but not limited to, the ability to sustain attention, divide attention, attend in the midst of distraction, follow group-based instructions, learn through observation, wait and inhibit behavior, and initiate and complete work independently. Mastering these skills can be a challenge for many children with ASD. When demands to learn academic content are added, many children with ASD have an uphill battle to fight. Teachers often introduce new concepts in a language-rich manner, include a great deal of discussion that is not always critical to the core meaning of the concepts being taught, and introduce a variety of different materials and concepts simultaneously. For many children with ASD, this can be overwhelming. While our goal is for

TABLE 15.1   Commonly Targeted Academic Lessons

Domains	Lessons	
Language Arts	Colors	Phonological awareness
	Letters	Sight words
	Community helpers	Decoding
	Handwriting and penmanship	Print concepts
	Listening comprehension	Spelling
	Phonics	Reading comprehension
	Phonemic awareness	Independent writing
Mathematics	Quantitative concepts	Addition
	Counting and quantities	Time of day and daily
	Shapes	activities
	Numbers	Sequencing numerals and
	Patterning	ordering groups
	Quantitative comparisons	Charts and graphs
	Calendar	Skip counting
	Ordinal numbers	Money
		Telling time
		Subtraction

the learner to acquire new skills directly in the classroom setting, we can help to prepare the learner for the initial school transition and promote long-term success by teaching some of the foundational academic skills before the learner enters the classroom setting. Our initial goal on entering a classroom setting is for the learner to generalize the foundational skills taught in the home program and to ensure that the learner demonstrates the prerequisite skills required to learn in the school setting. Providing the learner with a basic understanding of the some foundational academic concepts will increase his confidence and his likelihood of success and will enable him to focus on acquiring the prerequisite skills required for group-based learning.

ACADEMIC DOMAINS

The CARD Academic curriculum is organized into Language Arts and Mathematics domains, each consisting of multiple lessons. Appendix H provides an outline for the entire Academic curriculum.

Language Arts

Language arts lessons focus on teaching skills that will lay the foundation for reading and writing. For example: 1) the Letters, Phonics, and Sight Words lessons prepare the learner for decoding and reading comprehension; 2) the Listening Comprehension lesson is critical to the learner's ability to participate actively in classroom conversations related to written material; and 3) the Handwriting and Penmanship lesson is critical for the learner to complete in-class assignments that require written responses, as well as to learn to write about objects, events, and experiences.

The CARD approach to teaching any of these skills is to break them down into small, teachable components. For example, when teaching phonics, the following components are targeted:

- Single Letter-Sound Correspondence
  - "Give me (<u>sound</u>)." (in the presence of letter cards)
  - "What sound does (<u>letter</u>) say?" (in the presence and absence of the letter)
  - "What letter says (<u>sound</u>)?" (in the presence and absence of an array of letters)
- Initial/Final Consonants
  - "Match this letter to the object that starts/ends with it." (in the presence of an array of objects)
  - "Give me the one that begins/ends with (<u>letter</u>)." (in the presence of an array of objects)

- "Give me the letter that (<u>word</u>) begins/ends with." (in the presence of an array of letters)
- "What letter does (<u>word</u>) begin/end with?" (with and without letter options present)
- "Tell me something that begins/ends with (<u>letter</u>)." (with and without object options present)
- Short Vowels
  - "Match this (letter card) to the one where (<u>letter</u>) is heard in the middle of the word." (in the presence of an array of objects)
  - "Give me the one where you hear (<u>letter</u>) in the middle of its name." (in the presence of an array of objects)
  - "Give me the letter that you hear in the middle of the word (<u>word</u>)." (in the presence of an array of letter cards)
  - "What letter do you hear in the middle of the word (<u>word</u>)?" (with and without letter card options present)
  - "Tell me something where you hear (<u>letter</u>) in the middle of its name." (with and without object options present)
- Consonant Blends/Digraphs
  - "Give me (<u>consonant blend/digraph</u>)." (in the presence of an array of cards with consonant blends, such as "br" and "cl," or digraphs, such as "ch," "th," and "wh" written on them)
  - "Read this." (in the presence of a written consonant blend such as "sl" or digraph such as "ch")
  - "Match this (written card with consonant blend/digraph) to the one that begins/ends with (<u>consonant blend/digraph</u>)." (in the presence of an array of objects)
  - "Give me the one that begins/ends with (<u>consonant blend/digraph</u>)." (in the presence of an array of objects)
  - "Give me the card that (<u>object</u>) begins/ends with." (in the presence of an array of cards with blends/digraphs written on them)

Mathematics

Early math lessons, such as 1) Numbers and 2) Counting and Quantities, focus on teaching foundational skills that will help prepare learners for more advanced math concepts. As with language arts, math concepts are broken down into component skills. For example, the Counting and Quantities lesson is broken down into the following units:

- Rote Counting
  - "Count to (<u>number</u>)."
  - "Count from (<u>number</u>)" or "Count from (<u>number</u>) to (<u>number</u>)."
  - "Count backward from (<u>number</u>) to (<u>number</u>)."
- One-to-One Correspondence
  - "Match one (<u>object</u>) to each (<u>object</u>)." (e.g., "Match one spoon to each bowl.")

- Rational Counting and Cardinal Numbers
  - "Count the (<u>objects</u>)" and "How many (<u>objects</u>) are there?" (in the presence of an array of objects)
  - "Point to the group that has (<u>number</u>)." (in the presence of groups of objects)
- Representing Groups
  - "Show me (<u>quantity</u>)." (e.g., "Show me five blocks" in the presence of a pile of objects)
  - "I have (<u>base quantity</u>) (<u>objects</u>), but I want (<u>goal quantity</u>). Can you get me more (<u>objects</u>) so I have (<u>goal quantity</u>)?" (in the presence of a pile of objects)
- Matching Numerals to Groups
  - "Put with same." (e.g., in the presence of an array of grouped objects, the learner matches a card with the numeral 3 written on it to a group of three bears)
  - "Touch the number that tells how many (<u>objects</u>)." (in the presence of an array of numeral cards)

TEACHING PROCEDURES

Evidence-based procedures for teaching skills to learners with ASD are described in Chapter 4, but we briefly review the most useful ones for academics below, with specific examples from academic lessons.

Discrete Trial Training

When using discrete trial training (DTT) to teach academic skills, an instruction is presented, the learner responds, and a consequence is delivered indicating if the response was correct or incorrect (see Chapter 4). The instruction presented by the therapist states the skill to be performed (e.g., "Read"; "What sound does M say?"; "Trace the letter W"; "Count to 10"; "Touch 6:30"; "What is 4 minus 2?"). Then the learner provides a vocal or nonvocal response, depending on the instruction. Since the instruction of basic pre-academics starts early, the use of the DTT format is a natural choice, and it mirrors the format that an academic tutor would normally use with a typically developing child.

DTT has several advantages for teaching academics. One is that the instruction is specific, and another is that the feedback for the learner's response is clear and immediate. The DTT approach to teaching academic skills begins with breaking down a skill into its simplest components. The learner is then taught each component to mastery before progressing to the next skill target. Further, the stimuli used in DTT are clear and lack distractions. For example, when teaching letter identification in DTT, therapists typically teach one or a few letters at a time. Uppercase and lowercase letters are generally separated, and letters with a dissimilar appearance are usually taught first. Further, the stimuli used in DTT contain only a single letter, with no additional pictures or information. Let's contrast this with how letters might be introduced in a classroom setting where academic skills are usually taught in more complex ways. The teacher might introduce a single letter at a time. However, both uppercase and lowercase might be introduced simultaneously, and the letter sounds, as well as the name, are introduced. Additionally, the teacher may discuss different words that begin with the target letter, and different pictures of objects beginning with the letter may be included on the representation of the letter itself. Additionally, immediate individualized feedback is rare in a classroom setting, simply because teachers are responsible for too many students to be able to give each student immediate attention and feedback. While this method of instruction and the rate of feedback are effective with typically developing children, children with ASD may find them challenging. By breaking down the skills and also ensuring that the target is clearly defined in DTT, we can ensure success and then work to increase distraction and generalize the skill to the classroom. Our goal in behavioral approaches to teaching academics is always for the learner to be able to learn in a classroom setting eventually. However, we can increase the learner's opportunities for initial success by first teaching the foundational skills that allow for generalization of what is taught in the classroom, as well as acquisition of more advanced concepts.

Multiple Exemplar Training

Academics might be the one curriculum in which many targets need to be memorized; multiplication facts and sight words are examples of this. However, whenever memorization is not the goal, multiple exemplar training (MET) can assist with the generalization of academic skills. For example, a therapist may teach the learner to read and spell many different words that all contain the phonics being targeted, to skip count starting at various different numbers, and to add and subtract a variety of quantities. MET such as this encourages generalization of the skill being taught, so a learner does not merely memorize the correct answer to particular stimuli used during teaching but, rather, forms the generalized operant skill being taught.

Natural Environment Training

Academic skills can also be practiced as opportunities are captured and contrived in the natural environment. For example, when the learner shows interest during play in a particular item or activity associated with language arts or math concepts, the therapist might instruct the learner to identify colors, shapes, and numbers, count items, and/or sound out words. With typically developing children, many academic concepts become part of their language in daily life. For example, when playing hide and seek, the child must count to ten while the others hide. Highly preferred arts and crafts projects can also be great natural environment settings in which to practice basic academics. For example, when drawing, the therapist can have the learner name the shapes she would like the therapist to draw. Or when painting, the therapist can have the learner sound out the names of the colors written on the tubes of paint she wants before handing them to her. Regardless, the key to using NET effectively is to ensure that the natural environment activity is preferred by the learner and that the consequences that occur for the learner engaging in the behavior are preferred and meaningful. For example, the therapist who merely asks the learner to read random words that she sees while engaged in an unrelated activity is going to be far less effective than if he asks the learner to read the words printed on an item the learner wants and then receives after she reads the words. Utilizing NET procedures for teaching academic skills can be critical to ensuring that the skills taught become meaningful for the learner in that she learns to apply them to useful situations in everyday life.

Worksheets

Worksheets are also commonly used to target academic skills. A worksheet contains multiple opportunities for a learner to practice a skill while also targeting the learner's ability to complete work independently. Initially, prompts may be necessary, including reading the instructions to the learner, assisting the learner with difficult questions, providing reinforcement for each item on the worksheet, and encouraging the learner to stay on task. Over time, the learner will learn to follow the written instructions on the worksheet without the addition of vocal instructions from the therapist. The ultimate goal is for the learner to complete the worksheet independently, asking for help when needed, because the goal is always to prepare the learner for real-life situations, such as the classroom setting.

STRATEGIES FOR SUCCESS

Teach Independence

Sometimes great emphasis is placed on producing a perfect finished product that requires adult assistance rather than teaching the learner to complete assignments independently. If adults consistently help a learner to complete assignments without a plan to reduce and ultimately eliminate the additional assistance over time, the learner may become dependent on the extra help and struggle to complete assignments on his own. It may be helpful to target independent work completion as a separate skill in itself, providing reinforcement for independently completing assignments before teaching the learner to ask for assistance with particularly difficult tasks. To do this, start with small amounts of a mastered task, such as a worksheet with only a few easy problems that the learner has already mastered. Fade out adult presence and prompting, and make positive reinforcement contingent upon the learner's completing the worksheet accurately and without asking for assistance. As the learner becomes successful while working independently, gradually increase the size and difficulty of the tasks. Of course, don't forget to practice across multiple different types of tasks, different times of day, and different work areas (desk, kitchen table, etc.).

Teach Test-Taking Strategies

The assumption is often made that, if a child has mastered an academic skill, he should be able to demonstrate that mastery when he takes a test. From a behavioral perspective, a child does not automatically replicate a skill in an environment (i.e., classroom) that differs greatly from the one in which he learned that skill (i.e., home). Simply put, this assumption is relying on generalization of a skill without programming for generalization. Performing well on a test is a particularly stressful sort of generalization, and you may want to consider giving your learner explicit practice and reinforcement for taking tests. Simulating testing during therapy can help the learner adapt to the particular stimulus conditions present during testing.

Readiness to Learn in the Classroom

A successful early intervention program prepares a learner for continued learning in a classroom environment by teaching her the prerequisite skills that are needed for success in that environment. Many children with ASD, even after great success in home-based behavioral intervention programs, still do not develop many skills that are fundamental to success in the school environment. Some basic skills to consider targeting include:

- Responding to group instructions
- Completing assignments independently
- Understanding the meaning of grades
- Raising one's hand to get the teacher's attention (rather than speaking out)

- Responding to instructions delivered at a distance (e.g., a teacher standing at the front of class)
- Standing in line for recess or to participate in sports
- Responding to group instructions from the teacher (even though the teacher is not speaking directly to the learner)
- Looking to peers as cues for what to do in the moment when the learner misses the teacher's request

As with any other skill taught in an ABA program, the skills listed above can be taught through prompting, reinforcement, prompt fading and generalization training. Some creativity is needed to simulate classroom settings, and role-play may be needed to simulate situations involving teachers or peers.

In addition to teaching fundamental school-readiness skills, make sure to set the learner up for success by consulting with the school to determine whether it uses particular language arts or math procedures and incorporating those procedures into the learner's ABA program. By incorporating these variables into the learner's home-based therapy before she enters school, you can help ensure that the stimuli in the school environment will already cue the desired behavior when the learner arrives in the classroom.

Collaborate with the Academic Team

Before a learner enters school, it is helpful to meet with the school-based team to discuss the transition, including the learner's strengths and weaknesses, parent and teacher concerns, expectations for classroom behavior, teaching procedures, communication between the parent and teacher, and whether additional classroom support is needed. When the learner starts regularly attending school, frequent communication between the teacher and parent will allow the parent to provide supplemental reinforcement for the learner's classroom successes and rapid remediation of any weaknesses. See Chapter 24 on interdisciplinary collaboration and Chapter 8 on communicating between home and school settings.

Promote Generalization to the Classroom Setting

To promote generalization to the classroom, ask the classroom teacher how skills are practiced at school; then ensure that the instructions, stimuli, and responses used during therapy sessions are similar to those used in the classroom. For example, if the learner is expected to provide an oral response at school, practice an oral response in therapy, or if the learner is expected to complete a worksheet independently at school, practice independently completing worksheets during therapy. Other procedures that assist with generalization include practicing the skill in different settings, using variable instructions delivered by several different people, and using the skill to complete various types of assignments.

Perhaps the most important variable for ensuring generalization is teaching the learner to apply newly learned academic skills in ways similar to how they will be used in the classroom. All too often, poor-quality ABA programs use DTT to teach learners to memorize letters and numbers receptively and expressively without any concern for how and when the learner will actually use those skills in the classroom in the future. Care should be taken to identify how the classroom teacher teaches the skill and what the next several steps are in using that skill, so the learner can be taught to apply the skill in those ways. For example, perhaps a teacher in a mainstream classroom gives the students worksheets involving letters and asks them to write letters, match letters to pictures of objects that contain the letter, or respond in unison by labeling a letter to which the teacher points. After mastering letters receptively and expressively in DTT, a learner who is going into this classroom in the near future could practice using letters in all of these various ways as part of her home-based therapy program, thereby ensuring that the learner will actually have the opportunity to use the academic skills she has mastered at home.

Maintenance

Academic skills need to be fully incorporated into the learner's everyday life and practiced on an ongoing basis, as with any other skill – perhaps even more *because* they tend to be abstract and may not always be directly useful. Maintenance can be improved by implementing a variable reinforcement schedule (see Chapter 4), so the learner is not able to determine when a reinforcer will be delivered. When reinforcers are delivered less frequently, the learner is allowed to experience the naturally occurring consequences of the behavior. Consider blending traditional forms of reinforcement and feedback used in schools, such as letter grades, stickers, and stars, with other forms of reinforcement and feedback used during therapy sessions. For example, when a learner completes a worksheet with 100% accuracy, assign a letter grade of "A" and deliver a highly preferred item. Modify the value and magnitude of the preferred item with the accuracy of the assignment and letter grade. That is, if the learner completes an assignment with 70% accuracy, assign a letter grade of "C" and deliver a small amount of a moderately preferred item. Then begin delivering the preferred item intermittently while continuing to assign appropriate letter grades.

Fluency-Based Instruction

Fluency-based instruction is often incorporated into a maintenance and generalization plan to ensure both speed and accuracy of performance in reading, math, and handwriting. Fluency is critical across a variety of pre-academic skills, as the demonstration of fluent responding with basic skills sets the foundation for performance on later emerging and more complicated skills. For example, a learner may slowly count money with 100% accuracy, but if she is not fluent with basic counting, then any type of problem-solving or practical application that requires counting money will be more difficult for her. Further, consider how important it is for a learner to demonstrate fluent handwriting skills. If the learner is slow to write responses, it will take him longer to complete in-class assignments and tests, as well as make it difficult to keep up in small and large group lessons where written responses are required. Fluency-based instruction involves timing the learner for 10 to 60 seconds, recording how many items (e.g., words read, math problems completed, etc.) the learner completes accurately, and increasing the amount completed across timings until she is able to respond rapidly and without hesitation. See Chapter 4 for more on fluency (see also Kubina & Yurich, 2012).

COMMON PITFALLS

Progressing to Advanced Skills Before Foundational Skills Are Fluent

When a learner struggles to learn academic skills, the skills may be too difficult. Before introducing more advanced academic skills, it is important to ensure that the learner has mastered the necessary prerequisite skills and to monitor performance regularly with maintenance lessons. If a learner continues to struggle with prerequisite skills, delay the introduction of further academic skills. Also, consider increasing the mastery criterion for prerequisite skills (e.g., require 90% correct across 5 days, instead of 80% correct across 3 days), and run maintenance lessons more frequently.

Overfocusing on What Is Age Appropriate or Being Taught in Class

Avoid introducing skills solely because they are age appropriate, being taught in the learner's classroom, and/or a part of a standard curriculum. Instead, determine if the academic skills are functional for the learner and meet her individualized curriculum goals and whether the learner has the necessary prerequisite skills.

Irrelevant/Nonfunctional

Avoid teaching academic content for content's sake. In good-quality programs, each acquisition target should be logically and strategically linked to an outcome that will make the learner more independent and happier in the future. Unfortunately, poor-quality ABA programs (as well as non-behavioral special education programs) all too often attempt to make children with ASD memorize as many academic skills as possible without any meaningful plan for how the skills will benefit the child in the future.

Too Difficult or Too Easy

When the focus is on teaching age-appropriate or grade-level academic skills, you can easily fall into the trap of teaching skills that are either too difficult or too easy for the learner. A better approach is to determine the standard for the learner's grade level and then assess where he falls in relation to the standard. If the learner is behind grade level, it is necessary to work on prerequisite skills first. If the learner is above grade level for a given skill, the time you would have spent teaching that skill can be used to teach something else the learner needs to acquire in order to get caught up to grade level.

Difficulty with Handwriting and Written Assignments

Handwriting skills require the learner to grip a pencil and make small movements with his hand and fingers to create letters. If a learner is struggling with the acquisition of handwriting skills, ensure that he has sufficient fine motor strength and visual motor skills for proficient performance. Deficits in these motor skills can be remediated by introducing lessons that specifically target these skills (see Chapter 14 on motor skills).

When a learner struggles with handwriting, the learner is also likely to have difficulty with written assignments. For lessons that include a written response, first determine whether the written response is a necessary component of the target skill. If a written response is not essential, consider accepting an alternative response form, such as an oral or typed response, while the learner continues to work on handwriting skills.

Decoding Versus Comprehension

Do not assume that, because a learner can read words ("decode" them), she also comprehends what she is reading. Make sure that comprehension is targeted during reading instruction. Just as important, probe for comprehension by having your learner read new passages that she has never been taught and then asking comprehension questions that she could only answer if she actually comprehended what she just read (as opposed to repeating what she has been taught to say in the past).

Working on the Same IEP Goals for a Long Time

Individualized Education Program (IEP) goals are regularly monitored to assess learning gains, with data being collected on accuracy of the skill and prompts needed to assist the learner in making a correct response. It can be helpful to graph these data in order to visually inspect progress over time. If the learner is making slow learning gains, consider reviewing the teaching procedures to determine whether any modifications will accelerate her learning rate. If progress has ceased for a significant amount of time, it is necessary to review the IEP and assess whether the goal is still appropriate for the learner and/or whether the teaching procedures are adequate (see Chapter 19 on clinical problem solving).

SUMMARY

This chapter outlined several instructional procedures that are useful when teaching academic language arts and mathematics skills. Initial instruction focuses on discriminating among basic letters, numbers, colors, and shapes. Then these skills are used to develop more complex academic skills. Satisfactory acquisition of academic-readiness skills will assist learners in their transition to instruction in an elementary school classroom, providing the foundation for more advanced skills taught later in their educational careers.

Social

Jennifer Yakos

One of the core defining features of autism spectrum disorder (ASD) is impairment in the ability to engage in appropriate and meaningful social interactions with others. In fact, social skills are often among the most critical yet challenging repertoires for individuals with ASD to develop. Social skills instruction begins within the earliest therapy sessions and often continues through the very last stages of intervention.

The range and complexity of social behaviors across the span of childhood into adulthood are vast, and their development is also hugely dependent on the interplay of other skill repertoires, such as communication, play skills, cognition, perspective taking, and executive functioning skills. Deficits in any of these other skill domains will likely have an impact on an individual's ability to develop successful social skills. Additionally, social interactions are inherently unpredictable and are influenced by numerous variables that constantly change. The context of the situation, the physical location, the activity in effect, the people involved, and most important, the emotions, thoughts, and motivations of the participants have a significant impact on the dynamics of social interactions. It is impossible to teach any individual how to respond in every social situation that he may face.

Considering all of these issues, social skills training can be very complex and challenging to design and implement effectively. Despite the complexity and difficulty of the challenge, individuals with ASD who receive top-quality behavioral intervention make substantial progress in the area of socialization, allowing many to develop meaningful, reciprocal relationships. While the task of implementing effective social skills instruction may seem daunting, progress is attainable with every child.

COMMON SOCIAL DIFFICULTIES IN AUTISM SPECTRUM DISORDER

Before describing how to teach social skills, we briefly discuss what social skills deficits look like across the autism spectrum. The degree to which any child demonstrates these social challenges varies greatly across individuals, just as is the case for all other major skill deficits in ASD.

Developmentally Appropriate Relationships

Children with ASD often have difficulty developing successful relationships with similar-age peers. This does not necessarily mean that the child with ASD does not have friendly interactions with others. In fact, many children with ASD form strong attachments to family members and others. However, relationships with similar-age peers may not be reciprocal in nature, meaning that they may not be a two-way, interactive relationship in which both individuals are equal partners within the friendship. Also, it is often observed that some children with ASD tend to form bonds with individuals who are much younger or much older than they are. It is not uncommon that a child with ASD may seek out the attention and interactions of adults while appearing uninterested or aloof in interactions with same-age peers. For example, children who are more severely affected by ASD may be seen standing in a corner of a room, engaging in repetitive behavior, while all of the other children are playing together according to a common theme. Children who are very mildly affected by ASD and who have very well-developed language may be highly successful when interacting with adults, to the extent that adults may even find them to be socially advanced. Yet, these same children are often largely unable to make or maintain friendships with children their own age because their social language is so different from that of their peers.

Non-vocal Social Behaviors

Children with ASD often demonstrate impairments in the ability to use and recognize non-vocal communication within social interactions. Most children with ASD, across the spectrum of severity, demonstrate some difficulty with eye contact, varying from an overall lack of eye contact to only fleeting eye contact at select times. Many have difficulty showing appropriate emotional affect or facial expressions related to the context at hand. Others struggle with recognizing and responding to the facial expressions, gestures, and body language of others. The lack of use and understanding of non-vocal communication often lead to unsuccessful interactions with others. For example, if a highly verbal child with ASD is conversing with a peer and says something "overly honest" to the peer that hurts the peer's feelings, she may completely miss the look of surprise, anger, or sadness that her honest comment evokes from the peer, therefore completely missing the crucial negative social feedback that she should have received. Consequently, instead of noticing that making negative comments to peers results in an undesirable social consequence, the child with ASD may continue to behave in this way and continue to be unsuccessful in the future, thereby further socially isolating himself. Without the ability to recognize and respond appropriately to subtle non-vocal social cues, it is understandable that children with ASD struggle to navigate the social world.

Sharing Experiences with Others

Many children with ASD show limited interest in sharing experiences with others, often referred to as *joint attention.* This can be seen from early childhood, where a child may not spontaneously point out interesting objects, sounds, or events to other people. Also, many children with ASD do not show items to a parent or caregiver to share their delight or involve them in play, although they may point to or bring items to caregivers but only when they need the caregiver to give them the item or fix it for them. Seeking help from a caregiver is an important interaction, but it differs from the social function of pointing at or showing an item purely for the purpose of engaging the caregiver, as is often done by typically developing young children when initiating joint attention. In addition, many children with ASD do not respond reliably to bids for joint attention by others. For example, when a parent says a child's name and points vigorously at an object or event, a typically developing toddler or preschooler will usually engage with the parent in the interaction and look to see what the parent is looking at. Many children with ASD do not reliably respond to these attempts at social initiation by their parents.

Social Reciprocity

Social and emotional reciprocity refers to an individual's ability to return vocal and non-vocal social exchanges, as well as empathize with others and demonstrate appropriate emotional reactions within social contexts. Social reciprocity can be noted in very young children who smile when smiled at or respond with affection when given affection. In older children, social reciprocity also includes the ability to participate in social exchanges with others, including conversations. Emotional reciprocity involves identifying the emotions of others and matching one's emotional reaction appropriately to the situation, as well as empathizing and connecting the emotional experiences of others to their own personal experiences. Many children with ASD may struggle with one or both of these types of social relations.

DOMAINS OF SOCIAL SKILLS INSTRUCTION

Social skills encompass a very large repertoire of behaviors. In addition, social skills build upon and support multiple other repertoires, such as verbal behavior, perspective taking, executive function, and play skills, repertoires which are described in detail in other chapters of this manual. The Center for Autism and Related Disorders (CARD) Social curriculum, contained in the Skills® system (www.skillsforautism.com; see Chapter 26), consists of nearly 50 lessons across the following eight domains: 1) Non-vocal Social Behavior, 2) Social Interaction, 3) Social Language, 4) Social Rules, 5) Social Context, 6) Group-Related Social Behavior, 7) Self-Esteem, and 8) Absurdities. Appendix I provides an outline of the entire CARD Social curriculum. Space does not permit a description of how to teach the skills from every lesson in the Social curriculum. Instead, we provide practical descriptions of how to teach a few key skills in each domain.

Non-vocal Social Behavior

Non-vocal social behavior is a critical foundation for the development of more advanced social skills. Non-vocal behaviors, such as eye contact, joint attention, and imitation, are among the first skills to emerge in typical child development. Direct eye contact, which typically emerges between 6 and 8 weeks of life, is an essential skill that facilitates social and emotional bonding with others and provides the foundation for learning and imitating the actions of others. Early on, infants learn to discriminate the human face from other visual images and learn the importance of looking to others to gain important information about the world around them. Social skills training should target the improvement of eye contact, as needed, due to its importance in the development of many other necessary skills. Later, we will discuss ways in which to do so effectively and naturally.

The development of joint attention, described above, is just important as eye contact. Joint attention is essential in the development of social relationships with others and allows us to gain information about the environment, as well as share joint social experiences with others.

Non-vocal imitation, which is another core social skill in this area, allows individuals to copy the behaviors of others that they observe in order to learn effective ways to engage with their surroundings. The development of spontaneous imitation skills enables us to learn incidentally in the natural environment by watching how others move, use objects, play, and interact and then doing the same behaviors ourselves when opportunities arise.

Social Interaction

Examples of social interaction skills include gaining attention from others, demonstrating assertiveness appropriate to the situation, sharing and turn-taking, cooperating and negotiating, giving compliments, and apologizing. This subset of skills is especially important for individuals who are motivated to interact with others but experience difficulty doing so with positive results. For example, an individual who lacks appropriate assertiveness skills may either fail to speak up when someone takes his lunch money or may respond inappropriately by screaming and hitting the person. Both of these responses to the situation will not result in a positive outcome for the individual.

Another example of a social interaction skill is the ability to gain attention from others. Those who are unable to use a person's name appropriately or gesture to get another's attention oftentimes make requests or comments that go unnoticed by others. Examples of this include making a request to have a turn playing a video game or making a social comment about a new movie that no one is able to hear or to which no one responds. Further, many individuals resort to inappropriate means for gaining attention from others, typically in the form of inappropriate or challenging behaviors, such as screaming, throwing things, aggression, or even self-injurious behaviors.

Social Language

The social use of language is often referred to as *conversational language* or *pragmatic language*. The social language domain is comprised of a complex set of skills that work together to facilitate reciprocal conversations between two or more people. This skill set is especially important for individuals with ASD who have a solid foundation in communication skills but have a limited ability to engage in mutually rewarding conversations with others. Several common issues that arise include difficulties initiating conversations with appropriate and relevant detail, maintaining conversations through conversational turn-taking, discussing neutral or non-preferred topics, staying on topic, asking questions of others, and responding to non-literal language and social cues. Social language targets include listening to a conversation, initiating topics with appropriate opening phrases ("Hey, guess what?"), making relevant comments and questions about a topic, participating in conversational turn-taking, transitioning topics, responding to non-vocal social language (e.g., shoulder shrug, confused expression), and adjusting conversations to the audience and situational context. Social language instruction is most effective when targeted with individuals who are able to communicate easily with others, including making requests, making social comments, answering and asking questions, and using more complex sentence structures.

Social Rules and Rule-Governed Behavior

The ability to understand and follow social rules is another critical social skill domain. Much of our social behavior is, at least partially, "rule-governed behavior" in that our behavior is partially governed by our understanding of rules and consequences and our desire/decision to adhere to those rules to avoid negative consequences and to be rewarded by positive consequences. For instance, a child may know that if she asks politely for a turn with a toy, it will make others happy and likely result in getting access to the toy. However, if she yells and grabs the toy away from another person, she will likely be in trouble and not get the toy or even be punished. In cases of "purely" rule-governed behavior, a typically developing child need only hear a rule that describes these contingencies and can then respond successfully, even though she has never directly contacted the contingencies in the past. Of course, much social behavior is learned through direct contact with contingencies and rules are not required, but rules prepare us for future social interactions free of major errors that can result in negative outcomes. Therefore, the ability to follow social rules is critical to success in a wide variety of social situations.

Children with ASD often have difficulty understanding and detecting social rules and, therefore, are less likely to develop rule-governed behavior independently. That is, they may not possess a rule-following repertoire. Particularly if you begin incorporating social rules into early or intermediate stages of social skills training, you should not expect a rule-following repertoire to be present; you may well have to teach that. Research has demonstrated that children with ASD can learn the generalized ability to understand and follow the if/then contingency statements contained in rules (Tarbox, Zuckerman, Bishop, Olive, & O'Hora, 2011).

Early rule-governed behavior instruction often needs to incorporate practice and exposure to many examples of rules and the consequences the rules describe. At first, these experiences teach the learner through direct acting contingencies, but after sufficient exemplars have been trained, the generalized ability to follow untrained rules can emerge (see Chapter 7 on teaching generalized repertoires). Since it is impossible to contrive every situation that a learner may encounter in life, general rules regarding social behavior can be useful because they apply to numerous situations that share common features and allow the learner to be successful in a variety of settings. Instruction in this domain typically begins with following basic compliance instructions and later includes targets such as following basic rules, say-do correspondence (e.g., matching what one says he will do with what he actually does), rules for politeness and manners, and following community rules.

Group-Related Social Behavior

Many critical social skills involve successful participation in group interactions. Much of our social behavior occurs within group settings, including academic, extracurricular, and vocational environments. Specific behaviors are especially relevant to group situations, particularly those having to do with appropriate levels of participation, understanding one's role and responsibilities as a member or leader, participating in group discussions and sharing ideas with others, and making joint decisions that are mutually agreeable to all members. Individuals must learn how to participate at an appropriate level corresponding to their role in the group and must learn to respect the roles of others in the group. Being part of a group also involves balancing an appropriate level of assertiveness when sharing ideas and making suggestions while being respectful and willing to compromise and negotiate with others.

Self-Esteem

Self-esteem refers to having a positive yet realistic view of one's own abilities, which is important when trying new things, pursuing new social relationships with others, and being assertive in social situations. Individuals who have realistic views of their own positive traits may also be more able to accept constructive feedback from others, accept winning and losing appropriately, and deal with conflict appropriately. Noticing one's own strengths likely contributes to overall happiness. Although this may sound like "fluff," this is a very important consideration for children with ASD, especially in light of the many social and emotional challenges that face many young people in the autism population, such as bullying and depression.

Absurdities

Absurdities is an area of social skill functioning that focuses on humor, including jokes, puns, and figures of speech. Having a sense of humor is a popular characteristic, and many social interactions involve the use of humor. Individuals with ASD may have difficulty understanding the non-literal meaning of language, which facilitates the understanding of jokes and other funny stories. Being able to understand humor and puns is an important skill that is necessary for responding appropriately to a variety of social situations. Further, the ability to tell age-appropriate jokes and comical anecdotes and use figures of speech can help individuals successfully engage in natural social interactions and forge friendships with peers. Simply put, life is just more fun if humor is part of the daily experience.

TEACHING STRATEGIES

In this section, we discuss how teaching strategies based on applied behavior analysis (ABA) are used to teach social skills across a variety of domains, starting with beginning-level instruction and progressing to more advanced skills.

Beginning-Level Instruction

As we discussed earlier, it is critical for social skills training to begin during the very earliest stages of autism treatment, even with learners aged 2 or younger. Foundational skills, such as establishing eye contact, learning to follow instructions and requests, and developing basic imitation, serve as critical prerequisites to the development of other necessary social skills. Some would consider these skills to be "behavioral cusps," meaning that they have a far-reaching impact on the development of the learner beyond the actual skill itself because they open doors to the potential acquisition of other skills. For instance, a child's ability to make eye contact with others and to do so across a variety of people and settings serves as a prerequisite for multiple other skills, including identifying facial expressions, recognizing subtle social cues, and developing joint attention skills.

Beginning-level social skills instruction primarily involves contingency-shaped learning (as opposed to rule governance). That is, the child learns new behaviors through direct exposure to their consequences. For instance, a learner might learn to follow the instruction "come here" because it is reinforced by hugs and social praise from a therapist. Learning new basic social behaviors generally requires the direct delivery of reinforcers. While targeting these skills generally requires some structure, they should also be targeted in more natural situations. Many learners benefit from a combination of both Discrete Trial Training (DTT) methods and Natural Environment Training (NET) procedures. The structure of a DTT format provides clear messages to the learner about what is required, along with the repetition of learning opportunities to allow the learner to receive prompting and reinforcement at a high frequency. In addition, using NET to target these skills within natural learning opportunities helps with generalization and motivation. Let's take a look at some examples of how both DTT and NET can be used to teach the early social skill of imitation.

Imitation through DTT instruction. During basic imitation instruction, a learner is presented with a simple object, and the therapist uses the object in a particular way and presents the vocal instruction "do this." The learner is then prompted to perform the same action with the object and receives reinforcement when he complies. The trial is then repeated multiple times, and as the learner continues to perform the same action with the object, the prompts are gradually faded. Other actions, with and without objects, are taught in this manner until the learner acquires the generalized ability to imitate actions that were never directly taught. Thus, the child has learned generalized imitation. However, many learners with ASD will not automatically start to apply this skill in natural settings with various actions and people, unless they are specifically instructed to "do this." NET procedures should also be used very early on to aid in generalization.

Imitation through NET procedures. To use NET to teach imitation, the learner should be engaged in a preferred activity in the natural environment. For example, a learner might be playing with a musical keyboard during free play. To capture the learner's motivation, the therapist turns the power button on the keyboard to the off position, resulting in the keys no longer producing sound when pressed. The therapist then shows the learner how to push the "on" button on the keyboard. The learner then pushes the same button on the keyboard, and the power turns on, allowing him to hear music when the keys are pressed. Here, imitation is targeted during an activity that is motivating to the learner and produces a reinforcing payoff, specifically, being able to play with a desired toy. The learner should continue to be presented with opportunities to imitate various actions of therapists and parents across a variety of natural settings and during a variety of activities. Sometimes, it may be useful initially to include the instruction "do this" during these teaching interactions. The instruction should be faded as soon as possible, so the imitation skill generalizes across situations and does not come under the sole stimulus control of that particular instruction. Keep in mind that the learner will rarely be told directly to imitate others in the natural environment, especially by peers. Instead, the learner must imitate others without needing to be told to do so.

Imitation training may progress by teaching the learner to imitate multiple-step actions demonstrated by others, specifically action chains across a variety of skill areas. For instance, a child should be able to imitate the play actions of others, such as feeding a baby doll, building and playing with a train, or pretending to be a fireman. In the academic setting, learners should be able to imitate classroom routines, such as putting backpacks away and lining up at the door. Also, multiple-step imitation is important when learning how to write and draw, to engage in playground or group games, and other school-related activities. Further, the imitation of self-care chains, such as getting dressed or brushing teeth, is obviously a relevant target for many individuals. It may be necessary to teach multiple-step imitation within a structured DTT format first and then program for generalization across a wide variety of activities and settings within the natural environment using NET procedures.

Teaching eye contact through NET. Let's look at another example of teaching strategies for a beginning social skill: eye contact. Eye contact is an essential prerequisite skill for almost all other instructional targets within a comprehensive ABA intervention program. More importantly, it is a critical skill that facilitates success in practically all areas of life, including developing social relationships, participating in learning activities, and protecting one's well-being and safety in the natural environment. Making and sustaining eye contact are both necessary in order to attend and respond to most learning activities, as well as to be cognizant of relevant events happening in the world around us. Many ABA programs approach early instruction activities for eye contact using more structured teaching formats, such as DTT. While this approach to increasing eye contact may have its benefits, it can often lead to individuals only making eye contact when instructed to do so or using patterns of eye contact that appear unnatural. Many verbal individuals with ASD have commented that eye contact can be one of the more difficult social skills to master. For these reasons, it can be advantageous to attempt improvements in eye contact using more natural teaching activities first. Let's consider an example of how eye contact can begin to be taught using an NET approach. A learner and a therapist are playing together, with the therapist tickling the learner (and tickling is preferred by the learner). The therapist then pauses tickling and looks expectantly at the learner with an anticipatory expression and hands raised in the air. After several seconds, the learner looks in the direction of the therapist, who immediately resumes the tickling activity and praises the learner as soon as he makes eye contact. The therapist repeats this pattern of pausing tickling, waiting for the child to make eye contact, and resuming tickling for approximately 10 seconds as soon as eye contact is given. The therapist can then very gradually increase the duration of eye contact that she requires before resuming tickling. When this process works, the learner begins to give eye contact with greater ease and frequency during the tickling interactions. By frequent pairing of eye contact with reinforcement, eye contact begins to be established as a source of conditioned reinforcement, thereby further increasing the probability that it will maintain and generalize.

While it is critical to improve the spontaneous eye contact of individuals with ASD during play, it is also often necessary to teach the learner to make eye contact when requested to do so by another person. An example of this is learning to look at a person when called by name. Both NET and DTT formats can be used for this purpose, although many learners may require the more structured format of DTT to learn this skill. Let's look at an example of how this can be done.

Teaching eye contact through DTT. When teaching eye contact through DTT, the learner is sitting down across from the therapist, perhaps seated at a table with the therapist or sitting across from him on the floor. The therapist calls the name of the learner and immediately prompts her to look by pointing at his eyes. When the learner makes eye contact with the therapist, she immediately receives reinforcement in the form of social praise and whatever other powerful reinforcers are available. The activity is repeated multiple times within a short time frame, and prompts are gradually faded out until the learner makes eye contact with the therapist whenever her name is called. Once this begins to happen consistently, the therapist can start to expand upon the skill by increasing the length of the glance prior to giving reinforcement, increasing the distance between therapist and learner, conducting trials more intermittently during the session, and adding distractions to the environment to facilitate generalizing the skill to more natural situations (e.g., having music in the background, calling the learner's name while he is eating a snack, etc.).

Whether it is taught using NET, DTT, or a combination of both, consider several of the following guidelines for developing natural, socially appropriate eye contact. First, **eye contact should be taught within situations where it has a purpose**. When teaching learners to make eye contact, especially for extended durations, there should be a clear purpose for doing so. While teaching a learner to maintain eye contact for several seconds, the therapist should be engaging him in a social interaction, speaking to him, or showing him something of interest. For young learners, even just smiling or making silly faces while making eye contact gives them a reason to look and make eye contact. Therapists should avoid having the learner sit and simply stare. This does not teach a socially functional eye contact repertoire but, rather, rote compliance to a socially arbitrary demand.

Another guideline to follow is to **limit the duration of time the learner is expected to sustain uninterrupted eye contact to a duration that is reasonable**. It is unnatural for any person – especially young children – to sit and look continuously at another person for an extended period of time. Consider taking a measure of how long typically developing same-age peers hold eye contact, and use that as a realistic goal. Also, do not require learners to stare without intermittently glancing away from the person or object of interest. While speaking or listening to another person, it is completely natural and appropriate to look away occasionally and quickly look back. It would be unnatural for anyone, including an individual with ASD, not to break eye contact intermittently during a conversation and would likely make the learner's peer uncomfortable as well. Remember, facilitating natural social interactions – not rote compliance – is the goal.

Last, **make sure that eye contact is taught within a variety of practical and social situations**. For example, rather than teaching a learner to sit at one table and stare at a therapist, she should be taught to initiate and sustain joint attention in response to novel and exciting events, make eye contact during conversations, make eye contact during a variety of play activities, and so on.

Intermediate-Level Instruction

As learners progress beyond basic skill instruction, social skill targets become more complex and involve much more emphasis on peer interactions. As skills improve, learners are generally taking part in a wider variety of social contexts, including attending a classroom setting and participating in group activities, clubs, or community outings. Previously taught skills that were mastered with familiar adults need to be further generalized to peers and other, less familiar individuals. Learners who are moving into intermediate-level social skills instruction are often characterized by emerging communication skills (e.g., the ability to follow single- and multiple-step instructions, use simple phrases to make requests and some comments, answer simple questions), foundational play/leisure skills (e.g., the ability to engage in a variety of independent play/leisure activities, participate in simple games), and basic compliance skills (e.g., the ability to follow instructions with decreasing behavioral issues). Social skills instruction at this stage will generally involve both contingency-based instruction, as described above, and rule-governed behavior instruction. Let's take a look at how contingency-based instruction and rule-based instruction can be combined to teach several intermediate social skill targets.

Gaining attention using contingency-based instruction. Consider the following example of using direct-acting contingencies to teach a learner to gain the attention of others. The learner sits with the therapist, who is looking at a book that is known to be preferred by the learner. The learner has not looked at the book today and cannot see the pages from where he is sitting (i.e., he is motivated to obtain the book), so he asks the therapist, "Can I have the book?" The therapist is busy and pretends not to hear the learner. Another person (e.g., a second therapist, a parent, or a trained sibling) prompts the learner to gain the attention of the first therapist by using a shoulder tap or calling the person's name before asking for the book. The learner performs this action, and the therapist turns toward the learner and gives him the book. The learner's behavior of gaining the therapist's attention prior to requesting for the item is reinforced by getting access to the desired book. This activity is then practiced multiple times, across a wide variety of desired items, settings, activities, and people. After the learner has mastered this skill, it can be further expanded by teaching him to persist and to make several attempts at gaining a person's attention prior to requesting an item. Also, the skill can be expanded to gaining attention prior to making a social comment or asking a question for desired information.

In the example above, the new skill of gaining the attention of another person before making a request is learned through the repeated exposure to the direct consequences of that behavior. That is, the contingencies for the behavior are what shape the child's learning. However, many other variables should be considered when appropriately gaining the attention of others in social situations, including the setting, the relationship with the person(s) involved, the activities in place, and the emotions and physical state of the other person. For instance, a learner needs to use different strategies when seeking to gain the attention of someone sitting next to him at the lunch table versus gaining the attention of a teacher in class, gaining the attention of a parent who is on the phone, and so on. In order to teach these specific skill applications and many others that involve complex social conditions, the use of rules may improve effectiveness and efficiency. Rule-governed behavior instruction often includes the following steps: 1) introduction of the rule, 2) review and discussion of the rule, 3) role-play rehearsal, 4) practice in actual social situations, and 5) application to generalized situations.

Using rules to teach attention-gaining. To begin, the learner is presented with a social rule (e.g., a description of a situation, a specific behavior, and the likely consequence for that behavior in the situation) for gaining the attention of others within a particular situation. For instance, the rule could read, "If someone is busy, I should wait until the person is done with what he is doing and then get his attention. If I don't wait or I'm too loud, I might get in trouble and the person would feel mad." The therapist states the rule to the learner, and they both review it together. In addition, hypothetical situations are presented, and the learner is asked to identify if each would be an example of when the rule would or would not apply (e.g., teacher during math class, dad talking on the phone, friends at recess). Next, the therapist and the learner role-play one of the scenarios related to the rule, such as a parent talking on the phone. The learner practices waiting until his father (role-played by the therapist) is finished talking and then quietly tapping him on the shoulder to get his attention prior to speaking. If you think the learner will find it fun, you can switch roles, with the learner pretending to be the parent and the therapist gaining his attention appropriately.

The next step is capturing and contriving situations in the natural environment wherein the learner can apply and practice the new rule. For instance, the learner can be told to ask his mother for a snack when his mother is involved in a conversation with a sibling. The learner should wait until there is a pause in the conversation and then quietly get the attention of his mother. At this point, the therapist may need to remind the learner of the rule immediately prior to the contrived learning opportunity. Reminders, or priming, should eventually be faded out to promote independence over time. Further, multiple exemplars of relevant situations should also be practiced in this manner. Last, the new behavior should be observed to occur naturally in novel, everyday situations without priming. Throughout the entire process, the learner should receive reinforcement for demonstrating competency with the skill, and this, too, should eventually be faded out, so natural contingencies alone eventually maintain the behavior. Extensions of this rule might include how to get attention without interrupting and rules for gaining the attention of others in emergency/non-emergency situations.

Teaching learners with ASD to understand and apply rules can be time consuming, especially if they are new to the process. However, many intermediate- and higher level social skills are most effectively taught if a combined contingency-shaped and rule-governed approach is used. Let's look at one more example of instruction at the intermediate level using both approaches.

Teaching sharing and turn-taking with direct contingencies. The setup in this scenario includes a learner playing with a toy, for example, a remote control car. After several minutes, a therapist holds out a hand and says, "Can I have a turn?" The learner is prompted to give the controller to the therapist and is immediately given reinforcement for sharing the toy. After several seconds, the therapist returns the controller to the learner and says, "OK, it's your turn." The learner is allowed to play with the car, and again after a short period, the therapist asks, "Can I have a turn?" The process is repeated, and the learner is immediately given reinforcement for sharing the controller with the therapist. Following multiple opportunities, the prompts are gradually faded, and the learner shares the controller with the therapist for several seconds when asked. Once consistent, the therapist gradually increases the duration of her turn from several seconds to a more natural duration for the activity. The learner continues to receive reinforcement for sharing the controller; however, reinforcement is thinned out and faded to something more natural, such as, "Thanks for sharing." Throughout the process, the skill is practiced across a wide variety of activities and settings and with a wide variety of people.

Using rules to teach sharing and turn-taking. To begin, a rule about turn-taking is presented to the learner, such as, "If I am not ready to give other people a turn, I can say, 'Okay, as soon as I am done,' or 'in a minute.' Then I can finish what I am doing, and after a few minutes, I can give them a turn. They will be happy that I am sharing and want to share with me, too." The therapist and the learner review the rule, and the therapist discusses the rule using multiple examples. Role-play activities are conducted during which the therapist asks to have a turn with a desired item and the learner practices using the targeted phrases, which are then reinforced. Additionally, roles are switched, so the learner practices waiting to take a turn when the therapist tells him "in a minute," and the therapist delivers reinforcement if the learner waits patiently.

Following role-play activities, naturally occurring situations are captured or contrived in which another person asks to take turns with the learner immediately after the learner has gained access to the desired activity. During these activities, prompts are given, if necessary, including advanced priming of the rule, to apply the new skill within the natural situation. The learner receives reinforcement by appropriately using one of the phrases and then sharing the item with the other person. Eventually, prompting and reinforcement are faded until only the naturally occurring cues and reinforcement are left to maintain the behavior. Finally, the skill is generalized to other social situations with a variety of people and contexts.

The combination of both structured, contingency-based instruction and rule-governed procedures allows learners to acquire the foundational skill in a direct, effective manner and then apply those skills to a wider repertoire of social contexts. The balance between the two teaching approaches should be customized for each learner and for each skill. Some will need extended practice and reinforcement within structured ABA teaching strategies, while others will only require minimal practice and can more quickly begin to apply skills to other contexts according to various social rules. Regardless, within either approach, social skill targets should be selected that are meaningful and functional for the individual within her own respective situation, and instruction should be embedded within natural events as much as possible. Let's now look at examples of instructional procedures for teaching advanced social skills.

Advanced-Level Instruction

Children with ASD who are ready for instruction in advanced social skills are typically interacting with peers on a regular basis and may be participating in various general education settings with typically developing peers. These learners have strong communication skills but may have difficulty engaging in social conversations. Their ability to interact independently with peers is emerging; however, they may have difficulty maintaining the interaction or friendship for extended periods of time. Also, these learners can follow concrete rules regarding social behaviors but may have difficulty with more complex rules across different social boundaries, contexts, and relationships. Other common skill targets within this group of learners include recognizing and responding to subtle body language and social cues, understanding humor and non-literal speech, and resolving conflict situations using appropriate compromising and negotiating skills. It is during this level of instruction that cognition skills (e.g., perspective-taking skills, emotions and preferences of others, social cause and effect) and executive function skills (e.g., flexibility, problem solving) become increasingly important in the success of social skills training. Many of the lesson activities integrate concepts from these other domains to help the learner understand why targeted social skills are necessary, as well as how and when to use them.

At this point, instruction may primarily consist of rule-governed behavior approaches; however, role-play and active practice within the natural environment are still required to promote skill development. Let's look at a few examples of instruction at this level. In the first example, we will focus on social language, specifically rules regarding introducing a conversation. For the purposes of our example, we are assuming that the learner is already able to make statements and ask questions about given topics. Let's look at some instructional strategies for using appropriate introductory statements when introducing a conversation to another person.

Using rules to teach conversation introductions. The therapist might begin by presenting a rule to the learner, such as, "When you want to start talking to someone, it is helpful to use an opening question or comment. This lets the other person know that you are about to say something to him, so he can be ready to listen. Other people will like this and be more willing to talk to you." The rule is discussed, and the learner and therapist make a list of several opening phrases or questions that are commonly used to start conversations, such as, "Hey, (*name*), guess what?"; "Do you want to know something cool?"; or "(*Name*), check this out." Role-play is then conducted during which the learner is asked to introduce conversations about various topics using some of the conversation openers. Reinforcement is given and gradually thinned.

Following role-play, natural situations are captured or contrived to target more practical application of the skill. Prompting strategies can be used, such as posting visual cues on the wall that depict some of the opening phrases. Also, situations can be contrived that might evoke conversation, such as events occurring in the environment that remind the learner about some highly preferred topics. For example, if the learner just watched a new movie, the ticket stubs or DVD case can be left on the table within the learner's view. Other examples include bringing over a book about sea life shortly after the learner has visited an aquarium, or wearing a t-shirt that has a favorite character depicted on it. Before each opportunity, the learner can also be primed with particular opening phrases. Eventually, prompts and supplemental reinforcement should be faded until the learner is independently using appropriate opening statements to initiate conversations with others. All along, this skill should be practiced across multiple people, settings, and topics in order to encourage generalization.

Extensions of the skill described above could include selecting a topic of conversation that is relevant to the listener or context. For example, the learner can pick which topics of conversation may be appropriate for various situations, such as being at a birthday party, a football game, or the beach or while playing a video game. Appropriate topics may also be selected for specific people, such as a friend, sibling, or parent, according to her particular preferences. For instance, the learner can identify who would be interested in hearing about a new computer game, topics that his younger sister would be motivated to discuss, and so on. Here, perspective-taking skills from the Cognition curriculum, such as identifying the emotions and preferences of others, are integrated into the instruction of social language. This example illustrates the importance of developing both skill areas simultaneously and how the development of one skill set supports the growth of another.

Using rules to teach complex social cues. The therapist begins by introducing a rule to the learner, such as, "Sometimes, people tell us how they are feeling or what they are thinking by using their body or face or changing the way their voice sounds. When people feel bored, they might look away, roll their eyes, or sigh. They might start getting fidgety, and their voice may sound low or flat. When I notice someone doing these things, she might be telling me she is bored, so I should try to find something more interesting to talk about or play with. I can even ask her what she would like to talk about or do. When I do this, my friends will be happy and want to keep hanging out with me." The therapist and learner review the rule, including a discussion of situations in which someone might feel bored, as well as demonstrations of expressions and body language that might indicate boredom. Next, instruction moves to role-play activities in which the therapist pretends to act bored and the learner must adjust her behavior by changing the conversation topic or activity. Appropriate responding is prompted and reinforced, and as always, contrived prompting and reinforcement are gradually reduced until only naturally occurring cues and reinforcement maintain the behavior.

Other complex social cues can be taught in this same manner, including cues indicating preference, anger, frustration, confusion, excitement, or fear. Video modeling may also be used, as well as picture images of various facial expressions, to examine and discuss different emotional cues and features indicating the thoughts and feelings of another person. Another extension would be to have the learner practice demonstrating appropriate facial expressions and social cues appropriate to specific situations. This may be helpful for learners who occasionally demonstrate inappropriate reactions to social events (e.g., smiling when another person is hurt, lack of expression when another person is upset) or exhibit flat facial affect. Let's look at one final example for teaching a social skill from a different domain.

Using rules to teach good sportsmanship. As in the previous examples, teaching begins when the learner is presented with a social rule regarding appropriate behavior when losing a game or competition, such as, "Everyone experiences winning or losing a game. Sometimes I win, and sometimes someone else wins. When someone else wins, I may feel sad or even mad. I can still use nice words like, 'Oh, well, maybe next time,' or 'Good game!' and try to win the next time we play. My friend will be happy that I am being a good sport and will want to keep playing with me." The rule is reviewed, and situations are discussed where the learner has either won or lost a game. The therapist helps the learner identify how he was feeling in those situations and discusses the emotions of the other person involved in the activity. The therapist then discusses how the other person would feel if the learner reacted with anger or as a good sport and the likely effect that each response would have on future interactions. This could be illustrated using drawings or other visual images to facilitate understanding. Again, instruction in cognition skills (e.g., emotions, cause/effect, perspective taking) should be integrated into this activity for deeper meaning and comprehension.

Next, role-play activities are conducted to practice appropriate reactions to losing games or competitions. For many learners, this skill can be extremely challenging, and some may have difficulty at the role-play level. It may be helpful to practice losing silly or less-preferred activities at first and then gradually include games that are more highly desired by the learner. Using larger reinforcers may facilitate success in role-play when the target behavior is more difficult to perform. Consider teaching the learner alternative behaviors for "de-escalation" that the learner can do within these difficult situations, such as getting a drink of water or counting quietly to 10. Following role-play, implement plenty of practice opportunities with the learner in the natural environment, and fade supports gradually in order to foster independence.

Settings for Social Skills Instruction

As discussed in multiple sections above, instructional activities should not be limited to a structured therapy setting. On the contrary, social skills training should incorporate a variety of settings and situations from the learner's natural environment in order to promote generalization, as well as flexible, natural responding. While many social skills may need to be taught initially in a one-on-one setting with a therapist, attempts to target and generalize the skill to other environments should occur within the early stages of intervention. Additionally, natural social settings should increasingly become the backdrop of social skills training activities as the learner advances and skills become more complex in nature. Facilitated playdates with peers are an essential step in the process of generalizing acquired social skills from structured to natural environments.

Playdates

Structured playdates are an integral component of effective social skills instruction. They can provide one of the earliest opportunities for learners to practice their skills with other peers within a semi-structured environment. In home-based settings, play activities may first occur with siblings and then later involve one or multiple peers. In center or school-based settings, specific times can be set aside for semi-structured play activities with particular peers who are a good match. In either case, the learner can practice newly acquired skills within an environment that is still structured and familiar. It is generally easier for adults to control the conditions in place during the playdate in order to facilitate success for the learner, as opposed to completely unstructured play in a larger group. For instance, the therapist can determine the types of reinforcements to be used, the level of prompting that will occur, the selection of activities that will be available, the duration of the playdate, and the behavioral expectations that will be implemented during that time. Initially, it can also be easier for an individual with ASD to practice social skills with one person rather than within a group setting. Playdates are usually assisted by a therapist but can just as easily be conducted by a parent who has been trained in ABA techniques and social skills facilitation. Let's review some general guidelines for success within playdates.

Prerequisite skills. The learner should have certain foundational skills in place prior to commencing playdates with peers. For instance, learners should have the ability to functionally communicate with others. Whether using vocal speech, iconic exchange (e.g., pictures, icons), or an assistive communication device, it is important that the learner is able to express his wants, desires, and needs. Learners also should have emerging early play skills, including some independent and interactive activities. Additionally, the learner should be able to demonstrate basic compliance with instructions with little or no challenging behavior. There is no point wasting another child's time while you manage frequent challenging behavior. This does not mean that the learner must have perfect compliance, as that is not realistic for any child, and various behaviors often must be addressed and worked through during any playdate. However, if a learner is still engaging in high rates of tantrums or aggression on a regular basis, it may be advantageous to address those issues first, so as not to detract from the goals of the playdate.

Include siblings. If the learner has siblings who are similar in age, they should be incorporated into structured play activities with the learner prior to starting playdates. Siblings are a great resource for teaching social skills, as they offer ongoing opportunities for new social skills that have been learned with a therapist to be immediately generalized with peers. Also, siblings are generally accustomed to behavioral issues that the learner may exhibit and can use structured play activities to learn successful strategies for interacting with their brother or sister outside of the therapeutic setting. As appropriate social skills are prompted and directly reinforced, both the learner and siblings can practice targeted skills and receive reinforcement for engaging in positive interactions, with the hope that these interactions generalize to naturally occurring activities throughout the day. Facilitating sibling interactions is often a high priority for families and can have a tremendous positive impact on everyone involved. Empowering siblings with effective skills to use when interacting with their brother or sister often results in improved social interactions and attitudes regarding their relationship.

Preparation. Advanced preparation is key for conducting successful playdates with peers. Once you have the learner and a peer sitting together waiting for the next activity, it is far too late for you to do the prep work you needed to do earlier in the day. Downtime breeds challenging behavior and boredom. Ideally, the therapist should not have to think about what comes next or find the necessary materials. If you have done a sufficient job preparing, the children should be able to progress from activity to activity seamlessly. Planning out the structure of the playdate can help interactions run smoothly and can allow the learner to become familiar with the structure in advance. One successful strategy is the implementation of a turn-taking format. The learner and peer can take turns choosing the activities that they will play during the playdate. This allows each child to select activities that she prefers in a fair manner, which will help maintain interest and motivation for both during the playdate. It also provides clear expectations for both regarding participating in the selections of the other person. Having this structure can be equally beneficial to the peer who may not be accustomed to following directions or sustaining an activity for a specific period of time.

Preparing a highly rewarding activity at the end of the playdate can be a natural reinforcer (for both children) for participating cooperatively during the activities. Reward systems, such as tokens or points, can also be used during a playdate to promote specific social targets or general compliance, but they should be used for both children. Reinforcement systems are often equally helpful to encourage the peer to follow directions, cooperate, and participate in activities that are not always highly preferred.

Set the learner up for success. Make sure to include activities that are likely to be successful for the learner. Typically, it is a good idea to select a variety of activities with which the learner is familiar, that require little support from adults, and that are preferable. These could be set up around the room while other options that may not be good selections for playdates (e.g., solitary activities, toys that elicit stereotypy or perseveration) can be removed from the area. Another alternative is to make a list of all possible activities that are available during the playdate, and the children can take turns selecting activities from the list. However, it is still important to be flexible regarding the selection of activities, as there may be other fun ideas that come up naturally during the playdate that could be explored and may be highly successful and reinforcing for everyone. Also, there may be times when none of the activities selected in advance are motivating to the children, so it is important to have several back-up ideas prepared. Another approach is to have an open-ended activity in place when the playdate arrives, such as painting, coloring, or jumping on a trampoline. This will allow the children to warm up to each other in a relaxed way without immediately placing specific demands on them to interact. For more advanced learners, allowing the children to "hang out" during the first 5–10 minutes of the playdate without imposing a structure may be a good idea. This is often a more natural way to start the interaction and gives them the opportunity to start an activity together without assistance.

Consider using a combination of structured and open-ended activities for the participants of the playdate. For instance, a playdate might include a structured board game or group game that has set rules and can be easier for some learners; a pretend play activity, such as dress-up or superheroes; a gross motor activity outside, such as riding bikes or jumping on the trampoline; and a snack time. Each type of activity will target a different set of social skills and can offer a nice balance between the learner's strengths and areas that require more assistance.

Set realistic goals. It is important to have realistic playdate goals, especially during the early stages. At first, limit playdates to a shorter duration, possibly as short as 30–45 minutes. It is more likely that the learner will be successful within a shorter time frame during which he is less likely to become bored or fatigued. Shorter playdates are less likely to overwhelm the learner or evoke challenging behaviors, such as tantrums or noncompliance. As the learner develops more competence within social interactions, playdates can be lengthened, structure can be gradually faded, and other settings, such as public parks, can be incorporated. Also, have realistic goals in mind for skill targets. For instance, it may not be realistic or developmentally appropriate for a 3-year-old learner to interact cooperatively with another peer for the entire playdate. Instead, target skills that are currently in the learner's repertoire, and practice generalizing them to interactions with the peer. Examples of target skills could include imitating the play actions and sounds of the peer while playing in the sandbox, responding to greetings and simple questions, taking turns during a game, or sustaining pretend play with a peer for 5 minutes. Having specific, realistic goals promotes more effective social skill development and prevents the learner and the adult from becoming overwhelmed.

Fine-tuning your level of support. The success of playdates is highly dependent on the level of support being provided by the adult. Put simply, you can ruin the playdate if you are either too involved or not involved enough. Therefore, it is important for the therapist to monitor the playdate at all times in order to recognize moments when more direct support is required versus moments when facilitation is not needed. The role of the therapist often changes from activity to activity, depending on the learner's level of independence in the particular skill. Oftentimes, therapists can fade back during structured activities, such as games, and can step in to prompt the learner or peer at any particular moment, as needed. During open-ended activities, therapists may need to be more involved, either by offering ideas and instructions throughout the activity or as a direct participant playing alongside the children. Either way, the therapist should be available to offer the appropriate level of support to enable the learner's successful participation while allowing ample opportunities for the learner to practice skills independently with the peer.

Expanding group size. Playdates can eventually involve multiple peers, allowing the learner to practice group-related social skills within a semi-structured setting. Another option is to practice social skills within a small group environment, such as a social skills group or club. Skills that can be targeted within this type of environment include participating in group conversations (e.g., joining a conversation, taking conversational turns with multiple participants), compromising and negotiating group decisions, group-related social games (e.g., hide and seek, red light/green light, telephone), and coordinated group play (e.g., pretend play scenarios involving multiple people, group-related tasks, and sharing). The purpose of small group social skills training is to prepare the learner to participate in natural large group environments that occur on a daily basis in academic and extracurricular settings. School shadowing plays a large part in the successful transition of social skills into these environments and is often necessary to fully generalize the learner's skills to these environments. For more information in this area, see Chapter 8.

Don't embarrass the learner. This should go without saying, but it's easy for the therapist to embarrass the learner. Especially for older and more verbally developed learners, the mere presence of a therapist can make him seem odd to peers or neighbors. In these cases, make sure the therapist is not called a therapist; instead, the therapist can be referred to as the nanny, babysitter, or au pair. While the therapist does not want to let the learner do something that is socially unsuccessful, she must avoid intervening too much and making it seem as though the learner relies too heavily on an adult. A good tip for these types of playdates is to review any rules and instructions with the learner before the peer arrives and then review how the playdate went after the peer leaves. Another tip is for the therapist to contrive excuses to speak with the learner in a separate room briefly in the middle of the playdate (e.g., asking the learner to help carry something or get something from another location in the house). It is important to point out that peers will quickly detect that something is awry if therapists invent reasons to talk to the learner too frequently.

STRATEGIES FOR SUCCESS IN TEACHING SOCIAL SKILLS

Build Rapport

Successful social skills instruction is highly dependent on establishing positive rapport with the learner. Spend time pairing yourself with fun, highly reinforcing activities. This increases the learner's motivation to engage with you in social activities and is an important step in helping the learner experience the positive rewards of having social relationships. The more a learner finds other people reinforcing, the more likely she will be to find social interactions reinforcing, which is key to maintaining social skills outside of instructional activities. Without sufficient rapport, the learner will be less likely to put in the hard work that is required for social skills development.

Targets and Expectations Should Be Developmentally Appropriate

Oftentimes, therapy teams choose social skills targets that are too advanced or not developmentally appropriate for the learner. This can lead to high levels of frustration for both the learner and the treatment team and result in a lack of meaningful progress. Observe the social skills being exhibited by same-age peers or peers who are at the same developmental level as the learner, and use those findings to help establish realistic goals. For instance, it is unrealistic to expect 100% compliance from any child, regardless of diagnosis. Additionally, most children do not share or take turns with desired toys 100% of the time when they are asked. Set the learner up for success by selecting goals that are attainable and aligned with his developmental level.

Take Baby Steps

Approach social skills training using the same methodologies that apply to other skills in ABA programs. Many social skills are complex and multifaceted and can be overwhelming to learners and therapists alike. However, most social skills can be successfully taught if they are properly broken down into their component skills. For instance, when teaching conversation skills – in particular, how to join a conversation – the learner must 1) listen to a conversation between two people, 2) identify the topic, 3) identify something related to the topic that he can say or ask, 4) wait for a pause in the conversation, 5) use an appropriate opening phrase, and 6) state the comment or question relevant to the topic. Teaching all of these skills at once is not likely to be successful. Instead, each skill can be systematically taught to the learner. Gradually, they can be combined and practiced in natural settings, until the learner is able to perform the complex skill in generalized settings with peers.

Use Effective Reinforcement

Remember that social interactions are not as reinforcing to some individuals with ASD as they are to others. Naturally occurring social reinforcement may not initially be enough to motivate a learner. In fact, for individuals with ASD, social skills instruction can often be more challenging and less motivating than other types of skill targets. Therefore, social skills instruction may require larger amounts of reinforcement, especially at the beginning of instruction. Additionally, incorporate natural reinforcers specific to the learner as much as possible. For instance, if a learner really enjoys movies, they can be used as a context in which to practice conversation skills by having the learner engage in conversation about his favorite movies. Also, a learner who takes turns and behaves nicely when playing with a friend may learn that the friend will be more likely to accept an invitation to the movies over the weekend. Moreover, a trip to the movies with a friend can be a naturally motivating context in which to practice phone skills and social planning for an outing. In short, use what is naturally motivating for a learner and find a way to link it to social skills instruction.

Consider Cultural Perspectives and Differences

ASD affects people and families of all cultures and backgrounds. Clinicians need to be aware of any cultural considerations that may impact the content or implementation of social skills instruction. For instance, some cultures may have different beliefs regarding social boundaries and relationships with family members and others. Others may place a higher value on politeness and manners, especially toward adults. When teaching a social skill such as assertiveness with peers and adults, goals and social rules should be in line with the family's cultural values. Always make sure that the learner's family is in agreement with the social targets, and be prepared to engage in additional conversation and to compromise.

Be Proactive

Many times, social interactions may be less than successful due to a lack of sufficient planning. Many social situations can be successfully maneuvered with advanced practice. Proactive planning can include practicing and priming of social rules, setting up token systems or other types of reinforcements, gathering visual cues or supports, planning prompting strategies, and setting realistic durations and behavioral expectations. Whenever possible, plan for and practice related social skills prior to social situations. Additionally, these strategies can then be generalized to situations where advanced planning is not possible (e.g., the last-minute party for a family friend, the surprise visit from a neighbor). Have a token system or rewards stashed in the car for impromptu situations, or quietly pull the learner aside and write down the social rules or agenda for the activity; for example, 1) say "hi, (*name*)" when I see people, 2) watch and join in with my friends' activities, and 3) use my words to tell my friends what I want. The more prepared the learner is, the greater her chances of success in social situations.

Actively Program for Generalization

As with everything we teach in behavioral intervention programs, social skills do not automatically generalize from the one-on-one setting with a therapist to natural settings involving peers and siblings. Most individuals with ASD require assistance in transferring learned skills to novel, untrained situations with new people. Treatment programs must plan for this and include activities that systematically introduce the learner to new environments, people, and situations. This is critical for social skills instruction to be practical and meaningful. Without thoughtful planning for generalization activities, it is unlikely that newly acquired social skills will be used in natural settings.

Fine-Tune Prompting

Beginning social skills instruction most likely requires more direct forms of prompting, such as verbal, modeling, or gesture prompts. Once instruction advances and skills become more complex, it is important to move away from prompts that simply give the answer toward prompts that help the learner engage in reasoning and problem-solving behaviors to come up with the answer (see Chapter 18 on executive functions). Indirect prompting strategies should be included, such as asking leading questions (e.g., What is he doing? Where is he? Who can see what he's doing?) regarding critical information within the situation to indirectly help the learner to develop an appropriate response herself. Another effective method of prompting social skills is the use of visual prompts. Checklists, templates, drawings, or other visual displays are effective for presenting a complex or abstract concept in a more concrete form. For instance, a learner might be more likely to remember how to introduce a conversation if he can refer to a checklist, such as 1) think of what my friend would like to talk about; 2) gain my friend's attention; 3) use an opening phrase; and 4) ask a question or make a statement about the topic. Another prompt is to remind the learner of a previous social situation in which a target skill was needed, and relate it to the current situation. For instance, when learning to compromise, the learner can be reminded of a similar situation where compromise was effective in order to prompt him to use a comparable strategy in the current situation. Video modeling can also be effective to demonstrate targeted social skills, as well as to help the learner identify critical cues in depicted video scenarios. Other effective prompts that have been discussed in this chapter include advanced priming of social rules, modeling of key skills, and role-play. Prompting hierarchies can be developed using these types of advanced prompts in order to provide appropriate support and to plan for successful fading of prompts. Again, the goal of prompting for advanced social skills instruction is to promote the individual's ability to identify which social skills are required in any given situation and to use those skills with confidence. Advanced social skills often consist of the ability to figure out what to do given the idiosyncrasies of the current moment, rather than simply doing some "stock" appropriate behavior.

Integrate Skills from Other Domains

Flexible, adaptable social functioning depends on the interworking of skills from several other domains. For example, it is possible to teach an individual with ASD the rules for compromising and negotiating, as well as the strategies for doing so. However, it is unlikely that these skills will be used in naturally occurring situations with peers unless the learner can also take the perspectives (e.g., the emotions, desires, and thoughts) of peers, predict likely social outcomes, and be flexible enough to generate another solution to the problem. To maximize success, you need to constantly consider the interplay of the learner's social skills with those learned in the areas of play, executive function, and cognition (perspective taking).

Incorporate Self-Management Strategies

For intermediate and advanced instruction, it is critical for learners to develop independence in social situations for long-term success. Learners who acquire the ability to monitor their own social behavior can use this skill as a highly effective tool with which to facilitate their own ongoing social learning and success. By incorporating rules, checklists, priming, review, self-observation, and self-reinforcement strategies within advanced social skills instruction, learners will be able to manage their own social development, identify ongoing needs, and seek out appropriate levels of support when needed. Again, many skills within the executive function domain will be relevant here (see Chapter 18).

COMMON PITFALLS IN SOCIAL SKILLS INSTRUCTION

Memorization/Rote Learning

Rote memorization of social rules or other strategies will not result in social success. In fact, memorization of social skills may lead to awkward social interactions that are rigid and unnatural. Teaching strategies should incorporate generalization of social skills across a wide variety of situations and exemplars, and flexible responding within social situations should be taught and reinforced. Role-play and *in vivo* application are essential for social skills instruction to be meaningful. However, specific scenarios that are role-played should change constantly. Especially for more advanced social skills, there is no need to rehearse *particular* scenarios until the learner can go through them accurately; practice new ones constantly. Additionally, learners should not memorize how to respond in every social situation but, instead, should learn how to recognize the critical components occurring within any given social situation and how to respond accordingly.

Adult-Centered Social Interaction Styles

Avoid teaching the learner "adult-sounding" conversational language. For instance, a child responding to an unexpected event would typically use a phrase such as "No way!" or "Whoa!" instead of saying, "Well, that is surprising!" Incorporate slang and child-appropriate language into social language lessons. Additionally, therapists should model child-appropriate language in their social interactions with learners. If a child or adolescent uses language that is too formal, it is generally noticeable to other peers and can appear awkward or "nerdy." Also, therapists should occasionally respond to the learner in ways that a peer would respond. Children tend to be less accommodating than adults to the needs of others, which is often reflected in their reactions to requests, comments, and behaviors of others. Where an adult may not overtly show that he is uninterested in a one-sided conversation, children and adolescents will be fairly obvious about their feelings. In order to prepare the learner for interactions with peers, instruction should include practice in handling these situations and the use of compensation strategies that will facilitate successful relations with peers.

Targeting Too Many Skills at Once

Avoid having the learner practice too many skills at once, especially when you are working with younger learners. For example, during a play-date, it is generally more effective to target 3 to 5 social skills targets instead of 10 to 15 skills. This may be overwhelming for both the learner and the therapist who is responsible for creating learning opportunities for each of the targets. Learners often are more successful with a shorter list of targets that can be practiced thoroughly and with enough repetition to facilitate acquisition. As the learner progresses, the number of target skills can be increased according to his abilities. Remember, quality instead of quantity typically leads to greater social skill success.

Focusing on the Negatives

Best practice in ABA instruction is to focus interventions on positive reinforcement and the acquisition of appropriate replacement skills to address a learner's needs. This also applies to social skills instruction, particularly in the use of reinforcement and the phrasing of social rules. Try to avoid using negative statements, such as, "I will not interrupt my friends' conversation." Instead, focus on the positive replacement behavior, such as, "I will wait for a pause and then get my friend's attention by saying his name." This keeps the focus on rewarding adaptive behaviors.

Don't Worry About the Number of Friendships

Developing meaningful relationships is obviously a primary goal for social skills instruction. Some individuals with ASD may tend to have fewer friends, but this is not necessarily problematic. For many individuals, regardless of diagnoses, having several close friends can be just as gratifying – if not more so – than having a larger number of acquaintances. For children and teenagers, having even one or two good friends can make a tremendous difference in their social experience. It is important for the treatment team (and the learner) to avoid becoming discouraged if a learner has a small but meaningful social circle. Often, individuals will grow into other social relationships as they mature. Keep striving for social skills development, but remember that not every person needs a large group of social connections to be happy.

Confusing Verbal Behavior with Genuine Skill Proficiency

Being able to say what you should do is not the same as being able to do it when it counts. This point has been repeated throughout the chapter, but its importance to successful social skills instruction warrants repeating it yet again. Verbal behavior must be followed by actual demonstration and reinforcement of the target behavior. Instruction should always require a learner to practice the skill in a variety of situations with a variety of people, particularly peers. Structured practice should always be followed by actual demonstration in real life. It is not important what a learner can tell you about a skill but, rather, how well she can implement it with others. Being able to describe the rules is just the beginning.

Sabotaging the Social Environment

While preparing for social skills training, it is important for clinicians to consider how to avoid sabotaging the social interaction before it starts. Remove highly distracting things from the environment that will detract from the learner's attention and motivation, such as perseverative items that may provoke stereotypy. Choose locations that offer appropriate and fun activities for the individual, but avoid areas that may be distracting due to noise or visual stimuli. Also, decide whether an open area, such as a park, or an enclosed area, such as a house or back yard, would be more favorable for facilitating a playdate. When possible, schedule sessions during favorable times of day. Plan for issues such as fatigue or hunger by providing snacks before or during the interaction, or avoid scheduling sessions at the end of a long day. Avoid highly preferred activities immediately before social interaction sessions. For instance, if the learner is watching a favorite cartoon at the beginning of a playdate, he is not likely to be interested in doing other things and may engage in challenging behaviors when the cartoon is turned off. Also, schedule playdates with only one peer initially to avoid the learner being "left out" by the other children. Groups of three are notorious for excluding one person.

SUMMARY

Social skills deficits are characteristic of ASD. Therefore, social skills training forms a crucial foundation in any top-quality autism treatment program. Social skills training begins with the simplest social norms, such as sharing and turn-taking, and progresses to the subtlest and most complex social skills, which involve complex rules and perspective taking. Teaching social skills requires the full quiver of behavioral skill acquisition procedures, with a focus on role-play, feedback, rules, and generalization training.

Cognition

Adel C. Najdowski, Angela Persicke, Evelyn Kung

The Cognition curriculum gets its name from the traditional name for the skills it is used to teach, metacognition and social cognition. Metacognition consists of one's knowledge about one's own mental states, whereas social cognition refers to one's knowledge about others' mental states, that is, perspective taking. For example, individuals are using metacognition when they are able to identify mental states such as thoughts, emotions, beliefs, and intentions in themselves, and they are using social cognition when they are able to identify those same mental states in others. The field of study known as Theory of Mind (ToM) is by far the most active area of research on perspective taking in children with autism spectrum disorder (ASD). ToM is an evolutionary cognitive theory that states that, in order to understand someone else's mental states, one has to grasp the theory that one's own mind is distinct from the minds of others (Baron-Cohen, Leslie, & Frith, 1985). For example, the thoughts, feelings, knowledge, beliefs, and intentions of others are not necessarily the same as one's own.

The terms *cognition, metacognition, social cognition,* and *mental states* come from the cognitive literature and are therefore somewhat foreign to the field of applied behavior analysis (ABA). In the field of ABA, we deal only with things people do (behavior) and things that happen in their environment (antecedent and consequence stimuli). Much of what people do is observable by other people, and this is referred to as **overt behavior**. However, some of the things people do are not observable by others, and this is referred to as **covert behavior**. Covert and overt behavior are assumed to be the same, in principle, except for their availability for observation by others. For example, we assume that when one reads aloud and when one reads silently "in one's head," the two behaviors are fundamentally the same – they are both reading. Similarly, one may talk to oneself while planning a future event, or one may do exactly the same thing covertly by thinking about it. The ABA perspective on these two behaviors is that they are the same, except that one occurs covertly and the other overtly. Both are behaviors, and neither is a mental, cognitive, or brain process. Brain function is critical to both, but it is a substitute for neither. The role of the brain in behavior is interesting, but it is not part of the field of ABA; it is more usefully entrusted to behavioral neuroscience, a separate but related science.

Just as there are overt and covert behaviors, there are overt and covert stimuli. Much of a person's environment is observable by others, but much of it is not. For example, someone who daydreams for hours on end is experiencing a very rich interaction with her environment; it just so happens that many of the stimuli with which that person is interacting are not observable by anyone else. Again, covert stimuli are assumed to be the same as overt stimuli, in principle, except that they cannot be observed by others. Covert stimuli and behaviors are generally referred to as "private events" in ABA. *Perspective taking is the ability to infer and respond to the likely private events that others are experiencing,* and this chapter is about how to teach children with ASD the ability to do so.

Perspective taking is a complex topic, and it is therefore useful to be very clear about the terms we use and the ways in which we use them. We chose to use the term *cognition* when naming the Cognition curriculum in an effort to facilitate communication across disciplines. Very few researchers or practitioners outside of the ABA field are familiar with the term *private events*, and the purpose of this chapter – and the Center for Autism and Related Disorders (CARD) curriculum – is to promote interdisciplinary collaboration and to foster the broader dissemination of ABA for teaching higher order skills, not to alienate the non-behavioral world by using esoteric terms. Beyond the title of this chapter, there is nothing non-behavioral about the content of the Cognition curriculum – it's all behavior, whether covert or overt – and the teaching methods used to teach it are all ABA-based procedures.

In this chapter, the term *mental states* is used synonymously with the term *private event*. That is, every time *mental state* is written, it means covert behaviors or stimuli, and it never means mental constructs or brain structures. Similarly, the term *perspective taking* is used synonymously with *social cognition* throughout this chapter, and it always means some actual behavior (overt or covert) that a person is doing in response to someone else's mental states (or more precisely, some overt cue of what those mental states might be). In this chapter, perspective taking and social cognition do not mean mental processes or brain functions. What the brain itself is doing during instances of perspective taking is fascinating, but it is not the subject of this chapter. This chapter addresses what the child with ASD is doing and thinking and how these skills can be improved.

PERSPECTIVE-TAKING DEFICITS IN CHILDREN WITH AUTISM

Perspective-taking skills are critical for successful social behavior, as they allow children with ASD to infer others' private events in order to interpret their current behavior, predict their future behavior, and adjust their own behavior in order to be more effective socially. There has been a great deal of documentation, much of it coming from the ToM literature, that demonstrates that individuals with ASD have difficulty attributing and understanding their own private events and the private events of others and how these relate to overt behavior. For example, many children with ASD have difficulty interpreting body language and facial expressions; identifying and using deception, sarcasm, and other non-literal language; and inferring others' emotions, thoughts, intentions, desires, and preferences. In fact, research has demonstrated that many children with ASD perform significantly worse on tests of even basic levels of perspective taking compared to both typically developing children and those diagnosed with other developmental disabilities, such as Down's syndrome, general developmental delay, or specific language delays (Baron-Cohen et al., 1985).

Perspective taking is a critical component of successful social behavior, as the repertoire involves a complex set of skills that are needed in order to regulate social interactions appropriately, empathize with others, make appropriate social choices, demonstrate social reciprocity and interest in others, and ultimately develop and maintain friendships. Let's take a look at a few examples of how perspective taking is used in everyday social interactions.

Real-World Applications of Perspective Taking

First of all, perspective taking is used to infer the current private events of others. For example, if I see my spouse walking around the room with a frown on his face, furiously opening drawers and looking under the bed, I might infer that Adam has misplaced something he needs. I might also infer that his private events consist of thinking and worrying about the misplaced item, retracing steps, and so on. In addition to using perspective taking to infer current private events of others, it is also used to predict what a person's behavior and/or private events would likely be in a given future event, so one can take effective action. For example, let's say I know that my friend, Sara, likes to sit in the front row of a class we take together, so she can see the teacher better. If she sends a text message to let me know that she is running late and I see that the first row is filling up quickly, I might predict that she will be disappointed if she has to sit in the back, and I might then save her a seat in the front row. In many cases, this process also involves predicting the effect of one's own behavior on how others will feel and what they will think and/or do. In Sara's case, for example, I might predict that she will be happy that I saved a seat for her and that she might think I'm a good friend and save a seat for me the next time she gets to class before I do. In short, one uses perspective taking across a variety of everyday life situations, and one makes choices about how to interact with people based on predictions of how others will think, feel, and behave overtly under various conditions in an effort to avoid making others feel or think negatively about oneself.

When children do not develop an effective perspective-taking repertoire, they tend to engage in awkward social behaviors. Let's take a look at a few examples of how heavily this can impact their lives for the worse:

- **Consideration of others' thoughts, feelings, preferences, or desires**: When one doesn't consider the thoughts and feelings of others, one might engage in inconsiderate behaviors, such as telling someone that he is fat or that the cookies he made are disgusting.
- **Reading others' intentions**: If one can't read others' intentions, one may think that unintentional wrongdoings were done maliciously; for example, the child might overreact and call a peer a bully because he accidentally stepped on the child's foot.
- **Discriminating between what is said and what is meant**: If one can't discriminate truth from fiction, as in the cases of deception and sarcasm, one might interpret deceptive and sarcastic statements as being sincere.
- **Determining what others know**: If one can't identify what others already know, one might talk about unknown topics without giving background details, talk above others' heads, or tell peers something they obviously already know.

Social awkwardness such as that described above can result in the child's being labeled as weird, dorky, or rude and may lead to the child's being bullied, having low self-esteem, or feeling depressed, anxious, or even aggressive. In other words, deficits in perspective-taking skills may not seem to be as obvious a problem as tantrums or self-injurious behavior, but they can have very serious social consequences for the children who suffer from them.

Development of the Cognition Curriculum

The development of the CARD Cognition curriculum was highly influenced by the ToM literature. Hundreds of studies have been published on ToM in autism, and space does not permit a representative review here. However, one of the major accomplishments of the ToM literature has been to carefully describe a wide variety of perspective-taking skills that children learn in the course of typical development. In the development of the CARD Cognition curriculum, we reviewed this literature extensively in order to ensure that we comprehensively addressed all of the perspective-taking skills that a child might need to learn. Then we studied the behavioral literature to determine which studies had been conducted on how to teach the skills. Effective methods identified from these studies were incorporated into the lessons, which were broken down into over 300 ABA-based teaching activities.

General Teaching Methods

The general method for teaching perspective-taking skills involves first identifying the terminal desired goal for each perspective-taking concept. Perspective-taking concepts include desires, preferences, intentions, thoughts, feelings, and so on. (Each of the concepts touched upon in the Cognition curriculum is discussed in its own section in this chapter.) For each concept, there is one lesson with many different activities (see Appendix J). The activities teach the learner to recognize the concepts not only in others (perspective taking/social cognition) but also in themselves (metacognition). The terminal desired goal for each concept is for the learner to apply her knowledge about the concept to everyday social interactions. Thus, initial activities teach the learner to understand concepts in simple and contrived settings, whereas final activities expect the learner to use the information in real-life social interactions.

In all cases, concepts are taught as generalized operants, not specific behaviors under stimulus control (see Chapter 7 on generalization). The whole perspective-taking training process is conceptualized as the development of a larger, overarching operant repertoire of relating oneself to others (Hayes, Barnes-Holmes, & Roche, 2001). To achieve this, multiple exemplar training is used to ensure that the child is learning to respond to novel stimuli in novel situations and with novel people. This is done to establish flexible repertoires of perspective taking. In other words, rote learning and memorization are the enemy! The skills in this chapter are meaningless if the child cannot use them in a generalized, flexible manner across her life. Initially, prompts are provided to help the learner be successful, but they are always faded out rapidly. Mastery is determined once learners are able to respond to multiple novel exemplars without prompting across several people, settings, and teaching sessions. Let us now take a look at how to teach each of the various concepts in the Cognition curriculum.

Structure of the Cognition Curriculum

The CARD Cognition curriculum consists of lessons aimed at teaching children with ASD to understand their own and others' perspectives,

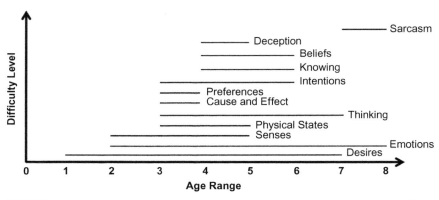

FIGURE 17.1   Cognition lessons by age range and difficulty level. *Reprinted from Skills®*
with permission from the Center for Autism and Related Disorders.

including: 1) desires, 2) preferences, 3) emotions, 4) sensory perspectives,
5) knowing, 6) beliefs, 7) thinking, 8) deception, 9) intentions, 10) and sarcasm. Figure 17.1 depicts the main lessons in the CARD Cognition curriculum. The horizontal axis depicts the age range in typical development
during which children begin to learn the concepts, and the vertical axis
depicts the relative difficulty of the concepts. Many concepts take years to
fully develop. Appendix J provides an outline of the lessons, sections, and
activities contained in these lessons. In what follows, we provide practical
recommendations for how to teach sample skills in all of these areas.

DESIRES

The ability to express one's desires and respond to the desires of others begins to emerge at a very young age. Typically, between 1 and 2
years of age, children use vocalizations and gestures to indicate what
they want when asked. They also extend objects to an adult in response
to a palm-up request and give an adult an object for which the adult
exhibits a facial expression indicating pleasure rather than disgust.
Between 2 and 3 years of age, children begin to request objects and
actions, and between 4 and 7 years, they understand and use indirect
requests.
The purpose of the Desires lesson is to teach the learner to identify
desires (e.g., things one currently wants) in himself and others and to
respond accordingly by requesting (for self) and offering (to others) the
desired item. The learner is also taught to infer others' desires by attending to their body language, facial expressions, and vocal language and to
find out others' desires by asking. Finally, this lesson teaches the learner to
respond appropriately to indirect requests, such as disguised mands (e.g.,

saying, "Mmm, those cookies look good," instead of simply asking for a cookie), and to use indirect requests to obtain desired items.

Learner's Desires

One of the first skills taught to children with ASD is how to directly express their own desires. This has been addressed at length in Chapter 11 on manding and will not be elaborated here.

Identifying and Inferring Others' Desires

The topic of desires becomes relevant to perspective taking when the child learns to identify and infer the desires of others. Begin teaching this skill by teaching the learner to respond to simple, obvious requests from others, such as "Can I please have...?" or "I want...." Also, early on, teach the learner that she can find out what others desire by asking them. For example, if a peer asks, "Can I have a car?," then prompt the learner to ask, "Which one do you want?" Train multiple exemplars and fade out prompts until the learner is spontaneously asking others what they want in socially appropriate circumstances.

People are usually not blunt when expressing their desires, so it is often necessary to teach children with ASD to make inferences about others' desires. For example, teach the learner to respond to indications of desire based on subtle cues, such as gestures, body language, facial expressions, and "disguised mands" (Chapter 11). Begin with concrete cues, such as someone holding his hand out or reaching for an object that is out of reach. Progress to more subtle cues, such as when a third person reacts differently to two or more different stimuli. For example, the therapist reacts positively toward one object (e.g., smiling and saying "yummy," etc.) and negatively toward a second object (e.g., grimacing and saying "yuck," etc.). Then the therapist asks, "Which one do I want?" In order for the learner to respond correctly to this question, she will need to attend to the therapist's subtle cues. Once the learner makes this basic inference, the therapist captures or contrives situations in the natural environment in which the learner should infer someone's desires and teaches the learner how to respond appropriately to this information. For example, while the child is on a swing at the park, the therapist might have a peer stand nearby, staring longingly at the child to indicate desire for a turn on the swing. The learner will be prompted to offer the peer a turn, and this skill would be practiced until no prompts are necessary and the learner is engaging appropriately during new situations in the natural environment. Make sure to teach the learner to detect and reinforce a variety of disguised mands from others. Disguised mands are indirect mands — for example, saying, "This is so heavy," rather than, "Can you help me carry this?" Teach the learner to detect and respond to a variety of disguised mands until you observe generalization to novel disguised mands.

PREFERENCES

In the ToM literature, the term *preferences* means essentially the same thing as desires – it's what someone wants. The difference is that the term *preferences* refers to longer term *preferences*, whereas the term *desires*, as discussed above, refers to what someone wants in the moment. For example, a person may have a lifelong preference for one basketball team over another, whereas she might have a momentary desire for either a sandwich or pasta, but that desire likely changes from day to day. The Preferences lesson teaches learners to identify and respond to the long-term preferences of others. Typically developing children between 3 and 4 years of age can often identify their own basic preferences and those of familiar people, and some time between 6 and 8 years, they begin to identify the likes and dislikes of others. Knowing and being sensitive to others' preferences allow the child to make appropriate suggestions for play, conversation, and other activities. A lack of response to others' preferences is usually interpreted as "inconsiderate" and is likely to have negative social consequences.

Learner's Preferences

The easiest skill to teach children with ASD about preferences is the identification of their own likes and dislikes. This can be done by asking them what they like and dislike, as in, "What toys do you like?" and "What toys do you dislike?" Once the learner can identify basic likes and dislikes across various categories (e.g., foods, activities, colors, etc.), the therapist brings in relative preference by asking questions such as, "What do you like/dislike more, ____ or ____?" The therapist also works on teaching the learner to identify the things he likes the most (favorite) versus those he dislikes the most (hate) by asking, "What is your favorite?" or "Which one do you dislike the most/hate?"

Others' Preferences

The first and easiest method to use to teach children to identify others' preferences is to ask others what they like/dislike in the appropriate context, such as while playing or eating. For example, if the learner is painting with a peer, the therapist should prompt the learner to ask the peer, "What is your favorite color?" However, asking people what they like out of context can appear weird or inappropriate. Thus, it is also necessary to teach the learner how to make inferences about others' possible preferences. The therapist should teach the learner that it is possible to guess what people like by observing them. For example, a therapist could say, "You can tell if people like something by watching how they react to it. If they smile or do something that shows they are enjoying it or are excited about it, then they like it. If they don't react much to it, then maybe they don't like it or they don't really care. If they frown, then they don't like it." Then the therapist contrives and captures situations to practice this across many exemplars, people, and settings. In addition to teaching the learner to identify others' preferences, teach her to predict another's behavior based on that person's preferences. Thus, after the learner has identified that Johnny likes to play with action figures, the therapist asks her, "What do you think Johnny will do during free play?," to which the learner will answer, "Play with action figures."

Social application. Being able to identify others' preferences and predict their behavior in various situations given their preferences is an important tool for effective social interactions with peers. As with all perspective-taking skills, the learner should be taught to apply the skill to real social interactions with peers. To teach this, the therapist should contrive or capture situations in social contexts for the learner to practice using his knowledge of others' preferences during social interactions. For example, the therapist should set up playdates for the learner and prompt the learner to identify preferred items that the peer is going to like. The therapist can also prompt the learner to initiate conversational topics that are preferred by the peer. When it is the learner's mother's birthday, the therapist should prompt the learner to identify a gift to get her mother that is based on the mother's preferences. Even if the child is simply going to make a card for her mother, she should think about her mother's preferred colors and objects when deciding what to draw on the card. As always, this skill will not be considered mastered until the learner is able to apply it independently to new situations as they arise.

EMOTIONS

Typically developing children begin to develop an understanding of others' emotions around 3 years of age, when children begin to label emotions such as happy, sad, and mad. At this time, they also begin to understand that emotions are caused by external situations and that there is a connection between desires and emotions; for example, when people get something they want, they are happy, versus sad or mad when they don't. Starting around 4 years of age, children express a range of emotions and also begin to understand that their beliefs can affect their emotions; for example, if I believe something to be true and find out it is false, I might be upset.

The Emotions lesson aims to teach learners to identify emotions in people, as well as the causal link between actions, desires, and emotions. The
ability to identify and express one's own emotions improves one's ability
to have needs and desires met, while the ability to perceive and react appropriately to others' emotional facial expressions and contextual cues is
necessary for successful social and communicative interaction. This lesson will teach the learner to infer others' emotions based on their desires,
preferences, and beliefs. The child will also learn that people can experience different emotions given the same situation and that one's actions
can cause others' emotions to change for the better or worse. When one's
actions cause others to feel bad or uncomfortable, the child will learn how
he can rectify the situation.

Emotion Identification

The first step in teaching children with ASD about emotions is to teach
them to identify emotions, both receptively and through the use of tacts.
This process is relatively straightforward and progresses in the same way
as any other receptive and tact training (see Chapter 11), so it is not elaborated further here. One aspect of emotions worth noting is that emotions are
something than can be acted out, so a receptive instruction such as "show
me happy," "show me sad," and so on, can be implemented in addition to
the usual receptive identification of picture cards.

Cause and Effect

In order for the learner to interact successfully in her social environment, it is very important for her to learn to predict how someone will feel
in a given situation (effect of that situation on emotion), as well as why
people have certain emotions (cause of the emotion). To teach the learner
to predict the emotional effect of given situations, the therapist should
begin by asking the learner to identify conventional emotions that are felt
in given situations. For example, most people feel scared when someone
jumps out at them and yells "Boo!," so the therapist might ask the child,
"How would Sara feel if I jumped out at her and yelled 'Boo'?" to which
the learner's correct response would be, "Scared."

To teach the learner to identify the cause of an emotion, the therapist
should begin by allowing the learner to observe a scenario depicting a
cause and an emotional effect and then asking, "Why is she sad?," to which
the learner is prompted to identify the cause ("because her toy broke"). As
always, the therapist will fade prompts and repeat this process until the
learner is able to respond correctly across multiple novel exemplars of untrained causes.

Desire and Belief-based Emotions

Once the learner can identify emotional cause and effect, the next step is to teach the learner the connection between desires/beliefs and emotions. Desire-based emotions refer to the concept that people will feel different emotions based on whether their desires are met. Belief-based emotions refer to the concept that the emotions of people are affected when they find out that something they believe to be true is actually false and vice versa. For example, if I think I have lost my bike, I will be happy when I find out that my belief about my bike being gone is false and that it was in the lost-and-found.

To teach the learner to identify desire-based emotions, the therapist should allow the learner to observe an event (either via video, using cartoon drawings, or *in vivo*) wherein a third person's desire is being met or unmet and the resulting emotional reaction occurs. For example, the learner might observe a peer at a birthday party start crying when she is given a vanilla cupcake even though she asked for a chocolate cupcake. The therapist then asks, "Why is she sad?" and prompts a correct response, such as, "Because she wanted a chocolate cupcake but got a vanilla one." It's important to note here that the learner is not being asked to identify the emotion conventionally felt in a given situation. Rather, the emotion of the third person is specific to his or her desires either being met or unmet.

The next step is to teach the learner to predict the emotion of a third person based on whether a desire is going to be met. Again, the therapist should present scenarios to the learner, such as, "He wants a turn with the toy. How will he feel if he gets a turn?" and then prompt a correct response, such as, "He will feel happy." Make sure to present many different scenarios wherein the third person's desires are met sometimes and not met other times and where the specific types of desires change frequently. Do not consider this skill mastered until the learner is able to respond correctly to novel captured situations in natural environment settings.

To teach the learner to identify belief-based emotions, the therapist should allow the learner to observe an event wherein a third person discovers his belief is true or false and exhibits the resulting emotional reaction. For example, the therapist might present a scenario to the learner about a sad boy who thinks his Nintendo DS™ is stored in his nightstand drawer where he always keeps it only to discover that he is wrong. The therapist then asks how the third person feels and why and prompts correct responding.

Application to Social Interaction

Once the learner is able to identify emotions and emotional causes and effects and is able to predict how people will feel based on desires and beliefs, consider moving on to teach the learner to think about the effect of his own behavior on the emotions of others when making daily decisions about how to interact with others socially. For example, the therapist might present a rule, such as, "When you do things that make people happy, they will like you and want to be your friend. When you do things that make them sad, angry, or upset, they will not like you as much and will not want to play with you as much." The therapist then presents and captures situations wherein the child has the opportunity to behave one way versus another and to predict how each option will emotionally affect others. The therapist might say, "Susie wants to play with one of your games. If you let her, how will she feel? If you don't, how will she feel? What should you do?" Naturally, practice this skill with siblings, family members, or carefully chosen peers, so the learner can come into contact with the consequences of failing to consider peers' perspectives but without actually endangering potential friendships!

PHYSICAL STATES

A physical state is an internal feeling, such as feeling hot, sick, or hungry. Physical states are similar to emotions in the sense that they are private events that cannot be directly observed by anyone else; they can only be inferred from overt cues. Typically developing children begin to understand others' physical states at around 3 and 4 years of age. For example, a child might identify that someone feels hurt when that person falls off a bike. Children also begin to identify what to do when someone is sleepy, cold, tired, hungry, and hurt around this age. As with the Emotions lesson, the Physical States lesson aims to teach learners to identify and respond to their own physical states and those of others. Because physical states cannot be directly observed, this lesson teaches the learner to make inferences from overt behavior and the context in which this overt behavior occurs relevant to internal states (Skinner, 1974). For example, when the learner encounters a sweaty person on a hot day, she should be able to infer that the person likely feels hot. In addition to inferring physical states, this lesson teaches the learner to infer cause-and-effect relationships between others' physical states and their behavior in both directions; for example, falling down (behavior) can cause one to feel hurt (physical state), and feeling hurt (physical state) can make one want to ask for a hug (behavior).

Identifying Physical States

Receptive identification of physical states can be taught using picture cards. Place multiple cards representing different physical states on the table and instruct the learner to touch a physical state, as in, "Touch hurt." This can also be taught using real people and instructing the learner to identify the person exhibiting a physical state, such as, "Point to hungry," or by telling the child to demonstrate a physical state, as in, "Show me tired."

Teaching learners to tact physical states involves showing the learner a picture card and asking, "How does he feel?," or demonstrating a physical state through actions and asking, "How do I feel?," to which the answer might be "sick," "tired," "hurt," or the like. The learner should also begin to be taught to label his physical states when actually feeling them in the natural environment. For example, when the learner is thirsty, the therapist might ask, "How do you feel?," to which the learner would answer, "Thirsty." However, be cautious; you never can be completely certain of the physical state that the learner is currently feeling, so be modest about your own ability to identify her physical states while teaching her to tact her own! You don't want to accidentally prompt the child to tell you that she is feeling something when she actually is not.

Cause and Effect

Physical states are particularly important socially because of the role they play in social interactions. Begin teaching the learner about cause-and-effect relations in physical states by asking the learner to predict the effect of an event on his own and others' physical states. For example, when asked, "How would he feel if he fell off his bike and skinned his knee?," the learner would be prompted to answer, "Hurt." He should also be taught to predict what people would do if they were experiencing a particular physical state, as in, "What would you do if you felt tired?," with one reasonable answer being, "Sleep." Prompts are faded, and multiple exemplars are trained for each physical state until the learner demonstrates generalization to novel scenarios with novel causes and effects. Move on to teaching the learner to identify the cause of a physical state and what can be done to change it. For example, ask the learner, "How do you feel?" to which the learner might respond, "Hot." Ask the learner, "Why?," to which the learner might respond, "Because I'm wearing a jacket." Then ask the learner, "What can you do to stop feeling hot?," to which the learner might respond, "Take off the jacket."

Social Application

The Physical States lesson becomes socially relevant when you teach the learner effective ways to interact with others who are experiencing various physical states. For example, teach her to make offers to people who indicate discomfort due to physical states: for example, if someone is cold, offer him a blanket; if people are hungry, offer food, etc. To teach these skills, contrive or capture situations where others are feeling physical states, and prompt the learner to talk through identifying the other person's physical state and a socially effective reaction to it. When the learner is ready, take this skill to a more advanced level by prompting the learner to predict another person's physical state in a future scenario and an effective action she can take to prevent it or prepare for it (e.g., having a snack ready for a friend who might get hungry during a playdate). As always, the skill is not considered mastered until the learner demonstrates generalization across novel exemplars, people, and settings.

SENSORY PERSPECTIVE TAKING

Around the age of 3 years, typically developing children begin to develop the ability to identify what other people can see, hear, taste, feel, and smell. Starting around 4 years old, children begin to have the ability to infer how an object appears to another person (understanding that people may have different views of the same object depending on where they are standing). The Sensory Perspective Taking lesson aims to teach children to understand others' senses, including what others can and cannot sense, why they are or aren't able to sense the items, and how to change current conditions in order to allow others to experience items they currently are unable to sense. All of this is important because once the child can engage in sensory perspective taking, she can begin to identify what others know through seeing, hearing, telling, and so on. The concept of knowing is addressed later in this chapter.

Learner's Senses

We generally start by teaching the learner to identify what he is able to sense. For example, the therapist will usually start by asking, "What can you see?" in various scenarios before moving onto other senses. When moving onto other senses, the therapist might ensure the object making the sound (or being smelled etc.) is out of sight or might put a blindfold on the learner to help him identify that he can no longer see something when blindfolded but can hear it. The therapist then ensures that the object makes its sound and asks, "What can you hear?" The therapist might then also follow this up by asking, "Can you see it?," and the learner will identify that he cannot see the item. At this point, the therapist takes the blindfold off and asks, "Can you see it now?" Another method for facilitating the learner's ability to attend to smell alone is to use cotton balls that have each been dipped in different scents and ask the learner to identify what he smells. Likewise, to block the learner's visual perspective when teaching the learner to identify what she can feel, the therapist might put an object in a bag or instruct the learner to close her eyes before the therapist asks, "What do you feel?"

Once the learner is able to identify what he can sense, the therapist asks questions, such as, "Can you see the book?" or "Can you hear the music?" when the learner can and cannot sense the item. Once the learner answers "yes" or "no," the therapist follows up by asking, "Why?" and then prompting a response, such as, "Because the table is in the way." Follow-up questions (e.g., "What can you do?") can then be used to further teach the learner cause-and-effect relations between physical proximity and the ability to sense something (i.e., what in the environment can be changed to allow the learner to sense the item).

Others' Senses

Being able to identify what other people sense is an important prerequisite skill for many other perspective-taking skills. When teaching the learner to understand her own senses, she may need to be taught to identify what others can see in fairly concrete situations at first (Gould, Tarbox, O'Hora, Noone, & Bergstrom, 2011). Begin by setting up situations that contain objects, as well as a third person whose perspective the learner is to take. For example, the therapist asks, "What can he see?" and "What can he smell?" and so on. Once the learner is able to identify what one person can sense, the therapist might ask in a room of people, "Who can see the book?" In this scenario, the learner will be required to take the unique perspective of each individual person and identify who can and cannot see an object based on where they are standing, the direction of their eye gaze, whether there are any obstructions, and so forth. When the learner identifies people who cannot sense the item, the therapist should present instructions such as, "Why can't he see the book?" and prompt appropriate answers, such as, "Because he is standing on the other side of the couch." The therapist can elaborate the lesson by asking the learner to show people items that they currently cannot see, so the learner is required to change the environment in order to allow the person to see the item. For example, the therapist hands the learner a book that is upside down and facing away from the person and says, "Show him what book you are reading," and the learner will need to make sure the book is placed right-side-up with the front cover facing the person in order for him or her to see it. All of these learning opportunities require the learner to attend to and discriminate between complex combinations of object locations, person locations, eye gaze, and locations of obstructions, and to switch between making these discriminations for each different person versus themselves, all the while discriminating cause-and-effect relations between all of these variables.

KNOWING

Around 4 years of age, typically developing children can explain how others know something using all of the senses; that is, people know something because they can see it, etc. Beginning around 5 years of age, they consider what listeners already know about a topic when speaking to them. The Knowing lesson teaches children to identify what others know and why they know it. Specifically, this lesson teaches the learner the concept of knowing and that our senses and interactions with others and our environment allow us to know things; that is, seeing leads to knowing. The child learns to identify what he and others know and how they know it. Considering what other people know is of vital importance in communicative and social interactions because it allows the speaker to judge the amount of information required by the listener in order to provide sufficient – but not excessive – background detail. An inability to consider others' knowledge may result in speech without context or redundant communication. Further, identification of what others know and do not know is required for other perspective-taking skills, including false beliefs and deception. This lesson aims to improve the learner's identification ("Does she know?") and application ("If she doesn't know, what do I do?") of others' knowledge during social interactions.

Identifying What the Learner Knows

The premise behind teaching children to identify what others know is that sensory experience and perception lead to knowing. For example, one knows something because one has seen, heard, tasted, smelled, touched, been told, read about, remembered, or in some other way experienced it. We usually begin by teaching the learner to identify whether she knows something and why. For example, the therapist asks the learner, "What kind of bike does Jimmy have?" When the learner answers the question (e.g., "a Batman bike"), the therapist then asks, "How do you know?" and the learner is prompted to refer to her sensory experience to answer the question, as in, "Because I can see it." Then the learner is asked a question about something she does not know, such as, "What song is playing?" while the therapist is listening to music with headphones. When the learner responds, "I don't know," the therapist asks, "Why not?," to which the learner is prompted again to refer to her sensory experience, as in, "Because I can't hear it." The therapist might then follow this up by asking, "How can you find out?" to which the learner again refers to her sensory experience, such as, "I can use your headphones to listen to it."

Identifying What Others Know

The therapist begins teaching the learner how to identify what others know by presenting something that is either able to be experienced or blocked from being experienced by a third person and then asking the learner if the person knows some aspect of it, such as, "Does Evelyn know what is in the picture?" If Evelyn does not know what is in the picture, the learner is asked, "Why doesn't she know?" and the learner is prompted to identify the sensory experience that is being blocked, as in, "Because she can't see it." Then the learner is prompted either to tell or show Evelyn what is in the picture, and the therapist then asks, "Does Evelyn know what is in the picture now?" Once the learner says "yes," the therapist asks, "How does she know?," to which the learner is prompted to identify the relevant experience that led to knowledge, such as, "because I told her" or "because she saw it." The therapist might also work on this skill is by having multiple people in a room and asking the learner, "Who knows ____?," to which the learner responds by identifying everyone who has experiential access to the knowledge. The therapist then follows this up by asking the learner why certain individuals do or don't know and prompting the learner to provide explanations based on sensory experience. For those who do not know, the therapist teaches the learner to give unknown information by first asking the learner, "How can you let him know?" Once the learner refers to the sensory experience needed to inform the person, as in, "I can show him" or "I can let him see it," the therapist prompts the learner to inform the person through the identified method. To ensure that this skill is used appropriately in social interactions in the natural environment, the therapist also contrives or captures situations for the learner to provide unknown information to others. For example, the therapist might present some candy to the learner and prompt the learner to ask a third person if he likes the candy. When the third person says, "I don't know. I've never tried it before," the learner is prompted to say, "Here, try some."

Conversation is a critical setting in which the ability to identify others' knowledge needs to be applied. The therapist can work on this by presenting a rule, such as, "If people do not know something, you can tell them or show them, so they will know; but if they already know, then you should not show or tell them because that is boring." There are many ways to practice this skill. The therapist can have multiple people placed in different locations throughout the house, so different people know different things based on what they can and cannot see. The learner will need to infer who knows what and then describe what is happening to people who cannot see while refraining from telling people who can see. The therapist might say to the child, "Tell Tim something he does not know because he cannot see." The goal is not for the learner to identify who knows what but for the learner to apply that knowledge to his social and communicative interactions.

Another activity might include having the learner make "introductions." For example, during a playdate, the learner might be instructed to tell the peer about the therapist. The learner should tell the peer only things about the therapist that the peer does not already know and should not tell the peer things that the peer does know (e.g., things the peer can see, such as gender, hair color, eye color, the color of the therapist's shirt, etc.). A third way to practice this skill is to have the learner go through old family photo albums with the therapist. Ask the learner to describe only the things that the therapist does not know by looking at the picture. For example, the learner is prompted to say, "This was the time we went to Mexico," rather than saying, "This is my brother" (since the therapist already knows the child's brother). Once the learner has taught the therapist something, the learner should refrain from retelling the same information to the same therapist if the photos are reviewed the next day, since he told him the day before and the therapist therefore already knows it.

It is equally important to consider what another person does not know because failing to do so will usually result in not giving the person sufficient background information to make sense of what you are saying. For example, children with ASD often jump into the middle of a story without including background details that provide the context and framework for the story. For these learners, the therapist can provide rules, such as, "When people aren't in the room, they don't know what happened while they were gone, so you need to tell them," and so on. As always, frequent practice across many different conversations, peers, and settings is necessary until generalization occurs. The following are two games that can be useful for this:

- **Blindfold Task**. The therapist is blindfolded, and the learner must guide the therapist through a series of obstacles. As an "experiential prompt," the therapist and learner can switch roles, so the learner experiences what it is like not to be able to see and to be given instructions that do not take that into consideration.
- **Barrier Games**. Place a barrier between the therapist and learner such that neither can see the other's materials. The therapist and learner each have an identical set of materials, and the learner is instructed to create anything she wants (e.g., a building, a picture, etc.) and to give the therapist specific instructions (e.g., "Put the small yellow circle on the string first" as opposed to, "Put this one on first") on how to construct an identical creation without seeing what the learner is doing. Once the learner finishes giving instructions, the barrier is removed and both products are compared. The two products should be identical if the learner gave clear instructions.

Knowing how. In addition to knowing "about" something, consider teaching your learner to identify whether others know "how" to do something. The therapist should start by asking the learner whether someone knows how, as in, "Do you know how to play hopscotch?" or "Does Joey know how to set up the train set?" Once the learner answers "yes" versus "no," the therapist asks, "Why?" or "Why not?," to which the learner is prompted to identify that the person has never done it before or has yet to learn how to do it and/or the opposite – the fact that the person has learned or done it before. When someone does not know how to do something, the therapist can follow up with instructions such as, "How can he find out how to do it?," and prompt the learner to identify the various ways that individuals can learn how to do something, such as watch someone else do it, ask someone how to do it, read instructions, try it and see what works, and so on. To ensure that this skill is used appropriately in social interactions in the natural environment, the therapist should contrive or capture situations in which others do not know how to do something and prompt the learner to give them the unknown information that they need, either through showing or telling (e.g., setting up for a preferred game, etc.).

BELIEFS

In the ToM literature, a belief is what a person thinks to be true, given his perception and interpretation of events. For example, if someone has seen or heard something, his interpretation of this event and what he subsequently thinks about it constitutes his beliefs about that event. If the person's perception is correct, he holds a true belief, and if his perception is not correct, then he holds a false belief. Between the ages of 4 and 5 years, typically developing children begin to understand that there is a connection between perception and beliefs and can identify what others will believe based on their perception of events. They also understand that beliefs cause actions: for example, if someone thinks her ball is in the closet, she will look for it there. The Beliefs lesson teaches children to identify and predict others' beliefs and to predict actions based upon beliefs. This includes situations in which either the learner's own beliefs or others beliefs are true or false based on what is known by each individual or what each individual has experienced.

Learner's True and False Beliefs

We generally begin with teaching the learner to identify her own beliefs and to label whether they are true or false. The following tasks can be used to practice this skill:

- **Deceptive container task**. To perform this task, the therapist shows the learner a clearly labeled container, asks her what she thinks is inside, and then asks the learner to explain her answer: for example, "What do you think is inside the box? Why?" At this point, the therapist reveals that, in reality, a random item is inside the box that does not correspond to the container's label (e.g., a pencil inside a candy box). Then the therapist asks, "Were you right?" to help the learner to identify whether her belief was true or false. The therapist should also randomly rotate trials where the child's belief is false with trials where it's true.

- **Appearance-reality task**. This task is similar to the deceptive container task, except that an object is used that looks exactly like a different object (e.g., a sponge that looks like a rock).
- **Unexpected transfer task**. This task involves moving an item from its expected location (sometimes with the learner watching and sometimes not) and asking the learner to identify where she thinks the item is located, only to reveal that it is not there (e.g., the Sally Anne Task).

Others' True and False Beliefs

The next step is to teach the learner to identify another person's beliefs and whether they are true or false. To teach this skill, the learner observes the therapist implementing any of the tasks mentioned above but with a third person. Using the "unexpected transfer task" as an example, the therapist starts by asking the child's sister, Megan, "Where do you think your bike is?" When Megan says, "In the garage," the therapist reveals that the bike has been moved to the back yard. The therapist then asks the learner, "Before Megan looked in the back yard, where did she think her bike was located?" When the learner says, "In the garage," the therapist then asks, "Why did Megan think that?" Once the learner identifies the reason (e.g., "Because that's where she keeps it"), the therapist asks, "Was Megan right?" As always, rotate belief-true and belief-false trials across multiple exemplars, people, and settings.

Predicting Beliefs and Belief-based Actions

Once the learner is able to identify the beliefs of another person and whether they are true or false, the next step is to teach the learner to predict what someone's beliefs will be in a given situation. For example, the therapist might ask the learner, "If I put a fake snake in your sister's bed when she is out of the room, what would she think is in her bed?" The correct answer is something like, "Nothing, since she didn't see it." Then the therapist should ask something like, "Would she be right?," and the learner would say that his sister would be wrong (holding a false belief). The therapist can incorporate predicting others' actions by asking questions such as, "What would your sister do if she saw a fake snake in her bed?" When the learner replies, "Scream," the therapist then asks, "Why?," to which the learner would say, "Because she will think it is a real snake." For application and generalization, make sure to actually practice friendly pranks such as these – ones that will not anger friends and family, of course!

Identifying beliefs leading to actions. Around the same time you are teaching the learner to predict beliefs and belief-based actions, consider teaching the ability to identify which belief has led to a person's actions. For example, the therapist might hold up a snowball and look at the learner's sister. When the learner's sister begins to run away, the therapist asks the learner, "Why is she running away?" to which he responds, "Because she thinks you are going to throw that snowball at her."

DECEPTION

According to the ToM literature, once the learner has developed an understanding of others' beliefs and false beliefs, she is said to have developed the most important core perspective-taking skills. Understanding deception takes false belief one step further in that it allows the child to understand how false beliefs are key to deceptive behavior, such as tricks, bluffs, white lies, and persuasion. Appropriate social behavior includes a large variety of deceptive behaviors and reasons that people engage in them, such as telling white lies to avoid hurting someone's feelings and bluffing or lying (or omitting information) to avoid getting in trouble, to obtain something one wants, to look cool, to keep a secret or surprise, or to tell a joke without giving the punch line away. Starting at around the age of 4 years, children understand that the false beliefs held by a person determine their behavior, and they begin to engage in deception. Later, starting around age 5, their deceptive behavior becomes more sophisticated, and they are able to play bluffing games. The Deception lesson teaches children to identify and use deception. This lesson not only teaches the learner to create false beliefs in others but also teaches the learner to keep secrets, identify the many forms of deception others use in an attempt to deceive the learner, and understand which forms of deception are harmless versus harmful.

Tricks

When it comes to teaching learners about deception, tricks are a good place to start. There are many good reasons that teaching children with ASD to play friendly tricks on others is a good idea. First, it's a fun way to teach them to understand deception and to experience it without hurting anyone's feelings. In addition, friendly tricks are a great way to teach humor and playful behavior, which is an attractive quality in a friend. Furthermore, since many children with ASD tend to think in black and white or to be extremely literal, it's common for them to misinterpret others' playful tricks as being malicious.

To teach trick playing, the therapist can start by teaching the learner to identify whether something is a trick. In doing so, the therapist first provides a description of a trick, such as, "A trick is something someone does to make you think that something is going on that isn't, and it's funny when you find out." Then the therapist engages in a behavior and asks the learner whether it is a trick. For example, the therapist might point while saying, "Look, there's a spider!," and then ask, "Is this a trick?" If there is a spider present, the learner answers, "No." However, if there is not a spider present, the learner answers, "Yes." The therapist should follow up with a typical trick-closing behavior, such as saying, "Gotcha!" while smiling and patting the learner on the back.

Once the learner can identify whether a behavior is a trick, the next step is to teach the learner to engage in playful (not hurtful) tricks. To teach this skill, the therapist leads the learner by saying, "Let's play a trick. What can we do?" At first, the therapist will likely have to provide the learner with some ideas (e.g., fake reptiles, made-ya'-look games, pretending to throw something) and let the learner choose one. Then the therapist should walk the learner through the process of coming up with a plan to carry out the trick, which sometimes includes a plan for how to keep it a secret (avoid giving the trick away). After talking through the plan with the learner (and possibly even role-playing, if necessary), the therapist instructs the learner to implement the trick. If needed, the therapist prompts the learner through the trick as it is occurring, including what to say and do, how to avoid giving it away, waiting to confess the truth, the appropriate language for confession (e.g., "Ha ha, made ya' look!"), and so on. With each new trick, prompts should be faded out. The learner should begin to come up with his own ideas for tricks and should start to lead the design of the plan, as well as its execution. The skill should be considered mastered once the learner can design and carry out novel tricks independently.

In addition to teaching the learner to play tricks, it is also important for the therapist to contrive and capture opportunities for others to play tricks on the learner and for the learner to practice learning to laugh and react good-naturedly to the trick without getting upset. To teach the learner to laugh and be accepting when tricked, the therapist might start by providing a rule, such as, "It's okay for others to play tricks on you as long as they are not making fun of you or hurting you. When they do this, you should laugh or say something like, 'That's a good one!' while smiling. This will show that you are a good sport and a fun friend." Then, if needed, the therapist should have the learner rehearse a reaction to a trick by playing a trick on the learner and modeling an appropriate response. This might then be faded to the therapist's saying, "Today, someone will play a trick on you. Remember what I taught you, and practice laughing." Eventually, this might be faded to, "Any time someone plays a trick that is not meant to hurt your feelings, remember to try just laughing at it." Then the therapist might have to provide reinforcement for responding appropriately; however, the ultimate goal is for the learner to actually learn to enjoy and find humor in others playing tricks on her, as well as to take turns playing friendly tricks on others. If this lesson is taught successfully, the learner and her peers are going to have more fun and laugh more than they did before – not a bad outcome!

Identifying Deception in Others

Two types of deceptions you should consider teaching your learners to detect are cheating and lying. To teach the learner to detect cheating, the therapist should start by giving the learner a rule that describes cheating, such as, "Cheating is when someone breaks the rules during a game. You should never cheat during a game unless that is the point of the game. If you see someone cheat, you can call them out on it." Then, the therapist will set up an opportunity for the learner to play a game. Even though the main goal here is to teach the learner to detect when others are cheating, the learner is prompted not to cheat (and provided praise for compliance), and situations where others try to cheat should be contrived. The learner is prompted to notice and call others out when they cheat.

To teach the learner to detect when others are lying, the therapist starts off by giving the learner a rule, such as, "A lie is when someone says something that isn't true. Sometimes people lie to _____." The various reasons that people lie include to obtain something they want, to look cool, to exclude you, to take your things, and so on. The therapist chooses which of these reasons might be relevant to the learner and includes them in the rule. Then the therapist contrives situations for the learner to detect a lie. For example, the therapist might play with the learner and every now and then say lies to obtain the learner's toy: for example, "Your mom said I could have this," "This is mine; I brought it from home," or "I'm the guest, so you have to give me one of your toys." The therapist could also say lies to exclude the learner: for example, "Only people with brown hair can play this game" or "You have to be older than 6 years old to play this game." The learner is prompted to identify when the therapist is lying, first by using leading questions, such as, "Hold on, why would I get to have three turns just because I'm a girl? Does that sound true?" If the learner cannot identify correctly that the statement is a lie, the therapist might then tell the learner it's a lie and give an explanation as to why that statement is a lie: for example, "The rules of the game don't say girls can have three turns – everyone only gets one turn." The therapist presents many different new lies and starts with allowing the learner to detect the lie on his own before prompting. If needed, prompts are provided, but as the learner becomes more independent, they will be faded. Once the learner is able to detect and respond appropriately to lies with the therapist, peers will be brought into sessions (Ranick, Persicke, Tarbox, & Kornack, 2013). As always, continue training multiple exemplars until you get generalization across lies, settings, and peers.

Using Advanced Deception

Many children with ASD are "overly honest" in that they do not know how to keep secrets or surprises, bluff during card games, or tell white lies.

Secrets. The therapist can begin teaching secret-keeping by providing an explanation of a secret, as in, "A secret is something that people tell you that they don't want you to tell anyone else. If anyone tries to get you to tell the secret, you need to make sure not to tell it, or you can tell that person that it's a secret and you can't tell." Then, to practice keeping a secret, the therapist tells the learner a secret (as an option, the therapist might ask, "Why is it a secret?" to help the learner talk through the reason the therapist doesn't want anyone to know) and instructs the learner not to tell anyone. At this point, the therapist sets up occasions for various people to ask questions in an effort to tempt the learner to tell the secret. In all cases, the learner is prompted to keep the secret by either not saying anything to give it away or by saying, "I can't tell you; it's a secret." Prompts are faded as the learner is successful and the length of time that the learner is able to keep the secret is gradually increased. Don't forget to teach the learner to distinguish between secrets that are okay to keep versus ones that must be told to an adult, such as those that involve harm or danger. To teach the learner to keep a surprise, the therapist uses a similar procedure as described above and explains that the reason for the secret is that it is a surprise, as in preparing gifts and so on.

Bluffing. To teach the learner to bluff during games, the therapist starts by having the learner play a game that requires bluffing. For example, the therapist might have the learner hide an item under one of three cups while a third person has to guess which cup contains the item. Before the game begins, the therapist reminds the learner how to bluff, saying "Remember, don't look at the cup that contains the item. You can even look at a different cup if you want to bluff." Once the game begins, the learner is prompted further, if needed. This process is repeated across various types of bluffing games, including ones where the learner has to lie (e.g., about the cards he has, etc.), and as the learner learns to bluff more effectively across games, prompts are faded out until the learner is able to bluff independently with new games.

White lies. To teach the learner to engage in white lies, the therapist starts by giving the learner various rules related to white lies, such as, "If someone gives you a gift you don't like, never say you don't like it. Always smile and thank the person who gave it to you. If that person asks you if you like it, tell him you like it, so you don't hurt his feelings" or "If someone looks funny – maybe his new haircut is weird or he is wearing a shirt for babies – never laugh at that person and don't say anything to suggest you think he looks funny. If he asks you what you think, say you think it's cool, so you don't hurt his feelings." After the rules have been provided, the therapist and learner practice using white lies. If needed, the learner is prompted to engage in the correct behavior. In addition to the learner saying the correct vocal response, the learner may also need to be prompted to use convincing facial expressions and tone. New situations in which the learner can engage in white lies should be contrived and captured with prompts faded out. In order to avoid increasing lying overall, consider also including a discrimination program in which you teach the learner to discriminate when it is and is not appropriate to tell a white lie.

THINKING

Emerging at around age 3 years, typically developing children begin to use the word *think* to denote uncertainty, as well as desires and preferences, and to describe the mental states of others. They understand that they cannot see or touch what others are thinking and that they can see their own mental images but others cannot. They also understand that they can think one thing, and someone else can think something else. Between the ages of 4 and 7, they begin to use language to state their opinions and – around 5 years of age – identify fact versus opinion. The Thinking lesson teaches children to express their own and infer and predict others' thoughts. The purpose of this lesson is to improve the learner's understanding and application of the word *think* and the concepts of "thinking" and "thoughts." Specifically, the child will learn that thoughts are intangible, and thus he cannot see or touch others' thoughts nor can others see or touch his thoughts. However, thoughts can be inferred based on others' behavior. Furthermore, future behavior may be predicted based on inference of others' thoughts. This lesson also aims to help the learner understand that, given similar situations, different people might think different things.

Using the Word *Think*

People use the word *think* in a large variety of situations in everyday conversational language. One example is to use it as suggestion for action, as when answering the question, "What do you think we should have for dinner?" The learner might say, "I think we should have pizza." The learner should also be prompted to use this language spontaneously when opportunities arise in the natural environment. For example, while playing, the learner might be prompted to say, "I think we should play soccer" when she wants to play soccer.

Another scenario in which the word *think* is used is when denoting uncertainty. To teach the learner to do this, the therapist might present an ambiguous picture, perhaps a drawing of a circle with small dots on it, and ask, "What do you think this is?," to which the learner will answer, "I think it's a ___." Given the ambiguous nature of the picture, the correct answer could be anything that the picture resembles, such as a cookie, pizza with pepperoni, golf ball, moon, etc. As before, the therapist teaches the learner to begin using this language when opportunities arise in natural, everyday interactions.

Thoughts as intangible. The abstract nature of thoughts can be a difficult concept to grasp. Thus, the child learns to distinguish between real things and thoughts and is exposed to the idea that thoughts are private or going on "in her head." To teach this concept, the therapist might present a visual of a face with a thought bubble, tell the learner to think about something, and then ask, "What are you thinking about?" The therapist might then draw what the learner is thinking about in the thought bubble and then ask the learner, "Do I know what you are thinking about if you don't tell me?" Once the learner answers "No," the therapist asks, "Why not?" and the learner is prompted to identify that the therapist cannot see what the learner is thinking. Once the learner begins to understand that thoughts are private events, the next step is occasionally to ask the learner, "What are you thinking?" in an effort to help the learner explain her current thoughts ("I am thinking about ___"). If the learner doesn't provide enough detail for the therapist to understand the thoughts, the therapist reminds the learner that he cannot see the learner's thoughts and prompts the learner to provide more background information, labels, time frame, attributes, etc. Of course, don't forget to be flexible here, as you truly don't know what the learner is thinking, so you can't really provide prompts to correct inaccurate descriptions.

Others' Thoughts

Inferring others' thoughts is something that most humans do on a daily basis in order to have successful social interactions. An easy way to begin to teach this ability is for the therapist to teach the learner to ask others, "What do you think?" or "What are you thinking?" The therapist might set up a situation wherein the learner presents an idea and then is prompted to ask, "What do you think?" Similarly, the therapist might contrive a situation to appear as if he or a third person is deep in thought (e.g., by placing one's finger to one's head and looking up, etc.) and prompt the learner to ask, "What are you thinking about?"

In addition to asking others what they are thinking, it is also important for children to be able to infer others' possible thoughts. One way that this is taught is by having someone suggest an activity or present an item and then having another person react either positively or negatively through facial expression (e.g., smiling, laughing versus scowling, furrowing brow, wrinkling nose, staring blankly) and then asking the learner, "Does she think we should do that?" or "What does she think about that?" This can also be done using pictures from magazines, drawings, or comic strips, through role-play with dolls and action figures, or through stories, as well as through contrived or captured situations *in vivo*. Another way this can be taught is by presenting a scenario with two people (either *in vivo* or in pictures) and asking, "Who is thinking (<u>thought</u>)?" For example, while observing two children in class, one is looking out the window and the other is watching the teacher, and the therapist asks, "Which student is thinking that he wishes he were outside playing?" The learner is then prompted to identify the person who is more likely to be thinking the thought. Multiple exemplars are presented and trained until the learner can do this activity with untrained novel exemplars.

Once the learner can identify who is more likely to be thinking a particular thought, the next step is to ask the learner what someone is thinking. The learner would need to attend to social cues, such as the person's eye gaze, to make an inference about what he might be thinking. For example, the therapist might stare at pictures of his puppy in a photo album and ask, "What am I thinking about?" to which the learner might guess, "Your dog." Obviously, reinforce a variety of reasonable answers since there is no "correct" answer.

Once the learner is able to identify what people are thinking in the present, she should be taught to predict what others will think or would think in specific situations based on their preferences. For example, the therapist might ask, "What would Sally think about playing tennis?" or "What would Sally think we should do during your playdate?" In this scenario, the learner has no overt cues to guide her inference about what Sally might think, so the learner should use her knowledge about Sally's preferences when answering this question: for example, the learner might say, "She would probably like to play tennis, because she loves tennis."

Facts versus Opinions

Many children with ASD could benefit from learning to understand the difference between facts versus opinions and that it's okay to let people think their own opinions, rather than arguing with them or insisting that they should change their opinions. Begin by teaching the learner to discriminate between facts and opinions. The therapist might start by explaining the difference between fact and opinion, such as, "A fact is something that everyone would agree is true and does not change. An opinion can change. With opinions, sometimes other people will think the same thing as you or they might think something different than you, but facts always stay the same." Then the therapist follows this up with a statement of either fact or opinion, such as, "Basketball is a sport," and asks, "Is that fact or opinion?"

The therapist might then say, "Basketball is the best sport," and again ask, "Is that fact or opinion?" Multiple exemplars will need to be trained until generalization occurs across novel exemplars. Once the learner can discriminate facts from opinions, she should be taught to accept others' opinions without arguing or attempting to make them change their opinion, if needed. The therapist might do this by first stating a rule, such as, "When someone gives an opinion, it is okay to say what you think, too, but don't try to change the other person's opinion." The therapist then follows this up by contriving or capturing scenarios *in vivo* for the learner to practice accepting others' opinions. The learner will be prompted through it until she displays the correct social behavior to new untrained scenarios. As the learner progresses on this skill, make it more challenging by introducing situations wherein the peer believes that his opinion is a fact, but the learner has additional information to help the peer realize that it is actually an opinion – that is, situations where it is appropriate for the learner to disagree with a peer's opinion by politely offering additional information about the topic.

Think-feel-say-do

One of the most difficult concepts to teach children with autism regarding others' thoughts is that sometimes what people say and do does not match what they are really thinking and feeling. Many children with ASD have difficulty with this concept because they have no separation between the literal truth of what they think versus what they say. Initially, it might be helpful to use a visual when teaching this skill and to provide an explanation, such as, "Everyone thinks thoughts, feels feelings, says words, and does actions. We will show what people might be thinking with this thought bubble, what people might be feeling with this heart, what people are saying with this word bubble, and what people are doing with this box. Sometimes, what people think, feel, say, and do all match. Let's look at this situation." The therapist might then present a drawing of a scenario, such as the top panel in Figure 17.2. The therapist might then say, "Sometimes, what people think, feel, say, and do don't all match. Let's look at this situation," and present something like the bottom panel of Figure 17.2.

The therapist might then follow this up with some questions, such as, "What is he thinking?"; "How does he feel?"; "What is he saying?"; "What is he doing?"; "Why is he saying, 'Look at the cool spider'?"; and "Why is he acting cool?" The goal here is for the learner to identify that the boy might be acting cool by *saying*, "Look at the cool spider," but he is really *feeling* scared and *thinking* that he doesn't want the girl to know that he's scared.

Once the learner is able to discriminate between thoughts, feelings, words, and actions, the therapist asks the learner to identify all of these variables in his own behavior during real-life *in vivo* scenarios. The learner can also be taught that there are times when it is more appropriate to think

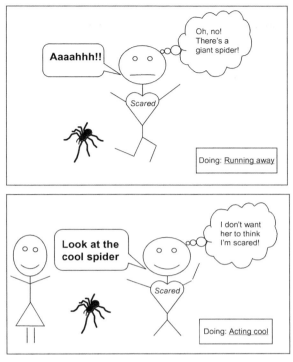

FIGURE 17.2 Sample visual supports for teaching the difference between thinking, feeling, saying, and doing. *Reprinted from Skills® with permission from the Center for Autism and Related Disorders.*

and feel something than it is to say or do something. For example, it is okay to *feel* bored and *think* the teacher is mean, but it is not okay to say, "This is boring" or "You are mean." During real-life social situations in which the learner exhibits socially inappropriate behavior or overreacts, the therapist might review what actually happened using the visuals in Figure 17.2 and discuss alternative methods for dealing with the social situation: for example, "What else could you/he say/do?"; "Why should you/he do that?"; "What would happen if ___?"

Once the learner can identify that some things we think and feel are inappropriate to say and do, the next step is to teach the learner to make inferences about what others might be thinking and feeling, given what they are saying and doing. This can be done using the same visual aids shown in Figure 17.2 by filling in the word bubble and box with what is being said and done but leaving the heart and thought bubble empty for the learner to fill in. The therapist then teaches the reverse by showing the same visual aid but with the heart and thought bubble filled in and the word bubble and box blank for the learner to fill in what someone might say and do, given what the person is thinking and feeling. In this scenario, the therapist has the learner infer what someone might say and do if he doesn't mind others knowing how he really feels and what he really thinks versus what he might say and do if he doesn't want others to know how he really feels and thinks due to embarrassment or some other factor.

Thinking Before Doing

Many children with ASD impulsively engage in actions without first thinking about the potential consequences of their actions, resulting in negative situations, such as hurting and offending others, and potentially resulting in the learner's being unable to make and maintain friendships. In order to help the learner to be more cautious and mindful in his social interactions, the therapist can teach the learner to think before doing. The therapist might do this by presenting a visual aid (Figure 17.3) combined with a rule, such as, "Before doing something, *stop* (represented by the color red) and *think* (represented by yellow) about what you want to do

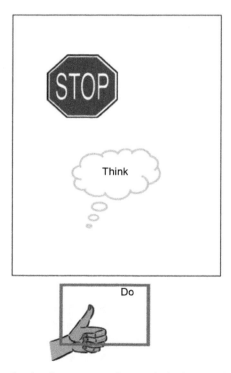

FIGURE 17.3   Sample visual support used to teach the learner the concept of stopping and thinking before acting. *Reprinted from Skills® with permission from the Center for Autism and Related Disorders.*

and if anything bad will happen if you do it. If nothing bad will happen, then you can *do* it (represented by the color green)." The therapist follows this up with role-play and rehearsal until the learner is making good choices in new situations without direct training. The therapist also contrives and captures instances for the learner to practice this skill in his natural environment until the learner demonstrates this skill independently in new situations. See, also, the Inhibition lesson in Chapter 18, as this is a very closely related skill.

DETECTING SARCASM

Starting at 7+ years of age, typically developing children begin to use sarcasm, and many children can respond appropriately to sarcasm even earlier. The Detecting Sarcasm lesson teaches children to detect and respond appropriately to sarcasm expressed by others. Sarcasm usually consists of saying the opposite of what is actually meant. For example, if two people are standing next to each other outside in the rain, and one says to the other, "Beautiful day out!" we can safely assume the person is using sarcasm because we normally reserve such statements for clear and sunny days. So, in this instance, the person is communicating the opposite of what is intended (i.e., that the weather is terrible). To understand sarcasm, the learner must be able to identify that what is actually said (a public event) is the opposite of what the person likely meant (a private event). This largely consists of the ability to infer the most plausible meaning of what was said and respond to the fact that it is in opposition to its literal meaning. The speaker's tone of voice, facial expression, and body language are often helpful. At first blush, this ability may seem obscure, but the inability to understand sarcasm can make a learner with ASD stand out. For example, if she shoots a basket and misses and a peer says, "Wow, nice shot," then the learner with ASD is going to look silly if she thinks the peer actually meant it and she therefore disagrees, as in, "No, it wasn't; I missed!"

To teach the learner to detect sarcasm, the therapist should begin by providing a rule, as in, "When people say the opposite of what is true, they are probably being sarcastic. They do this to be funny." After stating the rule, the therapist begins to insert sarcastic statements every now and then into everyday conversation. When a sarcastic statement is made, the therapist then asks the learner some questions to help the learner identify the statement as being sarcastic and how to respond appropriately to it: for example, "What did I say?" (the opposite of what you were thinking); "Why did I say it?" (to be funny); "What did I mean?" (the opposite of what you said); "What should you do?" (laugh, smile, say "That's funny," or provide a reciprocal sarcastic statement). The purpose of asking the learner these questions is to help her to begin to ask these questions covertly on her own. To ensure that the learner doesn't begin to expect all statements to be sarcastic, the therapist must make plenty of sincere statements during conversation, as well. In the beginning, when the therapist makes a sarcastic statement, she can use exaggerated facial expression (rolling of the eyes) and intonation. Over time, as the learner becomes more adept at detecting and responding appropriately to sarcastic statements, the therapist begins to fade out the questions, as well as the exaggerated sarcastic expressions (Persicke, Tarbox, Ranick, & St Clair, 2013). The skill is considered mastered once the learner is able to detect and respond appropriately to sarcasm in the presence of new people and new sarcastic statements in natural everyday conversation.

INTENTIONS

Between 3 and 4 years of age, typically developing children begin to infer the intentions of others through their emotional reactions to successes and failures of goal-directed behavior. Starting at around 5 years of age, children begin to make apologies for their own unintentional mistakes and infer the intentional versus accidental behavior of others. It's important to be able to infer others' intentions in order to respond to them appropriately during everyday interactions. For example, children need to be able to discriminate between accidental mistakes and intentional wrongdoings. They also need to be able to recognize and make apologies for their own unintentional wrongdoings. The Intentions lesson teaches children to identify their own and others' intentions and respond appropriately to their own and others' intentional and unintentional behaviors.

Inferring Intentions from Actions

Therapists can begin teaching the learner to infer the intentions of others by having the learner observe someone engaging in an action that is accompanied by an emotional response indicating the person's intentions. For example, the therapist might begin to build a tower with blocks and then knock the tower down. As the tower is falling, the therapist might make a crashing sound and smile versus scowl and say, "Shoot!" In either case, the therapist will then ask the learner, "What did I do?" After the learner identifies that the therapist knocked over the blocks, the therapist will ask, "Is that what I wanted to/meant to do?" After the learner answers "yes" versus "no," the therapist asks, "What did I want to do?" At this point, the learner identifies the intended action, as in, "You wanted to crash the tower" or "You wanted to build the tower taller." Trials of intentional and unintentional behavior should be rotated randomly.

Inferring Intentions of Current, Incomplete Actions

Around the same time that typically developing children learn to infer the intentions of others during previous actions, they also learn to infer the intentions of others' current, incomplete actions. To teach this skill, the therapist starts to engage in an action: for example, the therapist goes into the kitchen and takes out a butter knife, bread, peanut butter, and jelly. At this point, the therapist pauses and asks the learner, "What do I want to do?" and prompts and reinforces reasonable inferences. Another way this might be taught is to "try" to engage in a behavior. For example, the therapist might "try" to take the lid off of a jar but be unsuccessful in doing so. Then the therapist asks the learner, "What do I want to do?"

Responding to Intentional and Unintentional Actions

Therapists can begin teaching appropriate responses to intentional and unintentional behaviors by starting with behaviors done accidentally by the learner. For example, the therapist might ask the learner, "If you accidentally stepped on someone's toe, what would you say?" and prompt and reinforce a response along the lines of, "I'm sorry! I didn't mean to do that," or "Oops, I'm sorry. I didn't see you," or any other response that indicates the behavior was an accident. Once the learner is able to respond appropriately to questions about what he would do in hypothetical situations, the therapist should then contrive and capture scenarios for the learner to demonstrate the skill in everyday life.

At the same time, the therapist can begin teaching the learner what to do in response to others' intentional and unintentional behaviors. For example, the therapist might ask the learner, "If a kid came over and said, 'I don't like your picture' and ripped it up, what would you do?" In this case, the wrongdoing was intentional, and an appropriate response would be to stand up for oneself and/or tell an adult. The therapist should also counterbalance examples of intentional wrongdoings with unintentional ones, such as, "If a kid tripped and spilled water on your picture, what would you do?" In this case, the learner would respond to the wrong-doing as accidental and indicate that he would tell the kid, "It's okay. It was an accident." Once the learner is able to say what he would do given various possible scenarios involving both intentional and unintentional wrongdoings, the therapist begins to contrive and capture scenarios for the learner to practice the skill in the natural environment.

Inferring Intention in Scenarios Involving Others

A final step in teaching intentions is to teach the learner to interpret intention in interactions between others. To teach this, the therapist presents scenarios describing the interaction between two or more people and asks the learner to identify intention. For example, the therapist might say, "Billy's mom tells Billy that if he has a good day at school, he will get to have ice cream after school. When she picks him up, she asks whether he was good all day. He says he was good even though he got a time-out for being disruptive. Why did Billy tell his mom that he was good all day?" In this case, the learner is taught to identify Billy's intention behind his interaction with his mother by replying something like, "So that she would take him to get ice cream." As always, train across multiple exemplars until you see generalization to novel exemplars, settings, and people.

GENERAL TIPS FOR SUCCESS

Perspective taking is among the most challenging repertoires to teach children with ASD. However, we have found that the same principles and procedures used to teach simpler skills can effectively be modified to teach complex skills such as perspective taking. The following are some general tips to return to on a regular basis to ensure that this process is successful.

Identify Prerequisite Skills

First of all, it's important that prerequisites are in place before working on each content area. Given the scope of this chapter, it's impossible to list all of the prerequisites necessary for working on each of the skills described. However, generally speaking, it is important to ensure that the learner's spontaneous language is varied, detailed, and fluent before working on complex perspective-taking skills.

Pronouns. Understanding and using pronouns is not perspective taking, per se, but pronouns involve a critical set of prerequisites for perspective taking. The reason for this is that, in a large portion of perspective-taking situations, pronouns cue the learner to engage in perspective taking. For example, if a therapist merely said, "How feeling?" to a learner, no perspective taking would be necessary because pronouns are absent. However, if the therapist asked the learner, "How is *he* feeling?" this would cue the learner to engage in perspective taking with respect to the person to whom the pronoun "he" refers. An even more complex perspective-taking behavior would be cued if the therapist asked something like, "How would *you* feel if *you* were *he*?"

To teach pronouns, proceed through the same general phases of teaching as you normally would with other language lessons (see Chapter 11). You might begin by teaching the learner to respond to pronouns receptively, that is, as a listener. For example, you might present an instruction, such as, "Touch *my* shoe" versus "Touch *your* shoe," and prompt and reinforce correct responding. To begin expressive pronoun training, you might present instructions, such as, "What color is *your* shirt?"; "What color is *my* shirt?"; "Where am *I* sitting?"; "Where are *you* sitting?" and so on. Echoic prompts can be difficult to use when teaching pronouns because the correct pronouns reverse when acting as the speaker versus the listener, so written cues are often more effective. For example, a therapist who is wearing a red shirt might tape a card on his shirt with the word *you* printed on it and ask the learner, "Who is wearing a red shirt?" As with other language lessons, teach all of the different verbal operants that are relevant to the concept and appropriate to the learner's age and continue training until you observe generalization across untrained exemplars, therapists, and settings.

Cause and effect. The ability to causally relate events in one's environment is critical to many higher order perspective-taking skills. Early perspective-taking activities do not always involve causal reasoning (e.g., labeling a smiling person as "happy"), but later perspective-taking skills require it. For example, predicting how others are going to feel based on whether they get what they want amounts to predicting a future effect, given a known potential cause. When causal reasoning is not already acquired as a generalized operant, attempting to teach complex perspective-taking skills that require causal reasoning will likely be futile.

Teaching learners to understand cause-and-effect relations follows a similar progression to other language lessons, beginning with receptive and basic labeling and progressing through more complex inferring behaviors. According to Relational Frame Theory (RFT), relating events causally is, in itself, a generalized operant class of behavior that is acquired through multiple exemplar training (Hayes, Barnes-Holmes, & Roche, 2001). Therefore, to teach the skill, teach across multiple exemplars until you observe generalization across untrained ones. For example, identify a large set of scenarios where there is a clear cause and effect: for example, someone drops an egg and it breaks, touches a stove and gets burned, etc. Teach the learner to respond receptively and expressively three scenarios at a time until generalization is obtained to untrained scenarios. For more specific information on prerequisites for each lesson in the Cognition curriculum, see Skills® (www.skillsforautism.com; Chapter 26).

Use Naturalistic Teaching Procedures Across Multiple Exemplars

All complex skill acquisition depends on avoiding rote responding and, instead, focusing on establishing generalized, flexible repertoires. Multiple exemplar training is the surest teaching method for this (see Chapter 7 on generalization). Multiple exemplar training requires varying every aspect of the teaching situation as frequently as possible and not engaging in rote repetition. Many opportunities to practice the skill are critical, but each should vary, thereby requiring the learner to engage in the actual skill, not merely repeat what she did previously. Such training must continue until the learner is able to respond correctly and independently with novel untrained exemplars across various people and settings. That is, true mastery is determined by the learner's ability to demonstrate generalization.

To ensure that the learned skills generalize to the everyday natural social interactions in which the learner needs to use them, avoid overusing structured discrete trial formats for teaching. Incorporate as much natural environment training as possible (see Chapter 4). However, keep in mind that, even though natural environment training might be a better method for establishing flexible repertoires, it's also important to ensure that there are still plenty of practice opportunities. When therapists only focus on capturing real moments for teaching in the natural environment, they miss out on the benefits of practice. Thus, it is important to use role-play and rehearsal with the learner in addition to contriving opportunities for the learner to practice the skills in the natural environment.

Prompting

When teaching complex verbal and relational skills, such as perspective taking, the CARD Model makes heavy use of "leading question" prompts, which help guide learners to "discover" the answers to questions as opposed to providing immediate full vocal prompts that provide the learner with an answer to memorize. In addition, do not focus too much on the specific topography of a response you are teaching at any one time (e.g., saying, "Are you okay?" when someone cries). The point of all of these lessons is to establish much larger repertoires of perspective-taking behavior, not specific appropriate topographies. This is why most of the Cognition lessons teach the learner to talk through scenarios – this constitutes teaching thinking and reasoning skills, albeit at the overt level initially. However, it is important to remember that teaching cognition skills should not only involve talking and role-playing between the therapist and learner. In other words, it won't be beneficial to teach the learner to talk about and "understand" others' perspectives but never expect him to apply this information to everyday social interactions. Thus, it is absolutely essential that the learner practice application of perspective-taking skills to real-life social interactions with peers.

COMMON PITFALLS WHEN TEACHING PERSPECTIVE-TAKING SKILLS

Knowing the Response vs. Applying the Skill

One common pitfall in teaching perspective-taking skills is that some children will learn to understand another's perspective but still won't apply the skills to everyday social interactions. If application has been targeted and the therapist is sure that the learner knows how to apply the skills, then there is likely a motivational issue; the learner understands yet does not care and therefore does not apply the skills. In this circumstance, contingencies might need to be contrived in order to motivate the learner to actually act differently. For example, the learner may need to be given access to items that are actually reinforcing to him (tangibles, activities, etc.) if the natural social consequences are insufficient. Additionally, it is easy to train rules and specific responses to many of the skills taught in the Cognition curriculum, which frequently results in problems when the learner is required to apply the skill. Being able to talk about what one should or shouldn't do does not always result in one behaving appropriately in the given context.

Teaching Age-Appropriate Skills

It is tempting to pick and choose which skills you want to teach as a therapist without a systematic plan, but it is important to consider the learner's developmental age and current skills when determining which perspective-taking skills to teach or which scenarios to use for examples. You will want to target applications of these skills that the learner will actually encounter in her daily life. For example, you would not teach a 4-year-old to detect and respond to sarcasm because most children do not learn this until they are older, and people usually don't use sarcasm when speaking to a 4-year-old. It would be more appropriate to target other related or prerequisite skills, such as intentions, that the learner will likely encounter on a daily basis. This will result in more opportunities for the learner to practice these skills in contexts that are familiar and may provide more natural forms of reinforcement.

SUMMARY

Perspective taking is a critical component of successful social behavior that requires identifying and responding appropriately to one's own and others' private events, yet individuals with ASD demonstrate difficulty in this area. This chapter describes the CARD approach to teaching perspective-taking skills across 11 major areas: 1) desires, 2) preferences, 3) emotions, 4) physical states, 5) sensory perspective taking, 6) knowledge, 7) beliefs, 8) deception, 9) thoughts, 10) sarcasm, and 11) intentions. The strategies used are designed to produce generalized, flexible repertoires of perspective taking across real-life social interactions.

Executive Functions

Adel C. Najdowski, Angela Persicke, Evelyn Kung

The term *executive functions* refers to the hypothesized brain processes that control other brain processes. Metaphorically speaking, the executive functions are the brain's chief executive officer. Executive functions include, at a minimum, inhibition, memory, attention, flexibility, planning, and problem solving. Most researchers agree that the term *executive function* (EF) is exceedingly broad, and there is little consensus on a definition. Even so, it is widely agreed that the activities to which the term refers are critical to everyday functioning in life. People who have difficulty inhibiting themselves, remembering things, planning and problem solving, and/ or being flexible will present with major deficiencies in social, academic, and vocational functioning. Unfortunately, children with autism spectrum disorder (ASD) commonly suffer from deficits in many or all of these areas, yet there is very little agreement or clarity across the various disciplines involved in autism treatment regarding what executive functions actually are and how, if at all, they can be improved.

The Center for Autism and Related Disorders (CARD) approach believes that all humans are the sums of their brain functions, learned behaviors, and ever-evolving environments. When a person has a learning interaction with her environment, it affects her brain and produces changes in the future functioning of her brain, likely through alterations in neural networks. Equally true, every time a person has a learning interaction with her environment, she brings an always-evolving set of brain functions to that interaction, and every behavior-environment interaction is therefore affected by the previous development of that person's brain functions. In other words, every time a person behaves in her environment, that action is the manifestation of a complex interaction between behavior, brain, and environment. The processes of learning via behavioral principles of learning and motivation both depend on one's current brain functions and affect one's future brain function. Put simply, behavioral learning affects the brain, and the brain affects learning.

The CARD approach to teaching EF skills consists of prompting and reinforcing the behaviors involved in these functions. We believe that all brain functions involve behaviors that are learned during the lifetime of the individual and that the principles and procedures of applied behavior analysis (ABA) can be used to enhance the development of these functions, just as they can be used to advance the development of any other skill area. In this chapter, we use traditional EF terms to refer to the general skill areas that are deficient in many children with ASD whom we treat using ABA procedures. For each EF, we identify: 1) what is happening in the environment and 2) the behavior the learner must execute in these settings in order to function successfully. ABA procedures are then used to teach these skills and ensure that they generalize to all relevant settings.

As clinicians, we arrange the learner's environment to help her learn and be successful. EF skills enable the learner to do the same thing for herself. EF skills involve intentional manipulation of one's own environment to help oneself function more independently. Therefore, EF skills are closely related to self-observation, self-management, self-control, and self-help, as will be discussed later in this chapter. As an aside, B. F. Skinner talked about such skills as "secondary repertoires of behavior" because they are behaviors in which one engages to help one's normal ongoing behavior be more effective. People with these repertoires are commonly called thoughtful, considerate, mature, self-disciplined, organized, and so forth. We use many secondary repertoires of behavior in everyday life in an effort to help our primary behavior to be more successful (e.g., making a shopping list, telling oneself to calm down before saying something regrettable, talking oneself through solving a problem, using a highlighter to highlight important passages when studying, and being aware of one's workload when agreeing to take on new tasks). All of these are behaviors that help us be more successful in the near future. They are a means of controlling and organizing our own behavior, and they are key to success in everyday life. EF skills help increase self-determination and personal freedom for the child with ASD because, by definition, they help her become the master of her own environment. The traditional cognitive terms that encompass these behaviors include **inhibition, memory, attention, flexibility, planning, problem solving**, and **self-management**. The CARD approach treats these "higher order cognitive skills" as any other skill: They are behaviors that can be taught through the principles and procedures of ABA.

TEACHING PROCEDURES

The procedures used to teach executive functions are the same procedures that are used to teach any other skills; they are the procedures derived from the principles of learning and motivation from ABA. Since

Chapter 4 describes these procedures in detail, we will not do so here. However, three particular procedures are critical enough to teaching EF skills that they deserve to be pointed out. First, all higher order skills, including EF skills, should be taught using multiple exemplar training, not rote or repetitive learning. The reason for this is that EF skills are not particular behaviors that need to be performed at particular times. Instead, EF skills are overarching, flexible repertoires of behavior that can be applied in virtually any situation in one's life. For example, calling a car a "car" (i.e., labeling or tacting) is a behavior that only needs to happen in the presence of cars. Inhibiting onself from doing something regrettable (an EF skill) is a skill that, by definition, the child needs to be able to apply in new situations, in the moment, without any prior training or rehearsal in that particular situation. By definition, EF skills are generalized behavior; they cannot be memorized. Therefore, training across multiple exemplars, settings, and people is always critical. For a helpful list of exemplars to teach for each lesson, see the EF domain of the Skills® curriculum (www.skillsforautism.com; see Chapter 26). Second, task analysis and chaining are particularly useful for EF skills (as we will describe below) because many of them tend to be long and complex. Finally, behavioral skills training (see Chapter 4) deserves special mention because it, too, is highly useful for teaching EF skills.

STRUCTURE OF THE EXECUTIVE FUNCTIONS CURRICULUM

The CARD Executive Functions curriculum is organized into the following domains: 1) inhibition, 2) attention, 3) memory, 4) flexibility, 5) problem solving, 6) planning, and 7) self-management. Appendix K provides an outline of the entire CARD Executive Functions curriculum, including domains, lessons, lesson sections, and activities. In what follows, we provide practical recommendations for how to teach sample skills across all domains.

Inhibition

Traditional definitions of inhibition suggest that it involves constraint of one's impulses and desires. From a behavioral perspective, inhibition likely involves an individual who is highly likely to engage in a particular behavior under a particular circumstance but who engages in a second behavior that prevents that first behavior from occurring. In other words, inhibition, as a behavior, consists of behaving to "stop oneself" from engaging in other behavior that won't be successful. For example, covering one's own mouth prevents the behavior of saying something that will get punished; therefore, covering one's mouth is negatively reinforced because it allows one to avoid punishment.

The ability to prevent oneself from engaging in a behavior is used in many ways in our daily life. For example, it can involve telling oneself not to do something that will be punished (e.g., thinking to oneself, "The teacher asked me to stop calling out in class so much, so I won't call out this time"). It can also involve ignoring distractions or disruptions that might impede one's ability to perform in distracting environments (e.g., telling oneself, "I can't look out the window; I need to look at my worksheet").

Identifying Deficits in Inhibition Skills

When deciding whether to target inhibition with your learners, consider the following examples of children with deficits in inhibition skills:

- Engages in inappropriate behaviors despite negative social, health, or safety effects. For example, during downtime, the learner pulls his eyelashes, eyebrows, and the hair on the side of his head, resulting in bald spots;
- Engages in impulsive, consistent, or perseverative behavior. For example, Jack calls out answers when he is not called on, despite numerous teacher and peer admonishments; and
- Frequently speaks out of context when others are in the middle of a conversation. For example, Sam has appropriate conversational skills but does not use them; instead, he repeats information or phrases inappropriate to the context.

Teaching Inhibition

When teaching inhibition, the goal is not to establish a rote ability to inhibit a particular behavior, given particular instructions or situations. Rather, the goal is to teach the child a generalized ability to inhibit her own behavior when the need arises. Generally speaking, the CARD approach to teaching inhibition progresses through the lessons described below. Keep in mind that more than one lesson can be taught at the same time, and that the progression will need to be customized for each child.

Waiting

Teaching the learner to wait for a preferred item is a good place to start teaching inhibition and is a common lesson in behavioral intervention programs for children with ASD. To teach this skill, start by presenting preferred items or activities and instruct the learner to wait. Initially, only require the learner to wait for a second or two and then provide the reinforcer for waiting appropriately without engaging in challenging behavior. Across trials, increase the duration of the waiting interval until the learner is able to wait for the natural time length required to gain access to an activity in the natural environment across settings and situations. For example, when the learner wants a swing at school, she might have to wait for a duration specified by a school rule, such as counting to 50. Or when the child wants to swim, she might have to wait the length of the car ride to the public pool. Or if the child wants to eat dessert, she might have to wait until everyone at the dinner table has finished eating. Continue to practice waiting in all settings (e.g., home, school, community) as needed to teach the learner to wait across all situations relevant to her life. You will know this skill is mastered once the child can wait for the natural time length associated with new items and activities without prompting.

Simple inhibition instructions

Teach the learner to follow instructions that require a response to be inhibited. For example, say, "Draw a tree but don't use the color brown," "Draw a car with no wheels," "Count to 10 without saying 7," "Sing Twinkle-Twinkle without saying the word star." Teach many examples until the learner can respond correctly to new examples without prompting or errors across multiple settings and people. The reason for starting with simple, non-functional examples such as those described above is to begin to build success with instructions that are not likely to evoke challenging behavior or negative emotional responding from the learner. Move on to the inhibition of socially relevant responses as soon as the learner demonstrates an increased capacity to inhibit simple behaviors.

Role-play inhibition of highly probable responses

Present practice/role-play situations wherein a response is highly probable and in which the child needs to learn to inhibit it. Choose probable behaviors in which the learner engages in real-life home, school, and community settings. For example, the learner might wake up the sleeping dog all day long at home, call out answers in the classroom, and pick his nose in the community. Have the child practice not engaging in the probable behavior during role-play. Initially, keep the inhibition duration short, and systematically extend it to levels that would be expected of same-age peers. Role-play across many examples and people and in various settings.

Extend to the natural environment

Once the learner can inhibit a response during practice/role-play, begin to contrive or capture opportunities for the learner to practice inhibition of a probable response in the natural environment. To contrive a situation, present incidental situations in the natural environment where a previous response has been reinforced, and require the learner to inhibit the response. Initially, you may need to keep the inhibition duration short and systematically extend it until the learner is practicing inhibition of the response either for a time length natural to the situation (e.g., inhibiting making sounds until class time ends) or even altogether. That is, in some situations, it is never appropriate to engage in a behavior. For example, some parents will never be okay with their child using foul language. This skill is considered mastered once the learner can inhibit responses outside therapy in new real-life natural settings for the natural time length required and without prompting or errors.

Inhibition rules

For children who are able to follow rules, specific rules about when to inhibit behaviors can be taught. For instance, the learner can be given rules as to when and with whom it is okay to engage in a probable response. For example, when around adults, swear words need to be inhibited, but it's okay to use some of the milder versions (e.g., saying "damn") when hanging out with friends. Or it's okay to pass gas at home in the presence of Mom and Dad, but it's never okay to do so in the presence of other people or outside of the home. To teach this advanced repertoire, start by giving a rule, then use practice/role-play, and then capture and contrive situations for the child to apply what he has learned to the natural environment. Teach many examples in different settings and with various people, and consider this skill mastered once the learner is able to follow novel inhibition rules without prompting or errors.

Attention

From a traditional standpoint, attention refers to how individuals process information and involves the ability to concentrate selectively on important aspects of the environment while ignoring others. From a behavioral perspective, attention is not a construct but, rather, *attending*, *per se*, is a behavior just like any other. B. F. Skinner noted that attending behavior is largely shaped by one's learning history; for example, if a geologist and a biologist take a walk together in the woods, they will quite literally notice very different things in that same environment (Skinner, 1974).

The ability to attend to important stimuli and tune out unimportant ones at the right times and for extended periods is critical in daily life. For example, we notice when important things are happening around us, such as when there is a loud noise, the classroom teacher speaks, or someone yells, "Ouch!" On the other hand, we don't care or pay much attention when minor things happen, such as when a student sharpens his pencil in the back of the classroom or when an irrelevant conversation occurs in the background. We also pay attention to the important details when we read or listen to instructions or stories, and we can identify the main characters and main ideas but might not necessarily recall the details of what someone was wearing (as this is not important information). We know what to do when multiple important stimuli present themselves to us at once. We can shift our attention between them and hold our attention to the important aspects of each. For example, when driving a car, we attend to the traffic lights and cars around us at the same time (and we attend to the color of the traffic lights but *not* to the color of the cars). When having a conversation, we attend to the conversation and shift our attention if an important announcement occurs over a loudspeaker and then shift attention back to the conversation. We can also sustain our attention for lengthy periods of time when necessary (e.g., listening to a long lecture, working on an extensive task, etc.). For many children with ASD, these attending skills have never been learned and will not be acquired if they are not directly taught.

Identifying Attention Deficits

The following are examples of deficits in attending skills and the corresponding lessons in the Skills® curriculum that address them:

- Easily distracted when more than one activity or task is presented, if multiple stimuli are presented, or if an interruption occurs during the current task or activity. Target skill areas to address (you'll read about these soon): Divided Attention, Disengagement, Shifting Attention, and Determining Saliency;
- Difficulty maintaining attention to one task or activity for more than a few minutes. Target skill area to address: Sustained Attention;
- Lack of attention or response to typical social cues unless specifically called upon, especially when engaged in a preferred activity. Target skill areas to address: Orienting, Disengagement, Shifting Attention, and Determining Saliency; and
- Difficulty relaying information to others. Target skill areas to address: Paraphrasing, Summarizing, and Determining Saliency.

Teaching Attention Skills

The first step to improving the learner's attention skills is to identify the area(s) of attention that need to be addressed. Assess each of the target areas outlined below with the learner, and then use the guidelines to teach those that are needed.

Orienting

Typically developing children orient to the presentation of objects, people, environmental sounds, and voices before the age of 1 year, yet this skill is lacking in many children with ASD. To teach orienting to salient stimuli, start by making sure the environment is sterile and that the learner is not already engaging with something. Then present visual and/or auditory stimuli within and outside of the learner's field of vision to determine if the learner orients. Make sure to present both non-social (e.g., environmental sounds and salient objects, such as a train sound or an item falling off a table) and social stimuli (e.g., a person yelling, "Ouch!"). Continue to train orienting until the learner is able to respond to novel stimuli without prompting or errors. Beware of teaching the learner to respond to unimportant or non-salient stimuli. The goal is not to teach the learner to be easily distracted, so make sure that the orienting stimuli are those to which a typically developing, same-age peer would attend.

Disengagement

During infancy, typically developing children are able to disengage from one visual stimulus when another is presented, yet this is often not observed in children with ASD. If the child with whom you are working is able to orient to salient stimuli (described above), assess whether he is able to disengage from an object/activity/conversation/thought in order to orient to another stimulus. Unlike when teaching orienting, the environment when teaching disengagement should not be sterile. That is, the learner should be engaged in an activity when the orienting stimuli are presented. Make the task of disengagement easy, and set the learner up for success by initially requiring him to disengage from lesser preferred activities. As the learner is successful over time, move toward teaching him to disengage from more preferred activities in order to orient to salient stimuli. Before considering this skill mastered, be sure the learner is able to disengage from most highly preferred stimuli without prompting. As before, make sure orienting stimuli are salient and include auditory and/or visual non-social and social stimuli.

Sustained attention

Assess how long the learner is able to remain attentive to various types of tasks relevant to her daily life, including sustaining attention to visual stimuli, paper/pencil tasks, and daily living tasks/chores. If the learner is unable to sustain her attention to activities for age-appropriate lengths of time, begin to reinforce attending for lengthier periods of time until the learner is able to attend for an age-appropriate duration. Between 4 and 5 years of age, typically developing children can engage in a task for 10 to 12 minutes; at 5 years and up, children are better able to attend to a task until it is complete; and between 5 and 8 years of age, children are able to attend to a homework assignment for 20 minutes. When working with younger children, refer to the learner's same-age peers for age-appropriate attending lengths.

As you begin to increase the length of sustained attention, also begin to bring in distractions. Require the learner to continue attending even though distractions are present. Children between 6 and 7 years of age are able to remain on task in the presence of minor distractions. Start with minor distractions, and then make them more salient over time. It's perfectly fine for the learner to disengage from the sustained attention task to orient to the distracting stimulus to a small degree (glancing in its direction or asking a quick question such as, "Are you okay?" if someone trips in his field of vision) and then disengage from the distractor and re-engage in the sustained attention task. Continue to train sustained attention until the learner is able to sustain attention to new tasks without direct teaching. Make sure sustained attention tasks are relevant to the learner's real life and avoid teaching the learner to sustain attention to non-functional tasks.

Shifting attention

Once the learner is able to orient and disengage from stimuli, it's time to start working on teaching the learner to engage in multiple shifts of her attention between stimuli. The learner's ability to shift her attention among different sources of information, tasks, and various components of a single task is of critical importance in making sense of the mass of information presented in academic and social environments. Being able to rapidly make multiple shifts of attention between different sources of information and tasks will help to improve the learner's ability to notice, understand, and respond to multiple cues and information, thereby improving her adaptive, academic, and social functioning. For example, in an academic setting, the learner might be required to copy information from a whiteboard to a sheet of paper by making multiple shifts of attention between the whiteboard and the paper.

When teaching the learner to shift attention, make sure the learner practices across a variety of stimuli, including visual and/or auditory, nonsocial and social stimuli, and tasks. You can start by requiring the learner to shift attention simply by glancing or engaging in a vocal response (e.g., comment/question) in relation to the presentation of visual (e.g., objects, people, etc.) and/or auditory (e.g., an alarm clock, dog barking, etc.) stimuli. This approach was shown to produce generalization across multiple untrained examples in a recent study (Persicke et al., 2013). You should initially include simple social stimuli (e.g., a person sneezing or clapping) and then later include more sophisticated social shifts of attention. For example, while having a conversation, the learner might have to shift attention multiple times to salient competing stimuli but be able to shift back to the conversation each time. Let's also not forget that the child needs to learn to shift attention during and between tasks. For example, while engaged in making her bed, there might be multiple shifts of attention to other stimuli, but the learner always ultimately shifts back to making her bed until the task is complete. In other cases, attention shifts can be between tasks. For example, the learner might start an arts-and-crafts project involving making a bird, with the first step being to paint the bird. Then, while waiting for the paint to dry, she might shift her attention to a second arts-and-crafts project involving making a ladybug. Once the child paints the body of the ladybug and the bird is dry, the child might shift her attention back to the bird project by gluing feathers, an eyeball, and a beak to it before moving back to the ladybug project and finishing it off with a head, eyes, and antennae. These are just some examples of the infinite stimulus shifts you can teach the learner; be creative when coming up with ideas, but remember that the goal is not for the child to learn rote memorization of specific attention shifts but, rather, to develop a generalized operant ability to shift among any stimuli. Once the learner is able to do this with novel stimuli relevant to her daily life without errors or prompting, consider this skill mastered.

Divided attention

Divided attention is synonymous with multi-tasking. When teaching this skill, the objective is to improve the learner's ability to attend to two or more things at the same time. For example, to proofread this chapter, it was necessary to attend to the meaning of sentences while also noticing grammatical errors, misspelled words, and formatting. This is not an easy thing to do, but being able to attend to multiple things at once will improve the learner's ability to notice and respond to multiple cues in his environment, thereby improving his adaptive, academic, and social functioning.

To teach this skill, start by presenting two stimuli at once and asking the learner to recall what was presented. For example, present a sound of a dog barking while also holding up a picture of a fire truck. Then ask the learner to identify what he saw and heard. No time delay is necessary, as this is not a memory task. Rather, it's meant to teach the learner to attend to more than one thing simultaneously. As you present stimuli simultaneously, make sure to touch upon the various senses by presenting stimuli or tasks that require the learner to see, hear, feel, smell, and/or a combination of these. Once the learner can notice two things simultaneously, begin tasks that require him to attend to two or more things. For example, the learner should be able to hold a conversation while also exhibiting pedestrian safety or talk on the phone while writing directions down. These are examples of practical and functional tasks you can present that the learner actually has to carry out in his everyday life. However, for the sake of practice and exposure to multiple examples and teaching opportunities, you can also do less practical examples, such as having the learner rehearse spelling words while cleaning his room. Once the learner is able to do this with novel stimuli relevant to his daily life without errors or prompting, consider this skill mastered.

Determining saliency

The process of identifying and thinking about which information is most salient or important is referred to as "determining saliency." Children with a strong ability to determine saliency are better able to filter out distractions and focus on the most important, relevant, or necessary concepts and ideas from the mass of information presented in social and academic situations. Successful social, academic, and vocational functioning requires us to attend to the most relevant, salient stimuli at any given moment and not to attend to the hundreds of others that are present. In this section, we will focus on how you can teach the learner to identify saliency. The purpose is to teach the learner to focus on the most important information delivered during class, read in a book, heard in a conversation, or observed in social situations.

To teach a learner to determine saliency, present many different types of stimuli and ask the learner to identify saliency. Present visual and/or auditory stimuli (e.g., objects, pictures, sounds, video clips, oral stories, and picture books), and ask the learner to identify:

- the biggest thing;
- the thing in the center and/or front;
- the item that there is a lot of or the item that she sees most;
- the thing that is most noticeable, stands out the most, or seems most important;
- the item that keeps changing or the one that stays the same;
- the loudest sound or thing said the loudest;
- the thing said the most;
- the thing that is interesting, different, unusual, missing, or new; and
- the main character and main idea.

Social saliency is another target for the learner. Here, you might ask the child to identify the most important person in class (the teacher), leader of a group, summary, purpose, or most important piece of a social interaction. For example, you might say, "You went to math class, you had lunch, and Johnny fell off the swing and broke his arm. Which one is the most important?" and so on. Don't forget textual saliency. Here, the child will learn to identify saliency while reading text, such as which words or categories are repeated the most in sentences, the main character, and the main idea of a paragraph, passage, or story she has read.

When teaching the learner to determine saliency, teach her to recognize saliency across many different examples until she is able to do so with new examples without prompting or errors. Then work on applying her ability to recognize salient stimuli to her everyday interactions by contriving and capturing opportunities for the child to exhibit her ability to detect and respond appropriately to salient stimuli. For example, she should be able to recognize which person in a given social situation is most important to obey (the adult, not an older child) and do so appropriately. Or when out in the community, the learner should note that it is more important to evacuate the building when a fire alarm goes off than to finish a conversation with a peer or adult.

Paraphrasing and summarizing

Between 6 and 7 years of age, typically developing children are able to identify and describe the beginning, middle, and end of a story (summarizing), and between 7 and 8 years of age, they are able to paraphrase oral information. Children with ASD, however, often have difficulties doing so. Both paraphrasing and summarizing involve the ability to express another's idea in one's own words; however, paraphrasing may or may not shorten the length of a passage, while summarizing presents only the most essential points of the original passage in a more concise format.

Being able to paraphrase is especially helpful for everyday living tasks in the child's life and school activities, such as delivering oral messages, writing down oral messages (such as phone messages), answering open-ended questions in school, and explaining or discussing something read in a book. Likewise, being able to summarize is especially helpful for everyday living tasks in the child's life and school activities, such as writing notes, making lists, writing book reports, and taking phone messages.

When teaching the learner to paraphrase and summarize, teach the learner to respond not only to oral information but also to written information. Likewise, teach the learner to paraphrase and summarize vocally (in conversation and when giving oral reports or recounts of information) and through written expression (for book reports and writing notes). After the learner has listened to a conversation or oral story or read a book, teach paraphrasing by instructing the learner to describe what was just heard or read in a different way using his own words. For example, after hearing, "There was a huge dog," the learner could say, "There was a massive dog." The learner can do this vocally and/or through written expression. Teach summarizing by instructing the learner to identify what was most important or the main idea, as well as to identify what happened at the beginning, middle, and end of what was heard, and then ask the learner to repeat the information (either vocally or by writing) in a shorter way. When the learner is reading, teach her to highlight or underline important points that will be useful for summarizing. When teaching both of these skill sets, provide the learner with many examples until she is able to respond correctly to new stimuli without direct training. Also, contrive and capture opportunities for the learner to practice the skills in everyday life. For example, in school, the learner might need to retell a story that she read or write a book report using paraphrasing or summarizing. In social situations, the learner might need to recount a conversation or an overheard story. These are just some of the many possible examples that can be taught. Make sure the learner is able to exhibit skills across various settings, people, and situations before considering this skill mastered. Focus on teaching the concept, and avoid presenting the same item over and over again to the learner.

Flexibility

Traditional descriptions of flexibility include thinking about multiple concepts simultaneously, the ability to think flexibly and shift approaches, adjusting to the unexpected, and adapting to change. Flexibility is often contrasted to rigidity, which involves an insistence on doing things the same way from one time to another, despite changes that may have occurred in the environment. Flexibility is difficult to define from a behavioral perspective, but it likely involves variability in one's ongoing behavior, probably due to sensitivity to changes in one's ongoing environment. That is, as one's environment changes, one's behavior changes accordingly. A person who is described as flexible does things differently on different occasions as the environment changes and as the need arises to do things differently.

Being able to change one's behavior in order to adjust to ongoing changes in the environment is critical to success in many aspects of life. Typically developing children as young as 3 years old become aware of rules, and they report changes in rules. Rules change all the time at home, in school, and in social interactions, requiring individuals to adapt their normal responses to new conditions. For example, when playing "house" with a peer, the rules can change in the moment as to who is to play the role of "mommy" versus "baby," or when driving in the car with Mom, new routes might need to be taken when there is a roadblock or car accident. For some children with autism, change in the environment, *per se*, appears to be aversive, thereby leading them to resist change or even to engage in challenging behavior to escape or avoid change. Thus, flexibility can be an especially critical focus in treatment for children with ASD.

Identifying Inflexibility

The following are examples of flexibility deficits you may want to consider when evaluating whether your learner could benefit from flexibility training:

- Undue emotional reactions and resistance to changes in routine or schedule;
- Insistence on using specific methods for completing tasks and persistence using those methods even when unsuccessful (i.e., lack of problem-solving skills);
- Insistence on keeping items in specific locations and emotional reactions to moving them; and
- Difficulty adjusting to new people, environments, or rules, especially rules that conflict with previously known rules.

Teaching Flexibility

Variability, as a property of behavior, can be reinforced. Little research has evaluated whether children with ASD can be made more flexible overall, but CARD clinicians have been teaching flexibility to children with ASD for years. As with all higher order programming, the goal is not to teach the learner rote instances of flexibility to specific situations but, rather, to teach the learner to behave flexibly in new situations without training. In doing so, keep in mind that flexibility is closely related to inhibition, as the flexible child is often required to inhibit a prepotent response in order to allow change to occur. Thus, it might be helpful to work on both flexibility and inhibition at the same time. See the section on Inhibition above for some ideas. Likewise, being flexible can be very stressful for children with ASD, so see also the Emotional Self-Control excerpt of the Self-Management section of this chapter below.

In order to teach flexibility, the first step is to identify situations and events in which the learner exhibits inflexibility and target them. Children with ASD may be inflexible about many things, including non-social stimuli (e.g., wearing sandals without socks, performing routines out of order), social stimuli (e.g., play sequences, rules in games), language (e.g., always using the same phrases), and thoughts (e.g., thinking in black and white, with no "gray areas"). Make sure to cover everything that is relevant in your programming of flexible behavior. The general teaching progression is described below.

Hypothetical situations

If the learner has conversational skills, you can start by describing a hypothetical situation to the learner wherein she has a preferred response or where a previous response has been reinforced and then instructing the learner to identify an alternative way to respond. The alternative behavior will include whatever responses are associated with going along with the change in the environment. For example, if the learner is playing a game with peers and they change the rules, the alternative response would be changing her play behavior in accordance with the new rules. In some cases, the only alternative response is acceptance of the change as exhibited by absence of challenging behavior when the change occurs. In either case, it might be helpful to teach the learner to engage in alternative behaviors of the "coping" type, such as taking deep breaths, counting to 10, or thinking about something else. To learn more about teaching coping strategies, see the Self-Management section of this chapter. It is unlikely that teaching the learner to talk through how she *should* respond merely in hypothetical situations will have a significant effect on how she *will* respond to those actual situations in the future, but it likely provides a verbal foundation for the lessons that follow.

Role-play situations

Using role-play, have the learner practice an alternative response to the inflexibility stimulus. Start by presenting a small magnitude of the inflexibility stimulus. As the learner is able to tolerate and adjust his behavior to the inflexibility stimulus, gradually increase the magnitude of it. For example, if the learner has an issue with the rug being wrinkled, start by only wrinkling the edge of the rug. Once the learner is able to tolerate that without engaging in challenging behavior, begin to wrinkle it more. Another way to increase the magnitude of the inflexibility stimulus is to increase the duration of its presence. For example, if the learner dislikes it when you wear your hair in a ponytail, slowly increase the duration of time during which you are wearing a ponytail until eventually it can be done indefinitely. In addition to increasing the magnitude of the inflexibility stimulus, begin to increase the complexity of it. For example, the learner might be required to adjust her behavior eventually from one rule change during play (switching from using real food while playing "restaurant" to using blocks to represent food) to multiple rule shifts (switching items to represent food, switching who gets to be the chef versus the customer, switching the name of the restaurant, and so on).

Extend to the natural environment

Contrive and capture moments in natural environment settings (e.g., home, community, school) wherein the learner would normally engage in a particular response, and prompt the learner to adjust his behavior to various inflexibility stimuli. Reinforce instances when the learner exhibits flexibility, and fade prompts. Continue to present new situations incidentally in the natural environment until the learner is able to behave flexibly by engaging in a response that is an alternative to her normal response to any new situation presented across various settings and people.

Flexibility rules

For children who are able to follow rules, specific rules about behaving flexibly can be taught. For example, the following rule might be given to a learner who engages in challenging behavior whenever he makes a mistake: "Everyone makes mistakes; it just means that you are learning to do something that is difficult, and that makes you smarter. When you make a mistake, you can just fix it and move on." Keep the rules positive. Do not use rules that threaten punishment, or you risk increasing the learner's anxiety in that situation. To teach this advanced repertoire, start by giving a rule. Then use practice/role-play, and capture and contrive situations for the learner to apply what he has learned to the natural environment. Teach many examples in different settings and with various people, and consider this skill mastered once the learner is able to follow novel flexibility rules without prompting or errors.

When children with ASD exhibit behavioral rigidity, they can become highly upset during the process of changing their behavior to adjust to the presence of inflexibility stimuli. Above, we mentioned the idea of starting with a smaller magnitude of the inflexibility stimuli. In addition to this, you might also need to use some of the following strategies:

- Make flexibility seem fun or silly (e.g., backwards day, wacky Wednesday, etc.).
- Start with inflexibility stimuli that are not as emotionally charged, e.g., ask, "What do you think this could be?" of an ambiguous picture; present a nonsense word and ask, "What do you think this could mean?"; when playing with blocks, build new combinations of block structures each turn.
- Present the inflexibility stimuli to a third person, and have the learner identify what that person could do, or have the learner tolerate a third person being flexible to the situation.
- Present overly silly or nonsense flexibility stimuli (e.g., ask, "What color is the sky?" and have the learner tolerate the answer, "Green").
- Present the stimuli in a game format (e.g., if the child is inflexible about making mistakes, see who can make the most mistakes).
- Richly reinforce any spontaneous instances of variable responding!
- Have fun; be flexible yourself!

Memory

The behavior of remembering or recalling information is necessary in many aspects of everyday life and is important because it allows the learner to engage in behavior in the present with respect to stimuli that are currently absent. As the learner becomes better at remembering, she is able to imitate complex behavioral chains, recall details about past events, and behave in relation to covert behavior, such as visualizing, rehearsing, and thinking; for example, "Yesterday, my mom let me play a video game after I did my chores, so maybe she'll let me do that again today." In typical development, children as young as 2 years old can recall a string of three unrelated words, and by the age of 8, many typically developing children can recall a string of six unrelated digits.

Identifying Memory Deficits

The following are examples of challenging situations that traditionally might be labeled memory deficits. Consider these when evaluating whether your learners might benefit from learning memory skills:

- When more than one instruction is given or multiple materials are required to complete a task, the learner will only remember one instruction or will only get some of the necessary materials, even when told what to do immediately prior to beginning the task.

- The learner has difficulty locating familiar items that are always in the same place.
- The learner has difficulty recalling what occurred at an earlier time, such as activities engaged in at school and assignments to be completed at home.
- The learner frequently loses or misplaces personal items.
- The learner has difficulty establishing and using strategies to help remember things without others prompting him to do so.

Teaching Memory

When teaching children with ASD to recall information, we want to teach the generalized ability, not rote responses to particular tasks. To teach this skill, start with small, easy tasks, and teach the learner recall strategies, such as rehearsal and visualizing. At first, the learner will use vocal rehearsal overtly, but gradually prompt her to emit them covertly over time as she demonstrates success with overt recall strategies (Baltruschat et al., 2011). Use positive reinforcement for correct responding, and teach across many tasks, prompting the learner to engage in covert rehearsal if needed until generalization to untrained tasks occurs. Below are some examples of small, easy tasks for the learner to complete when you begin teaching memory. Ask the learner to:

- identify an object seen recently;
- repeat/identify/recreate a random string of words, numbers, letters, names of sounds heard or seen, forward or backward;
- identify the third and fifth (vary these numbers) thing heard or seen;
- identify how many times an action occurred or an item was presented;
- imitate sequences of behavior(s) forward or backward;
- answer questions about items seen (what was seen, spatial locations of items, etc.);
- identify what is missing, new, or different/changed;
- identify under which cup an item was placed;
- put object(s) back in the spatial location(s) seen;
- recreate a recently viewed picture or block structure; and
- recall items heard/seen in forward or backward order by size or other attribute.

In addition to teaching the learner to recall information using small, easy tasks, it's extremely important to teach the learner application of memory skills using real-life examples. Below are just a few of the many tasks that you could teach:

- Follow multiple-step instructions.
- Follow instructions delivered by a parent in the morning about what is to be done at school.

- Follow in-class teacher instructions for doing homework while at home.
- Recall location of seat or cubby in classroom.
- Put school supplies back in the locations where they belong in the classroom.
- Follow instructions after a delay.
- Remember to bring items home from school or to a friend's house.
- Recall an earlier conversation to relay information.
- Tell parents what happened at school (e.g., what, who, when, where, main events, etc.).
- Answer questions about a movie, conversation, oral story, or event.
- Answer comprehension questions after reading or listening to a story.

With all of the tasks above, the general teaching progression is as follows:

1. Present simple stimulus to the learner with no time delay between presentation and recall instruction.
2. Increase difficulty slowly by adding more stimuli to recall and by gradually increasing a time delay between presentation of stimuli and recall instruction.
3. Stop when the learner can recall at levels of same-age typically developing peers with untrained tasks that are relevant to the learner's daily life. Beware of having unrealistic expectations, and observe same-age peers to identify what is appropriate.

Commonly used memory strategies

Here are some common **verbal** memory skills to consider teaching:

- Rehearsal (e.g., saying something over and over to oneself);
- Verbal association with another item, word, or symbol;
- Mnemonic acronyms (e.g., "**E**very **G**ood **B**oy **D**oes **F**ine" to remember the notes on musical notation);
- Verbally grouping or "chunking" information by category;
- Verbally grouping information by shared location (e.g., all farm animals); and
- Making a song or story out of the information.

In many cases, it is completely acceptable to rely on visual, tactile, or auditory cues to remember information. In these cases, teach your learners to create their own cues. Here are some socially appropriate cues that you should consider teaching your learners to create:

- Making a list;
- Visualizing words or pictures;
- Making note cards for class presentations;
- Writing a note on one's hand;

- Putting a related object in a prominent place to jog one's memory;
- Texting or emailing oneself;
- Leaving oneself a voice mail or voice recording; and
- Setting an alarm or timer or an appointment on the calendar of a phone or tablet.

Consider the following phases when teaching learners to use strategies such as those listed above:

1. Explain and/or demonstrate the strategy to be used, and prompt the learner to use it.
2. Explain the rules for appropriate times and contexts to use the strategy.
3. Present something that needs to be remembered, and ask the learner what she can do to remember it; suggest a strategy, if needed. Prompt the learner to use the strategy.
4. Contrive and capture opportunities where the learner needs to remember information in her daily life. She should identify the appropriate strategy and implement it on her own.

As strategies approach mastery in the natural environment, only provide leading question prompts to help the learner identify what needs to be done. The skill is mastered when the learner uses various strategies to remember various things without prompting or feedback.

Self-Management and Related Skills

Self-management involves observing and responding to one's own behavior by intentionally manipulating one's own environment in order to bring about a change in behavior. This can involve management of covert behaviors, such as emotions (e.g., anger, fear) and thoughts (e.g., negative self-talk), as well as overt behaviors, such as yelling at others, nail biting, eating poorly, and so on. When one tracks one's covert and overt behaviors and sets contingencies for the behavior in an effort to effectively change the behavior in a desired direction, one is engaging in self-management (Cooper, Heron, & Heward, 2007). Self-management is equally applicable to typically developing adults (e.g., improving nutrition, increasing exercise) as it is to children with ASD (e.g., staying on task, decreasing outbursts). Being able to engage in self-management is critical for success in the school, vocational, and social environments, yet many children with ASD may not develop this advanced repertoire if we do not teach it to them.

Identifying Deficits in Self-Management Skills

Below are examples of challenges that are often related to deficits in self-management skills. Each involves a lack of awareness of one's own body and behavior and/or a lack of skills needed to act upon such an awareness:

- Frequently invades others' "personal space" by standing too close and touching others;
- Is unaware of own body appearance (e.g., food on face, pants unzipped, etc.);
- Has emotional overreactions to common situations; and
- Has contextually inappropriate emotional reactions (e.g., laughing at a sad story).

Teaching Self-Management

The following five steps are useful for teaching self-management:

1. Identifying one's own target behavior,
2. Self-monitoring,
3. Self-evaluation,
4. Self-reinforcement, and
5. Independent self-management.

We discuss each of these five steps briefly and then discuss how to enhance your self-management teaching programs by addressing self-awareness and emotional self-control.

1. **Identifying the target behavior.** Begin by talking with the learner and identifying the target behavior with her. Obviously, a socially relevant target behavior should be selected and the learner herself and the learner's parents should be involved in the selection. When identifying the behavior, make sure to provide a clear definition, including examples and non-examples of it.
2. **Self-monitoring.** Next, teach the learner to observe and record her own target behavior. This can be done by making tallies on a piece of paper, keeping a log/diary, or using a golf counter to record instances. Interestingly, some children are completely unaware that they engage in particular behaviors until they learn to observe and identify instances of them. Initially, provide frequent prompting and reinforcement for accurate observation and recording. Occasionally, merely teaching a child to monitor and record her own stereotypy (and providing reinforcement for accurate recording) results in a decrease in the behavior.
3. **Self-evaluation.** In this stage of self-management, the learner is provided a goal for her target behavior. You should involve the learner in determining an appropriate goal if she has the verbal abilities to set goals. After each period during which the learner is expected to record her own behavior, review the data with her and use prompting, reinforcement, and prompt-fading to teach her to determine whether she met her goal for that period. If the goal was met, provide reinforcement. If not, withhold reinforcement.

At this stage of self-management, the learner is being expected to engage in a lower rate of a behavior than she typically would; that is, the learner is learning to inhibit her own behaviors. If the learner is having difficulty during this stage, consider teaching specific inhibition skills relevant to the target behavior. (See the Inhibition section above.) Likewise, if the behavior that you are expecting the learner to manage involves emotional responding, consider teaching emotional self-control skills, as described later in this chapter.

4. **Self-reinforcement.** Once the learner is engaging in accurate self-monitoring and self-evaluation, you may want to teach her to engage in self-reinforcement. This involves the learner retrieving a reinforcer – or asking a caregiver for one – when the goal is met. As with all other steps, use prompting, reinforcement, and prompt-fading to teach this step to mastery.

5. **Independent self-management.** Once the learner has had ample experience engaging in self-management programs under your supervision and is able to engage in accurate self-monitoring, self-evaluation, and self-reinforcement, encourage the learner to begin to set up her own self-management programs. Start by asking her which personal goals she would like to meet. You can use leading questions to guide the learner to come to some ideas, such as, "Is there anything you wish you could be better at or do less?" or "Is there anything you'd like to change about yourself?" or "Is there anything that frustrates you at school?" and then "Let's figure out what you can do to make that work better."

Expanding self-awareness

Many children with ASD can be taught the first and second steps described above in the process of decreasing one or two particular behaviors, but this does not establish a larger, more general repertoire of self-awareness. Ultimately, for children to be able to expand and apply their self-management skills more broadly, they will need to become more self-aware overall. What this means behaviorally is that they observe their own behavior generally (not one or two particular topographies), the settings in which their behaviors occur, and the results that are produced. To establish this ability as a generalized repertoire, you will need to teach multiple examples of self-observation across many behaviors and contexts. Here are some practical examples to consider:

- Ask the learner to identify the presence and degree of a behavior in herself (e.g., Do you check your work for mistakes? Is your handwriting neat? Do you talk loudly?).

- Ask the learner to identify her strengths and weaknesses (e.g., What are some things you are good at? What are some things you know about? What is something you are not so great at? What is something you need to learn? How can you use the things you are good at to help yourself be more successful?).
- Ask the learner to identify her likes and dislikes (e.g., What do you like to do? What do you not like to do? What could you do to make it more fun?).
- Ask the learner to describe himself.

One thing that is very important to consider is that self-evaluative statements can have long-lasting and far-reaching effects on a person's quality of life, far beyond what you might expect when teaching them. For example, negative self-statements, as behavior, are clearly functionally related to depression and anxiety. Keep in mind that, by setting up contingencies for reinforcement in ABA programs – and the learner cannot possibly succeed every time – we are frequently showing the learner when his behavior did not meet the contingency. It is a short verbal distance from a learner saying something along the lines of, "I didn't do what I needed to do," to "I did bad," to "I am bad." Moreover, it is common to see highly verbal children with ASD make overly negative self-statements. Given that, when you teach self-awareness and self-evaluation, it is critical that you do not make the experience aversive and that you spend an equal amount of time teaching the learner to notice what he does well. Do not blindly reinforce positive statements. Rather, take the time to prompt and reinforce *accurate* positive self-statements that refer to what the learner truly does well. The point of teaching self-awareness is to establish an accurate and dispassionate repertoire of "noticing oneself," not to make the child overly self-critical or unrealistically self-praising.

Emotional self-control

Emotional self-control involves the ability to respond to one's own intense emotions (which are covert behaviors) by displaying overt behaviors that will help one achieve what one wants, as opposed to engaging in an overt emotional overreaction, thereby producing a negative outcome. In other words, emotional self-control refers to a special repertoire of self-management that is used directly for managing one's own emotional reactions in life. Emotional overreactions are commonly lumped into the category of challenging behavior because they are often accompanied by overt destructive behavior, such as screaming, tantrums, aggression, and self-injury. It is important to note, however, that having an intense emotion (covert event) is not the same thing as engaging in an intense overt behavior. People can be sad (covert) and smile simultaneously (overt), and they can be angry (covert) but walk away instead of hitting (overt). Unfortunately, society has taught us that our emotions often directly cause our overt actions, and children with ASD often believe this. This idea is not useful if one actually wants to behave more effectively. Teaching children with ASD emotional self-control skills does not involve teaching them to suppress their emotions or to have different emotions. It consists of teaching them skills to use *while* feeling negative emotions to help them engage in overt behaviors that will be more effective. Here are some skills targets we have found useful for this process:

- **Function-based alternative behaviors, especially communication.** Refer to Chapter 5 on challenging behavior. This step is somewhat obvious and should be a standard part of treatment for any child with ASD who displays challenging behaviors.
- **Coping strategies.** In real life, a child's function-based alternative behavior will often simply not be reinforced; e.g., the learner cannot have the thing she asks for because it belongs to someone else, etc. Coping strategies can be useful backups. At first blush, coping strategies might seem silly, but just consider what you do when you are really upset and it is impossible for you to get what you want – you probably do something else that makes you feel better. A short list of socially appropriate coping strategies includes:
  - Positive statements. Teach the learner to express what he *can* do or have; for example, "This is hard for me, so if I start to feel upset, I can ask for help"; "I don't get to do what I want this time, but it will be my turn next time."
  - Venting. Learners can be taught to initiate a socially appropriate conversation about the event or circumstance that is making them unhappy.
  - Burning off steam. Teach the learner to engage in a physical activity for a short period when he feels upset.
  - Deep and slow breathing. Teach the learner to count to 10 while taking 10 deep, slow breaths.
- **Identifying appropriate levels of emotional reactions to common situations.** Between 6 and 8 years of age, typically developing children learn to demonstrate a similar level of emotion as peers without downplaying or overdramatizing situations. You can start to teach the learner this by teaching him the continuum of emotions (i.e., from happy, to surprised, to sad/annoyed/slightly angry, to very angry). Visual supports can be useful for this (e.g., emotions charts using a thermometer or a strip of faces, going from full smiley face to full angry face, as depicted in the top panel of Figure 18.1). Role-playing each level of emotional reaction with the learner can be useful in combination.
- **Identifying the severity of various types of problems.** Teaching children with ASD to rank their problems in terms of severity can

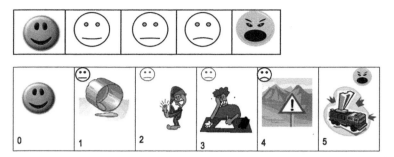

FIGURE 18.1   Visual supports for teaching learners to identify the continuum of emotional responses that are reasonable for common situations. The top panel is used to teach the range of emotions from happy to angry, and the bottom panel is used to teach the range of problems, from no problem to severe emergency. *Reprinted from Skills® with permission from the Center for Autism and Related Disorders.*

help them understand the scale of their problems. For example, the child might learn to rank problems from "0" (no problem) to "5" (emergency/severe problem). A problem ranked as "0" would be something negligible, such as spilling milk. An emergency/severe problem would be something that requires urgent attention, such as a broken leg. Visual supports can be useful here, as well. (See bottom panel of Figure 18.1.) The next step is then to teach the learner to identify which emotion goes with problems of various sizes. To help with this, you can cut out the emotion faces and have the learner match the appropriate face with the appropriate size of the problem. As always with these higher order skills, we are not trying to teach the child to memorize particular responses; we are trying to teach an overall repertoire of talking and thinking about the topic. Therefore, do not get hung up on whether the learner matches exactly the "right" emotional level for every single example (as if that even existed); the goal is to get the learner's responses into a reasonable range that is more likely to be socially successful.

- Don't forget to practice all of these skills across multiple exemplars in the natural environment. Consider the skill mastered when you see generalization to untrained and uncontrived examples.

Problem Solving

Problem solving is a complex and confusing topic, but B. F. Skinner (1974) provided a simple, practical foundation from which to begin treating problem solving as a skill that can be taught. Skinner described problem solving as a situation where a person desires an outcome that he can only attain if he has an appropriate behavior that would bring it about.

This situation is the "problem," and the unknown behavior that would bring about the desired outcome is the "solution." Problem solving, as a skill, includes all of the things the person will now do to help himself figure out the solution. In other words, merely doing the right behavior is not problem solving. If it were, then problem solving would not be needed. Problem solving is a complex repertoire of behaviors that help an individual identify the correct behavior that then solves the problem. A broken toy is a simple example. If a child picks up a preferred toy and begins manipulating it but it does not work, then she is faced with a problem: The toy functioning properly would be a reinforcer, if only she could identify the behavior needed to repair the toy. Problem-solving skills would include all of the different behaviors she would engage in to fix the toy (e.g., checking the batteries, checking for missing parts, talking to herself about potential solutions, asking an adult for help, etc.).

Problem solving is an essential life skill because children face all manner of problems in their daily lives. Problems include non-social problems, such as a book on a top shelf, a difficult lid, a locked door, a broken toy, a toy without batteries, an item too heavy to lift, and so on. Children will also face many social problems, such as a peer failing to share toys, a peer being given something the child wants, a disagreement, and many more. Social problem solving often requires the problem solver to put herself in the shoes of another person to see the problem from that person's perspective and explore why the issue became a problem (e.g., a peer does not like a particular movie, but the child loves it and wants to watch it with the peer). Refer to Chapter 17 on perspective taking. Problem-solving skills contribute to independence and success, both in terms of getting things done and in terms of maintaining relationships with others.

Identifying Deficits in Problem Solving

The following are common clinical examples that may be indicative of learners who could benefit from learning problem-solving skills:

- Children who "give up" immediately when something doesn't work. For example, instead of figuring out how to fix his favorite toy or locate his favorite snack item, the child might become angry and simply waits until others fix the situation for him.
- Children who do not persist socially when something does not work. For example, if peers want to play with something non-preferred, the child leaves. Or a child who wants to make friends with a peer gives up before trying because he can't identify how to approach that particular peer.

Teaching Problem Solving

A well-developed problem-solving repertoire includes the ability to identify a problem, identify possible solutions, consider the pros and cons of each potential solution, select the best solution, implement it, evaluate the effectiveness of the solution, and persist when the first solution fails by generating and implementing alternative solutions. The breadth of examples and situations you can use to teach these skills is practically limitless. The following are some commonplace scenarios encountered by young children that we view as useful opportunities for teaching problem-solving skills:

- Can't find an item;
- Can't obtain an item that is out of reach, stuck, or otherwise inaccessible;
- Makes a mess (e.g., wets her pants, gets paint on shirt);
- Breaks an item or has the wrong item (e.g., is given a fork to eat soup);
- Encounters a difficult task; and
- Experiences a social conflict (e.g., not getting a turn, peer took toy, etc.).

The following teaching steps provide a starting point for teaching problem solving:

- **Identifying a problem.** Contrive and capture problems. Do not mass trial particular problems; rather, present novel but similar exemplars to help generalization of previously successful strategies. Teach within motivating, functional activities that contact functionally relevant reinforcement (e.g., replacing batteries allows learner to play video game, fixing the tent allows learner and peer to play "camping" in back yard).
  - Ask the learner, "What's wrong?" or "What's the problem?"
  - Prompt at first and then fade out prompting, so the learner identifies problems independently when they arise, rather than having to be asked.
  - Gradually increase the complexity of problems as the learner generalizes correct responding to untrained problems of less complexity.
- **Identifying, considering, and selecting a preferred solution.**
  - Ask the learner what she can do to fix the problem, and encourage a variety of answers (i.e., avoid being rigid about right or wrong answers).
  - Provide solutions, if needed, but encourage independence.
  - As solutions are named, discuss the pros and cons using cause-and-effect language (e.g., "What will happen if we do that?").
  - If it's a social problem, prompt the learner to use perspective taking by considering the third person's thoughts, preferences, intentions, etc. (see Chapter 17).
  - Ask the learner which option she thinks will work the best and why.
- **Implementing and evaluating the solution.**
  - Prompt the learner through implementing the solution she selected with you.

- After she implements the solution, ask the learner if it worked. If it worked, celebrate. If not, discuss what went wrong and which other solution she should try.
- As the complexity of problems increases, prompt the learner several times while she is fixing it to monitor and state aloud whether the solution is working.
- Considering using visual supports (see Figure 18.2).
- For social problems, consider using role-play and rehearsal with feedback from the therapist prior to having the learner implement the solution with a peer.
- **Persisting when solutions fail.**
  - After identifying what went wrong and what can be done differently, prompt the learner to identify an alternative solution and implement it.
  - Continue this process until the problem is solved.

Planning

Planning is somewhat similar to problem solving in that there is a complex, multi-step process that needs to occur between now and some time in the future in order for future behavior to be successful. However, two differences are worth mentioning. First, when planning, one generally anticipates a future need and behaves in a specific way in the present to avoid future problems, whereas problem solving usually occurs in response to a problem

Problem Solving Visual Representation

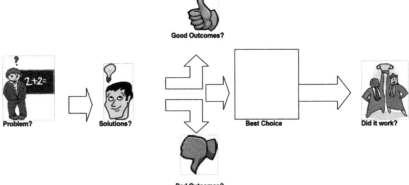

FIGURE 18.2   An example of a visual support for teaching problem solving. Depending on the verbal skills of the learner, have her point, vocalize, and write words in each area of the diagram. *Reprinted from Skills® with permission from the Center for Autism and Related Disorders.*

that is occurring at the present time. In short, planning is more proactive than problem solving. Second, planning often requires less creativity or novelty than problem solving. Sometimes, when people plan, they already know what to do and are merely making a plan to ensure that they actually do it in the future. Problem solving, on the other hand, often involves thinking of a new solution. All other things being equal, the more you plan, the less you should have to problem solve. However, both skills are critical for optimal functioning in everyday social, academic, domestic, and vocational life.

Generally speaking, planning involves a complex chain of behaviors used to accomplish a future goal, including 1) goal setting; 2) identifying materials, roles, and steps needed to achieve the goal; 3) implementing the steps; and 4) monitoring, evaluating, and readjusting the plan as needed until the goal is met. These skills can be critical to a variety of scenarios, including getting ready for school each morning on time, getting better at a sport or hobby, cooking a meal, organizing one's bedroom, designing a Halloween costume, or playing a card/board game. Planning might also involve academic goals, such as completing in-class and homework assignments and short-term and long-term projects. It is also relevant to our social lives in that we plan outings with friends, sleepovers, and birthday gifts/parties, as well as devise plans for how we will make friends with a particular social group, join a club, or get elected to student council.

Effective planning involves many of the other EF skills discussed earlier in the chapter. For example, the learner should be able to demonstrate sustained attention to the task at hand and practice inhibition when distractions arise. She should also demonstrate flexibility and problem-solving skills as necessary to identify solutions when problems arise and readjust the plan if an obstacle is encountered. Finally, the learner needs to have some ability to monitor and evaluate her own performance (self-management).

Identifying Planning Deficits

The following examples of common clinical observations may indicate that your learner could benefit from learning planning skills:

- Learner has difficulty determining the appropriate materials necessary to complete a task or prepare for an event (e.g., making several trips to a supply bin when one should suffice);
- Learner has difficulty succeeding on longer-term projects, such as book reports, because the learner procrastinates; and
- Learner has difficulty anticipating future consequences of her social behavior.

Teaching Planning

- **Goal setting.** At ages 5–7, typically developing children begin to identify goals with adult help.

- Prompt the learner to develop a goal by asking him goal-related questions for a particular task; for example, "What do you need to do to get ready in the morning?" or "What do you need to do for this assignment?" or "What should you and your friend do during your playdate this afternoon?"
- **Materials.**
  - Ask the learner to identify which materials will be needed to complete a task, and use leading questions if the learner has difficulty with correct identification of materials.
  - Begin to require the learner to gather the materials and gradually increase complexity and difficulty of getting materials.
- **Roles and steps.**
  - Teach the learner to identify potential role assignments prior to the event she is planning. For example, for a sleepover, certain tasks can be assigned to the learner (e.g., choosing play activities) while others are assigned to parents (e.g., shopping).
  - Have the learner describe the steps, including sequence and who should do them; for example, ask "What should you do first? Then what?".
  - If needed, create a visual aid. Starting around first grade, teachers start using weekly homework sheets. They may be prefilled or the student may need to write in them, but in either case, they can serve as visual aids for planning throughout the week.
- **Self-monitoring and evaluation.** See self-monitoring section earlier in this chapter.
  - Have the learner cross steps off the list as they are carried out.
  - When problems arise during the plan, ask the learner what she can do to fix them.
  - Prompt the learner to update the plan as new situations or problems arise.
  - After the activity is complete, ask the learner questions, such as, "What worked?"; "What didn't work?"; and "What could you do differently next time?"

GENERAL TIPS FOR SUCCESS

Teach Relevant and Practical Skills

It would be a mistake to assume that every domain, skill within a domain, or target of a skill mentioned in this chapter needs to be taught to every child with ASD. For example, some children have excellent abilities with recalling information and will not necessarily need to work on memory tasks, and other children might have great attention skills, inhibition, and flexibility. In other words, don't fall into the trap of teaching something just because it's in the curriculum or because it can be taught. In fact, most typically functioning adults could improve on most of the skills in this chapter! Just because ABA can be used to teach a skill does not mean that it should be.

Assess the learner by testing her abilities within each domain, and then develop a curriculum based on the learner's individual needs. When choosing targets to teach, make sure to choose those that will be relevant to the learner's real life. For example, if the learner is very young, avoid working on complex skills that develop at a later age. Instead, work on skills that are developmentally appropriate to the learner. Also, consider what the learner's caregivers would like her to learn and what will be maintained in her natural environment when the teaching phase is over. Choose skills that will be functional to the learner and used often. For example, when teaching the learner to sustain his attention to tasks, choose tasks that are required of him at home and school. When setting up self-management programs for the learner, choose target behaviors that matter to his caregivers, teachers, and – ideally – to him. When and if you encounter skill sets or targets in this chapter that you can't ever see benefiting the learner, skip them and move on to things that matter!

Make Sure the Child Has the Prerequisite Skills

The topic of prerequisite skills is challenging, especially when it comes to teaching complex and highly abstract skills, such as EF skills. As you are designing a learner's curriculum program and choosing activities and targets, ask yourself what other skills seem necessary to be in place before working on the current skill, and probe them to make sure the learner can already do them. If you are working from a curriculum that has prerequisite skills listed, such as the Skills® curriculum (see Chapter 26), be sure to consult it before introducing each lesson. The Skills curriculum has both prerequisite skills and age equivalents in typical development listed for all EF lessons. Be sure to teach only a particular lesson when the learner's chronological age is at or above the age at which that skill emerges in typical development, and always make sure the learner has the necessary prerequisites. Particularly when it comes to teaching skills as complex as EF skills, if there is any doubt whether the learner is ready to start working on the skill, you are probably better off waiting and building fluency with fundamental prerequisites first.

Use Rules

Rules can be particularly helpful for teaching EF skills. If the learner with whom you are working understands and follows rules, try adding them to various tasks to help him learn the concepts and contingencies faster. For example, when teaching him to inhibit a behavior, you might say, "If you keep your hands quiet until this timer goes off, you will get to play with your LEGOS®." When teaching the learner to attend to important stimuli, you might say, "When you hear someone yell, you should look to see if everything is okay" or "When your teacher talks in class, you should always stop what you are doing and listen." When working on strengthening a learner's sustained attention, you might say, "If you read for 5 minutes, you will get free time." When teaching flexibility, you might say, "Sometimes we don't like it when things happen in a new way, so we are going to practice being okay with change. I am going to crinkle your rug, and when I do that, I want you to practice using one of the coping skills I taught you before, like taking a deep breath and counting to 10." Consider inserting rules wherever it seems appropriate for establishing a new skill. Start with specific rules and work toward more general rules that the child will learn to apply himself; for example, "Sometimes it's fun to do things differently." Remember that a therapist-stated rule is a prompt, so remember to fade them out over time. Finally, remember that flexibility is key to all EF skills, so if you use rules, make sure your rules are flexible. By using rules, you do not want to inadvertently make the learner more rule governed overall – quite the opposite! You can avoid this by stating rules in different ways every time and by providing rules for being flexible and not always following rules. For example, "Sometimes there is no right or wrong way; you just have to do your best."

Use Visual Supports

Visual supports can be particularly helpful for teaching EF skills. Since visual supports are addressed at length in their own chapter (Chapter 6), we will only briefly mention some that are particularly useful for EF skills. Visual supports can be used to help a learner understand the passage of time. For example, when teaching the learner to wait or to inhibit a particular behavior for a period of time or to sustain attention over time, a visual timer can be helpful. Visual cues can also be provided to help organize long and complex chains of behaviors, as in self-management, problem solving, and planning. For planning, you might use a worksheet with a place to write down the materials needed, the steps and who is assigned to complete each step, and the deadlines for each.

Visual supports are prompts, but not all of them will need to be faded. It's standard for people to use visual prompts to help with many executive functions. For example, we all make to-do lists and track events in our calendars. We also draw things out in an effort to help ourselves solve a problem. Generally speaking, you should only need to fade out visual supports that are not typically used by others.

COMMON PITFALLS IN TEACHING EXECUTIVE FUNCTION SKILLS

Teaching Children to Memorize/Failing to Generalize

When teaching EF skills, it's easy to fall into the trap of teaching children to memorize answers to particular tasks because many memory and attention tasks are artificial, repetitive, and contrived. From the start, make an effort to think outside the box to identify creative ways to teach skills, so they will be applied to situations in the natural environment. If you need to start teaching the learner to respond while sitting at a table, figure out how you can eventually move practice of the skills into the natural environments where they will be useful to the learner in daily life. Also, capture opportunities in the learner's normal daily routine for her to practice EF skills. For example, when playing, have the learner help to prepare for the play situation (teach planning).

To avoid teaching the learner rote memorization of items, it is important to program immediately for generalization and focus on ways you can teach the learner to understand and apply concepts. Some learners are very good at acclimatizing to the requests of their therapists and learning the game of providing "surface responses" in which skills appear intact but really cannot be applied in new situations. To avoid this, make sure to teach multiple ways to use skills. Avoid repetition of the same target. Instead, use multiple exemplar training to teach the learner to use skills in a more generalized fashion with all sorts of new targets. The goal is to teach the learner a repertoire, not particular responses. For example, when teaching problem solving, you wouldn't want to present the same problem over and over. Instead, you would want to teach the process of problem solving across many different problems. Likewise, when teaching the learner memory skills, you wouldn't ask the learner to recall the same set of numbers (or other random stimuli) over and over. Rather, you would vary the stimuli each time they are presented.

Creating Prompt Dependency

For many EF skills, it will be helpful for the child to learn through experience or to be guided indirectly to correct answers rather than being directly told through model prompts. For example, when teaching the learner problem-solving and planning skills, avoid immediately prompting the learner with the correct responses. Instead, use leading questions and/or experiential prompts; for example, ask "What could you try? What are some other things you could do?" If the learner identifies a solution that you know will be ineffective, you might want to allow him to rehearse its implementation with you so he will directly experience how the solution did not work. Or you might ask a leading question, such as, "What will happen if you do that?," and if the child identifies an unlikely positive outcome, you could follow up with another leading question that will help the learner identify the negative outcome. There is nothing wrong with using vocal model prompts for correct answers, *per se*, but it is all too easy for children with ASD to fall into the trap of merely repeating what the therapist states, rather than engaging in the behavior of thinking and talking themselves through a solution to the problem.

Not Involving Parents

Executive function skills are life skills that need to be used all day every day in order to accomplish goals. For this reason, it is recommended that you get parents on board right away in any capacity possible to help facilitate maintenance and generalization of these skills in their children. Failing to involve parents will relegate the use of EF skills to therapy time only, which will hinder generalization to everyday life. As with any other skill area, give parents EF targets to work on to follow up on what you teach during therapy. For example, have parents require their child to help with cooking, chores, or other daily tasks that will allow the child to use planning and problem-solving skills. Consider teaching parents how to:

- make activity schedules for morning and evening routines,
- use leading questions to guide their children to find answers on their own, and
- use experiential prompts to guide their children to discover new answers.

Model these prompting techniques for the parents and help them identify where they can infuse EF skills into their daily routines.

SUMMARY

EF skills involve the intentional manipulation of one's own environment to help oneself function more successfully and independently. They include repertoires of behavior that are critical components of being able to control and organize oneself. The traditional cognitive terms that encompass these behaviors include inhibition, attention, flexibility, memory, self-management, problem solving, and planning, to name just a few. Using the principles and procedures of ABA, this chapter provides strategies for teaching these skills. The strategies used are designed to produce generalized, flexible repertoires across the learner's everyday life.

Clinical Supervision

Jonathan Tarbox, Adel C. Najdowski

In the Center for Autism and Related Disorders (CARD) Model, clinical supervision is the process of designing and overseeing the implementation of comprehensive behavioral intervention programs. This process may also be referred to as "supervision," "case supervision," "case management," and "program direction." Clinical supervision, as it is described here, refers to the activities of the clinical supervisor in overseeing the learner's treatment. As discussed in the job descriptions in Chapter 21, the activities of the clinical supervisor are perhaps the most important single component of the provision of behavioral intervention services. Indeed, it is probably not an exaggeration to say that entire service provision organizations will either rise or fall on the backs of their clinical supervisors. No matter how dedicated the frontline or administrative staff, no matter how much funding is available for treatment, and no matter how involved the learner's parents may be, comprehensive behavioral interventions will be of insufficient quality and effectiveness if they are not given high-quality and an adequate quantity of supervision.

This chapter describes our supervision model and offers lessons from the development of this model over the past quarter century. Surely, many other models of supervision may work, and regional differences in funding and regulations will undoubtedly require adjustments in the model, but we have found this basic model to be adaptable to the provision of top-quality behavioral intervention services in virtually every region of the world. As the primary person in charge of the learner's treatment program, the clinical supervisor performs many roles. In this chapter, we describe these roles in the following sections: Programming, Supervision Across the Treatment Life Cycle, Ongoing Clinical Problem Solving, Critical Repertoires of Supervisor Behavior, Common Pitfalls in the Supervision Process, Staff Management, and Parent Support.

SUPERVISING THE CHILD'S LEARNING: PROGRAMMING

Programming is the central foundation of comprehensive behavioral intervention, and effective programming is the true mark of a master clinical supervisor. Virtually every other part of autism treatment provision could probably be accomplished, to some degree, by individuals who are not truly experts in applied behavior analysis (ABA). Programming is the "secret sauce" that makes ABA work. It is the design process that determines how to make the learner with autism spectrum disorder (ASD) acquire skills rapidly and effectively. Many aspects and considerations go into programming effectively, including an understanding of ABA procedures versus principles, consideration of chronological versus mental age, and others, as discussed below.

ABA Procedures Versus Principles

Anyone with any degree of experience with learners with ASD has likely seen "ABA" implemented purely as a procedure, with no analysis. For example, poor-quality programs often implement the same set of five lessons with the same prompting and reinforcement procedures for all learners with ASD, regardless of age, skill level, and so on. "Doing ABA" does not mean implementing a list of procedures; it means fine-tuning every single aspect of a learner's teaching environment in every way imaginable in order to maximize that learner's skill acquisition during every waking moment. The vast majority of that fine-tuning is based on behavioral principles of learning and motivation. Thus, it's critical that clinical supervisors understand the basic principles of ABA and are able to individualize the use of the principles when programming ABA-based intervention. For example, a clinical supervisor must not only know how to carry out procedures (e.g., shaping, chaining, DRO, etc.) but must also have the expertise to identify which is appropriate, given the nature of the behavior, the characteristics of the learner, and other environmental factors.

Chronological Age Versus Mental Age

Chronological age is the age of the learner based on his birth date, whereas mental age is the age at which the learner is functioning, given his current skill level. For example, a learner might be chronologically 5 years old according to his birth date but be functioning at the age of a 3-year-old, given his current abilities. In typical child development, the chronological and mental age are the same. A good clinical supervisor considers both the learner's chronological and mental age when making programming decisions. Mental age will be used as a starting point. That is, if the learner is functioning at the age of a 3-year-old, then skills starting at that age range will be taught, and the clinical supervisor will continue to introduce and teach skills progressively until the learner is functioning at his chronological age for that given skill. That said, good clinical supervisors will not waste time teaching younger "disappearing skills." For example, toddlers who do not have bike-riding skills will learn to ride a tricycle, but a 7-year-old who cannot ride a bicycle can skip learning to ride a tricycle and go straight to learning to ride a bicycle. The good clinical supervisor will bypass teaching the older learner to ride a tricycle and will go directly to the more age-appropriate and functional skill of riding a bicycle. The clinical supervisor does, however, teach younger skills if they are considered prerequisites or building blocks needed for later developing skills. In order to maximize treatment gains, given the amount of treatment hours available, the clinical supervisor also avoids teaching skills that are above the learner's chronological age and, instead, focuses on a different curriculum domain in which the learner is delayed. Therefore, the overall goal of the CARD approach to behavioral intervention is to merge the child's chronological and mental ages.

Curriculum

The process of assessing skills deficits and choosing which skills to include in a learner's treatment program at any given time is complex and challenging. (For a chapter dedicated to this process, see Najdowski, Gould, Lanagan, & Bishop, 2014.) Below, we provide brief practical recommendations for the assessment and target selection process.

Assessment. The assessment process is probably one of the most overlooked and yet most critical stages of the skill acquisition process in autism treatment. The assessment portion is somewhat analogous to diagnosing a medical illness: You can have the highest quality medical treatment procedures in the world, but if you get the diagnosis wrong, the patient is less likely to benefit. The same is true for behavioral skill acquisition. The best ABA therapy team in the world is still not going to be able to teach a child with ASD successfully if they do not know *where to start, what to teach*, and *in what order*. Effective and comprehensive assessment ensures that the team teaches skills that are appropriate for the learner and that will help bring about meaningful change in the learner's life.

Thus, the first step to designing a learner's curriculum is to conduct an assessment that allows you to identify the learner's deficits and developmental level across all areas of human development. At CARD, skill deficits are measured in two different ways: 1) standardized psychological assessment (as discussed in Chapter 25) and 2) curriculum-based assessment. For the latter, clinical supervisors use the Skills® program (see Chapter 26 and www.skillsforautism.com; developed by top-level CARD researchers and senior clinicians), which provides a comprehensive skills-based assessment across all eight areas of human development (social, motor, language, adaptive, play, executive function, cognition, and academic skills) for learners with ASD from infancy to adolescence. In the Skills® assessment, people who know the learner well (generally parents or clinicians who have worked with the child for a year or more) answer questions across all skill domains in order to identify which skills the child can and cannot already do. In cases where the caregiver is not sure, a note is made in the Skills® system for the skill to be probed directly with the child.

Identifying which and how many activities. Once the skills assessment is complete and barriers to learning have been identified, the results of the skills assessment are examined to determine the learner's current strengths and deficits. The goal is for the learner to become well balanced in her repertoires across all areas of human development. Thus, more emphasis is placed on teaching in areas of greater deficit, and areas of strength are used to help teach skills in those areas. For example, if the learner is a reader, textual prompts might be used to teach other skills. Ultimately, the goal is for the learner to catch up with her same-age, typically developing peers across all developmental areas.

As you can imagine, when working with learners with ASD, deficits are global. Some learners may need to be taught literally hundreds or even thousands of skills in order to catch up to their typically developing, same-age peers. In this case, you need to prioritize which and how many areas to target. The number of activities to be included in a learner's curriculum program at any given time depends on how many hours of treatment the learner is receiving. There are no hard-and-fast rules for this, but our rule of thumb is to work on less than 10 activities at a time if the learner is receiving 15 hours or less per week of intervention; 15 to 20 activities if the learner is receiving 30 hours of intervention per week; and 20 to 25 activities if the learner is receiving 40 hours of intervention per week.

When choosing which activities to fill those placeholders, attention should be given to which skills are most functional for the learner, given the number of treatment hours and duration of treatment, as well as the learner's level of functioning and acquisition rate. Sometimes, limited treatment hours or funding will not allow you to maintain a balanced focus across all eight developmental areas. In this case, it is important to determine which emphasis will help the learner the most, given the resources available. The goal is to do your best to teach the learner the skills that are the most adaptive in his normal daily routine. The learner's parents should be involved in helping to determine this and in the development of overall goals. Once goals are developed, teaching progresses in order of typical child development, and prerequisite skills are addressed for each skill targeted. The Skills® program provides a great deal of guidance for this by including the typical age of development for each activity and their prerequisites, along with a typical treatment progression from easiest to most difficult skills within each of the curriculum domains.

Other assessment sources. Naturally, utilizing as many resources as you can to identify the best possible skills to teach is always the best approach, and the Skills® system is only one such source, albeit a very comprehensive place to start. Other very important sources are standardized assessments (see Chapter 25), parent opinion, learner opinion (if she has the verbal skills to indicate what she would like to learn), teacher input, and information from existing reports of past successes and failures.

SUPERVISION ACROSS THE TREATMENT LIFE CYCLE

In this section, we describe the activities of the CARD supervisor from the very beginning of treatment to discharge.

Intakes

The intake is the first step toward initiating treatment. The purpose of the intake is to determine if the learner is a good fit for CARD services and to provide recommendations for the learner's treatment. The process of the intake takes anywhere from 8 to 16 hours and occurs over the course of 1 to 3 weeks. It includes an initial 2-hour in-person meeting between the learner, parents, clinical supervisor, and, usually, a second clinician. It also includes one to two observations of the learner in home and school (if applicable) settings.

During the in-person meeting, the clinical supervisor reviews the results of a questionnaire that parents have completed regarding the learner. Using both this questionnaire and time during the meeting to ask questions, the supervisor obtains background information about the learner that includes information about pregnancy, initial signs of ASD, diagnosis, milestones met/unmet, medical information, current behavioral deficits, current challenging behavior, and other concerns. While the clinical supervisor talks to the parents, the second clinician spends time assessing the learner. The goal of both clinicians is to gather baseline information about the learner's current level of functioning across all domains. During home and/or school observations, the clinical supervisor gathers baseline information about how the learner is performing in her natural environment settings.

Based on the information obtained from the intake meeting and observations, general observations and recommendations are made to the family and presented in a report. The report summarizes the learner's background information and present levels of functioning, including challenging behavior. In addition, the clinical supervisor suggests whether CARD is a good fit for the learner. If so, recommendations are made regarding optimal services for the learner. Specifically, the clinical supervisor outlines general goals of treatment and recommends the number of 1:1 ABA intervention hours, as well as the setting in which treatment should take place (home, center, or both). The clinical supervisor also recommends a suitable school placement, the number of hours to be spent in school, and the amount of school shadowing support.

Service recommendations. One of the most important recommendations made is the intensity and duration of services. Right now, the only scientifically supported service recommendation for a learner under the age of 5 is 30 to 40 hours per week of one-to-one behavioral intervention, supervised for at least 1 or 2 hours per week by an expert ABA clinical supervisor. (See Chapter 27 for a summary of research that supports this recommendation.) Of course, each learner's program must be customized to his unique educational, social, and behavioral needs, but the research literature must serve as the primary guideline. Young learners should begin with high-intensity ABA treatment (30 to 40 hours per week) for the first few years; then, as the learner's functional skills develop and deficits diminish, the treatment intensity is faded, allowing the learner to assimilate into typical educational and social settings. Having said that, senior clinicians at CARD have found that the specific characteristics of each learner can lead to modifications in these requirements. Unfortunately, available funding resources may limit the intensity of services for some learners. In addition, CARD may recommend lower intensity services for learners with an advanced repertoire of skills or for learners who attend school full time. However, Granpeesheh, Tarbox, and Dixon (2009) noted that, even though significant progress has been achieved with lower intensity ABA treatment, these improvements are less than the improvements reported following high-intensity ABA treatment.

The duration of treatment is determined by the rate at which a learner progresses through the curriculum, with the optimal outcome being recovery. Most outcome studies have implemented treatment for 2 years, and researchers have documented substantial progress over the course of several years of ABA treatment (see Chapter 27). Given these results, it is usually recommended that a learner receive at least 2 years of ABA treatment. While some learners have achieved an optimal outcome in less than 2 years, it is more common for learners to continue ABA treatment for approximately 4 years.

Ongoing Clinical Supervision

The primary ongoing work of clinical supervision is carried out through regular meetings with the family and therapists (referred to as clinic meetings or clinics), observations during therapy sessions, consultation with teachers and other service providers, and curriculum development.

Clinic Meetings. During clinic meetings – or "clinics" – the learner's entire treatment team comes together to discuss current lessons, ways to elaborate upon recently mastered skills, and any areas where the learner is struggling. The clinical supervisor reviews the learner's data in his logbook to determine how much progress has been made with current lessons and to make data-informed decisions about how to move the learner's program forward. The clinical supervisor also asks therapists to perform lessons with the learner during the clinic. This gives the clinical supervisor the opportunity to observe the learner's and therapists' performance across the lessons in the learner's treatment plan. Based on logbook data and these observations, the clinical supervisor makes decisions about mastery, items to introduce next, items to put on hold, prompt modifications, and so on. Clinical supervisors also use clinics to train family members and therapists on current protocols, as well as to address any emerging needs of the family. Clinics perform a critical function for maintaining consistency across therapists (see the section on consistency later in this chapter). CARD recommends 2-hour clinics twice per month; however, the intensity of supervision for a client may be increased to ensure continued success.

In addition to the observations that occur during clinics, clinical supervisors and their support staff conduct home and school visits in an effort to observe therapy occurring in the typical environments in which it is carried out, as programming within all learning environments is critical to maintaining ongoing excellence. During these observations, the clinical supervisor or her support staff give feedback and continued training to the therapists, teachers/aides, and other persons responsible for conducting therapy with the learner.

Reports and Accountability

Reports serve several functions. The primary purpose of a report is to document and be accountable for the effectiveness of your treatment program. The documentation of effectiveness is necessary to obtain and maintain funding. Reports typically include the following sections: background, current treating clinicians, medical and other interventions, current academic placement, developmental history, current functioning level across each skill domain, challenging behaviors, summary of observations, review of assessments, and recommendations for content and amount of treatment. The initial report provides a learner's history and baseline levels of performance and is given to the funding agency in an effort to obtain approval for services. Once funding is authorized, progress reports occur on a variety of schedules, as dictated by the funding agency. From the perspective of the funding agency, the progress report holds the treatment provider accountable for the learner's progress by showing that the learner is benefiting from intervention. In many states with autism insurance mandates, the reports also comply with legal minimum reporting requirements which are delineated to ensure both that the provider is accountable and that the funding source doesn't implement burdensome reporting requirements. In order to receive continued funding, the report must provide information on how much progress has been made toward achieving current learner goals while also listing current needs, articulating future goals, and providing recommendations for the number of therapy, supervision, and parent training hours.

Discharge

When a learner's annual standardized assessments and Skills® progress charts suggest that the learner is fast approaching performance at typical chronological age level, the clinical supervisor begins to discuss a discharge plan with the learner's parents. This discussion involves setting up a projected timeline for discharge and future plans for school placement, as well as other potential support services, such as social groups, tutors, and so on. Then, once it is believed that the learner is functioning at age level, formal assessments are conducted. Assessments include diagnostic testing and functioning across cognitive, language, and adaptive skills.

It is important to keep in mind that, for many parents, the topic of discharge can be sensitive. Treatment programs often last 2 or more years, and parents may have become particularly attached to the therapy team and/or supervisor over that time. In addition, many parents may feel their child is not ready to transition out of treatment, regardless of the degree of progress he has made. Parents of a child who is being discharged because he has recovered may worry about whether treatment gains will be maintained and whether their child will continue to succeed in mainstream settings with less support. Parents of a child who is being discharged even though he still has significant deficits may understandably be distressed by the fact that their child still has more that he could learn in an ABA program. In these cases, logistical factors, such as discontinuation of funding, may necessitate discharge, and this can be particularly distressing for parents.

Regardless of the circumstances of discharge, it is the supervisor's duty to ensure that the process goes as smoothly as possible and that the parents feel supported. Even in the most difficult circumstances, parents should be involved in discharge planning months ahead of the discharge date, and every effort should be made to connect parents with other resources in the community and to set up systems to ensure maintenance of the learner's treatment gains (see Chapter 7 on maintenance).

ONGOING CLINICAL PROBLEM SOLVING

Ongoing clinical problem solving is a major portion of the clinical supervisor's daily job. Even in a top-quality intervention program, the learner's environment is constantly changing, she is always learning new skills, and new challenges and opportunities arise on a daily basis. Accordingly, the clinical supervisor is literally never done analyzing and problem solving. Put another way, an intervention program for a child with ASD never goes "on automatic pilot"; it is a never-ending fine-tuning process, from intake to discharge. Below, we describe some of the major areas to consider when fine-tuning each learner's program on a daily basis.

Motivation

As discussed in many places in this manual, reinforcement is the engine of behavioral intervention, and the effectiveness of a learner's program relies heavily on how powerful his reinforcers are at any given time. The first thing to check when you suspect that the learner's motivation is low is whether staff are conducting frequent preference assessments. CARD defines frequent preference assessments as at least one before each new lesson or block of trials. If the frequency of preference assessments is not the problem, check on the stimuli being used. If the same three stimuli are included in preference assessments all day, every day, for a month, then it doesn't matter how frequently the preference assessments are conducted because the stimuli they contain are likely no longer effective reinforcers. Consider the following factors:

- **New stimuli must be introduced in preference assessments frequently.** Research has shown that a good method for introducing novel stimuli is to pick new stimuli that are related to known reinforcers on some dimension (Kenzer & Bishop, 2011). For example, if a learner loves playing with a train puzzle, then perhaps a book about trains or a wooden train toy might be a good choice for a new item;
- **Preference assessments must offer real choices.** A common mistake is for a therapist simply to hold up one preferred item and ask the learner, "Do you want to work for this?" The learner may be likely to

respond positively simply because there is no other choice, whereas she might prefer a different item if she had a real choice;

- **Deprivation is crucial to maintaining reinforcer effectiveness.** As described in Chapter 4, reinforcers are only as effective as the motivating operations that are in effect at any given time. If a learner has frequent access to a particular stimulus, that stimulus is sure to decrease in effectiveness as a reinforcer. It is wise to make schedules for when stimuli are and are not available in order to ensure that the learner "takes a break" from each reinforcer on a regular basis;
- **Delivery of reinforcement.** Consider how reinforcement is currently being delivered. Is the schedule of reinforcement dense enough? Is the learner receiving reinforcement immediately after making a correct response? Is the learner receiving frequent reinforcement throughout teaching sessions?; and
- **Value of the reinforcer.** Reinforcers need to be high value. Merely offering choices and conducting preference assessments do not guarantee this if the items included in the preference assessment are not highly valued by the learner. Make sure that the pool of reinforcers from which the learner chooses is comprised of a large variety of items and activities that she genuinely loves.

Procedural Integrity and Consistency

One of the most common barriers to rapid learning in behavioral intervention occurs when therapists implement teaching procedures inconsistently. For many learners with ASD, learning language and other skills is truly nothing short of an Olympic challenge, so anything that makes it more difficult is going to slow progress considerably. Even when teaching procedures are implemented perfectly, learning can be a major challenge, so it is truly critical that therapists implement the procedures the same way as one another and the same way from day to day.

Inconsistent response requirements. A common error to look for is when different therapists accept different topographies of behavior as the target response. For example, if you are teaching a learner to ask (i.e., mand) for blocks (one of his highest preferred items), and he has few or no words, you may start by reinforcing any approximation of the word "blocks" by giving him blocks. At first, you might accept a vocalization that starts with anything resembling a "b" sound. After that is consistently occurring, you might increase the requirement for reinforcement to something like "buh." If one therapist accepts anything similar to "buh," and the other therapist only accepts a clearly enunciated "buh," the teaching procedure is going to be inconsistent, and you will get inconsistent results. Moreover, the therapists may potentially evoke challenging behavior. Inconsistent expectations are going to make the learner feel frustrated.

In terms of behavioral principles, you are going to make the learning environment less preferred, which is going to make escape from instruction more negatively reinforcing, thereby evoking escape behaviors.

Inconsistent prompting. Another common source of inconsistency is in selecting which prompts to use. Any prompt that effectively occasions a correct response and can then be faded out readily is likely to work; however, if different therapists implement very different prompts from day to day for the same behavior with the same learner, it can create problems. When one prompt works, by definition it has stimulus control over the correct response. The key to effective prompt fading is to transfer stimulus control from that prompt to the desired discriminative stimulus through gradual fading of the prompt. However, if an entirely different prompt is used on a different day by a different therapist, then that fading process is disrupted. Essentially, the learner has to learn the same skill in two different ways with two different people. To make matters worse, the learner also then has only half the total number of learning opportunities per prompting procedure, making it even less likely that either of the two prompting procedures will actually work.

Inadequate procedural detail. When problem solving procedural inconsistency, one factor to consider is the amount of procedural detail that has been given to therapists. Is the correct procedure clearly written down anywhere for the therapists to see? Has the treatment team inadvertently developed a habit of just orally telling one another what to do? This is common when staff have worked together for a long time, and therapists often get away with doing it if they have good communication skills. ABA teaching procedures, however, are complex, and small details can mean the difference between success and failure. Therefore, it is often necessary to write down procedures clearly, even if the team doesn't think it's necessary.

Insufficient training. Another factor to consider is whether every therapist has actually been trained sufficiently on how to do the particular components of the procedure that must be implemented. As described in Chapter 22, talking about a procedure is not sufficient. Excellent performance comes from practice and feedback, not merely vocal instruction. Regardless of whether a therapist thinks she knows how to do a procedure, make sure you actually watch her do it, and give clear, upbeat feedback on how to do it properly.

Unspecified exemplars. Failing to specify the particular exemplars to be taught is a common source of procedural inconsistency. Especially when teaching higher order skills and concepts, you may be tempted to have the therapists improvise by using whatever stimuli are on hand, so the teaching procedure does not become repetitive and establish rote responding. However, expecting therapists to improvise stimuli in the moment is often unrealistic. In practice, therapists often end up using the same stimuli that happen to be available, or they choose something that isn't really appropriate, just for the sake of using something different. For example, a girl named Delilah was working on a lesson that was intended to teach her to describe multiple features of objects. The therapist would hold up a picture or an object and say to Delilah, "Tell me three things about this." Because of inadequate supervision of Delilah's lesson, she had not made any significant progress on the program for several months. After careful examination of the case, we learned that the exemplars were not specified for the therapists. Instead, they were expected to improvise whatever they could on any given day. We discovered that the stimuli that the therapists improvised were highly inconsistent, with some being very complex and obscure and others being overly simple and repetitive. To fix the problem, we specified a large set of objects to be used. We dictated that Delilah work on a set of three particular stimuli until they were mastered, then three more, then three more, and so on, until she demonstrated generalization to untrained stimuli. Delilah mastered the skill and demonstrated generalization to new stimuli in 2 weeks after this change was made. What she failed to learn in several months, she learned in 2 weeks after the problem of inconsistency was solved.

The level of specificity that must be determined will vary depending on the concept you are teaching. You may need to specify the exact color, shape, function, and so on, of each exemplar in order to make sure it is an example of what you are trying to teach.

Prerequisite Skills

Neglecting to consider necessary prerequisite skills sufficiently is a common roadblock to learning in behavioral intervention programs. Just as you must learn to multiply and divide before you can learn algebra, the vast majority of skills we teach during behavioral intervention build upon earlier skills, and it is unreasonable to expect a learner to acquire a skill if he has not already mastered the necessary prerequisite skills. For example, if you are teaching a learner to categorize items, it is critical that the learner can already name the items (tact them) and respond to them receptively (as a listener). Before you teach a learner multiple-step instructions, he must be able to complete each step of the instructions individually, as a single instruction. Before a learner can be taught complex scenes and "themes" of pretend play, she must be able to play with each item individually. Finally, before a learner can be expected to respond to complex rules, he must be taught to understand basic if/then statements.

Identifying prerequisite skills can sometimes be difficult, but curricula exist that supply much of that information for you. CARD's curriculum, Skills®, lists prerequisite skills for each lesson, so this is a good place to start. If you check for mastery of a prerequisite skill and you find it lacking, then put the more advanced lesson on hold for a while until you train the prerequisites to fluency. Don't forget to put the prerequisite skills on some kind of maintenance schedule after they are mastered.

Skill Difficulty

Trying to teach a skill that is too difficult is another common roadblock to effective teaching and learning in behavioral intervention programs. This is not quite the same issue as prerequisite skills. A particular skill can be too difficult even when all apparent prerequisites have already been mastered. Oftentimes, a skill can be too difficult because it is too long or too complex to teach all at once. In other words, is the chunk of behavior you are trying to teach too large? Can it be broken down into smaller units to be taught more gradually? Consider how task analysis or shaping may be used to make the skill you are trying to teach easier to learn. For example, teaching a learner to put one piece into a puzzle is going to proceed much faster than trying to teach the entire puzzle at once. Starting an activity schedule with a single activity and gradually increasing the number of activities is going to work far better than starting with a schedule that is full of a long sequence of activities. Finally, teaching a learner to make individual social initiations or conversational exchanges and gradually increasing conversational complexity works much better than trying to teach complex conversational exchanges.

Challenging Behavior

Everyone involved in autism treatment already knows that addressing challenging behavior is crucial to treatment success. Yet, it is common, even in good-quality treatment programs, to see learners with ASD continue to display significant challenging behavior during therapy for months or longer. If a learner's progress is slow, and he is also engaging in challenging behavior, this may well be one of the causes of the slow learning rate. Challenging behavior, although sometimes difficult to treat, is not part of the autism diagnosis, and it is critical that the treatment team does not come to accept the occurrence of challenging behavior as inevitable with particularly difficult cases. If challenging behavior is occurring on an ongoing basis, it means one simple thing: The treatment team is not treating the behavior successfully. If this is the case, it is critical that the team pause and make an honest assessment of what is going on with the behavior and what can be done about it. It is often necessary to put educational lessons on hold or to decrease their intensity temporarily while challenging behavior is intensively treated. You may be reluctant to put skill acquisition on hold, but the long-term result if you do not do so can be less learning overall (due to never-ending difficulties with challenging behavior). Challenging behavior does not go away on its own; rather, it requires intensive, effective, and consistently implemented behavior intervention plans.

It is also important to keep in mind that you may not be an expert in decreasing severe behavior. Many of the world's best skill acquisition clinicians have never had top-quality training on how to decrease severe behavior. If this includes you, be honest with yourself and ask your colleagues for help or refer the learner to an expert for treatment of his severe behavior. Expert clinicians ask for help all the time; novices stubbornly refuse to ask for help when they need it.

Poor Data Collection

Accurate data are critical to supervising behavioral intervention programs, and sloppy, inconsistent, or subjective data can impair progress. Inaccurate data may make it look as though a learner has mastered a target when she actually has not. For example, if your mastery criterion is 80% correct and the therapist misses or forgets to record just one or two incorrect responses, a true performance of 60% may be recorded and depicted as 80%, thereby giving the impression that the learner has mastered a target when she may actually be performing at little higher than chance levels of responding. Similarly, if different therapists are not consistent with which topographies they are recording for a particular behavior, it may give the impression that there is a lot of variability in the data. This can easily be interpreted as evidence that the intervention is not working when, in actuality, one or more therapists were recording behaviors that were never intended to be changed.

If a learner is making slow progress, double-check the accuracy of the team's data collection. A great way to do this is by assessing **Interobserver Agreement (IOA)**. To assess IOA, a supervisor and the therapists on the treatment team record data at the same time without talking to one another while they are doing it. They then compare their data to see if it matches. Each therapist's data should match the supervisor's data at least 90% of the time (Cooper, Heron, & Heward, 2007). If the data do not match, the team discusses the reasons why and gives one another feedback. The process is then repeated until the data match 90% of the time or more.

Some poor-quality ABA programs rely primarily on narrative data. For the sake of treatment evaluation and documentation, narrative data are not data at all. It is good practice to record narrative notes of details that data do not capture, but these notes are not a substitute for data on learner performance during therapy.

Interference

Occasionally, something else is happening in the learning environment that interferes with the learner's ability to listen or focus or simply takes too much time away from the teaching and learning interactions with the therapists. In home-based therapy, this can consist of interruptions of therapy by parents, siblings, neighbors, television programs, and so on. In centers and schools, this can consist of excessive noise or visual distraction from other teachers or students or from having overcrowded classrooms. In many of these situations, you might feel apprehensive about telling the people causing the distraction that their behavior needs to change, but avoiding the issue will not make it go away. If parents want to observe therapy, it may be more productive to invite them to watch at particular times when they can be incorporated into the lesson, as during play lessons. Another great option is to have webcams or "nanny cams" installed so that they can watch and listen whenever they want without even having to ask the therapist. Such observation can be particularly helpful because it enables parents to feel more connected to their child's therapy, and it also reminds therapists to be on their best behavior since they could be observed at any time. Of course, effectively training and involving parents in therapy from the beginning will usually avoid this problem altogether (see Chapter 9).

Insufficient Learning Opportunities

Very often, treatment providers forget to provide a sufficient number of learning opportunities for a skill to be successfully learned. Particularly with lessons that are difficult for the learner or therapist, are confusing or unclear, or evoke challenging behavior, it is common for the lesson to be implemented with insufficient frequency. For example, when teaching higher order skills, one practice opportunity could require quite a bit of setup time, especially if the situation needs to be captured or contrived. When teaching a learner to predict how someone else is going to feel about a surprise the learner is planning, a large amount of time may be needed for preparation. Beyond the work to initiate the learning opportunity, the practice trial itself can sometimes take a few minutes to carry out (and that's only ONE practice opportunity!). Given the difficulty associated with such a trial, some therapists will conduct only one trial and then move on to something else, even though it's important for the learner to get more practice with the skill. In addition, it is common for therapists to implement their least favorite lessons at the end of the session. When unanticipated events arise – and they do – these lessons often get neglected. In such cases, simply require your therapists to conduct their least favorite lessons at the beginnings of sessions.

Ecological Variables

A variety of ecological variables can impact negatively on the child's ability to learn at her optimal rate. If she is sick, sleep deprived, fatigued, in pain, or hungry, learning is going to be more challenging. When troubleshooting lessons that are challenging for a learner, remember to check all of these potential complicating variables, and make the appropriate behavioral recommendations and/or referrals to other professionals to address them.

CRITICAL REPERTOIRES OF CLINICAL SUPERVISOR BEHAVIOR

Being an excellent clinical supervisor requires more than just implementing procedures and policies; it requires more general characteristics or repertoires of behavior that can be difficult to define and difficult to measure but are nonetheless very real. In this section, we attempt to identify and describe these characteristics as well as practical strategies for cultivating them. Unfortunately, more often than not, we have found that these characteristics are particularly difficult to teach and are either present at an acceptable level before training begins or they are not. We strongly advise practitioners to take each into consideration while hiring and recruiting potential staff into clinical supervisor positions. That being said, just because a trait is difficult to teach does not mean it should not be attempted. Through modeling, role-play, and feedback, even the most subtle and difficult supervisory skills can often be strengthened.

Confidence

Confidence is a difficult quality to define, particularly from a behavioral perspective, but it's real and it matters a great deal. Clinical supervisors need to behave confidently, and their ability to do so will affect nearly every aspect of their job performance. When a clinical supervisor is interacting with parents, her confidence shows the parents that they are trusting their child to someone who actually knows what she is doing. When clinical supervisors project confidence to parents, parents are inspired to have confidence in the treatment plan. It is equally critical for clinical supervisors to display confidence to other professionals during interdisciplinary meetings and Individualized Education Program (IEP) meetings. When many professionals vie for a treatment program's limited time and resources, it's critical that the clinical supervisor politely and professionally conveys her expertise to the entire team. Finally, clinical supervisors must project confidence to the therapists they supervise. This makes the therapists feel more supported and that they are part of a team that is competent and professional. Nothing is worse for therapists' morale than the feeling that they are unsupported or that they are being led by someone who is not an expert. Of course, confidence is no substitute for competence, so supervisor training is equally critical.

It is easy to get mixed up between *feeling* confident and *behaving* confidently. All clinicians get nervous, and all clinicians feel fear at some point, especially early in their careers or when confronted with new challenges. It's important to note that clinical supervisors do not need to *feel* confident; they simply need to supervise confidently. They need to project confidence and excellence to those with whom they interact. If clinical supervisors wonder why they don't necessarily feel confident all the time, it's because they are burdened with an enormously challenging and stressful task! They are entrusted with a disabled learner's well-being. They are trusted by parents to ensure the parents' dreams of a happy, well-adjusted, mature child. What could be more stressful? So, *feeling* nervous is normal and is not to be avoided. Instead, clinical supervisors should be trained to observe their inner feelings and *simultaneously* display the outward behavior of supervising confidently.

Humility

Although confidence is absolutely critical, *overconfidence* can be perceived as arrogance or conceit. Few things are more annoying than someone who acts as if he has all the answers when he clearly doesn't. Moreover, it's admirable for confident clinical supervisors to ask for the advice of other clinical supervisors or superiors. This type of attitude goes a long way to show the team that you are smart but possess a desire to learn more, and it encourages others on the team to demonstrate humility. A clinical supervisor who demonstrates humility creates a team whose members feel no competition to outsmart each other. Rather, everyone works together in a collaborative fashion and looks forward to benefiting from one another's strengths. Excellent clinical supervisors demonstrate a desire to learn, a willingness to accept constructive criticism, and the ability to ask for help. It's literally impossible to know everything there is to know about effective autism treatment. Since the learners' characteristics vary so greatly across the spectrum, even clinical supervisors who have treated hundreds of children with ASD still have something to learn.

Flexibility

When one has supervised quite a few cases with success, it's easy to get into a mindset of trying to fit every case into one of a few molds. However, given the broad autism spectrum and unique qualities of each learner, it's important to remember that things will need to be "tweaked" to work with various learners. No one curriculum can be followed from start to finish without making individualized adjustments. In order to avoid wasting the learner's time, for example, the clinical supervisor needs to think about each skill and whether/how it will benefit the learner, given the learner's number of treatment hours, goals, resources, and so on. Some activities will simply be skipped or ignored because there are other, more urgent, skills to learn. Once skills are chosen, no single way of teaching a skill, works for every learner. Some learners require activities to be broken down into smaller units, while others can skip building blocks and go straight to learning the fundamental skills that actually matter. Likewise, prompts and prompting hierarchies need to be adjusted according to the learner's needs. Furthermore, when a learner is not learning a skill, the clinical supervisor needs to know when to stop drilling in on it and put it on hold. The fact that one approach worked with another learner doesn't mean that the same approach will work with the current learner. The clinical supervisor needs to be creative and flexible as she works to problem solve for each unique learner.

Goal Oriented

Great supervisors need to look through a telescope and a microscope simultaneously. In other words, they need to be goal oriented while at the same time being obsessively focused on the daily details that make learning happen. Every day that a supervisor evaluates her learner's program, she should ask herself several questions to ensure the learner is on the right track, such as: Where will this learner be in 6 months? How does this particular lesson help get her there? What lessons are going to come next? Where is she going to be in 2 years (e.g., school, other placements, etc.)? What do we need to start thinking about to prepare for that? It is easy for supervisors to fall into the daily routine of working with children with ASD, but top-quality autism treatment has no standard daily routine. Good supervisors think about how every single day is strategically connected to the near, middle, and distant future for every single one of their learners.

Empathy

As discussed in Chapter 9 on parent involvement, families living with ASD experience a tremendous amount of distress. For example, parents often report that they literally felt as if they were dying when their child received the ASD diagnosis. As early intervention practitioners, we are often among the first people to talk to parents during this hugely trying time. Family members of learners with ASD deserve to be treated with empathy, not just because it will make the whole treatment process work better (and it will), but also because it's an ethical imperative. Until you are grappling with a serious diagnosis of a person you love, it's easy to lack empathy as a professional. But please indulge us and take a few minutes to do some imagining as you read this. Imagine your perfect baby and all the hopes and expectations you have for her. Imagine the purity of love and dedication you feel when you look at her. Then, imagine that a doctor tells you that she will never learn to talk, never make a friend, never tell you she loves you, never go to college, and so on. Imagine the fear and anxiety you would feel if you were to see all of those hopes and dreams shattered. If you can feel even a small fraction of that while you read this, then keep that feeling with you when you work with parents. Remember, that is likely the feeling they live with every day. They deserve your empathy.

Professionalism

The clinical supervisor is viewed as the expert, the leader, the person who is ultimately responsible for the learner's well-being. This position holds a great deal of responsibility, commands a great deal of respect, and, accordingly, requires a great deal of professionalism. Professionalism includes the manner in which the clinical supervisor presents herself to others both through her actions and her appearance. A professional clinical supervisor makes an effort to interact with others politely and positively both during face-to-face interactions and through telephone calls and email. Professional language is used; that is, the clinical supervisor avoids swearing, gossiping, and talking about confidential topics or subjects that are inappropriate for the work environment. She avoids dual relationships by keeping her relationships with families and staff focused on the job at hand. She follows the ethical code(s) of the certification and/ or licensure boards associated with her credentials (see Chapter 23 on ethics). In addition to following ethical codes, when a professional clinical supervisor finds herself in a difficult situation, she takes the high road and avoids causing conflict or engaging in childlike behaviors, such as yelling, crying, or otherwise showing negative emotions in the work environment. Likewise, the professional clinical supervisor makes an effort to dress in a professional manner and follows appropriate dress codes.

Urgency

Early intensive behavioral intervention is nothing less than an emergency. The research is not yet conclusive about how much time one has to make the largest impact possible in early intervention, but all major professionals agree that it is short, perhaps only a few years. Thus, it is important that clinical supervisors present themselves as taking the limited time they have very seriously, with the goal of doing everything in their power to help the learner achieve his greatest potential. If you supervise intervention programs all day long for years, it is easy to get into feeling that it is "routine," but there is nothing routine about it, at least not for any individual child. Each child's case should be treated as if it were an emergency. Each early intervention case should be treated as a 2- or 3-year sprint. There is no time for rest, and no rate of progress should ever be considered good enough.

Work Ethic

Autism treatment requires a tremendous amount of hard work, and this is as true for supervisors as it is for therapists and parents. Clinical supervisors who are lazy or appear to be working without a sense of urgency about their learners' progress are doing the learner and themselves a huge disservice. In order to make a large impact on the learner's progress, the clinical supervisor must evaluate the learner's program daily. This requires the clinical supervisor to observe the learner and therapists continuously in home, school, and community settings. The clinical supervisor must also review the learner's curriculum program often and make plans for how to carry out lessons and behavior intervention plans for challenging behavior. A clinical supervisor cannot do a good job making clinical decisions if she is only interacting with the learner, parents, and therapists once every 2 weeks during clinics. Productive clinical supervisors will spend many hours per week away from their desks because they will be actively out in the field, working in the trenches with the learners, families, and therapists. Furthermore, clinical supervisors who work hard and take an active role in interacting with the learner, the parents, and the team set a good example for the therapists and earn the respect of the parents.

Positive Attitude

At the end of the day, we all enjoy our lives a lot more if we have humor in them. This basic truth is equally applicable to clinical supervisors and the staff, learners, and parents with whom they work. Of course, ASD and the challenges that characterize it are no joke, but the ability to balance seriousness and professionalism with a healthy dose of humor and lightheartedness is crucial to maintaining an upbeat level of morale in the workplace and among the learners' families. This can be a difficult balance to strike, so it is important to identify staff who can achieve that balance and encourage them to model it for others. Those who are in leadership positions and are, therefore, models for others to imitate should model a serious yet upbeat attitude toward the work they do.

COMMON PITFALLS IN THE SUPERVISION PROCESS

No one is perfect. One of the greatest differences between average supervisors and excellent ones is that excellent ones identify their own deficits and take active steps toward addressing them. Below, we describe common pitfalls in the supervision process. We highly recommend that all supervisors, whether a new trainee or a seasoned veteran, take a long, hard look at these pitfalls and make an honest assessment of which ones apply to them. Don't beat yourself up; just make a practical plan to fix the problems you identify, and set tangible goals and deadlines to meet those goals.

Caseload

A common question up for debate is how many cases a clinical supervisor can handle in his caseload at any given time. Low-quality ABA programs commonly overload their supervisors with too many cases, which inevitably produces poor-quality treatment because the supervisors simply do not have the time to dedicate adequate supervision to each individual case. As with everything else in autism treatment, there are no hard-and-fast rules for how many cases one supervisor can handle. However, our rule of thumb is, if the clinical supervisor is providing supervision without help from other clinicians in managing the cases (e.g., case managers or senior therapists), for learners receiving full 30- to 40-hour-per-week programs, most clinical supervisors can handle about 10 cases. However, if the clinical supervisor has help in the clinical management of the cases, she can generally handle more. Granted, given the varying levels of supervisor expertise and the varying demands of each case, this can be adjusted accordingly. Some "superstar" clinical supervisors are capable of handling more cases than others. Another way to determine the appropriate size of the caseload is to base it on the rule of thumb that, for every 10 hours of therapy, learners should be receiving on average 1–2 hours of supervision. Then it's a matter of doing the math to determine how many cases the clinical supervisor should be able to supervise. With more focused programs, in which learners are receiving only 10–15 hours of intervention per week, supervisors can generally handle a larger number of cases. Again, the rough guideline of 1–2 hours of supervision for every 10 hours of therapy can be applied to lower intensity cases as well.

Inadequate Experience with Similar Learners in the Past

Given the broad autism spectrum, clinical supervisors are constantly challenged by new learners presenting with issues that they have never had to address. For example, clinical supervisors might have less experience with older learners or learners who are higher/lower functioning.

Likewise, they might find themselves presented with a challenging behavior that they have never treated (e.g., feeding or sleep disorders). In these cases, the wrong thing to do would be to take the case but choose to ignore the unfamiliar area (not provide treatment) or to attempt treatment blindly. In these cases, the clinical supervisor should consult the research literature and reach out to others in the field who have had experience treating such issues. Good clinical supervisors try to find evidence-based solutions that they can implement. However, in some cases, the clinical supervisor may not be able to obtain enough information to make informed treatment decisions. In these cases, the clinical supervisor is probably better off referring the case to another organization or professional who is an expert in treating learners with similar profiles. At CARD, because of the number of supervisors we have and because of their large range of experience, supervisors frequently turn to one another for guidance and advice. Obviously, if the learner is presenting with issues unrelated to ABA, the clinical supervisor should refer the learner to the appropriate specialist. For example, an ABA clinical supervisor is not a medical doctor and would do well to encourage the family to seek the help of a medical doctor when a learner exhibits medical symptoms.

Being Defensive

Clinical supervisors are frequently presented with situations in which they need to provide rationales for their treatment decisions. This happens when talking to parents, staff, superiors, and other professionals during clinic and IEP meetings. It is not uncommon for professionals from other disciplines, for example, not to understand or even to disagree with the treatments presented by the clinical supervisor. In these cases, it is best to present rationales with confidence, respect, and professionalism. Responding defensively only suggests to others that you are feeling threatened by them and are perhaps insecure and unconfident in your decisions.

Blaming the Diagnosis/Learner/Teacher/Parent

There is a time-honored saying in ABA that goes something like this: "The learner is always right." This means that we all do what we do because of our history of learning in our own environments. If we fail to learn something, it is because our environment has not been adequately set up to cause the necessary learning and motivation to occur. This is the only acceptable perspective to take while supervising behavioral intervention programs for learners with ASD. The clinical supervisor's job is to identify how to engineer the learner's teaching environment to cause maximal learning to happen. Therefore, if learning fails to happen or if problem behavior continues to occur, it is never acceptable to blame the learner or the diagnosis. Even when people do not point fingers intentionally, blame often comes through in subtle statements. The left column of Table 19.1 lists common statements that blame the learner or the diagnosis, and the right column lists reasonable behavioral interpretations of the same challenges.

All of the statements in the left column of the table, at their core, assign blame to the learner or her diagnosis. It is a critically important exercise for all of us to examine the language we use while supervising intervention programs and be aware of the source to which we are attributing blame. In ABA, there is only one real source to blame: the environment. Luckily, behavioral principles provide a small and very useful list of potential causes to investigate when we want to know why something is not working. For example, if a learner is "not trying hard," it is likely a problem of motivation. We have two simple principles that explain human

TABLE 19.1 When a Treatment for ASD is not Working well, Good Supervisors Should Blame the Treatment, not the Child or the Diagnosis. This Table Depicts Commonly Heard Phrases that Blame the Child or the Diagnosis (left column) and Examples of More Productive Ways to Look at the Situation (Right Column).

Blaming the Child or the Diagnosis	Blaming the Environment
"He is just a really tough kid. Some kids are just going to have severe behavior."	"He has had a very long history of reinforcement for that challenging behavior, so that means we need to be extra vigilant to make sure we are being consistent in his behavior intervention plan."
"He just has really severe autism. That's why he's not making much progress."	"He has significant skill deficits across all areas of functioning, so we have a lot to teach. Let's get busy and figure out what we can change to make him learn faster."
"It's not just autism; she has other undiagnosed conditions, too."	"She may well have other undiagnosed issues, but the only thing we can do is identify the behaviors that need improvement and work on improving them, so let's do it."
"He isn't trying. He just doesn't care. It's impossible to motivate him."	"We aren't doing well at maximizing motivation, so let's revisit our pool of reinforcers, do some new preference assessments, and review our establishing operation procedures for ensuring our reinforcers are potent during therapy."
"It's normal for children with autism to have repetitive behavior. There isn't much we can do about it."	"Our treatment for repetitive behavior isn't working. Let's make sure we are doing it consistently and then consider what other evidence-based treatment options are available."

motivation: reinforcement and the motivating operations that affect it. If a learner is not motivated, we are either arranging the wrong type, frequency, or amount of reinforcement, or we are failing to control motivating operations in order to make that reinforcement effective.

Clinical supervisors often unintentionally blame a learner's parents or teachers. They rarely do so overtly, but this erroneous perspective often comes across when problem solving a failed intervention and the conversation ends with something like "If his parents would only follow through..." or "How can we expect to make any progress when his teacher keeps...?" Of course, parent and teacher involvement is crucial, but if a learner is not making progress in the context of your learning environment, it is because of your learning environment, not something else. For example, if you are implementing extinction for a challenging behavior in your sessions and a parent is reinforcing the challenging behavior when you are not present, this sets up a clear discrimination training situation for the learner: Do the behavior and get the reinforcer when with parents; don't do the behavior because the reinforcer is not forthcoming when with the therapists. This basic discrimination has been demonstrated across dozens of different species of animals who have only a fraction of the learning capacity of even the most affected child with ASD. If your intervention is effective, you will see progress in your intervention, even if others outside of your intervention are not on board. Of course, this does not mean that parent consistency isn't critical; it simply means that parent or teacher behavior cannot be used as an explanation for why *your* teaching behavior is not working. Having said that, since the supervisor's job is to improve the learner's behavior across all settings, it is critical for the supervisor to help the parents arrange similar contingencies at home (see Chapter 9 for more on parent training and involvement).

SUPERVISING THE THERAPY TEAM: STAFF MANAGEMENT

It is easy to focus primarily on the learner's program and focus less on the fact that the supervisor needs to supervise staff. However, the therapists cause learning to happen, not the supervisor, so the job of managing therapy staff is equally important to that of programming the learner's curriculum and teaching procedures.

Staff Training

Chapter 22 on training and quality assurance describes in detail how to train staff, so that will not be repeated here. However, it is worth noting that it is often the clinical supervisor's job to train staff. Larger organizations may have entire departments devoted to training, but most smaller organizations rely on the clinical supervisors to conduct training. This should not be a problem as long as the clinical supervisors have the necessary time and resources and have themselves been trained on how to conduct staff training properly. At CARD, the Institute for Behavioral Training, a subsidiary organization, conducts all initial trainings. Clinical supervisors at each local office are then responsible for ongoing training and professional development of the staff at that location.

Staff Performance Management

A major part of the clinical supervisor's job is to manage the performance of staff, particularly therapists working directly with the learner with ASD. It is common for professionals to confuse staff training and performance management. They are very different things, however, and each must be done sufficiently if excellent quality therapy is to be delivered. Staff training teaches staff *how* to do their jobs. Performance management ensures that they actually do their jobs on a daily basis by providing motivation for doing them. The paycheck is ultimately the motivation behind why most of us have a job, as most of us would rather spend our days engaging in hobbies and recreation if we did not need a paycheck. However, paychecks do not ensure good performance. Since receiving a paycheck only depends on not getting terminated, paychecks only ensure that employees display performance that is good enough to avoid being fired. To supplement this level of performance, other sources of motivation are needed. For some, mere recognition by colleagues, friends, and family is enough to ensure high-quality and highly productive performance. These employees tend to be the "exemplars," the "over-achievers," and often the leaders in organizations. However, for the vast majority of employees, receiving paychecks and impressing others are not sufficient motivation to maintain high-quality and productive performance, and additional motivation is needed.

Feedback. One performance management tool that has been proven by decades of research and practice is performance feedback. Feedback is just a fancy term for the clinical supervisor telling the employee what she did well and what could be improved. For feedback to be most effective, it should occur frequently, and it should occur as quickly as possible after the performance occurred. As you know from the learners you treat, the longer the delay between the behavior and the reinforcer, the less powerful the reinforcer will be. The same is true for managing staff performance with feedback. At CARD, the higher level management are trained to use the following strategies to deliver effective feedback.

Be positive. Good managers use far more positive than corrective feedback. Just as good parenting should include about five times more positive interactions than corrective interactions, good management means using much more positive feedback than negative feedback. Positive feedback works much like positive reinforcement: it increases productivity, makes the worker feel good, and makes staff want to stick around. Corrective feedback, although necessary, can have the opposite effect. It can make the worker unhappy and produce *countercontrol,* a term used by B.F. Skinner that refers to the tendency of people to want to either attack or escape when they are excessively exposed to punishment and negative reinforcement. In organizational settings with excessive negative feedback, employees likely want to "attack" the organization by speaking negatively about it and its leaders to other employees and, worse, perhaps even to clients. Of course, any aversive environment produces a desire for escape from that environment, so excessive negative feedback will likely increase turnover among your staff, an outcome that is clearly not in your best interest. Good management requires frank corrective feedback, but the ratio of positive to corrective feedback should lean far in the direction of positive.

Be honest. Feedback needs to be honest. Workers can see right through fake praise. This is why attempts at "employee of the month" and similar programs in many organizations backfire – because it's clear to the employees that it's an empty gesture, that the management is merely making a gesture to look good and that they don't truly appreciate the employee's performance. For feedback to be maximally effective, the clinical supervisor needs to find something about the employee's performance that she genuinely appreciates and with which she is truly impressed. When praise is given – and it should be given frequently – it needs to be genuine.

Be clear. Feedback should be clear in that it should refer to specific behaviors that the employee can clearly discern. Feedback that refers to internal states should be avoided because it's difficult for the employee to know how to do what the clinical supervisor asks. For example, if a therapist is perceived as overly negative, a less useful piece of feedback might be, "I need you to be more positive about work." A more useful piece of feedback might be, "During team meetings, I want you to offer at least one possible solution each time you raise a problem or concern. It's great that you want things to be better, but I need you to offer solutions in addition to raising problems."

Public versus private. Research has shown that feedback is an effective performance management tool when given either publicly or privately. However, as a clinical supervisor, you should take care to consider whether the particular employee to whom you are giving feedback actually wants public recognition. For many, public praise is a powerful reinforcer, but for some "shy" employees, it might actually be aversive. Corrective feedback should almost always be done in private. Even if an employee is making an error from which the other employees need to learn, avoid singling him out with corrective feedback in front of the others, as this can be overly aversive. Instead, consider holding a training or meeting for all staff that addresses the topic in a more general way.

Goal setting. Research shows that feedback is highly effective when combined with goals. Clinical supervisors should include employees in the goal-setting process. Goals should be *clear, challenging but achievable, measurable,* and *under the control of the employee* expected to meet them. Clear goals are goals that are easily understood by the employee – there is no ambiguity about what they mean. An unclear goal might be, "I need you to try harder." A better goal might be, "I need you to run every lesson in the learner's logbook at least one time every session." Goals are challenging but achievable when they set a high bar but are still realistic. One hundred percent session fulfillment for an entire year is highly challenging but not very achievable. If one parent cancels a single session and it is not made up, even once in an entire year, then the goal has not been achieved. A better goal might be 99% or 99.5% session fulfillment. The need for goals to be measurable should be self-explanatory; there is no way for employees to know if they achieved a goal and no way for the supervisor to give them positive or corrective feedback if the goal is not measurable. Goals are under the control of the employee when they are a direct result of the employee's behavior and not a result of someone else's behavior. For example, it cannot be one therapist's goal to have all therapists do something. The one therapist is only in control of his own behavior, not that of the other therapists.

Annual evaluations. As a final note about staff performance management, if you are relying on a staff member's annual evaluation to give feedback and to manage performance, then it is already too late to supervise the staff member meaningfully. Annual evaluations occur one time per year and are therefore far too infrequent and far too delayed to have a meaningful impact on daily performance. As a general rule, annual evaluations should hold no surprises. If the employee does not already know what you are going to say when you evaluate her, that is a clear indication that you have not been giving her frequent and specific performance feedback.

PARENT TRAINING AND SUPPORT

Parent training is addressed at length in Chapter 9; however, it is briefly addressed here because it is such an integral part of the clinical supervisor's job. Parent training is an important part of treatment delivery, as it allows the entire family system to be addressed, rather than simply treating the learner's deficits and excesses and leaving the parents in a position to have to deal with their child's behavior "after hours" on their own. The amount and type of parent training, unfortunately, are often dictated by the intervention's funding source. Regardless of the number of hours allotted, the goal of parent training is to provide strategies and tools for the parents to use when they are with their child.

At the beginning of parent training, parents are consulted and asked which areas they find most concerning and challenging, and the clinical supervisor tailors her parent training to these topics. Parent training is conducted both during clinic meetings and in home and community settings where the challenges lie. For example, if the parents report that they can never take their child to a store without a tantrum, then training would begin in a controlled environment with developing, discussing, and role-playing a protocol for these situations. Following this, the training would move into the community setting where the protocol would truly need to be used in order to be successful and maintained.

Many parents can be resistant to parent training, and this is something that clinical supervisors need to assess. Initially, the clinical supervisor should work on building rapport and trust with the parents and then focus parent training on the parents' needs, rather than what the clinical supervisor feels is important. The clinical supervisor also needs to remember all of the other issues that impede a parent's ability to implement and adhere to parent training protocols. Often, parents are dealing with stress, depression, and limited time, among other issues that make it difficult for them to comply with protocols. The clinical supervisor needs to consider these issues and create buy-in on the part of the parents, not be dogmatic about following procedures exactly. This can be done by starting slowly and devising protocols that are easy and fit nicely into the family's values and regular routines. Once the parents see success, you can trust that they will ask for more! Establishing a trusting and collaborative relationship with the parents from the beginning will augment the treatment plan and, ultimately, lead to more positive outcomes.

SUMMARY

Clinical supervisors are well-trained experts in ABA-based intervention for ASD and have the role of designing and ensuring proper implementation of a learner's treatment program. In this role, clinical supervisors are responsible for leading effective treatment programs for learners with ASD by training therapists and family members, managing the treatment team both positively and professionally, and using expertise to design individualized curriculum programs based on each learner's unique needs. This is single-handedly the most pivotal role in helping learners to achieve their maximum potential. Thus, it must be undertaken carefully, precisely, and individually. It is our hope that this chapter will help clinicians become the best possible supervisors they can be.

20

Data Collection and Treatment Evaluation

Jonathan Tarbox

Collecting accurate data is a foundational part of any top-quality behavioral intervention program for children with autism spectrum disorder (ASD). Data are crucial for a variety of reasons. First, data enable a treatment program to be accountable for its effectiveness. A hallmark of applied behavior analysis (ABA) is that it must be effective, and it must be continuously modified and adjusted to maintain maximum effectiveness. Second, treatment decisions must be made virtually every day, and those decisions must be informed by data. Clinical judgment, experience, and hunches are all relevant, but they cannot supplant data in the decision-making process. Every aspect of behavioral intervention is iterative, which means that it is constantly building on previous treatment and the gains of that treatment. When teaching a skill, we are typically building on prerequisite skills that the child has learned in the past. Through data, the treatment team can determine whether the learner is actually ready to learn a skill or move to the next phase of learning a particular skill. Third, accurate data collection helps maintain consistency across a learner's program. If a learner's data are excessively variable, it is often a red flag that her therapists are implementing treatment inconsistently. Finally, data collection is often required to secure and maintain funding. Many funding agencies and state laws require that providers of behavioral intervention to children with ASD keep accurate data throughout the treatment process. If continued progress is not documented on an ongoing basis, many funding providers will try to discontinue funding for treatment. A learner will always be able to make progress in a top-quality behavior intervention program, and these funding issues underscore the need to collect data that demonstrate that progress and alert the supervisor when a treatment plan is falling short.

DATA COLLECTION

Discrete Trial Data

A substantial portion of behavioral intervention programs for children with ASD is dedicated to discrete trial training (DTT), so it follows that DTT data represent a large amount of the overall data that are collected. Generally speaking, data are recorded on the learner's response for every single trial. Specifically, for each trial, the learner's response is categorized according to one of several specific categories, the most common of which are **correct, incorrect**, and **no response**. It is also very common to keep a separate record of responses that are prompted, so responses can also be scored as either **prompted correct** or **prompted incorrect**. You might wonder why the category of "prompted incorrect" would be necessary, since a prompt should produce a correct response, particularly a physical prompt. Many times, however, a prompt fails to evoke a correct response, such as with gestural or partial physical prompts.

Discrete trial data should be summarized and graphed frequently, ideally after each block of trials (e.g., every 5–15 trials). To summarize the data, divide the total number of unprompted correct responses by the total number of trials and multiply by 100, yielding a percentage of correct responses. This percentage is then graphed for each block of trials, so it can be visually inspected on a daily basis. Skills LogBook™ allows the data to be entered and tracked electronically on an ongoing basis (Chapter 26).

Data on procedures used. Many clinicians find it useful to record various aspects of the teaching procedure on each trial as well. For example, they may record whether a prompt was used and, if so, which particular prompt. The particular stimuli presented and their respective locations are also sometimes recorded.

Data on correction procedures. Some clinicians believe that discrete trial data should include only the learner's initial response to each trial and should not include responses made during correction procedures. For example, if 10 trials were conducted and the learner made one error, the data would include nine correct responses and one incorrect response and would not include data on the learner's prompted response during the correction procedure, for a total of nine out of 10 correct responses (90% correct). Other clinicians believe that discrete trial data should include all responses made by the learner, regardless of whether they are the initial response to a teaching trial or whether they occur during a correction procedure. In the example above, the data would then include nine correct responses, one incorrect response, and one prompted response, for a total of nine out of 11 correct responses (82% correct). Both data collection procedures work well. The general approach of the Center for Autism and Related Disorders (CARD) is to collect data on all responses during correction procedures, as it is a more complete description of what the learner actually did and also leads to a somewhat more stringent measure in that errors result in a greater decrease in percentage correct. That is, each error results in two total trials being counted against the overall percentage correct: the initial incorrect response, plus the prompted response during the correction procedure.

DTT datasheets. At the very minimum, DTT datasheets must have one space to record data for the response on each trial. To make data collection faster, it is often convenient to provide different symbols that could be scored for each trial, so the clinician need only circle the one that applies. Figure 20.1 shows a standard discrete trial data collection sheet used in the CARD Model. The datasheet allows the therapist to specify which target is being addressed on each trial, which type of prompting is being used, what the learner's response was, and any other relevant notes. Of course, basic information, such as the learner's name, the date, the therapist's name, and time of day, should be recorded as well. Within the CARD Model, an integrated software application, SkillsBook™, which operates on iPads®, has been developed to make the data collection process electronic and to allow data to be wirelessly synchronized to the Skills® server (see Chapter 26).

First trial data. Instead of collecting data on every response by a learner to every discrete trial, some clinicians believe that it is only necessary to

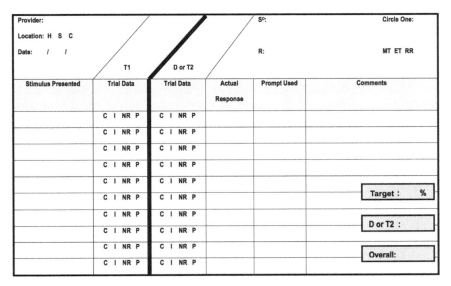

FIGURE 20.1 Standard CARD discrete trial datasheet. *Reprinted with permission from the Center for Autism and Related Disorders.*

collect data the very first time a particular trial is conducted each day. The rationale behind this practice is twofold. First, when the learner receives a consequence (reinforcement for correct, error correction for incorrect) for her first response to a particular trial at the beginning of the day, that consequence affects how she will respond to repetitions of that same trial later in that trial block and even later in that day. This may be especially true when the learner makes an error on the first trial. If she receives a correction procedure and then manages to respond correctly throughout the rest of the block of trials, it may appear as though she has responded at or above the mastery criteria and, therefore, may be thought to have mastered the lesson. In rare cases, a learner may not have actually mastered the skill; she may simply be doing what she was corrected to do a short time ago. If the only data that are counted are those from the very first trial, they will show that very same learner as not yet having mastered the skill, and teaching will continue until she responds correctly to the first trial on two or more consecutive days. A second rationale for collecting data only on the first trial of the day is that less data collection requires less of the therapist's time, thereby potentially freeing him to conduct more teaching in the same amount of session time. A small amount of previously published research has directly compared outcomes of collecting first trial data to outcomes of collecting data on all trials, and the preliminary results suggest little difference in outcome, thereby implying that, perhaps, first trial data collection is adequate (Najdowski et al., 2009). However, at the time this book was written, no studies had compared the implementation of the two types of data collection across a learner's actual whole therapy program, and no studies had evaluated whether first trial data collection actually allows clinicians to conduct more teaching.

Probe data. Often, you may want to conduct a brief probe of a particular skill with a learner outside of trying to teach the skill. This may occur before teaching begins, as a sort of abbreviated baseline measurement. For example, if you want to teach a learner to recognize emotional facial expressions, you might run through a stack of emotion flashcards, delivering one trial per card and simply recording a "correct" or "incorrect" for each card. Cards to which the learner responds correctly may not need to be taught, whereas cards that result in an incorrect response may go in a different stack to be probed again for potential inclusion in teaching. Some clinicians believe that no consequences for learner responding should be given during probing in order to ensure a purer test of the learner's skill. For example, if the learner makes a correct response, even by chance, and you reinforce it, then she might be more likely to make another correct response to the next probe of that skill, thereby producing a "false positive" result, suggesting that the child already has the skill when she actually may not. However, other clinicians believe that feedback during probing is important because you should try to capitalize on any additional learning that might occur during this process. In any case, you would do well to intersperse probe trials with trials of mastered targets to make sure that the learner has the opportunity to be correct and receive reinforcement for responding to you.

Task Analysis Data

When implementing chaining, data are generally collected on the steps in the task analysis. Data are generally collected both on whether the step was performed correctly and on what level of prompting was implemented. The data can be summarized as the percentage of the total steps that are being implemented correctly each time the task analysis is conducted. Take care to note on the datasheet the percentage that indicates correct responding at the current level. For example, if you are only teaching one step at a time (i.e., either backward chaining or forward chaining), and you are currently teaching the first step of a 10-step task analysis, then perfect responding would only represent 10% of the entire chain.

Free Operant Data

Many critically important behaviors occur outside of discrete trials, task analyses, or other structured, teacher-initiated opportunities. Behaviors that are not restricted in their rate of occurrence by teacher-controlled opportunities are referred to as "free operant." For example, the total number of times a learner independently asks for an apple per day would be the learner's "free operant rate" of manding for apples. In contrast, if you wanted to measure how often a learner says "apple" in response to a teacher asking, "Name a fruit that is crunchy, sweet, and red," the behavior is not free operant because, by definition, it can only occur in response to opportunities that are controlled by the teacher. This behavior would be measured as per-opportunity accuracy data, as in discrete trial data described above. Below, we describe the most common methods for collecting data on free operant behavior. While there are many variations, for the sake of space, we describe how to use the methods that we find the most commonly useful. Figure 20.2 is a standard behavior tracking form used in the CARD Model, allowing the user to specify the type of measurement used and providing a space to summarize the data when recording is complete. Skills LogBook™ replaces paper free operant datasheets and allows these data to be collected and tracked electronically.

Frequency/rate. The most basic and fundamental way to measure a behavior is simply to count how many times it happens. This is referred to as frequency data. Generally speaking, frequency data collection is considered the gold standard because it is usually the most direct measure of the

Behavior	Meas.	Initials_____ Date____ / ____ / ____ Duration(s) of Recording _____		Initials_____ Date____ / ____ / ____ Duration(s) of Recording _____	
		Raw Data	Conversion	Raw Data	Conversion
1.	F R D L % IRT				
2.	F R D L % IRT				
3.	F R D L % IRT				
4.	F R D L % IRT				
5.	F R D L % IRT				

FIGURE 20.2   Standard CARD free operant behavior tracking form. *Reprinted with permission from the Center for Autism and Related Disorders.*

behavior. Therefore, you should always consider frequency data collection first and determine whether it is practical and whether it captures the aspects of the behavior that matter the most in your particular clinical situation. When collecting frequency data, you simply count the number of times the behavior happens during your observation. If there is any possibility that the clinicians on the team will make observations of different length, you may need to correct for this by converting the frequency data into rate. To do this, you divide the frequency of the observation by the number of minutes or hours that the observation lasted. For example, if you observed the learner for 10 minutes and the behavior occurs 20 times, you would summarize that as a rate of two times per minute. Frequency data may be impossible to collect when behaviors occur at particularly high rates, especially if the clinician collecting data is also responsible for working with the learner, which is usually the case.

Duration. Duration data involves recording the total amount of time that elapses from the beginning of the behavior to its end. For example, when a learner begins a tantrum, a clinician may press start on a stopwatch and then press stop when the tantrum is over. The duration of time is then recorded from the stopwatch onto the datasheet. Duration data occasionally reveal the effects of an intervention when frequency data do not. For example, a learner may have approximately one tantrum per day before treatment begins, and the tantrums may last up to an hour. After an effective behavior intervention plan is put into effect, she still may have about one tantrum per day, but the duration of tantrums may gradually decrease to 30 minutes, then 20, and then 10, stabilizing at one tantrum per day lasting 6 minutes. If you only recorded frequency data, the data would show that the intervention had no effect, when, in reality, it produced a 90% decrease in the amount of time spent tantrumming.

Latency. Latency is used far less as a measure of behavior and involves measuring the duration of time that elapses between an event and the time the learner begins responding. For example, if a teacher asks, "What's five times five?" and the learner thinks about it and responds 5 seconds later with "25," then the learner's latency to response would be 5 seconds. Latency can be particularly important for social behavior, where a slow latency can make a child seem awkward or "weird" to other children.

Partial interval. Partial interval data is an indirect measure of behavior that can be useful for obtaining an estimate of how much a behavior is happening. In partial interval data, an observation is divided up into many intervals of equal length. Figure 20.3 is a sample interval datasheet with 60 intervals that can be used for partial interval, whole interval, or momentary time sampling. The observer scores a plus or minus for every interval. For partial interval, a plus is scored if the behavior happened at all during the interval. A minus is scored if the behavior never happened during the interval. Therefore, a plus means one or more occurrences of the behavior, and a minus means zero. The data are then summarized as the percentage of intervals during which the behavior occurred. Note that

Interval Recording Data Sheet

Client: _____ Therapist: _____ Date: _____ Target behavior: _____

Setting: _____ Partial / Whole / Momentary Time   Interval Duration: _____

+ / −	+ / −	+ / −	+ / −	+ / −	+ / −	+ / −	+ / −	+ / −	+ / −
+ / −	+ / −	+ / −	+ / −	+ / −	+ / −	+ / −	+ / −	+ / −	+ / −
+ / −	+ / −	+ / −	+ / −	+ / −	+ / −	+ / −	+ / −	+ / −	+ / −
+ / −	+ / −	+ / −	+ / −	+ / −	+ / −	+ / −	+ / −	+ / −	+ / −
+ / −	+ / −	+ / −	+ / −	+ / −	+ / −	+ / −	+ / −	+ / −	+ / −
+ / −	+ / −	+ / −	+ / −	+ / −	+ / −	+ / −	+ / −	+ / −	+ / −

Summary: _____ / 60 x 100 = _____% of intervals

FIGURE 20.3   Sample interval datasheet with 60 intervals. The user specifies the interval length. If each interval was 10 seconds, the total observation time would be 10 minutes. If intervals were 1 minute, the total time would be 1 hour, and so on.

partial interval data collection provides a very rough estimate of the behavior because, on any given interval, the behavior could occur once or 50 times and still only be scored as a plus for that one interval. All other things being equal, the longer the duration of your intervals, the easier data collection will be but the more inaccurate your data will be. In research, intervals of approximately 10 seconds are common. In practice, intervals of 1–10 minutes are more common. A very crude but sometimes useful method for collecting data across an entire school day is to divide the entire day into consecutive 15-minute intervals. It is worth noting that partial interval data tend to overestimate the occurrence of a behavior because if the behavior happens even once in an interval (even a very long interval), that whole interval is counted as a "plus." For that reason, be aware of the possibility of overestimation when interpreting partial interval data.

Whole interval. Whole interval data is the opposite of partial interval data. An interval is only scored as a plus if the behavior occurs for the *entire duration* of the interval. This system is used much less frequently than partial interval, likely because it requires the data collector to stare at the behavior for the entire duration of every interval. Also, it tends to underestimate the occurrence of a behavior. For example, a behavior could occur for 59 seconds out of a 60-second interval, and it would still be scored as a minus because there was just one moment in the interval when it did not occur.

Momentary time sampling. Momentary time sampling is an interval data collection procedure that requires far less time and focus from the data collector than partial or whole interval. To collect momentary time sampling data, the data collector only observes the behavior at the very moment that an interval elapses and scores a plus or minus for that very moment only. The data collector then waits for the next interval to elapse and then again records data only for that very moment. Momentary time sampling data can be very useful in situations where staff simply cannot collect data in a more direct and continuous manner. For example, a teacher who is responsible for teaching a classroom of 20 children does not have time to collect continuous data on any one student. However, the same teacher probably could take momentary time sampling data on one particular behavior (e.g., on-task), using 15-minute intervals.

TREATMENT EVALUATION AND DATA ANALYSIS

In their seminal article on the defining characteristics of ABA, Baer, Wolf & Risley (1968) discussed how ABA is "analytical." They meant that careful evaluation of the effects of procedures is at the heart of ABA. One of the features that distinguishes ABA from virtually all other autism treatments is the insistence that each individual component of a learner's treatment program needs to be evaluated using objective data. Behavior analysts believe they are accountable for the effectiveness of their treatments. Data must be collected and graphed on a daily basis, so they can be visually inspected and treatment decisions can be made on the basis of the data. When treatments are not working, it is not a failure; it is an opportunity to change aspects of the learner's environment until the desired result is produced.

Logbooks. Each learner has his own treatment logbook that contains all of the learner's lesson activities, behavior intervention plans for challenging behavior, acquisition datasheets, challenging behavior datasheets, and data analysis graphs. Essentially, the logbook is the place where the learner's entire treatment plan and accompanying data are stored. Each session, therapists use the logbook to determine what needs to be taught and which challenging behaviors need to be tracked, as well as to keep track of what happens during therapy sessions. Traditionally, ABA programs have used three-ring binders to store all of this content in paper form. In the CARD Model, Skills LogBook™, a computer application that operates on tablets, is the logbook in electronic form.

Graphs. Data are recorded onto datasheets in the logbook and then plotted onto data analysis graphs, both for skills in acquisition and for challenging behavior. Data are tracked using whatever measurement the clinical supervisor puts in place for the lesson. Once the data are recorded, therapists convert the data into a form of measurement as indicated by the clinical supervisor and then plot the data onto the data analysis graphs. Depending on what the data are tracking, this could include plotting a percentage correct for a block of trials, frequency of a behavior, rate per minute/hour for a behavior, and so on.

Figure 20.4 is a sample skill acquisition graph, with each critical feature labeled. The graph contains a **vertical axis**, which depicts the measure of the behavior. The **horizontal axis** depicts the passage of time, which generally consists of sessions or days. Each axis has **tick marks**, which demarcate each unit on that axis. Each axis also has **tick mark labels**, which give the tick marks meaning. Each axis is described by an **axis label**, so the team knows exactly what the axis is depicting. Each line of data has **data points** that depict the data for each session. Data points are connected by lines across time. Changes in phases are indicated by **phase lines**, which separate each phase from one another. Data points on either side of phase lines should not be connected. Each phase is clearly described with a **phase label**. If there is more than one type of data point or path of data in the graph, a **legend** is used to label them.

The clinical supervisor reviews these graphs to make data-based decisions for advancing the learner's curriculum program. When the graphs indicate that the learner's performance is improving, treatment

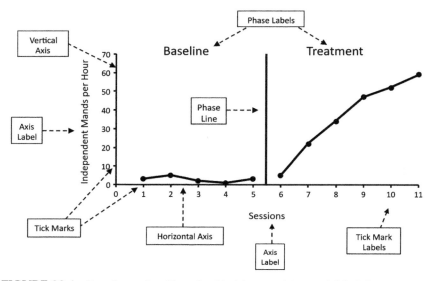

FIGURE 20.4   Sample graph, with each critical feature of the graph labeled.

continues until mastery, and then new targets are introduced. However, when a learner's performance is not improving, adjustments to the teaching procedures are made. This might include changing the target, modifying the response requirement, changing prompts, and so forth. In some cases, the clinical supervisor might also decide to put the target on hold. This could happen if there is a prerequisite skill that needs to be addressed first, if the amount of effort going into teaching the target is not worth the anticipated skill acquisition, or if other, higher priority, issues arise. Data are graphed in the data analysis graphs of the logbook in the following format.

Baseline. This is the first phase of the graph for each target. The purpose of collecting a baseline measure of a skill or challenging behavior is to identify what the status of that behavior is before an intervention is introduced or changed. Without a baseline, one cannot honestly know if a treatment has had an effect, as it is possible that the behavior was getting better or worse anyway and that one just happened to start the new treatment when behavior was already changing, therefore producing a false impression of treatment effectiveness. In research, the minimum number of measurement periods or "sessions" included in baseline is usually three, provided that the data are reasonably stable. This minimum is probably reasonable for most challenging behavior reduction interventions, as long as the challenging behavior is not producing a crisis for anyone involved. For skill acquisition interventions, three data points are usually more than is really required, particularly if it is a skill that the learner clearly does not know and has never demonstrated in the past according to those who know her well. In such cases, one baseline measurement is likely sufficient, particularly if one is measuring accuracy and the learner scores at or near zero percent correct. On the other hand, if there is great variability in the performance of a skill, baseline may need to be longer.

It is also worth noting that baseline does not necessarily mean lack of treatment. If your team has been implementing a particular treatment for a while and it is not working, then the ongoing data that you are currently taking can be used as the baseline against which your next intervention will be compared.

Phase changes. After a stable baseline is observed, the clinical supervisor draws a vertical phase line on the graph, indicating the phase change, and labels each phase at the top of the graph to name the intervention being evaluated in this phase. In order to judge whether the treatment is working, the supervisor evaluates three aspects of the data: 1) *level*, 2) *trend*, and 3) *variability*.

Interpreting Data

Level is obvious – it simply means how high or low the data are. A rapid change in the level of the data – in the direction that the treatment intends – is the strongest indication that the intervention is working. Figure 20.5 depicts a clear change in level from baseline to treatment.

Trend refers to the slope of the data – whether the data are heading in an upward or downward direction. Many effective interventions do not produce an immediate change in level, but they do produce a positive trend that is detectable within a few sessions of intervention. Figure 20.6 depicts such a result.

Variability refers to how much "bounce" there is in the data – how much the data go up and down. Flat lines have zero variability and make the data easiest to interpret. Real data are rarely flat, and

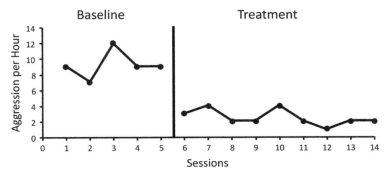

FIGURE 20.5   A clear change in level from baseline to treatment.

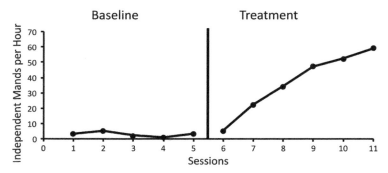

FIGURE 20.6 Independent mands (requests) per hour. A positive change in trend from baseline to treatment, without an immediate change in level.

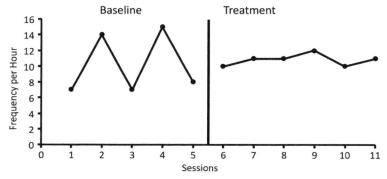

FIGURE 20.7 Rate of spontaneous vocalizations per hour. High degree of variability during baseline and no variability during treatment, yet the mean rate is equal in both phases.

it is assumed that some amount of variability is inherent in behavior. However, the more variable the data, the more difficult it is to evaluate an effect. Figure 20.7 depicts hypothetical data wherein the mean levels of behavior in baseline and intervention are the same, but one phase has a high degree of variability and the other has none. It is far easier to see a change in level when there is lower variability. In practice, it is good to continue collecting data in a phase until variability has either decreased to a reasonable level or you have a good reason to believe it is not going to decrease any further – that is, you have observed the real degree of variability that is present in that phase. Occasionally, an effective treatment may not produce an obvious change in level, but it does produce a very clear change in variability in a desirable direction.

Figure 20.8 depicts hypothetical data on stereotypy in a learner with ASD where an intervention produced a strong decrease, but the most obvious effect on the graph is a decrease in variability, not level. Too much

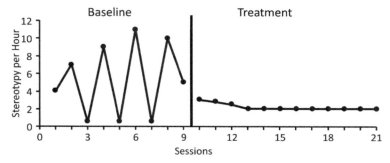

FIGURE 20.8 Rate of stereotypy per hour. High degree of variability during baseline with a large decrease in variability, but only a small decrease in level, during treatment.

variability could imply that numerous other variables are affecting your intervention, and those should be identified to the greatest degree possible. The ideal outcome produced by an intervention would be an immediate change in level, a positive trend, and minimal variability.

When is it time to change something? Poor-quality ABA programs are distinguished by the presence of graphs that show no positive trend and no phase changes for long periods of time. In other words, the treatment is not working, and no one is doing anything about it. Figure 20.9 depicts hypothetical data of teaching a skill for 3 months to a learner with ASD where no change in the treatment program was made. It is clear that, after 2 weeks, the treatment was not producing a change in behavior, and therefore the subsequent 2.5 months were simply a waste of the learner's

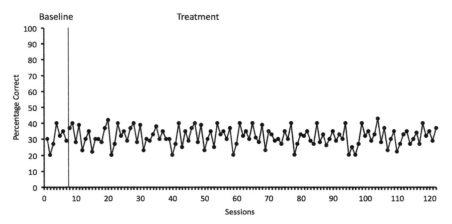

FIGURE 20.9 No change in level or trend for 3 months of treatment. Data like this clearly demonstrate the lack of a treatment effect, as well as the lack of an adequate response by the clinical supervisor. A program change should have been made months earlier.

time. The treatment was not working, and it should therefore have been changed long before 2.5 months elapsed.

No hard and fast rules dictate how frequently failing treatments should be changed. As a general rule, if the treatment team honestly believes enough evidence has been collected to show that an aspect of the treatment plan is not working, then it is time to make a change. Do not "run it out" longer just to see if it might change if it clearly is not changing. Do not simply "give the learner another few weeks to see if he gets it" if there has been no discernible effect of treatment for a while. If a treatment is going to work, you should see at least some change in behavior relatively immediately. If you are using prompting to teach a skill, you should see the intrusiveness or amount of prompting decreasing relatively rapidly, certainly within the first week or two. Many behavioral intervention programs are supervised every 2 weeks by a Board Certified Behavior Analyst (BCBA). This level of supervision may be sufficient, but components of the treatment program will likely need to be adjusted much more frequently, often every day. If a child is learning effectively, she should be mastering content on a regular basis, and new content will therefore need to be introduced regularly. If a new treatment is being implemented for challenging behavior, you should see a change in behavior in well under 2 weeks if the treatment is actually going to work. Often, an effective treatment for challenging behavior will produce a noticeable change in behavior in the first day, sometimes even in the first hour. If your behavior intervention includes extinction for the target challenging behavior, you will often see an immediate worsening of the behavior in the form of an extinction burst. This is actually a sign that your treatment is working and is not a bad thing, as long as the team can avoid reinforcing the behavior during the burst.

Mastery. As with everything else in ABA-based treatment for ASD, mastery criteria are individualized for each learner. A general guideline that works for many skills is 80–100% correct across two or three consecutive sessions. This criterion will need to be adjusted for learners for various reasons. For example, some learners will regress and fail to maintain skills with this criterion, requiring a stricter criterion, such as 90–100% across three or more sessions. Other learners might also require the mastery criterion to include a correct response on the first trial of each block of teaching trials. This is the case for learners who tend to fail on the first trial and then, after receiving one prompt, respond correctly on the remaining trials, yielding a 90% correct. In these cases, learners aren't truly "getting it," as they always get the first trial wrong during each initiation of the activity. You will also want to consider the skill being taught. In some cases, nothing less than a perfect 100% correct is acceptable, such as when teaching safety skills that address how to respond to strangers or what to do when lost. In other cases, responding as high as 90% correct might almost be atypical, such as when teaching the learner to bluff during games.

Typically developing children aren't perfect bluffers, so why would we expect our learners to do anything more than what their typical peers are capable of doing? The best strategy when choosing a mastery criterion for a particular skill and a particular learner is to think about what the behavior looks like in typical development, as well as the learner's historical record of being able to maintain skills that have been "mastered" in the past.

Thus far, our discussion of mastery has been at the level of the individual target. For example, when teaching colors, the targets are "blue," "red," "yellow," and so on. However, the goal for many skills is not to generate rote memorization of how to respond to particular targets, but rather to learn a generalized repertoire centered on a concept. For example, when teaching a learner to detect sarcasm, it is not good enough for the learner to be able to respond appropriately only to the sarcastic statements to which the learner has been exposed during therapy. Thus, the clinical supervisor will not consider the ability to detect sarcasm to be mastered just because the child has learned to detect a short list of specific sarcastic statements. Rather, the clinical supervisor will continue to introduce a variety of sarcastic statements into treatment while testing new ones that have not yet been taught. These probes are conducted to determine whether generalization has occurred to untrained sarcastic statements. Not until the learner is able to respond to novel sarcastic statements without training is the learner said to have "truly mastered" the ability to detect sarcasm. Thus, you will want to make sure that the learner is acquiring a generalized repertoire of behavior using this "test and train" method.

SUMMARY

Top-quality autism treatment depends heavily on therapists collecting accurate data on an ongoing basis, as well as supervisors basing their treatment decisions on those data. Human memory and clinical judgment are not adequate for making decisions regarding the effectiveness of autism treatment. A hallmark feature of ABA is a reliance on data-based decision making and data-based accountability for treatment effectiveness.

21

Organizational Structure

Jonathan Tarbox

Delivery of top-quality comprehensive autism treatment requires a tiered service delivery model, as it is truly a team-based approach that cannot be accomplished by one professional alone. Single applied behavior analysis (ABA) consultants can work alone and deliver direct service to achieve very targeted goals, such as toilet training or decreasing self-injury. To provide comprehensive behavioral intervention, however, a team of individuals is inevitably required.

Treatment teams include, at a minimum, individuals who work directly with the learners and the individuals who supervise them. In this chapter, we will refer to the former as *therapists* and the latter as *clinical supervisors*. Other names for the therapist position that are common in the ABA field include tutor, instructor, teacher, and technician. Clinical supervisors are sometimes referred to as case managers, clinical specialists, or behavioral specialists, depending on the region, treatment funding entity, and particular organization. As treatment is scaled up in larger organizations, more levels of management become critical to maintain treatment quality, and we will discuss several of these other job descriptions below. This chapter will describe the duties of each professional at each level, as well as how these roles can be customized to accommodate the size and location of the ABA provider's organization.

Naturally, very little research has been done on the optimal clinical structure of an organization, so we provide advice based on our quarter-century of clinical experience. Other formats may also be effective, and care should be taken to customize the job descriptions of any organization to the unique logistical, legal, and cultural requirements of each individual region and organization. In addition, job descriptions are highly influenced by local billing requirements. For example, in one state, Board Certified Behavior Analyst (BCBA) certification may be sufficient for billing third-party funding for clinical supervision, whereas in another region, state licensure as a psychologist may be required.

Therefore, job descriptions should be considered somewhat flexible and must be adapted to local logistical and legal realities.

CLINICAL JOB DESCRIPTIONS

Therapist

The therapist is the professional who works directly with the learner with autism spectrum disorder (ASD) and, therefore, has the greatest direct impact on the learner. Therapists provide the majority of the ABA treatment hours. They are responsible for directly implementing a learner's treatment plan, organizing and updating a learner's lesson materials (e.g., recording lesson data and graphing daily progress), writing detailed notes during clinic meetings, making instructional materials, communicating with other team members to ensure consistent implementation of procedures, and helping train new therapists.

Generally speaking, therapists are responsible for implementing treatment and collecting data. A good therapist needs to be adept at implementing all possible ABA-based treatment techniques (see Chapter 22), so she can readily and rapidly adjust to the unique needs of each learner. A good therapist also familiarizes herself with each learner's program, unique traits, pool of reinforcers, and so on, so she does not need to take an excessive amount of therapy time to consult written documents to identify which procedures to use. Good therapists are ambitious but humble, are open to feedback, and change their behavior readily when they receive feedback.

A good therapist knows she is the eyes and ears of the supervisor, but she is not the supervisor herself. A good therapist knows that her job is to implement a learner's therapy program, not to design or change it; that is the job of the clinical supervisor, as described below. This is not to say that creativity and initiative should not be encouraged – quite the contrary – but therapists should communicate their ideas of how to modify or enhance the learner's treatment program to the clinical supervisor. The clinical supervisor then decides whether to test the idea. This rule is in place to ensure consistency, not to discourage therapists from being professionally invested in the learner's outcome. If therapists were given the authority to try out whatever they thought might be a good idea, then far too much "experimentation" would likely ensue across the various therapists on a team, and it would be all but impossible to identify what was actually working and what was not. By definition, therapists do not have the necessary training and experience to make expert supervisory decisions. Good clinical supervisors encourage therapists to make observations, generate ideas, and offer their ideas to their clinical supervisor.

Clinical supervisors often receive multiple ideas from different therapists related to the same clinical issue and then choose which, if any, of the ideas should be tested with data.

Therapist credentials. The question of what previous experience, credentials, and education are necessary for newly hired therapists is one that is still debated. In many outcome studies (e.g., Lovaas, 1987), therapists were undergraduate college students whose experience was comprised of approximately two university courses and a small amount (e.g., 10 weeks) of previous practical experience working with learners with ASD. The outcomes of these studies were robust, showing that therapists are effective with no substantial previous experience or level of education. However, therapists in these studies were provided with fairly intensive clinical supervision by graduate students and doctoral level behavior analysts. At the time this book goes to press, there is still no standard as to what background and education level are necessary for new therapists. Many service provision agencies require at least a bachelor's degree, but very few agencies require any substantial amount of previous experience working with learners with autism, and many agencies do not even require a bachelor's degree.

From a purely behavioral perspective, there is no reason to believe that an average undergraduate college education would help prepare one to be a better ABA therapist. The vast majority of undergraduate students do not take a single course in behavioral psychology and do not receive any experience working with children of any kind. The outcome studies have shown that, given proper training and supervision from expert behavior analysts, no particular previous experience or credentials are necessary for someone to perform well as a therapist.

In reality, the experience and credentials that are required for entry-level therapists are often influenced more by the requirements of funding agencies and/or legislative mandates than by anything else. Some funding agencies require a minimum of a bachelor's degree. Some require a bachelor's degree, plus a minimum number of months of experience working with learners with autism and/or implementing ABA procedures. Some require all of the above, plus some minimum amount of undergraduate coursework in ABA. While each of these funding agencies may have its own justifications for its requirements, the truth is that few or none of these requirements are supported by research. Although it has rarely or never been proven, consumer advocates often note that funding agencies appear to make credential requirements more demanding when they need to decrease the amount of funding they provide for treatment. That is, strict requirements for therapists regarding credentialing, licensing, and/or experience can limit access to treatment by narrowing the pool of individuals who meet the requirements to provide treatment. For example, some insurance plans require the therapist to be a BCBA. Since BCBAs supervise multiple learners, they would rarely have sufficient time in their schedules to provide the one-to-one therapy. With few or no qualified individuals to provide therapy, the insurance plan's requirement effectively puts therapy out of reach. While inappropriately demanding standards should be challenged and overturned, the current system of no consistent standards is not acceptable because it essentially leaves it to the individual service providers to take the responsibility to hire good people and to train them properly, with no real checks on quality.

A credentialing process for newly hired therapists that is based on the competencies that actually matter for the job would address this problem. This process will need to balance two conflicting priorities: 1) ensuring high standards and 2) not restricting the number of therapists who can be trained and hired quickly to meet the demands for therapy. The Behavior Analyst Certification Board (BACB) has taken a promising step in the right direction with its newly created Registered Behavioral Technician™ (RBT) credential (www.bacb.com). The RBT credential requires that therapists receive 40 hours of training and demonstrate competence on a list of basic ABA-based procedures. The RBT program is an exciting development and represents a significant step forward for the field of ABA in ensuring competence at the therapist level. However, like the BCBA and Board Certified assistant Behavior Analyst (BCaBA) certifications, the RBT credential is not specific to autism, so it will be possible to become an RBT without ever having worked with children with autism. While the BACB's RBT program offers a potential framework for ensuring a minimum level of therapist competency, the Center for Autism and Related Disorders (CARD) approach to training therapists, as described in Chapter 22, is substantially more comprehensive than the RBT program and is specific to ABA-based intervention for autism.

Another development that would be highly helpful to the field of autism treatment is the expansion of therapist training at the 4-year and 2-year college levels. Many disciplines, such as nurses, physician assistants, dental hygienists, and others, have efficient and cost-effective training programs at 2- and 4-year colleges, thereby speeding up the training process and taking much of the training burden off of the organizations that provide services. Such programs would also offer an opportunity to standardize training to ensure a minimal level of therapist competency that is elusive when adequate training is defined differently from one provider to the next.

Senior Therapist

As organizations scale-up, they often find it useful to give particularly competent senior therapists a slightly elevated degree of responsibility. Senior therapists at CARD receive additional training and assist the clinical supervisor by helping oversee the delivery of treatment. In discrete trial training (DTT), each lesson needs to be advanced on a regular basis, either from one phase of teaching to another within a particular acquisition target (e.g., from mass trial to random rotation), from one exemplar to another within a particular instruction (e.g., from teaching "blue" to teaching "red"), or from one instruction to another within the same lesson (e.g., from teaching receptive identification of the color "blue" to tacting blue objects). As described in Chapter 4 on teaching procedures, it is critical to have objective criteria specified for each of these transitions. It is the job of the senior therapist to "check up" on a case on a regular basis in order to assess when such transitions should be made and to implement them. To be clear, senior therapists are still therapists and do not use or replace supervisor hours. Ideally, each learner works with a senior therapist at least twice per week to ensure that progression within lessons is on track.

Another critical responsibility of senior therapists is to help in training and oversight of entry-level therapists. When a new therapist is first being trained and acquiring field experience, a senior therapist should be present as often as possible to model correct implementation of therapy and to give immediate feedback to new therapists while they perform therapy. Depending on the experience level, senior therapists may be trusted to help with *in vivo* performance evaluations of entry-level therapists as well. In addition, when a therapist is first added to a learner's treatment team (even if she is a seasoned therapist), she should be given child-specific training. Senior therapists should be physically present for at least a few hours to overlap with the new therapists during these transitions.

Senior therapist credentials. No additional credentials are required of a senior therapist above those required for a therapist. Promotion to senior therapist should be purely competency based. However, if the senior therapist position is considered part of the track toward eventual promotion to the clinical supervisor position, candidates for the senior therapist position should be working toward attending graduate school, since a master's degree will be required of them and it generally takes 2 or more years to complete it. The BCaBA certification is particularly well suited to professionals working at the senior therapist level. However, many senior therapists are also attending master's programs and looking forward to pursuing their BCBA. In those instances, the BCaBA certification is not always the most efficient option, since it does not help the professional progress toward becoming a BCBA. Therefore, such professionals usually opt to enroll in a master's program and begin their BCBA coursework as soon as possible.

Case Manager

Case managers are BCBAs or are professionally licensed in a related discipline and are in the process of being trained to be supervisors.

Case managers are also sometimes referred to as case consultants or supervisor trainees. Case managers should begin to take on as much of the clinical supervisor duties as their qualifications allow, always under the careful mentorship of qualified clinical supervisors. Chapter 22 includes a detailed description of the many tasks that case managers should complete under the supervision of a clinical supervisor during their mentorship process.

Care Coordinator

Care coordinators work under the direction of the clinical supervisor assigned to each case. Care coordinators assist with writing reports, updating learner curriculum programs, collecting data, organizing and maintaining programs, scheduling, and coordinating calls and meetings with parents and therapists. Care coordinators also perform client observations and provide observation data to the supervisor.

Care coordinator credentials. Care coordinators are required to have a minimum of a bachelor's degree and several years of experience delivering top-quality behavioral intervention to children with ASD. Care coordinators generally have the same minimum credentials as candidates for the clinical supervisor position, except that they do not have a master's degree.

Therapist Liaison

As described earlier, the therapist position is absolutely critical to the success of treatment for children with ASD. All top-quality ABA service provision organizations will rise or fall on the quality and performance of their therapists. Therefore, it is sometimes useful to take extra steps to ensure that therapists are well trained and have easy access to resources and to experienced individuals who contribute to their effectiveness. Some agencies find it useful to appoint a specific person to ensure this, sometimes as a smaller portion of their overall job as a senior therapist or case manager. At CARD, this role is taken by the therapist liaison, who helps with training newly hired therapists by performing the didactic portion of training. The therapist liaison also functions as a mentor to new therapists (e.g., being present to answer questions, give advice, etc.).

Maintaining high therapist morale is also an important role of the therapist liaison. Activities that can contribute to this include holding regular therapist meetings, during which individual therapists are acknowledged for exemplary performance and therapists have opportunities to socialize with one another and receive praise from clinical supervisors. Particularly when treatment services are delivered in the home setting, therapists can feel detached from one another and can therefore benefit from more frequent contact with each other and from enthusiastic support from the organization.

Clinical Supervisor

The clinical supervisor is the professional who is ultimately responsible for the clinical quality of the learner's treatment program. CARD clinical supervisors manage the design, implementation, and evaluation of their learners' individualized treatment plans. They also train therapists and family members to implement treatment protocols and collaborate with other service providers (e.g., speech and language pathologists, occupational therapists, and classroom teachers).

It is probably not an exaggeration to say that the clinical supervisor position is the single most important professional position in the treatment of learners with ASD. Therapists are the ones who do the treatment, but there would be no treatment to do if a clinical supervisor had not first designed it. Moreover, the quality of the treatment would be sorely lacking if it were not monitored and adjusted by an expert clinical supervisor on an ongoing basis. In addition, a good clinical supervisor can take virtually any enthusiastic, hardworking person and train him to do therapy in a matter of months. On the other hand, even the most intelligent, hardworking person can take years to become an expert clinical supervisor. The entire process of clinical supervision is so complex and so central to the outcomes of autism intervention that an entire chapter is dedicated to it (Chapter 19), so we will not describe the supervision process further here.

Clinical supervisor credentials. At CARD, professionals are not considered for a supervisory position until they have had at least 2 years (and usually even more) of experience implementing top-quality autism intervention. The training process is intensive and comprehensive and is described in Chapter 22. In terms of professional credentials, clinical supervisors are required to pursue master's degrees and to have their BCBA certification or licensure in a related field. The insurance laws in many states require a supervisor to have either a BCBA certification or a professional license in a related discipline. Many other funding agencies, aside from insurance, also have similar requirements, and the requirements vary from state to state and from region to region within each state.

HIGHER LEVEL CLINICAL LEADERSHIP

Clinical Manager

In the CARD Model, each clinical site or school that has two or more clinical supervisors specifies one of them as the leader for that location. In other words, one person must ultimately be held accountable for the clinical quality of services provided in each center or in the homes serviced by each clinical site. The clinical manager's responsibilities include mentoring case managers and new clinical supervisors, holding regular staff meetings with clinical supervisors and therapists, providing clinical staff trainings in that office and/or overseeing other clinical supervisors who do so, and meeting with representatives from local funding agencies, to name a few. Depending on the size of the clinic, clinical managers may supervise a reduced caseload of their own (perhaps 30% of the caseload of a regular clinical supervisor), or they may spend 100% of their time supervising the clinical supervisors, who, in turn, do all of the clinical supervision. The clinical manager works closely with the operations manager (see below) in that they are the two directors of that site – one clinical and one operational. Furthermore, clinical managers are responsible for conducting regular evaluations of the clinical supervisors at their site. The clinical manager reports to the clinical director.

It is common in organizations of all types for people who are good at their current job to be promoted to the next level. This makes sense intuitively, but people often continue to be promoted until the demands of their position exceed their ability. That is, they are no longer doing what they are good at; they are, instead, managing others who do so. This has been called being "promoted to incompetence" and is a very real problem in many organizations. Keep in mind that people who are excellent clinical supervisors will not necessarily be excellent leaders and managers of other clinical supervisors. Promotion to clinical manager must be made on the basis of the competencies that will be involved in the job.

Clinical managers must be organized, proactive, great leaders, positive, hardworking, optimistic, and very approachable. Clinical managers set the tone for their entire clinic. If they demonstrate a genuinely positive attitude, the rest of the staff will do the same. If they demonstrate negativity, the staff will mimic that, too. Junior-level staff in any organization want solid leaders who deserve their respect. Junior-level employees imitate senior-level employees; whether they realize it, it's a fact of human behavior.

Regional Clinical Manager

Any organization that has more than several locations may need to begin to consider designating one clinician as the regional clinical manager for each region in which there are several clinics or schools. The regional clinical manager's job is to supervise the clinical managers of each location.

Clinical Director

In all organizations, across any discipline, the buck must ultimately stop somewhere. In autism treatment organizations, the clinical buck stops with the clinical director. It is crucial to have one expert clinician who is responsible for ensuring the provision of top-quality services across the entire organization. There is no research on the ideal background or credentials of a clinical director, but there is some consensus within the field of ABA that the person should be a BCBA or licensed in a related discipline (clinical, developmental, or experimental psychology or education) with perhaps 5 or more years of experience treating learners with ASD. As with any job, the most important qualification is a demonstrated track record of excellent performance with the particular skills required for the job. The clinical director meets with clinical managers (or the regional clinical managers who supervise them) on a regular basis in order to ensure that they are doing their utmost to maintain the highest clinical quality at their sites. In addition, the clinical director serves an important problem-solving function for all clinical supervisors in that she is available for consultation on individual cases that are particularly unique or challenging.

MANAGEMENT AND ADMINISTRATION

All organizations require the same administrative staff, including human resources, finance, and so on. In the CARD Model, the majority of management and administrative work occurs at corporate headquarters, so clinicians at each site can be left to work as clinicians. Just as we would not expect a businessperson to start implementing ABA therapy with a learner with ASD, it is not reasonable to expect an expert ABA clinical supervisor to start running the business side of operations in an ABA clinic without any training in business operations, yet that is exactly what is often done! Many ABA clinics start small and unintentionally put ABA clinicians into positions of managing finance, payroll, billing, human resources, and so on, despite a total lack of expertise in these areas. This is a recipe for disaster, and it will eventually catch up with you if this is how you are running your organization. The corporate management and administration side of CARD is too large to describe in this chapter, but we have found that two particular administrative positions are so critical for allowing clinicians to do their jobs that they deserve to be described here: scheduler and operations manager.

Scheduler

Home-based ABA service provision is notorious for being a scheduling nightmare. Family illness, therapist illness, traffic accidents, inclement weather, the learner's extracurricular activities, and a myriad of other factors collectively make it difficult to maintain staffing for home-based intervention services. The fact that every learner's family schedule is different and that many therapists are college students who work part time also make it challenging to maintain complete schedules and thereby provide a learner with 100% of the therapy hours to which she is entitled. For this reason, many organizations find it useful to dedicate a specific full-time position just to this task.

Although scheduling is not a clinical job, the impact that it has on clinical quality cannot be overstated. For example, when a therapist calls in sick and another therapist must be scheduled to fill in, many factors contribute to the decision of which therapist should be chosen. Significant variables include geographic area of the learner, potential fill-in therapists, and therapist availability, at a minimum. In addition, fill-in therapists should ideally have previous experience working with that learner. If that is not possible, the experience level of each potential fill-in therapist with other similar learners in the past must be considered. Ideally, any therapist should be able to work with any learner, but the reality is not always that simple. For example, if a therapist has never worked with a learner with particularly severe challenging behavior, then a fill-in is probably not the best time to do so for the first time. Similarly, a therapist who has only worked with very young, minimally verbal learners in the past would not be the best choice for a fill-in with a highly verbal 10-year-old who is primarily working on complex perspective-taking skills. The gender of the client or therapist may also play a role in the therapist selection process. For example, if you have a female client who is learning skills related to menstruation, a male therapist would not be an appropriate choice. You would be wise to choose good people to schedule your sessions, train them extensively, and make sure you support them – they have a very stressful job!

Operations Managers

We have found that operations managers can be particularly helpful in running the business and operations aspects of each office location. Operations managers' duties include such tasks as locating new office space, negotiating leases, undertaking local marketing and outreach efforts, and dealing with building facilities and maintenance staff, among many others. One of the most important functions of the operations manager is to oversee the financial viability of the individual site. Regardless of whether your site is for profit, nonprofit, a private school, a public school, or any other format of service delivery, someone needs to manage the financial side of operations, so the lights stay on and the rent gets paid. If this job is not specifically assigned to an administrative staff member, such as an operations manager, then someone else is going to have to do it. All too often, the clinical supervisor or clinical manager is expected to perform these duties, and in many cases, clinical staff are perfectly capable of learning these skill sets. However, keep in mind that is not what they were hired to do and not what they are trained to do. The more time clinicians spend on operations, the less time they can spend helping learners and training others to help learners. Many expert clinicians will burn out if they are given excessive operations responsibilities.

SUMMARY

Comprehensive autism treatment is a complex process that cannot be carried out by one person alone. Treatment teams require therapists and senior therapists who provide the treatment directly, as well as clinical supervisors who train and supervise them. Clinical supervisors, in turn, must be supervised by clinical directors and/or clinical managers who are ultimately responsible for the quality of treatment provided at their clinic.

Training and Quality Control

Cecilia H. Knight

The process of training clinical staff has always occupied a critical role in the Center for Autism and Related Disorders (CARD) Model. When CARD was founded in 1990 by Dr. Doreen Granpeesheh, the first staff who were hired were therapists who had been trained at the Lovaas Young Autism Project at the University of California, Los Angeles (UCLA). At that time, the training process for new therapists at the Young Autism Project began with a two-course sequence on applied behavior analysis (ABA), with the first being taught by Dr. Ivar Lovaas and the second by Dr. Granpeesheh. The best students from these courses were then invited to enroll in a practicum course, also taught by Dr. Granpeesheh. The practicum course consisted of a 10-week practicum during which college students worked with children with autism under the close supervision of Dr. Granpeesheh and Dr. Lovaas's other graduate students. Students who excelled in the practicum course were then invited to apply for a therapist position at the Young Autism Project. Therapists received intensive, ongoing supervision while they worked at the clinic. Given that the first 25 therapists to work at CARD had each participated in this rigorous training process, CARD, as an organization, benefited enormously from having extraordinarily well-trained therapists who provided a strong foundation for the training of future staff. As the scale of the organization grew from one or two clinics in the same region to multiple clinics across the United States and abroad, a formalized system of training was developed for every job description.

The CARD Model is infused with top-quality training at every level. The general philosophy behind the CARD approach to staff training is that comprehensiveness and rigor cannot be compromised. In fact, the length, scope, and rigor of the CARD training process are sometimes characterized as "unreasonable." A number of individuals decline to work at CARD because of the demanding nature of the training, a number of trainees terminate their employment because of the demands of the training, and a number of trainees are involuntarily terminated when they repeatedly fail to demonstrate required competencies during training. At CARD, we believe unequivocally that clinical quality is the highest priority and that it cannot be subjugated by convenience or financial pressures. As a rule of thumb, we believe that, if the training process seems reasonable, then it's not good enough. Top-quality training in ABA is expensive, time consuming, and irreplaceable. Having seen the impact of CARD's highly trained professionals on the lives of countless children and their families, we are confident that CARD training equips staff with the skill set required to excel at their jobs. Knowing that short-falls in training would manifest themselves in diminished outcomes for the families we serve, we are committed to investing both the human and financial capital required to produce the most qualified professionals in our field, and we believe this is the only acceptable approach to training.

This chapter describes the training and evaluation process for every clinical job in the CARD organizational system. CARD training programs are, first and foremost, fueled by our desire to provide training that improves clinical excellence at every level. As such, all aspects of CARD training are continually being evaluated and updated to meet the ever-changing demands of our field, integrating new information from research and incorporating professional standards as they continue to evolve. At each level, the training system uses a combination of evidence-based staff training procedures, including web-based eLearning, in-person lecture, in-person discussion, lecture and discussion via videoconference, role-play, feedback, and *in vivo* practice with feedback. To track and ensure effectiveness, written, oral, and hands-on competency evaluations are incorporated at every level.

THERAPIST TRAINING

The foundation of the CARD approach to therapist training has not changed since 1990. A new therapist must still be trained on the behavioral deficits and excesses typical of autism spectrum disorder (ASD), as well as the fundamental principles and procedures of ABA. However, diagnostic information, prevalence, the body of research that supports ABA, the various other treatments available to families, and training media continue to evolve and inform our training process. See Table 22.1 for an outline of therapist qualifications and training. (Qualifications for each job are discussed in detail in Chapter 21.) Therapist training is an interactive and comprehensive training process that prepares its participants to provide effective, evidence-based, 1:1 intervention to learners with ASD. Participants alternately view eLearning modules, role-play various

TABLE 22.1 Therapist Training

Training Component	Requirement
Qualifications	Bachelor's degree or current enrollment in a program that culminates with an associate's or bachelor's degree, experience working one-to-one with learners (children, teens, or adults), no criminal record, and a clear tuberculosis test
Length of training program	Approximately 6 weeks or as mandated by applicable state law
Classroom	40+ hours (15 hours eLearning and 25 hours lecture and role-play)
Overlaps and fieldwork	24–36 hours (12 2- to 3-hour sessions) working with a learner, under supervision of a trainer
Field evaluation	2- to 3-hour session; trainee conducts therapy while trainer observes and evaluates
Final written exam	2-hour written exam

therapy scenarios, and participate in class discussions to underscore important principles, revisit the content of previous modules, and solidify critical points.

Initial Training

Classroom Training

Therapist eLearning. Entry-level therapist training begins with the Therapist eLearning module, a web-based course that is approximately 15 hours long. Each lesson in Therapist eLearning lasts from 30 to 90 minutes and includes:

1. Introduction to ASD and ABA
2. Introduction to Skill Repertoire Building
3. The Discrete Trial
4. Skill Repertoire Building Procedures
5. Behavior Management: Assessment and Interventions
6. Skill Repertoire Building: Data Collection
7. Behavior Management: Data Collection
8. Graphing Behavior Change
9. Generalized Behavior Change

Table 22.2 displays the topics covered in the training. Research has shown that Therapist eLearning effectively establishes academic knowledge of ABA principles and procedures (Granpeesheh et al., 2010). CARD's Therapist eLearning is a product that is commercially available through

TABLE 22.2   Content Topics of Didactic Training for All Major Clinical Positions

Position	Content of Didactic Training
Therapist	Introduction to ASD and ABA, introduction to skill repertoire building, the discrete trial, skill repertoire building procedures, behavior management: assessment and interventions, skill repertoire building: data collection, behavior management: data collection, graphing behavior change, and generalized behavior change
Senior therapist	Initial clinic, preparation for the first session, preparation of a logbook, role of the senior therapist in clinics, general format and process of clinics, advanced topics in discrimination training, probing for generalization and mastery, managing therapist performance, conducting overlaps with new therapists, conducting field evaluations for therapist trainees, conducting ongoing drop-ins with therapists, school shadowing, functional assessment, function-based behavioral interventions, emergency interventions for challenging behavior, data collection, introduction to B. F. Skinner's verbal behavior, brief review of the CARD curriculum, picture communication systems, teaching sight reading, toilet training, prompting for teaching higher-order social and language skills, review of outcome research, introduction to the Individualized Education Program (IEP) process, and parent training
Therapist liaison	Reviewing résumés, how to interview, qualities to look for in a therapist candidate, Health Insurance Portability and Accountability Act, conducting therapist field evaluations, conducting therapist yearly evaluations, conducting therapist mentor meetings, professionalism, and avoiding dual relationships
Clinical supervisor	Outcome research on ABA treatment for children with ASD, how to handle non-evidence-based treatments, understanding and interpreting standardized assessments for learners with ASD, laws related to individuals with disabilities, educational practices across the United States, the Individualized Education Program (IEP) process, data and graphs when making treatment decisions, indirect functional assessment, descriptive functional assessment, experimental functional analyses, all major evidence-based interventions for challenging behavior, writing the BIP, teaching families and staff to implement BIPs appropriately, the client intake process, school placements, managing a school shadow, dealing with conflict with employees, parents, and other professionals, and intensive training in the eight CARD curriculum areas: 1) social, 2) motor, 3) language, 4) play, 5) adaptive, 6) executive function, 7) cognition, and 8) academic skills, designing comprehensive skill acquisition programs that incorporate all

the Institute for Behavioral Training (IBT; www.ibehavioraltraining.com) and is also discussed in Chapter 26.

Therapist eLearning begins with the most fundamental material, such as a basic understanding of ASD, and progresses to more complex topics, such as the principles and procedures of ABA. Throughout the eLearning, a narrator integrates questions from previous lessons into new subject matter, ensuring that the trainees retain the material as they progress through the course. Before providing the correct answer, the narrator reviews potential answers and then reveals the correct answer. Each answer is accompanied by an explanation as to why that answer is the best choice. For example, in the Introduction to ASD and ABA module, one question involves the statement "ASD is likely to be diagnosed more often in boys than in girls." The narrator asks, "Is it a) three times more likely, b) four times more likely, or c) five times more likely?" The narrator pauses and gives the participants time to consider the answer. Then, the narrator supplies the correct response, saying, "The answer is b) four times more likely." At the end of each lesson, trainees take a multiple-choice quiz. Once the therapist trainee completes all of the lessons, she takes a final test that covers the entire Therapist eLearning module. In order to pass the eLearning portion of the training, participants must pass every quiz and the final exam with at least 80% correct.

Role-play and feedback. To supplement the eLearning training, CARD instructors pause the program at multiple points to model therapist roles in various therapy scenarios, guide the trainees through role-play, answer questions, and provide individualized instruction and feedback on the role-playing. For example, after the therapist trainees watch a module on providing reinforcement, they role-play reinforcement with other trainees, breaking into groups of two and alternating the therapist and learner roles. The instructor provides a scenario, models the correct response, and then asks each trainee to practice the same activity. The instructor gives feedback during the role-play, which continues until mastery. The amount of time spent on role-play and feedback is approximately 25 hours, depending on how long it takes trainees to demonstrate mastery in each competency. Thus, with the eLearning video time of approximately 15 hours and the approximately 25 hours of role-play and feedback, the total initial therapist training lasts approximately 40 hours.

Final written exam. After therapist trainees complete the training described above, they must take a written exam comprised of 39 short-answer questions. Trainees have 2 hours to take the exam. They are proctored and must take the exam without notes or any other materials and must score at least 80% in the exam to pass. If a trainee fails the exam, one opportunity is given to retake it. Prior to retaking the exam, trainees have the opportunity and are encouraged to review their initial exam, identify the answers that they missed, meet with the instructor or a clinical supervisor for assistance, and then reschedule the exam within 1 week. Therapist trainees who do not pass the test on the second attempt are not allowed to move forward in the training process.

Field Training

Overlaps. Once therapist trainees pass the written exam, they begin the overlap process. During an overlap, the therapist trainee accompanies a seasoned therapist to a therapy session and observes all aspects of that therapist working with the learner. Therapist trainees are required to attend approximately 12 overlap sessions, depending on the time it takes for the trainee to demonstrate mastery of all therapy competencies while working with learners. In the first session, the trainee is expected to observe and take notes. Gradually, across subsequent sessions, the trainee becomes more involved in the therapy session, until – by the end of the 12th overlap session – the trainee is completing the entire therapy session with a learner while the seasoned therapist observes.

Trainees receive feedback across the 12 overlap sessions. They are given verbal feedback in the moment, as well as written feedback that delineates 84 component competencies required during each session. These components are described in greater detail in the **Field Evaluation** section. For example, when learning to collect data, the trainee is provided with blank datasheets and then uses them to take data while the seasoned therapist conducts therapy. When the learner is given a break, the seasoned therapist reviews the data taken by the trainee, compares the data with her own, and gives the trainee feedback. For example, the therapist might say, "Great job with data on items 1, 3, 4, 5, 6, and 7. You marked item 2 as incorrect, but it was really a non-response. Does that make sense?" The process repeats multiple times per session, thereby providing many opportunities for performance and feedback.

During early overlap sessions, therapist trainees are required to perform only a few competencies. The number of tasks required of them gradually increases across overlaps, with feedback given throughout the process. Each overlap session is 2–3 hours in duration, so the total overlap portion of training typically lasts 24–30 hours. Therapist trainees cannot move on from this portion of the training until they demonstrate competency on all skills. The vast majority of trainees master all competencies within 12 overlaps.

Field evaluation. During a trainee's potential final overlap session, the therapist trainee undergoes a field evaluation. A senior therapist, therapist liaison, or clinical supervisor (see Chapter 21 for job descriptions) conducts the field evaluation. The evaluator observes the therapy session and scores the trainee on a field evaluation form. All competencies being evaluated are objectively defined and include all of the competencies that were trained during the overlap process. The field evaluation form contains 84 items that evaluate the therapist across the following areas: initiative, professionalism, arranging the teaching situation, discrete trial training, teaching during downtime, use of log notes, and behavior management. An example of an item on the evaluation is, "The therapist observes the confidentiality of all clients" or "The therapist fades prompts as the learner gains independence with the target response effectively." Each of the items are scored on a scale from 0 (never) to 4 (always). The scores of all 84 items are then averaged, and a trainee must receive an average score of 3 or higher to pass the field evaluation.

If the trainee scores below 3 on one or more items, she must retake the field evaluation within 1 week. In the interim, the trainee continues to overlap with a trained therapist, and the trained therapist targets the items on which the trainee received low scores during the initial field evaluation. If the trainee scores below a 3 on any item during the second field evaluation, she is not allowed to continue training. After the therapist trainee passes the written exam and the field evaluation, she is no longer a trainee but is a full-fledged therapist, and she is allowed to work with learners without another therapist present. For a full-time employee, the training process usually takes approximately 3 weeks from the time she is hired to the time that she passes the field evaluation and formally becomes a therapist.

Ongoing Training

Clinics. After therapists begin work on their own, they continue to receive training and support from more experienced staff. Each learner has a clinic meeting that typically takes place every 2 weeks (see Chapter 19 on clinical supervision). At clinic meetings, the learner, the learner's parents, all of the therapists who work with the learner, and the clinical supervisor meet to review the learner's progress. Each therapist has a chance to ask questions of the clinical supervisor at this time. Also, the supervisor asks each therapist to demonstrate her skills by conducting lessons with the learner in front of the treatment team while the more experienced clinicians give the new therapists feedback about their performance.

Minor feedback is given during clinics. For example, the supervisor might tell another therapist, "Sally, it may work better if you slide the picture cards closer to Freido, so we are sure that he sees them each time you present them. On the next try, do that and let's see what happens." Then, later in the clinic meeting, the clinical supervisor might say, "Thank you for implementing my feedback. I think it worked better that way. What do you think?" More in-depth feedback, which may be embarrassing or inappropriate to give in a group or in front of the learner's parents, is provided privately. This might occur directly after a clinic meeting in the clinical supervisor's office or on the telephone. For example, the supervisor might say, "Randy, I am noticing that you frequently dress very casually for therapy sessions and clinics. It's important that you are comfortable, but ripped jean shorts and flip flops aren't really appropriate. It's important to dress less casually, so we demonstrate a professional image to parents."

Many teams have senior therapists who also serve an important feedback function for therapists. This feedback can be written, verbal, or both. The senior therapist may observe the therapist working with a learner in his home. In this setting, the senior therapist may give feedback to the therapist by saying, for example, "Great job increasing David's vocalizations today; the target for vocal mands is 20 per session. Make sure you are contriving situations throughout the session to keep him asking for things." Specific feedback of this nature is also accompanied by examples of how to implement it. For example, the senior therapist in this scenario would also suggest a few situations to contrive in order to increase the opportunity for the learner to provide vocal mands.

Mentor meetings. Therapists are assigned a specific supervisor who serves as their mentor. Generally, the mentor is also a supervisor of one of the therapist's learners. Therapists meet with their mentor each month during mentor meetings. During these meetings, mentors discuss ongoing progress, set performance goals, and provide direct feedback to therapists. This time is also used for therapists to discuss employment goals, professional development goals, and their interest in further education (e.g., pursuing a master's degree, Board Certified Behavior Analyst [BCBA] certification, and so on).

Monthly staff meetings/professional development. Each month, a staff meeting is held at the CARD clinic to review policies and procedures and to conduct continued professional development for therapists on a specific topic that is relevant to the therapist's job duties. The 1-hour trainings include topics such as graphing session data, iconic communication systems, behavior management, and so on. Professional development trainings do not duplicate the content of the initial therapist training, but rather build on it.

SENIOR THERAPIST

If a top-performing therapist has worked at CARD for more than 6 months, he may be eligible to enter senior therapist training. First, he must be nominated by his clinical supervisors as someone who would make a good leader on the therapy team. Next, he must pass a "drop-in" by one of his clinical supervisors, and lastly, he must pass a written qualification exam, as described below.

Drop-in. During a drop-in, a clinical supervisor observes a regular therapy session between the potential senior therapist trainee and a learner, taking data using a "general therapist drop-in" form. Eighty-four items are measured during the drop-in. The items are divided into the following categories: professionalism, arranging the teaching situation, discrete trial technique, pacing and inter-trial interval, teaching during downtime, familiarity with and adherence to log notes, and management of challenging behavior. The clinical supervisor rates the potential senior therapist on each item with a score between 0 and 4, with 0–1 meaning "poor" performance, 1–2 meaning "below average," 2–3 meaning "average," and 3–4 meaning "above average." The total score on all 84 items is then divided by 84 to give the therapist a mean score of 0–1, 1–2, 2–3, or 3–4. An average score of 0–1 is "poor," and the supervisor should schedule another drop-in within 1 week; 1–2 means that the therapist is "below average," and another drop-in should be scheduled in 1 week; 2–3 is "average," and another drop-in should be scheduled within 2 weeks; and 3–4 is "above average," and the therapist will not need a drop-in for another 1–2 months. Employees who receive an average score below 3 are provided written and verbal feedback about their performance. For any skills marked as needing improvement, clinical supervisors provide further training (modeling, rehearsal, and feedback).

Qualification exam. Potential senior therapists who receive a passing average score of 4 (i.e., "above average") are recommended for the next phase of the senior therapist qualification process: the qualification exam. Senior therapist candidates have 3 hours to take the qualification exam in front of a proctor and are not permitted to use notes. The exam has 30 questions that range from appropriate teaching methods to challenging behavior scenarios with learners. When candidates pass the exam with a score of 80% of higher, they are invited to enter senior therapist training.

Initial Training

During the first 4 to 5 weeks of initial training, senior therapist trainees attend both self-paced, web-based eLearning training and live web classes. Table 22.3 outlines the overall course and duration of senior therapist training.

TABLE 22.3 Senior Therapist Training

Training Component	Requirement
Qualifications	Bachelor's degree, 6 months of experience working one-to-one with learners diagnosed with ASD, successful completion of therapist training, passing a therapy session "drop-in" and a written qualification exam
Length of training program	Approximately 6 weeks
eLearning	16 hours (four sets of 4-hour sessions, one per week)
Web classes	8 hours (four sets of 2-hour video conferencing sessions)
Homework	Four homework assignments that cover various aspects of training
Final written exam	2-hour comprehensive written exam

eLearning. Senior therapist trainees take an initial 16-hour eLearning module, consisting of self-paced, prerecorded PowerPoint lectures on advanced topics. Table 22.2 lists the topics covered in the training. The training topics include the initial clinic, preparation for the first session, preparation of a logbook, the role of the senior therapist in clinics, general format and process of clinics, advanced topics in discrimination training, probing for generalization and mastery, managing therapist performance, conducting overlaps with new therapists, conducting field evaluations for therapist trainees, conducting ongoing drop-ins with therapists, school shadowing, functional assessment, function-based behavioral interventions, emergency interventions for challenging behavior, data collection, introduction to verbal behavior and review of B.F. Skinner's analysis of language, brief review of the CARD curriculum areas, picture communication systems, teaching sight reading, toilet training, prompting for teaching higher-order social and language skills, review of outcome research, introduction to the Individualized Education Program (IEP) process, and parent training. The eLearning module is broken up into 4-hour sessions, with trainees completing 4 hours per week during their first month of training. For the most part during this process, they continue with their regularly scheduled therapy sessions.

Web classes. To attend the web classes, senior therapist trainees log on to a web-based video conferencing system that has live video feed and audio. The classes are spaced across 4 to 5 weeks and take approximately 2 hours per week. The instructor lectures in real time over the web, and the trainees answer questions, provide examples from their local offices, and engage one another in discussion. Topics include new client startup; role and responsibilities of a senior therapist during clinics; introduction to the Skills® system (see Chapter 26) and data entry; advanced topics on discrimination training; probing skills in baseline and for generalization; senior therapist's role in training, evaluating, and managing therapists; school shadowing; advanced topics on functions of challenging behavior and function-based interventions; advanced topics on data collection and measurement; introduction to verbal behavior and review of the echoic, mand, tact, and intraverbal; overview of the CARD curriculum and introduction to the eight curriculum areas within the curriculum; iconic communication training; toilet training; prompting while teaching higher-order skills; review of outcome studies on early intensive behavioral intervention; overview of the senior therapist's role in the IEP process; and overview of the senior therapist's role in parent training.

Homework. Trainees complete homework that relates to the weekly eLearning and web classes. For example, trainees review learner logbooks and prepare written critiques and recommendations. The homework is graded each week, and written feedback is given. Successful completion of the homework is required in order to continue in the training program.

Final written exam. After trainees have completed the eLearning, web classes, and homework, they are required to take a written exam. The exam is paper and pencil format and is comprised of 35 short-answer questions. The questions range from "Name two ways you can use behavioral procedures to train therapists" to "What should you say to a parent who is asking you for feedback regarding his learner's prognosis?" Questions are graded by a senior instructor according to a rubric that indicates content that constitutes a correct answer. Trainees must receive a score of 80% or better to pass the exam. Once trainees pass the written senior therapist exam, they are promoted to senior therapist and begin working in that capacity.

Ongoing Training

Clinics. Relative to therapists, senior therapists take more of a leadership role in biweekly clinic meetings. They often meet briefly with the therapists immediately before the meeting and give them feedback about which lessons should be demonstrated with the learner in front of the family and the clinical supervisor. The clinical supervisor often looks to the senior therapist for specific insight as to what is and is not working for the learner. The senior therapist demonstrates therapy techniques with the learner, giving the clinical supervisor the opportunity to give feedback to the senior therapist. The clinical supervisor often asks the senior therapist to test new lessons and/or demonstrate or perform probe sessions and typically asks the senior therapist for feedback about the learner's progress and therapy targets in an effort to develop the senior therapist's skill set. For example, the clinical supervisor might ask, "Based on what Giselle has done here in the clinic meeting today and her performance at home, what do you think is the best next step in this lesson?" The supervisor and the senior therapist then discuss the pros and cons of the senior therapist's ideas.

Monthly staff meetings. The senior therapist's experience in the monthly staff meetings is similar to that of the therapists. The exception is that, in some monthly meetings, the material presented to the senior therapists is tailored to a higher level than the information presented to the therapists. Also, senior therapists often have the opportunity to help demonstrate competencies to the other therapy staff during the trainings. When senior therapists have an opportunity to assist in training, the clinical supervisor gives them feedback and direction on their training abilities, generally in one-on-one meetings following training.

Mentor meetings. As with therapists, senior therapists have the opportunity to meet monthly with a clinical supervisor. During this meeting, the mentor gives direct feedback to the senior therapist about her work with learners, and goals are discussed for future performance. The senior therapist can also use this time to discuss educational opportunities with the mentor.

THERAPIST LIAISONS

Therapist liaisons have previously served in the roles of therapist and senior therapist at CARD, and they have a thorough understanding of what it takes to be a great therapist (see Chapter 21 for further descriptions of this position). Table 22.4 gives an outline of the therapist liaison's qualifications and training. In order to qualify to enter therapist liaison training, a senior therapist must be nominated by a clinical supervisor to sit for a qualification exam. The therapist liaison qualification exam comprises 35 short-answer questions that review common terminology and case examples. When taking the exam, the candidate must explain the most appropriate techniques to use, strategies to implement, or course of action to take. The exam is graded by a clinical trainer using a written exam key. The employee must pass the exam with an 80% accuracy rate or higher. Candidates who do not pass the exam must wait to be nominated for the position again before being given the opportunity to take the exam. In addition to the qualification exam, the employee must pass a drop-in evaluation during which she demonstrates that she is an exceptional senior therapist and excels with learners in the field. After employees are nominated and pass the qualification exam and drop-in, training begins.

Initial Training

Web classes. Candidates receive live web-based training in groups where they can see and hear their peers and their instructor on the computer screen. Table 22.2 lists the topics included in the training. Classes are 4 hours each, and employees meet once per week for 4 weeks to complete their training. Topics in the therapist liaison training include:

1. Hiring (reviewing résumés, how to interview, qualities to look for in a candidate, and making job offers);
2. Health Insurance Portability and Accountability Act (HIPAA);
3. Evaluating therapists (how to do a drop-in, mentoring meetings, and therapist evaluations);
4. Professionalism; and
5. Avoiding dual relationships.

Courses consist of lecture and discussion.

Homework. After each class session, the therapist liaison trainees are given homework based on course material. The instructor grades the homework and provides feedback to the therapist liaison in written form. The homework consists of a variety of tasks related to training therapists (e.g., creating PowerPoint presentations for training therapists). Employees must successfully complete all of the homework in order to take the final exam.

TABLE 22.4   Therapist Liaison Training

Training Component	Requirement
Qualifications	Successful completion of therapist training and senior therapist training; passing a therapy session "drop-in" and a written qualification exam
Length of training program	Approximately 5 weeks
Web classes	16 hours (four sets of 4-hour video conferencing sessions)
Homework	Four homework assignments that cover various aspects of training
Final written exam	2-hour comprehensive written exam

Final written exam. Therapist liaison training culminates in a written 2-hour final exam, consisting of short-answer questions. An example question from the exam is "List two questions that you would ask a therapist in an interview" or "Give an example of a boundary violation with a learner's family." Candidates must score at least 80% to pass the exam.

CLINICAL SUPERVISOR TRAINING

Most candidates for the clinical supervisor position have been employees for 2 or more years or have equal or more experience proving top-quality behavioral intervention at other agencies. Table 22.5 provides an outline of the clinical supervisor qualifications and training.

Qualification Exam

Individuals who are being considered for entrance into the clinical supervisor training program must first take a 2-hour qualification exam consisting of short-answer questions. The exam topics include the diagnosis of ASD, writing a behavior intervention plan (BIP) when given specific scenarios, and the difference between discrete trial training (DTT) and natural environment training (NET), to name a few. The test is written in such a way that candidates do not need to have knowledge of procedures specific to the CARD Model, but rather general knowledge of how to implement evidence-based treatment for ASD. Candidates must score an 85% or better to pass the test. Employees who do not pass the exam must wait until the next clinical supervisor training is scheduled before retaking the exam. Candidates who pass the qualification exam are promoted to the position of case manager (see Chapter 21), and they hold this title until their successful completion of clinical supervisor training.

TABLE 22.5   Clinical Supervisor Training

Training Component	Requirement
Qualifications	Master's degree, BCBA or professional license (LMFT, LPC, etc.), any and all credentials required by governing state law, successful completion of therapist training and senior therapist training, nomination from the local office, passing a written qualification exam
Length of training program	Approximately 6 months
eLearning	15 hours
In-person classroom	10 full days at headquarters office
Web classes	36 hours (six sets of 6-hour classes)
Local mentorship	Approximately 24 hours (1 hour per week for 6 months)
Remote group mentorship	Approximately 36 hours (1.5 hours each week for 6 months)
Remote individual mentorship	Approximately 12 hours (1 hour every 2 weeks for 6 months)
Practicum	Written demonstration of clinical skill
Oral examination	6- to 8-hour oral examination in front of a panel of senior supervisors

Initial Training

eLearning. Training begins with eLearning modules and reading assignments. The reading assignments include several of the most commonly cited articles related to ABA and ASD treatment. The eLearning modules cover evidence-based treatment for ASD, comprising approximately 15 hours of training. The end of each eLearning module concludes with a short quiz that must be passed before continuing.

In-person classroom training. Employees who pass the qualification exam and enter the clinical supervisor training program come to the CARD headquarters office in Tarzana, California, for 10 days of in-person training. Table 22.2 lists the topics included in the training. Trainees learn about research that supports ABA for learners diagnosed with ASD, alternative treatments that are not evidence based, understanding and interpreting standardized assessments for learners with ASD, laws related to individuals with disabilities, educational practices across the United States, the IEP process, legal and ethical issues that arise when treating individuals and their families, data collection and graphing, using data and graphs when making treatment decisions, functional assessment, writing function-based BIPs, teaching families and staff to implement BIPs appropriately, managing challenging behavior, the client intake process, school placements, managing a school shadow, and how to address conflicts involving employees, parents, and other professionals.

The classroom training then progresses to the eight CARD curriculum areas: 1) social, 2) motor, 3) language, 4) play, 5) adaptive, 6) executive function, 7) cognition, and 8) academic skills. (See individual chapters on each curricular area for additional details.) Trainees first receive intensive training on how to design programs to teach learners with ASD skills in each curriculum area. Later, the focus shifts to how the eight areas work together to help clinicians develop a comprehensive ABA program. Trainees work with case studies to develop curriculum programs. The practical application of the training involves classroom presentations, role-play, question and answer, and group brainstorming. Trainees are given vignettes and then asked to make clinical recommendations. For example:

> Timmy is 3 years old and was recently diagnosed with ASD. His parents are seeking treatment. They have researched ABA and have decided to pursue early intervention services. They have an employee-sponsored insurance policy that will cover 90% of their son's treatment. Dad works, and Mom has stopped her part-time job to be involved with Timmy's program. Timmy has limited language, makes very little eye contact, and is very rigid about the color blue. He demands blue shirts and socks and always chooses blue toys over any other color.

Trainees are then asked to describe the next steps for developing a treatment plan. Each trainee presents suggestions to the group, the trainer provides feedback, and the entire group engages in discussion. During discussion, the group problem-solves the most difficult aspects of the case and comes to consensus on recommendations for how to proceed.

Vignettes progress from relatively simple to relatively advanced, requiring trainees to create solutions to increasingly complex real-world challenges that practitioners face in the field. For example:

> As recommended, Timmy has been receiving 35 hours per week of one-to-one early intervention services. His parents are very involved, and Timmy seems to be responding well to treatment. Unfortunately, Timmy's father just lost his job. He will be able to keep his insurance until the end of the year. That leaves 1 month for us to propose an alternate plan to Timmy's parents. Timmy's grandparents have agreed to pay for Timmy's treatment for 10 hours per week.

Trainees are asked various questions such as: What changes would you make to Timmy's treatment? Which lessons would you keep, and which lessons would you eliminate? How can you address Timmy's most pertinent needs? What ethical discussions should you have with Timmy's parents?

As vignettes become more complex and more difficult, trainees continue to identify the best courses of action. The instructors guide the trainees through conversations on prioritizing treatment targets for patients, how to make the best clinical decisions, how to address major skill deficits with limited resources, and so on. The trainees provide their suggestions, and the instructors shape their responses with specific guidelines from the previous classroom training.

In-person training exit exam. In-person training culminates in a written final exam. The exam takes place on the final day of training, and trainees are given 5 hours to complete it without the use of notes. The final exam is comprehensive and covers all material from the 10-day training, as well as concepts presented in the eLearning modules. Trainees must pass this test with a score of 90% or higher in order to progress to the next stage of training.

Web classes. After the in-person classroom training is complete, trainees return to their local CARD clinical sites and begin to attend web classes. The classes use technology that includes web cameras, audio (either connected through the phone or the computer), and a projection screen (to show slide presentations, graphs, etc.). These classes are led by an instructor who teaches topics from the syllabus, leads discussion, presents case reviews, and monitors the discussion and interaction of the group. The classes are typically once per week, 6–7 hours per class, and last 6–7 weeks. The web classes are primarily devoted to further development of skill acquisition programming across all curriculum areas, with an emphasis on designing teaching programs, integrating skill acquisition programs with behavior intervention plans for challenging behaviors, and adjusting programs as needs arise.

After the web classes, the trainees take another written test to ensure they have mastered the material presented in the classes. The trainees are given 5 hours to take the exam, which covers material presented in the web classes. The exam also provides scenarios/case reviews that require the trainees to apply their knowledge and decision-making skills. The exam is graded by a clinical instructor who uses a written answer key. Trainees must achieve a score of at least 90% on this written exam in order to progress to the next stage of training.

Mentorship

Local individual mentorship. Each local CARD clinical site has a clinical manager who has demonstrated expertise and has been supervising treatment for several years. At this point in the training process, trainees take on the duties of supervisors under the mentorship and guidance of a clinical manager. Each trainee has regular meetings with the clinical manager who mentors her throughout the training experience. The clinical manager walks the trainee through the entire process of being a clinical supervisor, detail by detail. The clinical manager also assists the trainee with the daily requirements of the job, such as managing local employees, handling schedules, working with funding sources, communicating with parents, writing reports, completing timesheets, and so on. The clinical manager meets with the trainee at least once a week for an hour to discuss progress, give feedback, and identify goals.

Remote individual mentorship. Trainees are assigned an individual mentor from the training department. The mentors in the training department are all seasoned clinical supervisors with a minimum of 10 years of experience supervising behavioral intervention for learners with ASD. Trainees meet with their mentors via videoconference once every 2 weeks for 1 hour to review the trainee's progress and discuss any challenges that may have arisen.

Remote group mentorship. In addition to individual mentorship, trainees are assigned to a group, and each group is assigned a training department mentor. The training department mentors hold group mentorship classes for the trainees once per week over a web conferencing system with video and audio. Here, trainees are able to present questions relating to the experiences that they are having in their local offices. They can also discuss ideas for treatment and problem-solve with their peers and the training department mentor. In addition to discussing ongoing clinical experiences, mentors present vignettes to set the occasion for further discussion and training. For example:

> I met a new learner at intake last week. He is four-and-a-half and just got a diagnosis. Mom and Dad brought both his brother and him to the clinic room for our meeting. I spent most of my time assessing him. However, I couldn't help but notice that his 3-year-old brother did not speak the entire session. He also made no eye contact, and he spun a toy on the floor for the entire one-and-a-half-hour meeting. What should I do if I suspect that the little brother may need to be evaluated, too?

Throughout the group mentorship, trainees share their experiences, receive feedback from their training department mentor, and connect with their peers. They attend this class until they pass their oral exam (described below). Trainees are encouraged to continue to participate in web-based group mentorship meetings for the first year after they pass their oral exam, but attendance is not required.

Co-supervision. As the trainee is assigned learners whose programs she will supervise, a trained clinical supervisor works with her on each case. The trainee designs and supervises the implementation of the treatment plans; however, she has a trained clinical supervisor working beside her during the entire training period. There are natural and planned opportunities for a trainee to receive feedback from the clinical supervisor. First, the trainee provides the treatment plan to the clinical supervisor in advance. Then, during the weekly mentorship meetings, the clinical supervisor gives the trainee feedback about the planned goals and objectives of the treatment plans as they relate to particular learners. Also, the clinical supervisor accompanies the trainee to all of the clinics that the trainee supervises. During the clinics, the trainee leads treatment planning, gives feedback about the BIP, and proposes goals for the next 2 weeks. This gives the clinical supervisor the opportunity to observe the trainee working directly with the learner and the family. The clinical supervisor has the opportunity during this time to provide feedback and make any needed adjustments to the planned treatment. This process continues until the trainee passes the oral exam and no longer needs feedback or support to maintain her learners' programs.

Practicum. Clinical supervisor trainees must complete a written practicum to ensure that they are able to write reports, document learner progress in writing, follow appropriate operations procedures, and communicate in writing with funding sources and other third parties. It is important that supervisors excel at corresponding effectively with different audiences. For example, writing a letter to a family is quite different from writing a letter to a funding source. Furthermore, we find that practitioners need training to communicate goals and objectives effectively to different funding sources, for example, writing behavioral goals for school districts versus for medical insurance companies. The practicum process also requires the trainee to overlap with a clinical supervisor on several different types of cases (e.g., a learner with only mild deficits in social skills, a learner using an augmentative device to communicate, a teenager on the spectrum, etc.) in order to ensure a broad supervision skill set. When all practicum assignments are complete, the trainee's local mentor must "sign off" on the practicum work. That signature indicates that the local mentor participated in, supervised, and approved all of the work that the trainee completed at the local level to complete the training exercises. When the practicum is complete, the trainee may take the oral exam.

Oral exam. The final step in the supervisor training process is the oral exam. The oral exam lasts 6–8 hours and consists of a panel of three senior supervisors presenting questions to the trainee. Questions consist largely of vignettes wherein trainees are given hypothetical cases and asked how to proceed. The trainee discusses learner treatment options and answers questions about treatment plan targets, learner progress, and other issues related to designing, implementing, and supervising treatment plans. The panel of examiners listens and responds to the oral answers and probes the trainee for elaboration where necessary. Here is a partial example of a vignette:

> Billy is a 9-year-old learner diagnosed with PDD-NOS. He is placed in a fourth grade classroom with his neurotypical peers. He has a classroom aide who is assigned to him each day at school. Billy's testing indicates he is at grade level in mathematics. However, he is significantly delayed in language arts skills. Billy has problems at recess and lunch, and at your last observation you noticed that this is the time of day when the classroom aide is on "break." Billy is obsessed with video games, and his parents reward him weekly with new games. Billy is protesting lately about going to school, he is acting out on the school bus, and he is alienating the few friends he has with his repetitive conversations about particular video games.

The trainee must prepare a plan of action that includes general impressions of the learner, program recommendations, a plan for intervention, recommendations to parents, recommended treatment hours/services, "red flags" or concerns about the learner, and legal or ethical issues that may need to be addressed. Here are some examples of the kinds of questions that the panel might ask the trainee during the oral exam:

- **Examiner**: "You mentioned that you would recommend 15 hours per week of one-to-one treatment for Billy after school each day. What is the basis of this recommendation? Can you reference research that supports this recommendation, or can you speak to Billy's progress or lack of progress on a certain assessment that supports this recommendation?"
- **Examiner**: "How do you plan to address Billy's social issues on the playground and at lunch?"
- **Examiner**: "Based on the information that you have been given, do you think that Billy's classroom placement is appropriate? Why or why not?"

The panel of examiners includes the trainee's mentor from her local office, as well as one or two senior clinicians with a combined experience of more than 20 years working with learners with ASD. It is important that some of the panel members know the trainee well and know the exact learners with whom the trainee has been working. However, it is also important that at least one panel member not be familiar with the trainee and the learners with whom the trainee works. This ensures a greater degree of objectivity in evaluating the trainee's responses. It also helps test whether the trainee can perform at a high level in the presence of authority figures with whom she is not familiar, as she will certainly be required to do in her future work as a clinical supervisor in IEP meetings and so on.

Scoring the oral exam. For each vignette, trainee performance on the oral exam is evaluated in the following competency areas: behavioral assessment, crisis management, designing the treatment plan, supervising the implementation of the treatment plan, laws, ethics, and policies and procedures. Each area receives a score from 0 (unqualified) to 5 (excellent) for each vignette. Trainees must complete multiple vignettes and receive no less than a score of 3 on each vignette and no less than a total average score of 3 in any one competency area. The vignettes vary in difficulty and focus on learners of varying ages, backgrounds, and presenting symptoms. The panel continues to ask trainees questions until they receive a passing score of 3 in each area or until time expires. Because each trainee requires varying amounts of time to answer the questions, the oral exam can last anywhere from 6 to 8 hours. Many times, oral exams have to be scheduled across 2 or more days because time does not permit the team to complete the exam in 1 day.

If a trainee does not receive a minimum score of 3 in each area, the trainee fails the exam. The panel then recommends specific goals and objectives for the trainee, so he can eventually retake the exam. For example, a trainee may receive a passing score in every area except for ethics. The team will then recommend that the trainee go back and attend a training session on ethics, review practical applications with the local mentor, role-play scenarios with the training department mentor, and then return in 1 month for further questioning on the area that previously proved difficult.

Case managers who pass the oral exam graduate from the training program and are promoted to the clinical supervisor position. They are then allowed to supervise cases independently and are no longer required to receive ongoing co-supervision from a more experienced supervisor. All supervisors are encouraged to maintain close contact with their training department mentor, so they can continue to seek assistance when issues arise in the future.

Ongoing Training

Monthly continuing education (CE) events. Clinical supervisors have the opportunity each month to attend CE events on topics related to the treatment of ASD. These events are commercially available through the website www.ibehavioraltraining.com and are often available through online webinars that allow staff to log on via computer. Participants can see the presenter live, and the presenter can see them. In-person training events are also offered on a regular basis. These CE events are provided at no charge to employees. Events address advanced topics across all areas of treatment provision for learners with ASD.

Biannual CE events. Every 2 years, CARD offers a weeklong training retreat for supervisors. CE events are offered live, and all supervisory-level staff attend the event together at a designated location. The CEs are offered at no charge and cover the latest developments in autism treatment.

Drop-ins. Clinical supervisors are encouraged to request assistance on challenging cases. When they request assistance, a more experienced clinician attends a clinic or home session to observe, problem-solve, and/or make suggestions. After that meeting, the more experienced clinician provides training and feedback to the clinical supervisor on areas that need to be addressed. Similarly, surprise "drop-in" sessions also take place wherein experienced supervisors observe lesser-experienced supervisors. The more-experienced supervisor then provides feedback to the clinical supervisor in order to strengthen relevant skills.

CLINICAL SUPERVISOR ONGOING QUALITY ASSURANCE

There is a common misconception within the autism treatment field that quality assurance and training are essentially the same thing. In other words, many people believe that, if the quality of a supervisor's treatment programs is not high enough, then the supervisor needs training. However, learning what to do and then actually doing it on a regular basis are not the same thing. In other words, even after receiving the highest quality training, supervisors will not always implement treatment at the highest level of quality if there are not ongoing systems in place to ensure that they do. The CARD Model of treatment includes rigorous measures to ensure that the highest quality standards for treatment are upheld on an ongoing basis.

Supervisor Performance Evaluations

Clinical supervisors are evaluated by their clinical managers every 6 months in order to ensure that they are continuing to supervise treatment at the highest level of quality and/or to identify any clinical supervisor performance deficits that may require additional training or performance management. For evaluations that occur at the 6-month mark, the clinical manager attends two of the supervisor's clinics. During these clinic observations, the clinical manager does not participate in the clinic, but rather observes and rates the supervisor's performance. The clinical manager uses a 51-item form to rate the supervisor's performance in each clinic across the following eight categories: 1) professionalism; 2) challenging behavior program design; 3) challenging behavior program implementation; 4) skill acquisition program design; 5) skill acquisition program implementation; 6) program modifications; 7) data collection; and 8) data organization. The clinical manager rates each of the 51 items from 1 to 5, with 1 being defined as "poor" and 5 being "exceptional." After the clinical manager conducts and scores the two clinic observations, she meets with the clinical supervisor for 2 hours to review the results of the evaluation. If any of the items on the observations receive an average score lower than 3, the clinical manager and clinical supervisor create a performance improvement plan. The plan generally incudes additional training tailored specifically to the performance deficit. The two will then meet again 3 months later, and the clinical manager will again evaluate the supervisor but only on the specific items contained in the performance improvement plan.

Supervisor evaluations that occur at the 12-month mark of each year follow the same process but are more comprehensive. In particular, the clinical manager bases her evaluation on four clinic observations, rather than two.

Program Reviews

Treatment programs for some learners are evaluated by senior clinicians, including the clinical director, on an as-needed basis. These reviews can be triggered by a request from the clinical supervisor if, for example, she is facing a particularly difficult clinical challenge. Program reviews can also be requested by funding providers, parents, or the clinical supervisor's manager. Depending on the concerns raised, the review can be done in a variety of formats. The senior clinician can observe the supervisor conducting one of the learner's clinics, she can meet with the supervisor or parents in person or on the telephone, she can review charts and written documents (e.g., BIPs, etc.), or some combination of these. After reviewing the learner's program, the senior clinician meets with the clinical supervisor to review her assessment and recommendations and makes plans and goals for any additional training or support for the supervisor, if needed.

Yearly Clinic Attendance

Clinical supervisor evaluations and program reviews, as described above, ensure high-quality performance on the part of the supervisor. However, in order to ensure that each individual learner's treatment program is being implemented with high quality, clinical managers also perform one clinical observation per year for each learner, above and beyond the clinic observations conducted for supervisor evaluations. After each clinic observation, the clinical manager meets with the learner's clinical supervisor to review the performance ratings and provide feedback. Just as with supervisor evaluations, if this process reveals any supervisor performance deficits, the clinical manager designs a performance improvement plan with the supervisor.

SUMMARY

The CARD Model of staff training and quality assurance is a formalized system for therapists, senior therapists, therapist liaisons, and clinical supervisors. Training is provided using a variety of methods, including lecture, discussion, role-play, eLearning, field training, web classes, homework, competencies, practicum, mentorship, clinic meetings, written exams, and oral exams. Training never ends for CARD staff, as subsequent to their initial training, there are many continuing education opportunities and events, as well as ongoing quality assurance. The training process in the CARD Model is an evolving system that is continually reviewed and refined to ensure that learners with ASD receive top-quality treatment based on the latest research and that treatment policies meet or exceed professional guidelines and legislative mandates as they emerge.

Ethics

Megan Maixner, Elizabeth Meshes

The term *ethics* commonly refers to a system or code of moral principles of a particular person or group. In other words, ethics are a set of rules regarding the correct way to behave given certain conditions. From a general perspective, ethics serve as a guide for determining whether actions are right or wrong and for identifying what action to take in a particular situation. A commonly held belief is that there is only **one** right way to behave in any given situation. In reality, people's ideas about the right way to act in a situation often differ and, at times, conflict. From a behavior analysis perspective, a person acts and thinks in particular ways because of his particular learning or reinforcement history. Therefore, most people live according to a set of rules that develop over the course of their lifetime.

Conduct in a professional situation may require behavior that differs from the way that an individual would behave in a personal or social situation. Therefore, professional ethics describe a set of rules for how to act as part of a particular group or culture, that being the group of professionals who make up one's discipline (e.g., applied behavior analysis [ABA], psychology, medicine, and so on). Professional ethics specify behaviors that will produce outcomes to benefit and, in some instances, protect the group of professionals, consumers, and the cause or purpose for which the group was formed. Defining a standard of conduct for a group has many advantages: It allows for others to have clear expectations; it makes it easier to identify inappropriate behavior; and it establishes accountability for actions of professionals.

Why Do ABA Providers Need Professional Ethics?

The role of ethics and values in behavior analysis, as with any other discipline, is complex. Delivering services based on the principles of ABA requires an individual to make frequent decisions that affect other people, including colleagues, learners and their families, other service providers, and school staff, to name just a few. Given that the goal of such services is to change the probability that individuals will behave in particular ways, ethical issues occur frequently. ABA practitioners should be aware of and adhere to the published ethical guidelines and professional codes of conduct of relevant professional organizations. The primary organizations are the Behavior Analyst Certification Board® (BACB®) and the American Psychological Association (APA). Licensed professionals in other disciplines, such as licensed clinical social workers and marriage and family therapists, have their own set of ethical guidelines for their respective disciplines and we strongly recommend that such professionals consult those. The remainder of this chapter presents scenarios that providers of behavioral intervention to children with autism spectrum disorder (ASD) may encounter, the potential ethical issues presented in each scenario, and a recommendation as to the best courses of action in each. To get the most out of this chapter, we recommend that you have the guidelines of the BACB (2012) and APA (2010) on hand. Space does not permit comprehensive coverage of all ethical guidelines, and the readers are referred to Bailey & Burch (2013) for a book-length treatment of the topic.

Scenario: Integrity

Joe works for a large agency providing services to individuals with ASD. Late one afternoon, as Joe is leaving the office to go to a therapy session, his supervisor calls out to him, "Stop. This report has no signature, and it needs to be submitted by 5:00 pm or this kiddo will not receive funding for services." Joe, always precise and thorough in his work, doesn't recall a report due for any of his learners for at least 3 more weeks, but ambitious and eager to please his supervisor, Joe takes the report from the supervisor. Joe glances at the client's name on the report and doesn't recognize it. Joe tells his supervisor that the report is not for one of his clients. His supervisor replies, "Yeah, this is my client, but I am not an authorized treatment provider for this funding source. I've worked with this child for over a year, so when the funding source changed a couple months ago, I just kept him. You have been authorized as a treatment provider for them, so no big deal. The report is all finished; you don't need to do anything except sign it." Joe replies, "Are you sure this is a good idea? I've never met this kid, and I don't even have time to read the report." Joe's supervisor asks, "Don't you trust me?"

Potential ethical concerns. Joe is in a difficult position because his direct supervisor has asked him to engage in unethical and potentially illegal behavior. Joe's signature on the report indicates that he is aware of and approves of the contents of the report, presumably a safeguard implemented to ensure that the learner is receiving appropriate and quality treatment. By signing the report, Joe would be bypassing an important treatment safeguard and potentially committing fraud. In addition, Joe would be violating BACB® guideline *1.04 Integrity:*

> (a) Behavior analysts are truthful and honest. The behavior analyst follows through on obligations and professional commitments with high quality work and refrains from making professional commitments that he cannot keep.
> (b) The behavior analyst's behavior conforms to the legal and moral codes of the social and professional community of which the behavior analyst is a member.

Potential courses of action. Joe should not sign the report. This is understandably a difficult position for Joe. He most likely feels that his job will be compromised if he refuses to do this. However, the ethical and legal consequences could be more severe. It would be in Joe's best interest to state that he is not comfortable signing the report at this time and ask if they could discuss transferring the case to him if he has the appropriate credentials to oversee the case.

Scenario: Dual Relationships

Richard, a therapist, has been working for about 6 months with Lucy, a 4-year-old girl diagnosed with ASD. Lucy's mom, Sharon, asks Richard many questions about his personal life. Initially, he did not think much about the questions beyond establishing a warm working relationship with the family. However, Sharon recently began asking Richard questions about his dating life. She also has increased working out and frequently wears form-fitting workout clothes around him. She has begun asking Richard's opinion on her physique, and he generally answers politely and makes short but relevant comments about the importance of physical activity. Sharon's behavior has been escalating to where she has now propositioned Richard with a sexual advance. She has also threatened him, implying that she will complain to his supervisor about his job performance if he does not respond to her advances.

Potential ethical concerns. Richard has unknowingly entered into a dual relationship with Sharon. BACB guideline *1.06, Dual Relationships and Conflicts of Interest,* gives guidance for what behavior analysts should do in such instances:

> (c) If a behavior analyst finds that, due to unforeseen factors, a potentially harmful multiple relationship has arisen (i.e., one in which a reasonable possibility of conflict of interest or undue influence is present), the behavior analyst attempts to resolve it with due regard for the best interests of the affected person and maximal compliance with these Guidelines.

Richard is facing an ethical dilemma. He can either engage in a sexual relationship with Sharon, which would be highly unethical, or potentially have a false accusation made that can jeopardize his career and overall future.

Potential courses of action. Richard should immediately report Sharon's statement to the designated human resources (HR) representative or other appropriate staff member where he works and request to be removed from the case. He should not compromise his career and future by considering her offer or failing to report her behavior.

Scenario: Dual Relationships

Pam has provided ABA services to Doug, a 3-year-old boy diagnosed with ASD, for about 7 months. Doug's parents have been struggling with the news of his diagnosis for almost a year and have spent little time or energy thinking or talking about anything else. They are grateful for the services that Pam provides for Doug and have come to rely on her a great deal. One evening, Doug's parents invite Pam to stay for dinner after Doug's session. Pam knows that she shouldn't accept the invitation but feels bad turning it down, so she accepts and enjoys an excellent dinner with Doug and his parents. The next time Pam arrives for a session, Doug's mother again asks her to stay for dinner. Pam, having missed lunch because a meeting ran late, again accepts the invitation and enjoys another dinner with Doug and his family. Doug's parents appear to relax during the dinners with Pam. Pam finds that she has a lot in common with Doug's mom, and the food is much better than the fast food that Pam usually picks up on the way home from sessions. After the next session, Doug's mom asks Pam if she wants to go out to dinner with her. Pam thanks her for the invitation and declines. Doug's mom starts crying and tells Pam that she really needs a night out and doesn't have anyone else to ask, so Pam agrees and has an evening out with Doug's mom. At successive sessions with Doug, Pam now spends the first 15 to 20 minutes chatting and catching up with Doug's mom. Pam knows that this is taking away from Doug's therapy time but justifies it by telling herself that she is helping the family and really making a difference in their lives.

Potential ethical concerns. By accepting the initial offer for dinner, Pam took the first step toward establishing a dual relationship, and it is not surprising that their dual relationship further developed. Again, BACB guideline *1.06, Dual Relationships and Conflicts of Interest*, recommends against entering into dual relationships and encourages guarding against situations such as these. In this case, the substantial amount of time that Pam now feels she needs to spend socializing with the learner's mother during each session clearly takes away from time she should be working directly with the child and is therefore a good example of how a dual re-lationship can "interfere with the behavior analyst's ability to effectively perform his or her functions as a behavior analyst."

Potential courses of action. At this point, Pam should refer to the sec-tion of BACB guideline *1.06* on dual relationships that recommends that *"behavior analysts attempt to resolve [the dual relationship] with due regard for the best interests of the affected person."* Pam should consider if she would like to be friends with Doug's mom or a service provider for Doug. If she chooses to be a friend, she should request to be removed from Doug's case immediately. If she would like to continue to provide services to Doug, she needs to have a conversation with Doug's mother, explaining that their friendship is getting in the way of her effectively treating Doug. She can ask that they put their friendship "on hold" until Doug's treatment is over, and Doug's mom can be referred to other sources of social support, such as support groups, listservs, social networks, and so on.

Scenario: Professional Relationship

Lindsey, a therapist for the past 3 years, recently had to take a few days off work to undergo emergency dental treatment. She discovered that an unintended side effect of her prescribed medication is that it decreases her anxiety and makes her feel happier overall. Although she is no longer in pain, she called her doctor and had her prescription refilled. She has since returned to providing direct services. One of her client's caregivers contacts Lindsey's supervisor to inform the organization that Lindsey has not been acting like herself since she returned to work. The caregiver is concerned about Lindsey's well-being. Lindsey's supervisor observes her in therapy and sees that Lindsey appears sluggish and confused and is speaking slowly.

Potential ethical concerns. Lindsey is not performing to the best of her abilities while on her pain medication. Although her medication is pre-scribed legally, it may compromise her ability to provide the best services, especially in the case of emergencies. By choosing to continue to provide services to learners while under the influence of narcotics that impair her effectiveness, Lindsey is likely violating BACB guideline *1.05, Professional and Scientific Relationship:*

> (f) Behavior analysts recognize that their personal problems and conflicts may interfere with their effectiveness. Behavior analysts refrain from providing services when their personal circumstances may compromise delivering services to the best of their abilities.

Potential courses of action. Lindsey's supervisor should immedi-ately seek guidance and consult with her company's HR staff. HR is best equipped to determine how to provide support to Lindsey until she can competently provide services again. The supervisor must also find appropriate replacement staff to provide services to Lindsey's clients and to comply with guideline *2.16, Interrupting or Terminating Services:*

> (f) Behavior analysts do not abandon clients. Behavior analysts terminate a professional relationship when it becomes reasonably clear that the client no longer needs the service, is not benefiting, or is being harmed by continued services.

Lindsey also should consider if her use of pain medication is becoming an addiction for which she should seek professional help from someone who is an expert at evidence-based treatment for addiction.

Scenario: Professional Development

Jennifer, a BCBA and supervisor, has been working with children diagnosed with ASD for nearly 2 decades. When she was new to the field, she was eager and excited to learn. She would regularly attend conferences and read behavior analytic journals to see what she could incorporate into her practice. These days, she feels she already knows everything that is presented at conferences and published in scientific journals. For the past year, Jennifer has taken only online continuing education (CE) modules. She usually skips through the presentation to the end, takes and passes the quiz, and prints her confirmation for CEUs.

Potential ethical concerns. Jennifer is likely doing a disservice to her clients and herself. By actively avoiding opportunities to continue to learn, she is failing to identify and utilize the most recent research to support her clients' progress. She should consult BACB guideline *1.03, Professional Development:*

> Behavior analysts…maintain a reasonable level of awareness of current scientific and professional information in their fields of activity, and undertake ongoing efforts to maintain competence in the skills they use by reading the appropriate literature, attending conferences and conventions, participating in workshops, and/or obtaining Behavior Analyst Certification Board certification.

Potential courses of action. If Jennifer has a difficult time accessing new and interesting research on ASD, she should pursue research and training in different but related areas. For example, she could seek out information on staff training, performance management, ethics, and so on. Many other areas of research and practice within the field of ABA are not directly related to autism but may still be relevant in that they address duties and responsibilities not specific to autism treatment that behavior analysts undertake on a daily basis.

Scenario: Competence and Consultation

Laura, a recent graduate of a master's program with a BCBA course sequence, has been promoted to a supervisor position within her agency. She has worked with children diagnosed with ASD for the past 3 years. She is excited and nervous to be the one making recommendations. Her most recent client, Fred, is diagnosed with ASD and obsessive compulsive disorder (OCD). The caregivers are concerned about his locking and unlocking of doors, which are symptoms of his OCD diagnosis. Laura recognizes that this is outside of her area of expertise and decides to seek consultation. She recalls that a fellow student, Bob, did really well in classes and is now working in organizational consulting. When Laura contacts Bob, he recommends that she provide the learner with something else to do with his hands, such as putting together puzzles, and then remind him to do it on a regular basis.

Potential ethical concerns. Laura knows that she does not have adequate training and experience to treat OCD, and she is therefore appropriately sensitive to BACB guideline *1.02, Competence:*

> (a) Behavior analysts provide services, teach, and conduct research only within the boundaries of their competence, based on their education, training, supervised experience, or appropriate professional experience.

When behavior analysts recognize that a learner has a problem that they are not competent to treat, the appropriate course of action is to seek consultation, as described in BACB guideline *2.04, Consultation:*

> (a) Behavior analysts arrange for appropriate consultations and referrals based principally on the best interests of their clients, with appropriate consent, and subject to other relevant considerations, including applicable law and contractual obligations.

Laura made an attempt to follow the guideline above by consulting her friend Bob. However, she did not seek appropriate consultation. Rather than seek consultation from someone who is an expert, she sought help from Bob because she perceives Bob as intelligent and respects him as a good behavior analyst. While Bob may excel in his area of expertise, organizational management, he does not have sufficient experience working with children with ASD or individuals with OCD. If Laura proceeds with Bob's recommendations, she is likely in violation of BACB guideline *1.01, Reliance on Scientific Knowledge:*

> Behavior analysts rely on scientifically and professional derived knowledge when making scientific or professional judgments in human service provision, or when engaging in scholarly or professional endeavors.

Potential courses of action. Laura should seek consultation from a clinician who is an expert in treating ASD and OCD. It is recommended that she speak with her supervisor at her current place of employment and reach out to professional networks. To learn more about the issue, she also can read peer-reviewed behavior analytic journals to determine what the research has demonstrated to be an effective intervention in similar circumstances. Merely reading articles, however, will not make her competent in implementing treatment procedures with which she has had no practical training and experience.

Scenario: Functional Assessment and Punishment

Ellie is a BCBA who has been supervising autism treatment for 15 years. She has found that token systems can be a useful way of using conditioned reinforcement to increase a variety of adaptive behaviors across many different learners. However, she has also found that, when a learner begins to display a new inappropriate behavior (e.g., a new form of stereotypy), it is usually most efficient to implement a response cost immediately. For response cost, she usually tells the learners' therapists to take a token away from the learner as a consequence for an inappropriate behavior.

Potential ethical concerns. It is good that Ellie uses tokens for positive reinforcement, but she has likely formed a habit of moving straight to punishment too quickly when a new inappropriate behavior arises. When a new inappropriate behavior appears, the behavior analyst should first consider the function of the behavior and try to identify it by conducting a functional assessment, as described in BACB guideline *3.02, Functional Assessment:*

> (a) The behavior analyst conducts a functional assessment…to provide the necessary data to develop an effective behavior change program.

By skipping straight to a treatment procedure, Ellie may well be missing the reason that the behavior is occurring, and her treatment is therefore less likely to be effective. Equally as concerning, Ellie's first resort in treating a new behavior is punishment. It is universally agreed in the field of behavior analysis, as well as in virtually every other helping profession, that the least intrusive treatment that is likely to be effective should be tried first. Ellie should consider BACB guideline *4.05, Reinforcement/Punishment:*

> The behavior analyst recommends reinforcement rather than punishment whenever possible. If punishment procedures are necessary, the behavior analyst always includes reinforcement procedures for alternative behavior in the program.

Potential courses of action. Ellie needs to remind herself that, even though it might be efficient to punish new inappropriate behaviors immediately, it is not the most ethical choice. She needs to begin with a functional assessment. Very rapid options for functional assessment exist, including indirect and descriptive assessment (see Chapter 5), so functional assessment need not slow treatment substantially. Additionally, Ellie needs to try multiple reinforcement-based options before resorting to punishment procedures such as response cost. For example, she could try teaching and reinforcing an alternative behavior that produces the same functional reinforcer as the inappropriate behavior. If that does not work, she could consider *giving* the learner tokens when she does not engage in the inappropriate behavior (i.e., differential reinforcement of other behavior; see Chapter 4), rather than *removing* tokens, as is done in response cost. Many reinforcement-based treatment options have been validated by research and should be tried before resorting to punishment.

Scenario: Integrity and Harmful Reinforcers

Caitlin has been working with Samantha, an 8-year-old girl diagnosed with ASD. Samantha does not have many items that are effective reinforcers. She enjoys watching movies but engages in aggression when they are interrupted. She likes to be picked up, spun, and carried around. She also enjoys several salty foods and an array of candy. Samantha's mom has expressed concern because Samantha has become considerably overweight, and the doctor has recommended restricting the sweets and salty foods to address concerns about her overall health. In fact, Samantha's weight has made it difficult for the 1:1 staff to use physical interactions as reinforcers. Caitlin has begun hiding her use of candy and salty foods from Samantha's mother in order to keep Samantha progressing in her treatment.

Potential ethical concerns. First, by deceiving the learner's mother about which reinforcers are being used, Caitlin is violating BACB ethical guideline *1.04, Integrity*:

> (a) Behavior analysts are truthful and honest.

It is not acceptable to deceive a learner's parents. In addition, by continuing to use reinforcers that may be causing unwanted weight gain and other health problems, Caitlin may well be violating BACB guideline *4.06, Avoiding Harmful Reinforcers*:

> The behavior analyst minimizes the use of items as potential reinforcers that maybe harmful to the long-term health of the client or participant (e.g., cigarettes, sugar or fat-laden food), or that may require undesirably marked deprivation procedures as motivating operations.

Potential courses of action. Caitlin needs to stop hiding her reinforcers from Samantha's mother. In addition, she likely needs to get more creative with reinforcer identification. Another potentially helpful strategy might be to implement an exercise program, which should help guard against unwanted weight gain.

Scenario: Data Collection

Judy has been treating individuals with ASD for decades. She takes pride in the fact that she has been trained by some of the best in the field of behavior analysis. For her, behavior analysis is not something that you do but, rather, a world view; it is how you live your life. She believes that behavior analysis is so ingrained in her that she almost has a "sixth sense" for determining appropriate treatments and when to make treatment changes. She finds that taking data takes away from her time helping learners meet the desired outcomes, so she rarely, if ever, collects data anymore.

Potential ethical concerns. It is common for very experienced clinicians to develop highly accurate skills at recalling learner performance. However, this does not excuse treatment providers from the obligation of documenting and evaluating learner progress with data. By eschewing data collection, Judy is likely in violation of BACB guideline *4.07, Ongoing Data Collection:*

> The behavior analyst collects data, or asks the client, client-surrogate, or designated others to collect data needed to assess progress within the program.

Potential courses of action. If Judy wants to minimize the amount of therapy time that is taken for data collection, there are methods for doing so that still meet the behavior analyst's obligation for collecting data. For example, first trial data collection during discrete trial training DTT and time sampling (see Chapter 20) are two methods for rapid data collection that can still yield accurate, useful data.

Scenario: Data-Based Program Modifications

Colette has been in a supervisory position for 12 years. She has demonstrated excellence across all of her cases. She is frequently cited as the "go-to person" for all clinical questions. She not only oversees a number of cases herself but is frequently called upon to consult on others' cases, as well. Needless to say, she is very busy. Recently, one of her therapists informed her that a learner is excelling in one particular skill acquisition program. Colette has no time to look at the graphs and believes she can trust the therapist's anecdotal report, so she changes the program without looking at the program data.

Potential ethical concerns. It is entirely possible that Colette's intuition is right and that the therapist's anecdotal report is correct, but there is no way for Colette to know this if she does not look at the data. Human memory and anecdotal observation are simply not reliable enough when a child's treatment success is at stake. BACB guideline 4.08 is very clear about the need to make treatment decisions based on data: *Program Modifications.*

> The behavior analyst modifies the program on the basis of data.

Potential courses of action. Colette should take the time needed to look at the data. Data can be exchanged electronically in order to aid in efficiency, and/or web-based data tracking and management systems, such as Skills® (see Chapter 26), can be used, so any team member can access treatment data at any time using the Internet.

Scenario: Consent for Program Modifications

Melissa has been asked to take a new case for her agency. The child is bilingual, but the caregivers only speak Spanish. Melissa does not speak Spanish, but she knows that there are limited individuals in the agency who speak Spanish and a large Spanish-speaking population that needs services. Her agency has offered the services of the Spanish-speaking receptionist, if needed. Due to the learner's high rates of aggression, Melissa decides she would like to stop all active programming while her 1:1 English-speaking staff re-establish rapport with the child. Melissa has her staff implement the changes immediately, and no one follows up with the caregivers to explain the changes until they call the office 2 weeks later because of a lack of progress in skill acquisition.

Potential ethical concerns. Melissa made a very significant change to her learner's program without talking to the learner's parents first. It is entirely possible that the change was a good decision and clinically appropriate for the learner, but this does not obviate the need for Melissa to discuss major program changes with the learner's parents before implementing them. She should consider BACB guideline *4.09, Program Modifications Consent*:

> The behavior analyst explains program modifications and the reasons for the modifications to the client or client-surrogate and obtains consent to implement the modifications.

Potential courses of action. Melissa should seek the help of someone who can translate for her when she interacts with the learner's parents, and she should apologize to them for not discussing their child's program changes with them prior to implementing them. In the future, Melissa should obtain the help of a translator, so she does not make the same mistake again.

Scenario: Medical Consultation and Least Restrictive Treatments

Jimmy, a 12-year-old boy diagnosed with ASD, has begun stealing items from the school cafeteria following the death of his dog. Nick, a behavior analyst, is the supervisor on the case, and he believes that Jimmy is stealing because he has become depressed. He recommends that Jimmy see a psychiatrist as soon as possible to be placed on antidepressants.

Potential ethical concerns. At this point, it is highly premature for Nick to recommend that Jimmy see a medical doctor. Nick has not seen any evidence that reasonably suggests that Jimmy is suffering from a medical problem. He should consider BACB guideline *3.0*, which states:

> Behavior analysts recommend seeking a medical consultation if there is any reasonable possibility that a referred behavior is a result of a medication side effect or some biological cause.

In addition, even if medication might be appropriate for Jimmy at some point, it is absolutely not appropriate to recommend medication as a first choice for treatment of a behavior problem. Behavior analysts must recommend the least restrictive procedures that are likely to work, and medication is almost always more restrictive than reinforcement-based behavioral intervention. Nick should consider BACB guideline *4.10, Least Restrictive Procedures*:

> The behavior analyst reviews and appraises the restrictiveness of alternative interventions and always recommends the least restrictive procedures likely to be effective in dealing with a behavior problem.

Potential courses of action. If the stealing behavior is a clinically significant problem, then Nick should conduct a functional assessment and design a function-based behavior intervention plan to decrease the behavior and replace it with a more adaptive, functionally similar behavior.

Scenario: Treatment Efficacy and Third-Party Relationships

Sally is the clinical director of a small ABA service provision agency that is relatively new and still trying to establish itself financially. Sally is approached by a major funding source in her area. The funding source tells Sally that it is difficult for them to provide funding for more than 5–10 hours per week for young children with ASD, even though this is far less than what is scientifically supported. The funding agency tells Sally that ABA providers create problems when they recommend 30–40 hours per week because parents then become upset when the funding provider only authorizes funding for 10 hours per week. The funding provider tells Sally that, if Sally's recommendations are closer to 10 hours per week, then they will be able to refer at least five new clients per month to her for treatment. Sally knows that 10 hours per week of behavioral intervention for young children is not the optimal treatment approach, nor is it the approach that is most supported by scientific research. Still, she reasons that, in the real world, you can't always get what is ideal. She decides that, if she wants to be able to treat children in that area at all, she needs to "play ball" and set her recommendations at a level that will please the funding provider, therefore positioning her to help more children overall access services. In the future, Sally recommends 5–10 hours per week of behavioral intervention for families of young children with ASD and does not inform the families that her recommendations are not supported by scientific research.

Potential ethical concerns. The scenario described above sounds terrible, but it is unfortunately quite common. Funding providers continue to try to make these deals because they have found treatment providers who will accept such terms. In other words, when treatment providers take this deal, they are effectively reinforcing the unethical – and often unlawful – behavior of the funding provider. Just as important, they are violating their own ethical obligations. All treatment providers have an ethical responsibility to their clients to recommend the treatments that they know are the most effective and supported by scientific research. Two ethical guidelines are relevant to the scenario above. First, behavior analysts have an ethical obligation to recommend treatments that are shown to be effective in scientific research, as described in guideline *2.10, Treatment Efficacy:*

> (a) The behavior analyst always has the responsibility to recommend scientifically supported most effective treatment procedures. Effective treatment procedures have been validated as having both long-term and short-term benefits to clients and society.
> (b) Clients have a right to effective treatment (i.e., based on the research literature and adapted to the individual client).

In addition, the BACB gives useful guidelines for how third-party relationships should be handled. In this case, Sally should not recommend a level of treatment that she knows is not shown to be most effective. However, if she decides to provide treatment for the reduced hours because that is all that the funding agency will authorize, she has an ethical responsibility to fully disclose all details of the third-party relationship to the parents of the children she treats, as described in guideline *2.05, Third-Party Requests for Services:*

> (b) If there is a foreseeable risk of the behavior analyst being called upon to perform conflicting roles because of the involvement of a third party, the behavior analyst clarifies the nature and direction of his or her responsibilities, keeps all parties appropriately informed as matters develop, and resolves the situation in accordance with these Guidelines.

SUMMARY

Evidence-based treatment for children with ASD is a highly complex process that involves many thousands of interactions among treatment providers, learners, their parents, third-party funding agencies, and other professionals over long periods of time. Complex interactions of this sort inevitably create the potential for ethical challenges. The question is not *if* you are going to face ethical dilemmas; it is *when*. Be prepared for potential ethical concerns by reviewing the suggestions here, as well as the ethical guidelines of the BACB and APA, and try to stay "in front" of any problems by following ethical guidelines to the best of your ability before problems occur. Keep in mind that behaving ethically does not merely depend on being a good person; it consists of actively, thoughtfully, and intentionally considering ethical guidelines when making decisions on an ongoing basis.

Medical Treatment and Interdisciplinary Collaboration

Megan St. Clair, Doreen Granpeesheh

Autism spectrum disorder (ASD) is a whole-body condition, and most children with ASD experience challenges across many different domains, including behavioral, educational, communication, and medical. It is no surprise, then, that autism treatment involves the participation of many different disciplines, including behavior analysts, licensed psychologists, speech-language pathologists, occupational therapists, physical therapists, special educators, school psychologists, nurses, and medical doctors. Since ASD affects the whole family system, it is not uncommon for social workers (LCSWs) and marriage and family therapists (LMFTs) to be involved in treatment as well, and parents and other family members are, of course, also core members of the treatment team.

It is widely acknowledged that effective autism treatment depends on healthy and productive collaboration across disciplines. It is also widely known, however, that interdisciplinary collaboration can be challenging at best, and interdisciplinary relations can be downright confrontational at their worst. In order to help maximize every child's treatment gains, it is critical that the professionals on the treatment team work together smoothly and help, rather than hinder, one another's efforts.

There are two primary reasons that establishing productive interdisciplinary collaboration is critical. First, it is more efficient. Time and resources are limited, and every available moment should be spent planning and executing treatment. Any time that is taken up by disagreements between professionals is wasted. Worse still, when the various members of the treatment team are not collaborating productively, then they are less likely to implement each other's suggestions consistently, thereby resulting in the child with ASD actually receiving less of each treatment component. In short, confrontation breeds inefficiency.

The second – and equally important – reason that establishing productive interdisciplinary collaboration is critical is that no one person knows everything about autism treatment. Regardless of how well trained you are and how much experience you have treating children with ASD, other team members will have ideas that haven't occurred to you. Behavior analysis is a comprehensive science of all behavior, but that does not mean that every single behavior analyst has experience and expertise in every area of human functioning. The other professionals sitting around the table have specialized training in their own respective disciplines – training that is different from that which behavior analysts receive. Healthy, productive interdisciplinary collaboration results in every team member learning and becoming more effective, ultimately leading to better treatment outcomes for the child with ASD.

The purpose of this chapter is to give guidance on how to build collaborative relationships between all members of the treatment team. We begin with a discussion addressing the medical treatment of ASD and, as a practitioner of evidence-based treatment for children with ASD, how to interact with parents and medical doctors on the topic of medical treatment. The remainder of the chapter is then dedicated to giving practical advice on how to build collaborative interdisciplinary relations, regardless of the disciplines of the various professionals.

MEDICAL TREATMENT FOR AUTISM

At the time this manual goes to press, there is no medical treatment for ASD that has been supported by replicated research showing clinically significant effects on alleviating ASD symptoms as a whole. Risperidone is approved by the Food and Drug Administration for the treatment of irritability (aggression, self-injury, tantrums, etc.) in individuals with ASD, but it is not approved for the treatment of any of the core symptoms of ASD. A thorough review of research on other medical treatments is beyond the scope of this chapter. Instead, we describe the perspective of the Center for Autism and Related Disorders (CARD) on the medical treatment of ASD and provide recommendations for how to collaborate with medical doctors who treat the learners with whom you work.

Medical Treatment for the Pathophysiology of Autism

There is currently little scientific agreement on the pathophysiology (underlying physiological cause) of ASD, but many theories abound. Hundreds of treatments exist that are claimed to treat the many potential pathophysiologies, but, to date, none have been proven to do so with any significant degree of scientific support.

Some unproven treatments are based on theories for which there is indirect scientific evidence. For example, several unproven treatments for ASD decrease inflammation, and several studies have found inflammation in the gastrointestinal tracts and/or brains of individuals with ASD. No research has yet proven that inflammation leads to ASD, but there is significant indirect evidence. Similarly, several unproven treatments exist that attempt to improve the functioning of the methylation pathway in individuals with ASD, and several studies have been published that document dysfunction in this system in the autism population. Again, no studies have shown that methylation dysfunction causes ASD, but there is a significant amount of indirect evidence. In summary, there are several theories of the pathophysiology of ASD for which there is, at least, preliminary scientific evidence.

In any discipline, research on new treatments generally progresses from case studies to single subject experimental designs and, eventually, to clinical trials. Most unproven biomedical treatments for ASD are still in the case study phase of development. Virtually all have some type of theory behind them, but little or no scientific evidence supports the theories, and no research has been done on the effectiveness of the vast majority of these treatments. Most of these treatments are probably best categorized as "fad" treatments because they change almost every year and are based more on Internet chatter and marketing than on any real evidence of merit.

Interacting with Parents over Unproven Treatments

The vast majority of parents of children with ASD choose to try a variety of unproven biomedical treatments with their children. This practice is somewhat akin to taking a daily multivitamin: No research supports that it actually improves health, but most people do it or think it's worth doing. Given the popularity of biomedical treatments among parents of children with ASD, it is probably not reasonable for you to expect that you can prevent the children with whom you work from receiving some of them.

A small minority of applied behavior analytic treatment providers have taken the extreme measure of threatening their learners' parents with termination of their child's behavioral treatment if they use biomedical treatments. We believe this constitutes client abandonment and is unethical. And, realistically, it doesn't work anyway. Parents will still do what they want in their own homes, but they will merely hide it from the behavioral provider. Other behavioral providers do not threaten termination, but they strongly admonish parents for using biomedical treatments, to the point where parents feel compelled to hide their use. Again, the result is simply that parents will do what they want in their homes, and the behavioral provider will merely be kept in the dark about it. This is an unfortunate outcome, because if the biomedical treatments have any effect at all – positive or negative – the behavioral provider will be unaware of it and will be left to guess at which aspect of behavioral treatment was responsible for the effect.

The CARD approach acknowledges that many parents of children with ASD choose to use unproven biomedical treatments. Given that this is the case, we recommend that parents be very judicious about which, if any, unproven treatments they choose to use. We provide the following recommendations to parents:

- Consider very carefully whether the monetary expense and risk of potential side effects are justified, given the lack of scientific evidence to suggest that the treatment is going to work.
- Do not begin a biomedical treatment for which there is no research support if there are significant potential side effects.
- All other things being equal, if you feel compelled to try something, try a treatment that has no conceivable side effects first. For example, ensuring that your child eats a healthy, balanced diet and giving her daily multivitamins have no possible negative side effects, whereas chelation or vitamin megadoses could have serious potential side effects.
- Do not begin an unproven treatment to solve a problem for which there is a proven solution. For example, rather than giving a drug or vitamin supplement to improve attention, use proven behavioral techniques for increasing attention (see Chapter 18).
- Do not begin an unproven treatment that directly interferes with another treatment that is proven to work. For example, for early learners for whom food is among the only powerful reinforcers, do not introduce a diet that takes all effective food reinforcement away (see the discussion of edible reinforcement in Chapter 4).
- Introduce only one unproven treatment (or any other treatment change, including behavioral) at a time, so the effects, if any, can be measured and documented without being confounded by multiple treatments being changed at once.
- Tell your child's applied behavior analysis (ABA) supervisor about all biomedical treatment changes before you do them. Tell her what behavioral changes you expect to see, so the supervisor can have her therapists begin collecting data on these behaviors to evaluate the effectiveness of the treatment.
- Do not tell your child's ABA therapists about biomedical treatments. The therapists are the ones collecting data on your child's behavior, so we want them to remain objective.
- If you believe an unproven treatment is working, consider stopping it for a brief time to see if the positive effects diminish. If the data show that the effects diminish, then reintroduce the treatment. If the effects

do not diminish, then perhaps the treatment never really produced them. Even if the treatment did produce the initial effect, but the effect does not reverse now that the treatment has been withdrawn, then the treatment is no longer necessary and is therefore not likely worth the expense and risk of side effects.

The recommendations above, if implemented consistently and judiciously, will help families sift through which unproven treatments they feel are right for them. Ultimately, you cannot make choices for the learner's family, but you can give guidance based on data that evaluates effectiveness, rather than on personal opinion and emotion.

Medical Treatment for Comorbid Medical Conditions

Many children with ASD suffer from comorbid medical conditions, e.g., seizure disorders, chronic constipation, diarrhea, skin rashes, sleep disorders, ear infections, and acid reflux, among others. Some people believe that some or all of these comorbid conditions are partially responsible for causing ASD, so treatments for them are sometimes falsely represented as treatments for ASD. Regardless of the accuracy of these claims, all children who have legitimate medical conditions have a right to effective medical treatment, irrespective of whether they have a diagnosis of ASD. Unfortunately, many children with ASD have significantly impaired abilities to communicate, and they are often, therefore, unable to tell others when they are ill and where they hurt. The unfortunate result is that, all too often, children with ASD suffer from chronic, untreated medical disorders. At the very worst, medical doctors have been known to say something along the lines of, "He has autism; it's normal for him to have gastrointestinal difficulties/poor diet/poor sleep/etc." We believe that this attitude is unacceptable. Anyone who is sick, regardless of whether she has ASD, deserves to be treated effectively.

Effect of Comorbid Medical Disorders on Learning

Everyone is likely to have more difficulty learning when they are sick. If a child is having diarrhea five times per day, it is not reasonable to expect him to be able to pay attention and learn at his optimal rate during ABA therapy. If you were that sick, you would likely stay home and lay on the couch. The unconscionable reality is that many children with ASD remain that sick for weeks or months without effective medical treatment. These children must receive effective treatment for their medical disorders before we can expect our treatment to reach maximum effectiveness. Put simply, a healthy child learns faster. If a learner presents with significant medical symptoms, we strongly recommend that the parents take her to a medical doctor. If the doctor does not take the symptoms seriously, the parents should consider choosing a new doctor.

Research on Medical Factors in Autism

We sincerely hope that a "magic bullet" pill will be invented one day that prevents ASD from ever developing. It seems unlikely that something that simplistic will ever be created, but we do believe that future research will identify the pathophysiology of autism and that biomedical treatments will be invented that directly address it, not merely cover up particular symptoms. We believe that there is a very strong possibility that more than one etiology of ASD will be discovered, all of which likely will consist of complex interactions of multiple genetic and environmental factors. It seems likely that separate biomedical treatments will need to be developed for each of these. Top-quality research will need to evaluate the effectiveness of these treatments at putting children with ASD back on the course of typical development. Such research will reorient the discussion of biomedical treatment of ASD away from anecdotes and toward science.

BUILDING PRODUCTIVE COLLABORATIVE RELATIONSHIPS

Most of the ethical guidelines for behavior analysts and the many other professionals with whom they work include guidelines on interdisciplinary collaboration. Most of these guidelines emphasize at least two basic suggestions that form the foundation of the CARD Model for building collaborative working relationships:

1. Treat others with whom you work respectfully, and
2. Cooperate and communicate continuously.

Being Respectful

Treating others with respect is fundamental to healthy interdisciplinary collaboration. The following is a list of practices that demonstrate respect for others:

- Accepting and valuing the differing opinions of others;
- Using discretion when disagreeing, especially in front of others;
- Remaining conciliatory;
- Acknowledging the personal and professional rights of others;
- Allowing other professionals to work within their respective professional boundaries;

- Establishing trust among colleagues through integrity and honesty;
- Promoting fairness;
- Publicly acknowledging the knowledge, skills, and expertise of others;
- Providing encouragement and support to other professionals; and
- Asking others for their input, even when you think you have it all figured out.

The following is a list of practices that are all but guaranteed to make other professionals feel disrespected by you:

- Making disparaging comments about others' recommendations or theoretical viewpoints;
- Expressing overly harsh or indiscreet criticism;
- Demanding conformity or compliance;
- Coercing people to get what you want; and
- Undermining other professionals' authority or positions, especially in front of third parties.

In some sense, being respectful is a matter of common sense. Virtually any professional can identify the difference between respectful and disrespectful behavior. Yet, knowing how to be respectful is clearly not enough, as is evidenced by the fact that many professionals fail to behave respectfully. In order to get the most out of reading this chapter, it is probably worth your time to think about difficult interdisciplinary interactions that you have experienced in the past and try to identify examples of when you or others engaged in behaviors such as those listed above, both good and bad. For many professionals, their first reaction in interdisciplinary settings is to behave defensively rather than respectfully. In addition to knowing how to be respectful, one must actively observe and evaluate one's own collaborative behavior and *practice* being respectful during every professional interaction.

Cooperative Communication

Interdisciplinary collaboration, by definition, involves cooperation between different professionals who speak different professional languages and have different viewpoints. It is virtually impossible for this process to work well unless communication is done efficiently and cooperatively. The following is a list of behaviors that are helpful for establishing effective communication in the context of collaboration:

- Making others aware of useful resources and sharing them;
- Frequently exchanging relevant information as it arises (at least every week but more often is better);
- Attempting to make group decisions by consensus, that is, withholding conclusions until all team members agree on the proposed action;

- Actively listening – when you respond to someone, your response should be directly related to what the person just said, not merely a change of topic to your preferred point;
- Communicating patiently;
- Demonstrating flexibility and a willingness to learn new ideas and understand others' positions;
- Negotiating differences, rather than arguing them; and
- Asking other professionals for help when issues arise outside of your area of expertise.

The following is a list of behaviors that happen all too often in interdisciplinary settings and which are sure to ruin any communication you are trying to build with other professionals:

- Being argumentative;
- Using profanity when disagreeing;
- Acting in a passive-aggressive manner;
- Ignoring others;
- Pressuring others;
- Being overly stubborn; and
- Having ulterior motives.

As a rule of thumb, good-quality communication is difficult. Put another way, if you are simply doing what comes naturally to you when talking to other professionals about a disagreement, you are probably not doing the best job at building cooperative communication. Productively communicating with others, even when you are sure they are wrong, requires patience, self-control, and deliberate practice. To be successful, when your viewpoint is in opposition to another professional's, you should be actively thinking about how to articulate your position in a way that will help establish common ground, rather than fuel the disagreement.

While the general ethical guidelines of being respectful and communicating cooperatively offer a helpful starting point for paving the way towards collaborative working relationships, they are not sufficient to resolve some of the fundamental impediments to effective, efficient, and successful collaboration for a variety of reasons. First, some professionals are bound by the standards set by their treatment methodology, and simultaneous implementation of other interventions may, in fact, have adverse effects by undermining preexisting interventions already put into place. If the behavior analyst perceives that the treatments instituted by others are impeding the progress of the child with ASD, it can be challenging to treat the other professionals respectfully by valuing their differing opinions, providing encouragement, and offering support in an effort to work collaboratively. Professionals from diverse backgrounds often have very different and conflicting ideas about what is "best" for a client. A major challenge for interdisciplinary collaboration, then, is the question of how various professionals reach consensus regarding what is best for the client without sacrificing the standards of their respective professions. These are all complex questions unanswered by the published ethical guidelines of various helping professions, which provide general guidelines rather than identifying specific strategies. In other words, these ethical guidelines may be good in theory, but putting them into practice can be difficult.

In the remainder of this chapter, we provide practical recommendations for addressing this challenge, including modeling good collaborative behavior, using a behavior analytic perspective, assessing and evaluating the behaviors of other professionals, finding the behavioral functions that maintain collaborative and noncollaborative behaviors, implementing preventative and protective strategies at the professional level, taking turns with treatment approaches, being a translator of behavior analysis and interpreter of mentalistic language, and, finally, remembering to self-check.

Modeling

The Golden Rule applies very well to interdisciplinary collaboration: If you want other professionals to treat you well, you should treat them well. Many clinicians feel reticent to show vulnerability or weakness first when interacting with other professionals. Clinicians sometimes think they need to arrive at interdisciplinary meetings with "guns blazing" in order to show everybody else that they "mean business." In some situations, it may be effective for some team members to be particularly assertive (e.g., parents being aggressive when trying to obtain funding for their child's treatment). Generally speaking, however, being aggressive only works if you can imply a real threat of aversive consequences for others if they do not go along with what you say. In reality, no professional on an interdisciplinary team has the power or authority to punish the other team members for noncompliance. Therefore, the end result of acting aggressively is to give the other professionals yet another reason not to do what you want them to do.

Modeling good behavior is generally much more likely to be effective than being overly assertive. If you want the other team members to behave reasonably toward you, then you should be the first one to behave reasonably toward them *before* the group even has the opportunity to become confrontational. More often than not, if you behave reasonably and show a willingness to compromise, other professionals will perceive this as professionalism, not weakness, and they will be more likely to reciprocate. In the CARD Model, we emphasize to clinical supervisors that they have the responsibility to model good collaborative behaviors throughout their working relationships with professionals from all disciplines.

Use a Behavior Analytic Perspective

Behavior analysts believe that all behavior, regardless of whether it is the behavior of children with ASD or their parents, of other professionals, or of the behavior analyst herself, is equally subject to the same basic principles of learning and motivation. As such, other professionals can be appreciated as individuals who possess their own unique behavioral repertoires that are ultimately affected by reinforcement (Bailey & Burch, 2013). Therefore, using a behavior analytic perspective when working with professionals of diverse backgrounds means applying the basic principles of behavior analysis to maximize the effectiveness of your collaboration with them. This involves identifying adequate reinforcers, assessing antecedents and consequences in order to determine environmental variables maintaining another professional's collaborative and noncollaborative behaviors, and then doing your part to build a strong collaborative relationship with that professional. Bear in mind that conducting interventions on another professional's behavior without her informed consent or knowledge would be unethical, and this is not what we are suggesting here. Rather, we suggest that you use your behavioral expertise to alter your own behavior in ways that will best facilitate productive collaboration with other professionals.

As we discussed earlier in this manual, an old saying in behavior analysis goes something like "The learner is always right." In other words, people do what they do because of their learning history and their current environments. Therefore, if a child is not learning effectively, we blame the teaching procedure; we do not blame the child. To a large extent, the same is true with interdisciplinary collaboration. If you are having a difficult time working with other professionals, blaming them is not going to help. Your behavior is part of their environment. Blaming them for what you perceive as their bad behavior is not going to help change their behavior. If the collaboration isn't working, then blame the collaborative procedures you have been using, try to identify what could work better, and keep trying new approaches until you find one that works. In short, you cannot control their behavior, but you can control your own, and your collaborative behavior (or lack thereof) has an important effect on the collaborative behavior of others.

Most professionals think that collaboration primarily depends on how "good" or "bad" their colleagues are. That is, if you have to work with someone who is not good at his job or does not have the ideal personality, then there is nothing you can do about it. This perspective is popular but not helpful. If you believe this, then you have already accepted that you are powerless to make effective collaboration happen. We suggest that you think of building effective collaboration in the same way that you approach anything that you teach a learner. Make it your goal to forge effective, upbeat, efficient collaborative relationships. When you teach a learner with ASD to communicate, your job is to do something effective to produce that outcome. In the case of building interdisciplinary collaboration, we suggest you view producing that outcome as a normal part of your job, too. If it's not working, it's your job to figure out how to make it work.

Assessment and Evaluation

When initially building relationships with other professionals, plan on scheduling individual meetings with the team members with whom you anticipate collaborating. These initial meetings can be brief and should be used as an opportunity to:

- ask open-ended questions in an effort to learn more about the background of the other professionals and their approaches to treatment;
- provide information about behavioral intervention approaches;
- exchange pertinent client information; and
- decide how and what, if any, additional information will have to be collected before moving forward and who will collect this information.

It may be helpful to create a checklist of information that you hope to obtain in order to guide the meeting most efficiently. Throughout each of these meetings, carefully observe and be mindful of your interactions with the other professional, that is, ask yourself the following questions: Were there any "red flags" regarding collaboration? Was the other professional open-minded and flexible or resistant and rigid? Is there anything he is particularly opposed to or in favor of? During these initial meetings, focus on gathering information, inspiring camaraderie, foregoing ego, and encouraging everyone involved to come together as a team.

Observing other professionals when they are working with the learner in their natural work environment can also be an important source of information useful for forging strong collaborations. This is an important additional step because professionals often behave differently under different circumstances (e.g., meetings with other professionals versus teaching the learner). Consider the following questions while you gather information:

1. Does the professional get along well with others?
2. Is she respectful and does she respect professional boundaries?
3. Do others in the environment seek the professional's opinion and initiate conversations, or do they avoid her?
4. How does the professional respond to the learner's behaviors?
5. Does she use a "hands-on" approach, or is she more distant?

Also, try to identify potential reinforcers for the professional. For example, do the professional's collaborative behaviors increase with feedback and praise from others? Does she seem to do whatever it takes to make the learner happy? Does she primarily seem to be responding to avoid punishment from her supervisor? Following each observation, review and examine the notes from your observations, and begin to formulate hypotheses about what maintains any collaborative and noncollaborative behaviors of the other professional. Identifying potential barriers to collaboration early on can help pave the way towards more coordinated care. Let's take a look at an example:

> **Pamela.** *Pamela is a boisterous and overbearing teacher who usually gets her way in Individualized Education Program (IEP) meetings. In the event that anyone politely disagrees with or questions Pamela, she becomes increasingly abrasive, argumentative, and even downright verbally abusive. She can be condescending and tends to resort to public humiliation. In addition, meetings have a tendency to run late, and consensus is rarely reached. As a result, most of the other members of the child's treatment team generally choose to sit in silence. Whenever Pamela offers a suggestion, everyone nods in agreement without verbally expressing their own respective positions, whether conciliatory or divergent. In return, Pamela speaks well of her colleagues to other school faculty and personally praises them for being so "easy to work with." Ultimately, in exchange for the silence of her colleagues, confrontation is avoided, team members are praised, and meetings end earlier.*

Let's consider how Pamela's professional behavior affects her colleagues and how her colleagues' responses affect her behavior. When her colleagues disagree with her, their behavior is effectively punished, so they are less likely to do it in the future. When they remain silent, they avoid the punishment from Pamela (their behavior of remaining silent is negatively reinforced), and they get the positive reinforcement of Pamela praising them (Table 24.1). Pamela's aggressive professional behavior is also being strongly reinforced here. When she was not aggressive in the past, other professionals voiced their opinions, and she had to compromise with them – something that is apparently aversive

TABLE 24.1   Hypothetical Contingencies That Have Taught Pamela's Colleagues Not to Contradict Her Professional Opinions, including Antecedents, Behaviors, and Consequences Affecting Colleagues' Behavior

Antecedent	Behavior	Consequences
Pamela speaks during IEP meetings.	Other professionals respond.	Pamela punishes their speaking by becoming abrasive, argumentative, and verbally abusive; meetings end up running late and everyone goes home late.
Pamela speaks during IEP meetings.	Other professionals remain silent.	Pamela reinforces their silence by speaking highly of them to the principal and praising them personally; confrontation is avoided, and meetings end early.

to her. When she was aggressive, the other professionals reinforced her aggression by remaining silent. Given these respective histories of reinforcement, how could the other team members alter their behaviors to successfully change Pamela's? The other team members could use shaping and differential reinforcement to increase Pamela's nonaggressive verbal behavior (e.g., gradually differentially reinforcing any and all of Pamela's collaborative/nonargumentative behaviors). In addition, they could stop remaining silent in response to her aggressive behaviors (i.e., extinction).

Let's briefly consider some other common noncollaborative behaviors and potential corresponding functions. Consider a professional who repeatedly takes credit for others' work because doing so has consistently led to high marks on employee evaluations and incremental raises in salary in the past. The reinforcing consequences here are likely praise from others and access to money. Consider an arrogant behavior analyst who is so certain of the superiority of her principles that she makes unsubstantiated claims of the effectiveness of her procedures because doing so has continually led to the praise of others and an esteemed, unquestioned reputation. The reinforcing consequence here may be attention and approval from others. Consider a nonconfrontational teacher who almost always agrees with recommendations for students' behavior intervention plans during IEP meetings but generally disregards the plans completely when teaching in her classroom because doing so allows her to do what she believes is right for her students without having to experience professional disagreements during the IEP meetings. The reinforcing consequence here appears to be avoidance of professional disagreement. None of these professionals are necessarily malicious people; they may simply be doing what has worked in the past.

Implementing Preventative and Protective Strategies at the Professional Level

The following questions can be helpful to ask yourself when making a plan for effective collaboration with another professional:

1. Which learner behaviors does the other professional want to increase and decrease?
2. Do these goals differ from your goals?
3. Which treatment strategies does the other professional recommend?
4. Do these strategies differ from yours?
5. Can the strategies that you believe are critical be effectively implemented in combination with the other professional's proposed strategies, or must they be implemented in isolation of one another?

Consider questions 1–5 above as you read the next hypothetical example:

> **Christian and Emily.** *Christian is a professional with a background in child-centered therapy who has been asked to attend an IEP meeting for a child with extreme tantrums that occur during classroom instruction. Christian's theoretical orientation advocates for the use of unconditional positive regard during times of emotional instability. As an intervention for this child's tantrums, Christian suggests pulling the child out of whatever activity she is engaged in when the tantrum happens and playing with her to help her explore and express her emotions before returning her to the regular classroom routine. Emily is a Board Certified Behavior Analyst (BCBA) also in attendance at this IEP meeting and, after conducting a functional assessment of the child's tantrums, has determined that the behavior is maintained by escape from nonpreferred classroom tasks. Emily recommends teaching the child to ask for a break and giving her a break when she asks for it but not removing any task demands when she tantrums.*

In the vignette, both professionals want to decrease the same behavior, tantrums. Now, let's sort out some of the differences. The procedures that the two professionals recommend are in opposition to each other. One professional wants to remove all demands and let the child play as a consequence for tantrums, whereas the other wants to prevent escape from task demands when tantrums occur. One strategy would be for Emily simply to argue until her suggestions are adopted by the team. Another strategy would be to suggest calmly and professionally to the team that evidence-based strategies be used and point out that communication training and extinction of challenging behavior are supported by a large amount of research, whereas removing work contingent on escape-maintained behavior is not supported by research. This strategy might be a reasonable option, but it is also possible that the team members do not value scientific evidence and that they think that their own personal experience and values are more important. A third strategy is to compromise by finding something about Christian's recommendations that can be accommodated without compromising the quality of the behavioral recommendations. For example, if Christian thinks that positive regard and playing are critical for the child, then perhaps Emily could pose the idea of implementing play breaks on a noncontingent schedule, so the child can still receive large amounts of positive regard but not as a consequence for tantrums. If Emily is especially inflexible, she might point out that increasing the overall amount of attention that the child receives may not decrease her tantrums because the tantrums are escape maintained, not attention maintained. However, pointing this out will do little to foster collaboration. Noncontingent attention cannot possibly hurt the child and is well worth giving, especially if it can convince the team to adopt the evidence-based recommendation of preventing escape during tantrums and teaching the child to communicate for a break before tantrums occur.

Taking Turns with Treatment Approaches

Although it would be ideal for professionals of diverse backgrounds to compromise by combining treatment approaches for the benefit of a shared client, this is not always going to happen. In the last vignette, if Christian is unwilling to compromise by allowing his recommendations to be implemented noncontingently, rather than contingent on tantrums, then some other course of action must be taken. If compromise is not possible and Emily cannot persuade the team to adopt her recommendations, then the team needs to agree on a method for choosing between the two opposing recommendations. One option is to try both interventions and see which one works best, with the agreement that the team adopt whichever is shown to be most effective.

In directly comparing two interventions, each professional has the opportunity to implement her intervention in isolation of other interventions (i.e., take turns) while data are gathered to determine which intervention is most effective in creating the desired behavior change. At first, data collection may seem intimidating and unwarranted to professionals who are not behavior analysts; you can ease this initial resistance, however, by explaining that data collection is merely a concrete method by which to measure the effectiveness of each intervention to determine whether one addresses the client's needs better than the other or whether both require refinements and additional test trials. Moreover, use this opportunity to describe the benefits of data collection in clinical decision making.

After emphasizing the need for data collection, the team should agree on a reasonable length of time for testing each intervention. At this stage, consider thoroughly describing any aspects of your intervention that may appear strange or disturbing to the other professionals. For example, if you are going to implement extinction, explain that extinction often causes behaviors to get worse (e.g., extinction burst) before getting better. You would do well to point out that this is, in fact, a sign that the intervention is working. You can supplement your explanation with a presentation of how the extinction burst would be reflected in the data (edifying your earlier assertion about the importance of data collection) and emphasize that the extinction burst is temporary.

Due to an ethical obligation to provide learners with the most effective evidence-based treatments (and, perhaps, a bit of arrogance), behavior analysts often struggle with the concept of allowing other professionals to have a turn at implementing their interventions (*especially* when the behavior analysts are fairly certain, based on the principles of behavior analysis, that those interventions will not work). However, it is critical to demonstrate flexibility in this regard in order to show respect to the other professionals. Additionally, this turn-taking arrangement offers you the opportunity to implement and modify your interventions in the absence of other interventions and often ultimately reveals the effectiveness of behavior analytic interventions to other professionals. If another professional's intervention proves to be more effective than yours, use the data that you acquire to broaden your own knowledge base. Throughout the process of establishing collaborative relationships, do your best to let your guard down, and in doing so, you may be surprised by how much you have in common with professionals from other disciplines.

Be a Translator and an Interpreter

The field of behavior analysis has its own unique, precise, and technical language to describe the principles upon which the science is based, the domains that characterize treatment approaches, and the interventions used to reliably influence socially significant behavior. This language was developed alongside a commitment to a scientific approach to the study of human behavior. It has aided in the conceptual understanding of behavior analysis and facilitated the development of an empirical foundation from which research, training, education, and treatment have grown. As with any other natural science, however, the technical scientific language of behavior analysis is not useful for communicating with professionals from other disciplines. In fact, differences in language between disciplines can create barriers to professionals relating to one another. This is because the words that compose a language can have varied evocative effects. For example, behavior analytic terminology can evoke warmth, pride, and unity among behavior analysts whose use of this language with one another is mutually reinforced. On the other hand, the same behavior analytic terminology can evoke hostility, opposition, or shame among professionals whose understanding of and exposure to the language is limited. This language barrier might accentuate the perception of behavior analysts as arrogant. It is also possible that the professionals with whom you are attempting to communicate today have had negative experiences in the past with arrogant behavior analysts who used technical terminology to demonstrate their vast knowledge, rather than to try to communicate effectively. Given that language is the primary mechanism that people use to communicate, language barriers between behavior analysts and professionals from other disciplines should be mitigated.

Ironically, the development of a mutual client's language skills often offers behavior analysts and other professionals common ground on which to base a multidisciplinary approach. However, remediating communication differences and altering behavior analytic language in an effort to promote alliances with other professionals can be complicated and can pose unique problems and concerns. The primary challenge is to "tone down" behavioral language without sacrificing its meaning. Behavior analysts can become active translators and can use the process of translation as an opportunity to teach and disseminate behavior analysis to other professionals. In addition, behavior analysts can take active steps in advancing their own knowledge of the language typically utilized by the other professionals with whom they work.

As active translators, behavior analysts should start by finding a way to describe the basic principles of their field in ways that will be welcomed by their audience. In other words, behavior analysts must modify behavior analytic terminology to fit more conventional ways of speaking. This involves identifying shared goals and desires for behavior change. For example, instead of saying, "Let's use positive reinforcement in the form of access to preferred tangibles contingent on occurrences of on-task behavior," you might say, "Let's use rewards to help the learner stay on-task and feel pride in a job well done." When talking about a functional assessment, instead of saying, "We conducted a functional assessment and determined that the learner's aggressive acts serve a negative reinforcement function by allowing him to escape from nonpreferred task demands," you might say, "Our functional assessment showed that the learner uses aggression to communicate that he is getting frustrated with work or wants a break." Translating complex technical terminology (i.e., talking like a normal person) is a skill that will take substantial practice, especially if your previous mentors have punished your use of nontechnical language. Your input will be better received by other professionals, though, if you cultivate the ability to describe behavior analytic concepts in more universal terms. In turn, these professionals will be more likely to seek further recommendations from you in the future. Put simply, no one likes a "know-it-all," and needlessly using overly technical terminology will only make you look like one. In the end, you can call it whatever you want to call it, as long as the interventions designed and implemented are functionally appropriate and effectively modify the behavior. Table 24.2 depicts commonly used behavioral jargon and some suggestions for how to translate it into everyday language.

Self-Check

If you want to be good at collaborating – or anything, for that matter – you will need to perfect the skill of self-checking. Self-checking consists of regularly asking yourself the following questions about your performance – in this case, about your collaborative behavior:

- What are you doing that works and doesn't work, and how can you change your behavior to be more effective?
- In the context of collaboration, are you the professional who is being difficult?
- Are you being fair?

- Are you being flexible?
- Are you failing to explain interventions clearly enough for others to implement them or understand them?
- Are you taking other professionals' questions and concerns seriously?
- Do your colleagues have any useful observations about your collaborative behavior?

Self-checking is not about regretting or harping on your own wrong-doings, and neither is it about self-congratulation. Good self-checking is a dispassionate process of identifying what you did well and what you could have done better. When you identify collaborative behaviors that

TABLE 24.2   Examples of Commonly Used Behavioral Jargon and Translations into Everyday Language

Behavioral Jargon	Everyday Translation
Positive reinforcer or preferred stimulus	Reward, motivator, incentive, outcome, getting something good, getting something that is worth it, what the person wants, what he cares about, what he's interested in, what he values
Prompt	Cue, reminder, help, assistance
Discriminative stimulus or S^D	Cue, instruction, signal
Motivating operation/ establishing operation	Motivation, want, desire, wish
Abolishing operation	Ruining, wrecking, or removing motivation; already has what he wants; doesn't need any more of it; doesn't want it; isn't interested in it; isn't trying to get it
Function of behavior	Reason, cause, purpose, what the behavior gets the person, what the person wants when he does the behavior, what the person is trying to get, what the person is trying to tell you when he does the behavior
Functional replacement behavior	Alternative behavior that gets the person what she wants, making a better choice
Pure mand	Spontaneous request, independent request, asking for something when he wants it, asking for something without having to be reminded
Pure tact	Naming things independently, spontaneous labeling, noticing things and pointing them out, commenting on things independently
Echoic	Vocal imitation, mimicking
Joint attention	Sharing experiences with others, noticing when others want to share their experiences

you can do better, take the same approach with yourself that you would when training someone else: Set goals for yourself that are clear, challenging, and achievable. Then, the next time that you have the opportunity to interact with other professionals, try to meet those goals, and then repeat the self-check process, giving yourself honest feedback.

SUMMARY

Collaborating with all of the various professionals involved in autism treatment can be challenging. Some topics, such as unproven biomedical treatments, can be controversial and emotionally charged for many people. However, the basic principles of being respectful, modeling cooperative behavior, and acting reasonably can serve you well. By modeling good collaborative behavior, using self-checking strategies, clearly showing an open-minded perspective to others, and conveying a genuine appreciation of what other professionals might have to offer, behavior analysts will find themselves accepted by some, welcomed by others, admired by many, and rejected by few. The strategies described in this chapter are important not only for establishing individual collaborative working relationships but also for playing a part in reconstructing the reputation of the field of behavior analysis as a whole.

Standardized Assessment

*Hilary Adams, Paige Cervantes, Jina Jang,
Dennis Dixon*

A standardized assessment is a way to gather information about an individual that is uniform across subjects, settings, and administrations. Such measures strive to provide consistency of testing, allowing comparisons to be made between the people to whom the assessment has been administered and the general population. Accumulating information about people in a uniform way allows the identification of average patterns of functioning across the general population, which in turn allows one to compare a particular child's development to the course of typical development.

Standardized assessments do not normally play a large role in behavioral intervention. Therefore, most behavior analysts have not been trained in their potential utility and limitations. Standardized assessments play a small but important role in the Center for Autism and Related Disorders (CARD) Model of treatment for children with autism spectrum disorder (ASD), and they can be useful to behavioral interventionists in a number of ways. Prior to the initiation of treatment based on applied behavior analysis (ABA), it is common for children with ASD to undergo a thorough psychological evaluation. A child typically undergoes this type of evaluation when her parents notice what they believe may be a deviation from typical development or behavior. The resulting evaluation may consist of standardized (e.g., intelligence and achievement testing) and unstandardized (e.g., unstructured interview and observation) assessment techniques. Taken together, the outcomes provide information for the professional to use – along with his or her clinical judgment and expertise – to assign a diagnosis, if warranted. Additionally, the professional is likely to provide recommendations and referrals to other service providers, including for ABA services. As a result, ABA providers often have access to the outcomes of standardized assessments in reports that the learner's family may provide. These reports may include a wealth of information that can help to inform treatment, but most ABA providers have not had the proper training to interpret them in a useful way. In this chapter, we provide an overview of the general categories of standardized assessments, describe the types of psychometric research that are usually done in the development of standardized tests, and give more in-depth descriptions of a small selection of standardized assessments that are included within the CARD Model of assessment. Finally, we provide guidance on how the results of standardized assessments can be useful in planning treatment.

CATEGORIES OF STANDARDIZED ASSESSMENT

Norm-Referenced Tests

Norm-referenced tests are pencil and paper tests that have established norms. That is, the performance of the individual tested can be compared to other individuals included in the *norm group*, the population of individuals who were administered the test and whose results were analyzed in order to establish a representative average (see further description of norms below). This category includes intelligence tests, achievement tests, and other tests of skills or knowledge that require the individual to complete tasks or answer objective questions. This category also includes statewide or district-wide academic achievement tests.

One challenge to the administration of norm-referenced tests is the motivation of the client. Especially for younger clients, sitting and being tested for an extended period of time may be difficult. Children may often put forth less than their best effort, resulting in scores that are not a true representation of their actual skills. Furthermore, children with ASD can be especially challenging to assess due to their low frustration tolerance, social difficulties, and limited understanding of assessment purpose and procedure. Test protocols are often precisely standardized, which may not allow for typical techniques used to increase motivation in children (e.g., edible or tangible reinforcement or praise). On the other hand, older school-age children sometimes better understand the purpose of testing and implications of their performance, resulting in increased motivation and leading to more representative scores. Overall, caution should be exercised when interpreting scores on norm-referenced tests. Quality reports by professionals are likely to include notes on observed behavior during testing or even actual statements regarding the representativeness of the client's score on the test, for example, "The client refused to answer the questions as their difficulty increased, and thus the scores should be interpreted with caution."

Structured Interview

A structured interview is a method of gathering information from an informant using a standardized set of questions. Many structured interviews are designed so that if a respondent endorses a screening question, follow-up questions are asked to obtain more data about a certain set of symptoms. If the screening item is denied, the administrator of the interview can forgo the remaining follow-up questions and proceed to the next screening question.

Structured interviews can be administered to the client or to a client's caregiver, should the client be unable to answer the questions appropriately or accurately due to factors such as age, verbal ability, or intellectual level. Obtaining information directly from the client allows the administrator to use a firsthand source to identify the symptoms that cause the most distress and interference. This report of subjective experience of distress or interference allows the service provider to pinpoint what is most problematic among the client's symptoms, leading to a more useful prioritization of treatment goals.

However, one major risk associated with this method is what is known as the *social desirability response bias,* that is, when the respondent gives answers based on what she thinks the administrator wants to hear or what she thinks is the "right" or "healthy" answer. This trend generally results in underreporting of symptoms. On the other hand, some respondents may overreport their symptoms in order to gain a diagnosis, sympathy, or treatment.

Structured Observation

A structured observation is a technique that allows a trained professional to watch and record the specific behaviors of a client in a specified manner. The observer may take note of the presence and/or absence of particular behaviors in order to gauge adaptive skills, incidence of behaviors characteristic of a certain disorder, etc. During a structured observation, the amount of interaction between the clinician and the child being assessed varies. For some measures, the clinician may observe the child interacting with a caregiver. Other protocols involve the clinician prompting the child to perform actions with items included in the test kit. For example, the *Autism Diagnostic Observation Schedule* (ADOS) (Lord, Rutter, DiLavore, & Risi, 1999) requires the trained administrator to set up various situations (e.g., pretend birthday party) using items from the test kit. These situations aim to evoke particular behaviors that a child with ASD may not display (e.g., joint attention). As such, the administrator can assess the child's functioning in a systematic way, rather than merely providing a "free play" setting, which may create opportunities for the assessor to see the behaviors she needs to see.

Because they are norm-referenced, structured observation measures allow the behavior of the client to be compared directly to the behavior of a representative norm group. For instance, the behavior of a child suspected to have developmental delays could be compared to typically developing same-age peers in order to determine the degree of difference between the two.

Personal bias of the observer must be taken into account when considering the results of a structured observation. Although structured observations are meant to be objective, bias can still affect ratings, and the influence of subjectivity cannot be completely avoided. Personal experience, knowledge of prior diagnoses, knowledge of implications of a diagnosis, and many other factors can influence the observations of even the most experienced professional.

PSYCHOMETRICS

Psychometrics consists of evaluating the instruments used for psychological measurement. Standardized assessments are evaluated in terms of their construct validity and reliability, aspects to be discussed in depth in subsequent sections. It is important for a standardized assessment to have good psychometric research supporting it because it helps to assure the clinician that the information the assessment produces is both reliable and valid. In order to be considered a good instrument, an assessment should have representative norms for its target population, as well as satisfactory reliability and validity.

One common problem is the inappropriate use of an instrument based on its available norms. For instance, in the past, the common belief was that individuals with intellectual disability could not have emotional problems or comorbid psychological disorders (Matson, Belva, Hattier, & Matson, 2012). Thus, until recently, measures of psychopathology intended for use with people with intellectual disability were not available. If a clinician wanted to assess in a standardized manner for psychopathology in individuals with intellectual disability, the only option was to use instruments developed for use with people without intellectual disability. Thus, the use of the available norms would not provide accurate comparisons. Fortunately, instruments intended to measure symptoms of psychopathology among individuals with intellectual disability are now available (e.g., *Diagnostic Assessment for the Severely Handicapped II* [*DASH-II*], Matson, 1995).

Norms

In the context of standardized assessment, the term *norm* means the average performance demonstrated by a specified group of individuals on a particular psychological instrument. To identify norms, researchers create a *norm group,* which is the researchers' best attempt at creating a group that is as representative of the measure's target population as possible. For instance, suppose a clinician wants to create an instrument that assesses inattentive behavior among school-age children. The clinician should then create a norm group using school-age children with both genders and all races represented. The people included may be similar in a specific way, such as being the same age or in the same grade in school. The instrument is then administered to everyone in the group, and the average performance of the group is analyzed, yielding the group norm. Theoretically, if the norm group is reasonably representative of the target population, then each child who is given that test can be compared to the average by comparing his results to the group norm.

Reliability and Validity

In psychometrics, *reliability* refers to the ability of an instrument to produce consistent results, whereas *validity* refers to the ability of an instrument to measure what it intends to measure (i.e., accuracy). Consider the analogy of a dartboard. If a dart player hits the bull's-eye, his hits are valid. That is, he is hitting where he is aiming, as the bull's-eye is what he intends to hit. On the other hand, if a dart player hits the right edge of the board, his hits are less valid. Say the dart player hits the right edge of the board every time he throws the dart. His hits are reliable (because they are the same every time) but not valid (and you probably do not want him on your team!). If a dart player hits the bull's-eye the first time, then the right edge of the board, and then the left edge of the board, his hits are less reliable. Finally, say the dart player hits the bull's-eye over and over, time after time. Then his hits would be considered reliable *and* valid. These are characteristics of a good dart player and a good standardized assessment. For example, a good autism measure is valid if it indicates the child has autism when she actually does. The measure is reliable if it is consistent in assigning diagnoses; for example, if the same child were assessed using the same measure several times, the measure would indicate the same result. It is important to keep in mind that a measure, like a dart player's hits, can be reliable but not valid.

Types of Reliability

Inter-rater reliability. Inter-rater reliability is the extent to which an assessment produces the same results when two different people administer it. Inter-rater reliability is calculated by quantitatively comparing the scores of assessments conducted by two different raters. Having multiple raters is useful in decreasing the influence of the individual bias of each rater.

Test-retest reliability. Test-retest reliability is the agreement between the results of an assessment administered at one point in time and administered again at a later time. Each administration should be as similar as possible (e.g., same location, same administrator) to make an accurate comparison. This measure of reliability should not necessarily be used for measures in which a change is likely or expected. For example, test-retest reliability need not be considered in a progress monitoring situation in which a depression scale is used each week of therapy. Presumably, therapy is decreasing levels of depression, so good test-retest reliability should not be present on a depression scale that is to be used frequently. Test-retest reliability is more likely to be useful in the measurement of more stable variables, such as the intelligence of a typically developing adult.

Types of Validity

Concurrent validity. Concurrent validity indicates the amount of agreement between two different assessments. Generally, one assessment is new while the other is well established and has already been proven to be valid. An author of a new assessment would want her assessment to have high concurrent validity with well-respected, well-established assessments.

Construct validity. Construct validity is the ability of the assessment to represent or evaluate the construct in question. This statistic answers the question "Does this assessment tool truly measure what it says it measures?"

Content validity. Content validity refers to the ability of the instrument to measure or evaluate all aspects of the construct it intends to assess. For example, an assessment that examines only socialization or communication would have low content validity for the assessment of autism because the measure ignores repetitive behavior, one of the core domains of impairment found in autism.

Predictive validity. Predictive validity indicates the ability of a measure to predict performance on some outcome variable. For instance, an autism screening measure utilized for infants and toddlers (e.g., *BISCUIT – Part 1*; Matson, Boisjoli, & Wilkins, 2007) should have good predictive validity for future autism diagnoses based on full evaluations. That is, infants and toddlers deemed "at risk" should be more likely to receive an autism diagnosis later when they receive a full diagnostic evaluation.

INTERPRETING STANDARDIZED ASSESSMENT SCORES

Behavior analysts often do not receive training on interpreting standardized assessment scores. These scores can be interpreted in a multitude of ways, so it is critical to know what the scores can and cannot tell you.

BELL CURVE

The bell curve refers to a normal probability distribution with a mean of zero and a standard deviation of one. When plotted on a graph, the distribution looks like a bell, hence its name. A standard deviation is how much a score differs from the mean, or average, score. In a normal distribution, about 68% of individuals fall within one standard deviation of the mean, an additional 26% within two standard deviations (for a total of 94% within two standard deviations), an additional 4% within three standard deviations, and so on. In other words, standard deviation in this context means how much different a child is from the average child in the typically developing population. Generally speaking, as one moves farther from the mean, there are fewer and fewer children who function at that level. For example, in any given population, very few people are geniuses or have profound intellectual disability (the two far ends of the bell curve of intelligence).

The bell curve can be a useful way to look at a child's performance because it allows clinicians and parents to visualize the child's scores compared to those of her peers. A visual representation can sometimes be easier for a parent or staff member to understand than a number, such as a percentile or standard score.

RAW SCORES

Raw scores are the total points scored on an assessment, either for the entire assessment or for subdomains. Raw scores cannot be directly compared between measures. Instead, their primary utility is for score conversion; raw scores can be translated into standard scores, percentiles, and age and grade equivalents, all of which facilitate understanding of performance.

Percentile

A percentile ranks the percentage of individuals in the norm group that scored at or below the score attained by the individual being assessed. For example, a percentile of 71, or scoring "in the 71st percentile," means the child scored the same as or better than 71% of individuals his or her age. Percentile does *not* mean percent correct on the test or percentage of development that a child has achieved.

Standard Score

The standard score is calculated from the raw score. It indicates how many standard deviations an individual's score is above or below the population's mean. Standard scores are most often reported in t-scores in standardized testing. These scores are useful for comparison and are especially useful for complex statistical comparisons. However, utilizing percentile ranks or age or grade equivalents to compare individuals may make more sense to most people.

Age and Grade Equivalents

Age and grade equivalents are included in the score reports or manuals of a variety of measures, such as IQ and achievement tests. Age and grade equivalents are probably easier to understand for those people who are less familiar with standardized assessment. An age or grade equivalent is defined as the age or grade level that corresponds with the score of an individual being assessed. For example, if a 7-year-old child receives an age equivalent of 5, that means that his performance on the assessment was similar to the average performance of a 5-year-old.

Cut-Off Scores

Cut-off scores are used to determine whether an individual "passes" a test. In psychological evaluation, these scores usually signal different levels of clinically significant impairment based on some norm-referenced or criterion-referenced research. For example, a child's results on a diagnostic scale may fall below or above the cut-off that suggests a diagnosis of autism spectrum disorder.

ASSESSMENTS

In this section, we provide brief descriptions of one or two of the standardized assessments that we find most useful in each major domain of assessment.

Adaptive Measures

The term *adaptive skills* concerns an individual's ability to be self-sufficient in multiple domains. Adaptive domains include self-care, communication skills, social skills, leisure skills, community use, vocational skills, and health and safety skills. A variety of adaptive measures are available, but the **Vineland Adaptive Behavior Scales, Second Edition** (Vineland-II; Sparrow, Cicchetti, & Balla, 2005) is the one that is probably the most highly regarded standardized measure of adaptive skills, and it is the one that we find most useful. The Vineland-II has been shown to have very strong psychometric properties and is used to measure adaptive skills in individuals from birth to 90 years of age. One of its main uses is to detect and diagnose intellectual disability from the adaptive skills side. (A diagnosis of intellectual disability requires cognitive *and* adaptive skill impairments, so the Vineland-II covers only the latter domain of deficits.) In addition to aiding in diagnosis, the Vineland-II is a good measure to inform treatment plans as well as track progress of development over the years. The current edition of the Vineland offers two survey forms (one interview and one rating scale), an expanded interview form, and a teacher rating form. The parent/caregiver rating form is especially useful in that it allows the clinician to assess key behaviors and skills that indicate appropriate or inappropriate adaptive ability based on age in the form of an easy and quick-to-administer rating scale. The Vineland-II also includes an optional maladaptive behavior index that addresses internalizing and externalizing problems. Percentile ranks, adaptive levels, and age equivalents are provided.

The assessment contains socialization, daily living skills, communication, and motor domains. The communication domain contains receptive, expressive, and written subdomains. The daily living skills domain contains personal, domestic, and community subdomains. The socialization domain contains interpersonal relationships, play and leisure time, and coping skills subdomains. Finally, the motor domain contains both fine and gross motor subdomains. Scores on the Vineland-II contain a mean of 100 and standard deviation of 15 for both the total score and each of the four subdomains.

The time required to administer the assessment varies from 20 to 60 minutes for survey interview and parent/caregiver rating forms, 25 to 90 minutes for the expanded interview form, and 20 minutes for the teacher rating form. Clinicians who administer the assessment should be professionals who are licensed or certified to practice in a healthcare field or who have received formal supervised mental health, speech/language, and/or educational training specific to working with parents and assessing children.

Intelligence Testing

Beyond its value to behavior analysts, the clinical utility of intelligence testing has been debated for years. Perhaps the largest question is simply how intelligence tests might be useful for treatment providers. The belief that intelligence could be measured and transformed into a number to be compared with others' numbers emerged in the 20th century, first in attempts to account for individual differences using evolutionary terms and then as a school readiness test (White, 2000). More recently, IQ measures have been criticized as culturally biased, as well as biased in relation to socioeconomic status. Despite the controversy, IQ tests do measure important cognitive abilities and can be useful in recognizing the strengths and deficits of individuals relative to same-age peers. IQ testing is commonly used to identify learning and intellectual disabilities in order to make decisions about student placement and supports in school systems.

Wechsler series. We have found the Wechsler series of IQ tests to be the most useful for individuals who have some language. Wechsler IQ tests are widely utilized and have strong psychometrics. The Wechsler series of IQ tests for children consists of the two tests described below.

Wechsler Preschool and Primary Scale of Intelligence – Third Edition (WPPSI-III). The WPPSI is an individually administered test that measures the cognitive abilities of children between the ages of 2 years, 6 months, and 7 years, 3 months (Wechsler, 2002a). It measures both verbal and nonverbal reasoning skills. These two areas are then combined to form the Full-Scale IQ, a number that represents overall cognitive functioning, with a mean of 100 and a standard deviation of 15.

Wechsler Intelligence Scale for Children – Fourth Edition (WISC-IV). The WISC is an individually administered test that measures the cognitive abilities of children between the ages of 6 and 16 years (Wechsler, 2003). The WISC-IV contains 10 core subtests that are organized into four cognitive domains (also referred to as index scales): Verbal Comprehension, Perceptual Reasoning, Working Memory, and Processing Speed. When combined together, these indices yield a Full-Scale IQ score. Composite scores have a mean of 100 and a standard deviation of 15 points. Individual subtest scores are reported as scaled scores, which have a mean of 10 and a standard deviation of 3.

Nonverbal intelligence tests. For learners who have little or no language, a nonverbal IQ test is likely to give more valid results. We have found the most useful nonverbal IQ test for children to be the **Leiter International Performance Scale – Revised (Leiter-R)**. The Leiter-R is an individually administered test designed to assess cognitive functions in children and adolescents ages 2 years, 0 months, to 20 years, 11 months (Roid & Miller, 1995, 1997). The test includes measures of nonverbal intelligence in fluid reasoning and visualization, as well as appraisals of visuospatial memory and attention. The Leiter-R includes two groupings of subtests:

1. The Visualization and Reasoning (VR) Battery with 10 subtests of nonverbal intellectual ability related to visualization, reasoning, and spatial ability and
2. The Attention and Memory (AM) Battery with 10 subtests of nonverbal attention and memory function.

Subtests from the VR Battery are used to estimate intellectual ability, and subtests from the AM Battery are used as a comprehensive assessment of attention and memory domains. Scales have a mean of a 100 and a standard deviation of 15 points. **The Merrill-Palmer-R Scales of**

Development is another widely regarded test that can provide useful results for nonverbal children. The Merrill-Palmer-R provides standard scores, percentiles, and age equivalents for children from infancy through 6 years of age across the following domains: cognitive, language, motor, self-help, and social-emotional (Roid & Sampers, 2004).

Social Skills

Social Skills Improvement System (SSIS): Parent Form. The SSIS provides a comprehensive evaluation of a child's social behaviors across two domains: Social Skills (communication, cooperation, assertion, responsibility, empathy, engagement, and self-control) and Problem Behaviors (externalizing, bullying, hyperactivity/inattention, and internalizing) (Gresham & Elliott, 2008). Standard scores on the SSIS have a mean of 100 and a standard deviation of 15. While a high standard score on the Social Skills portion of the assessment is desirable, a high score on the Problem Behaviors scale is undesirable. For example, on the Problem Behaviors scale, a percentile ranking of 84 would indicate that 84 percent of same-sex students at the same educational level in the standardization comparison group exhibit *fewer* problem behaviors than the rated student. Since each subscale represents a specific behavior, subscale scores are translated into Behavior Levels (below average, average, and above average) that refer to the level of particular behavioral characteristics compared to the child's same-age peers.

Language

Preschool Language Scale – Fourth Edition (PLS-4). For measuring early language learning, we have found that the PLS-4 is a useful standardized assessment. The PLS-4 is an individually administered test that is composed of two subscales: Auditory Comprehension and Expressive Communication (Zimmerman, Steiner, & Pond, 2002). The Auditory Comprehension subscale is used to evaluate how much language a child understands, while the Expressive Communication subscale is used to determine how well a child communicates with others. This test is constructed with a mean of 100 and a standard deviation of 15.

Test of Language Development – Primary: Fourth Edition (TOLD-P:4). The TOLD-P:4 is a language test designed for children ages 4 to 8 years, 11 months (Newcomer & Hammill, 2008). The TOLD-P:4 is intended to (1) measure receptive, organizational, and expressive competencies in the major components of linguistics; (2) determine the presence of strengths and weaknesses among linguistic abilities; (3) document progress in prescribed remedial or therapeutic programs; and (4) provide researchers with a statistically sound measure for use in studying children's language.

Composites have a mean of 100 and a standard deviation of 15 points, while subtests have a mean of 10 and a standard deviation of 3.

Clinical Evaluation of Language Fundamentals, Fourth Edition (CELF-4). The CELF-4 is an individually administered test used for the identification, diagnosis, and evaluation of language skill deficits in individuals between 5 and 21 years, 11 months (Semel, Wiig, & Secord, 2003). The CELF-4 provides standard scores for receptive language, expressive language, language structure, language content, language memory, and working memory. With a mean composite score of 100 and a standard deviation of 15, scores equal to and above 85 are considered within normal limits of language fundamentals.

Test of Pragmatic Language – Second Edition (TOPL-2). To measure a child's ability to use language socially, we have commonly used the TOPL-2. The TOPL-2 is an instrument used to evaluate the effectiveness and appropriateness of pragmatic or social language skills in children from 6 to 18 years of age (Phelps-Terasaki & Phelps-Gunn, 2007). The TOPL-2 has five principle uses:

1. To identify individuals with pragmatic language deficits;
2. To determine the individual's strengths and weaknesses among the different types of pragmatic skills;
3. To document an individual's progress in pragmatic language as a consequence of special intervention programs;
4. To measure pragmatic language in research; and
5. To address the needs of specific populations.

Individuals are asked questions intended to provide information on six core subcomponents of pragmatic language: physical setting, audience, topic, purpose (speech acts), visual-gestural cues, and abstraction. This test is constructed with a mean of 100 and a standard deviation of 15.

Neuropsychological, Executive Function, and Problem Solving

Behavior Rating Inventory of Executive Function – Preschool Version (BRIEF-P). We commonly use the BRIEF-P as a quick and efficient measure of executive function. Parents, teachers, and daycare providers complete the 63-item form to rate a child's executive functions within the context of his everyday environments (home and preschool). The BRIEF-P measures the following aspects of executive functioning: inhibition, working memory, shifting, planning/organizing, and emotional control (Gioia, Espy, & Isquith, 2003). T-scores at or below 59 are considered to be within the typical range. T-scores of 60–64 are in the mildly elevated range, and scores equal to or exceeding 65 are considered to be significantly elevated.

Developmental Neuropsychological Assessment – Second Edition (NEPSY-II). The NEPSY-II is a child-friendly neuropsychological instrument that provides a means of assessing six domains in children ages 3 to 16 years old (Korkman, Kirk, & Kemp, 2007). The six domains are Social Perception, Attention and Executive Functions, Language and Communication, Sensorimotor Functions, Visuospatial Functions, and Learning and Memory. Due to the length of time needed to administer the entire test, single domains are often selected and administered alone.

Test of Problem Solving 3: Elementary (TOPS-3). The TOPS-3 is an assessment that measures the ability to think and reason in children ages 6–12 (Bowers, Huisingh, & LoGiudice, 2005). The test specifically addresses a child's language strategies using both logic and experience. Questions assess critical thinking skills, such as inferring, predicting, determining causes, sequencing, answering negative questions, and problem solving. Questions relate directly to photographs shown to the individual. The pictures are intended to reflect common, everyday situations. Additionally, children are presented with information to answer the question regardless of their level of experience with the situation. The TOPS-3 has a mean of 100 and standard deviation of 15.

Achievement Tests

Achievement tests are designed to measure skills and knowledge learned in a given grade. Achievement tests may be used to identify the academic strengths and deficits of a student; to decide eligibility for educational services, placement, or a diagnosis of a specific learning disability; and to help plan instructional objectives and interventions. The most commonly used achievement tests include the Woodcock Johnson Tests of Achievement III (Woodcock, McGrew, & Mather, 2001) and the Wechsler Individual Achievement Test, Third Edition (Wechsler, 2002b).

Developmental Assessments

Developmental assessments are useful to assess a young child's current skills relative to where they should be compared to typical child development. A curriculum assessment that has age equivalents, such as Skills® (www.skillsforautism.com; see Chapter 26 for more about Skills), provides more specific information, making it more likely to be useful for identifying treatment targets. However, standardized developmental assessments, such as the Mullen Scales of Early Learning (Mullen, 1995) or the Bayley Scales of Infant and Toddler Development, Third Edition (Bayley, 1993), have the benefits of being standardized and faster to implement (because they are less comprehensive).

USING THE RESULTS OF STANDARDIZED ASSESSMENTS

Standardized assessment results can be useful in treatment in a variety of ways, including helping to identify skill areas to target, identifying other related disorders, and tracking treatment progress.

Identifying Targets for Treatment

The information obtained from standardized assessments can help identify each learner's strengths and deficits, so you can fine-tune your treatment programs to focus on improving deficit areas while capitalizing on strengths. Most intelligence tests result in both a full-scale IQ score and separate index scores. Each index represents a distinct construct (collection of skills). Intelligence tests can, therefore, guide the identification of skills that need development and indicate how to adapt the teaching of such skills for the individual learner. For instance, imagine that a significant weakness in the working memory subscale was observed in your 6-year-old learner after administering a test of executive function. Given this deficit, he is likely to have difficulty with instruction that requires attending to longer strings of stimuli and responding to them a short time later. For example, when teaching categories, you might ask, "Which one is an animal – cat, boat, yellow, or pizza?" For a learner with working memory deficits, it may be challenging to attend to the initial category question as well as the long string of potential answers, thereby resulting in an incorrect response. Therefore you may need to modify your presentation of the question and answers. For example, you could initially present the potential answers as written or picture stimuli, or you could consider specifically targeting working memory as a skill in itself (see Chapter 18).

Consider another example of a learner whose IQ test shows deficits in the Processing Speed subscale. For this learner, you may need to work on rate-building in order to increase the overall speed and fluency of responding (see section on fluency in Chapter 4). For example, using flashcards to teach labels, you could set goals for how many flashcards the learner needs to answer correctly in one minute and then deliver reinforcement when she meets or exceeds the goal. Fluent responding is important in discrete trial training (DTT), as well as imperative for success in a mainstream academic or social setting because interactions in these settings occur rapidly and require rapid processing.

The results of achievement tests can be helpful in identifying particular academic areas in which the learner could use additional practice during DTT tutoring outside of school and/or more support in the classroom setting. For example, a learner may have particular difficulty with literacy skills, so additional support in that area may be helpful.

Adaptive assessments, such as the Vineland-II, can produce results that are helpful in identifying areas of self-help skills on which to focus with particular learners. In particular, if you have access to the individual answers to individual questions, you can identify specific targets, such as tying shoes, making a snack, brushing teeth, and so on.

It is also useful for you to be aware of the results of any standardized assessment of psychopathology that your learner has undergone. It is very common for older children with ASD to suffer from comorbid psychopathology. For example, Simonoff & colleagues (2008) found that 70% of their sample of individuals with ASD had at least one comorbid diagnosis. It is also quite common for individuals with ASD to score high on assessments of attention deficit hyperactivity disorder (ADHD), and treatment programs may be more effective if they accommodate hyperactivity. For example, sitting at a table to complete DTT may be particularly frustrating for a learner with ADHD, so therapy can be conducted in a more natural environment (see section on natural environment training in Chapter 4), or the learner may simply be allowed to stand during instruction, rather than sit.

It is also very common for children with ASD to have social anxiety or specific phobias. Being aware of these conditions can help you modify therapy to be less anxiety provoking. Furthermore, if you have the proper training, desensitization and graduated exposure procedures can be incorporated into your behavioral intervention program.

Progress Tracking

Implementing a battery of standardized assessments at regular intervals can be useful in monitoring and documenting treatment progress, both at the level of the individual and against population norms. ASD severity measures have a fairly obvious use in terms of progress monitoring. If your treatment is effective in alleviating the overall symptoms of ASD, such scales should reflect improvement in core deficit areas (i.e., problems with socialization and communication) and/or reduction in behavioral excesses (i.e., repetitive behaviors and restricted interests). The use of standardized ASD severity measures differs from graphing progress in the programs that target core deficit areas over time in that it provides standardized norms; a child's symptom severity can be compared to a large population of same-age children with ASD. Results of standardized assessments of language, daily living skills, and socialization can, of course, be used to document progress in those domains, as well. In addition, standardized assessment results are more highly respected by people outside of the behavior analytic community when compared to actual data on specific behaviors.

SUMMARY

Standardized assessments are a means by which an individual child's functioning can be measured and compared against the general population of same-age children. Standardized assessments provide general, global information that is useful in obtaining a bigger-picture view of a child's strengths and challenges. The CARD Model of autism treatment includes comprehensive batteries of standardized assessments at regular intervals before, during, and after treatment. Behavior analysts generally are not trained on how to administer or interpret standardized assessments, and they would benefit from further training in this area. Standardized assessments are not a substitute for direct measures of behavior and skills used for treatment programming but, rather, complement direct measures by providing a broader scope and a form of measurement that are more widely accepted by those outside of behavior analysis.

Technology

Jonathan Tarbox, Adel C. Najdowski

The information technology revolution has changed virtually all aspects of modern society, and autism treatment is no exception. The adoption of technology in autism treatment, however, has lagged behind the adoption of technology in many other disciplines, such as education, medicine, and business. This chapter will provide a discussion of currently available technology solutions and the likely future development of technology in areas such as assessment and curriculum, data collection, training, and telemedicine, among others.

ASSESSMENT AND CURRICULUM

Assessment

Several advantages of technology-based assessment are worth discussing. First, assessment data are stored electronically, which allows results to be automatically updated and an assessment report to be produced to illustrate a learner's strengths and needs. If the assessment is linked directly to a curriculum, then the assessment results can help with the treatment planning process in an even more efficient manner. If the assessment is connected to the Internet, then it can allow multiple assessors to log in from their own locations and input data into the same assessment. Likewise, multiple people can log in and view the results of an assessment from various locations. Finally, the capacity of technology to reduce paperwork and eliminate the need to carry around the assessment documents further increases efficiency and improves mobility.

Curriculum

Most curricula for autism treatment are still distributed in traditional paper, hard-copy format. These curricula have served practitioners reasonably well, but their format is inherently limiting. First, since the discipline of autism treatment is always evolving, paper curricula should be out of date within a few years after being printed. Of course, new editions can always be printed, but this has occurred, in reality, on such an infrequent basis that most curricula remain outdated. A major advantage of web- or cloud-based curricula is that they can truly be "living documents" that are updated on a continuous basis to reflect the most current evidence base.

Second, lessons in paper format are difficult to adapt. As has been made clear in this manual, the *analysis* portion of applied behavior analysis (ABA) is absolutely critical, and teaching lessons must be customized to meet each individual learner's needs. Paper lessons need to be retyped and edited (and reprinted) in order to be customized, a waste of time and effort that can be avoided by using editable electronic formats. Given that professional communication often occurs nowadays via electronic formats, information from an electronic curriculum can therefore be copied and pasted into electronic mail to facilitate much more rapid communication among treatment team members.

Third, particularly large curriculum books can offer too much information for the practitioner to sift through efficiently at any one time. For example, if a paper curriculum contains hundreds of potential lessons, clinicians must ensure that they consider every possible lesson sufficiently, so they do not miss important lessons that should be taught but get "lost in the shuffle." Additionally, clinicians may pore over hundreds of pages of curriculum every time they consider what to teach their learner next (i.e., every 2 weeks), but this process robs the clinician of precious time that would be better used treating children. As an alternative, well-designed electronic curricula can solve these problems by organizing and presenting a more streamlined, relevant, and user-friendly amount of information targeted to what the clinician likely needs to see at any given time. For example, if an electronic curriculum is linked to an assessment, then only lessons that the learner has not already mastered are presented to the clinician. In addition, lessons can be sorted by difficulty, prerequisite skills, age of emergence in typical development, and so on, as is done in the Skills® curriculum (see description below).

Fourth, comprehensive curricula are massive, and the sheer weight and size that they occupy in paper form make them unwieldy and not amenable to travel or broad dissemination. If ABA is to be disseminated globally, coordination and consultation need to occur across vast distances – perhaps even across continents – in real-time, and the need to have multiple copies of the same paper curriculum in different places around the world for a team to collaborate effectively is unreasonably cumbersome.

Fifth, electronic curricula allow for web- or cloud-based progress tracking. Data from a single learner's treatment program can be tracked and graphed in a single place, making it easily accessible by multiple team members from different locations, thereby greatly enhancing interdisciplinary collaboration. Online real-time progress tracking can also greatly enhance a clinical supervisor's ability to stay abreast of her learners' progress in home-based programs because it obviates the need to physically bring paper copies of data sheets to the supervisor's location.

Sixth, electronic curricula, if they include progress tracking, hold tremendous potential for research on autism treatment simply because of the data that can be collected. A significant challenge of research on autism treatment is the very large individual differences between children of the same age who receive the same treatment. Very large samples are therefore required to find meaningful relationships between variables of interest and treatment outcome. The need for very large sample sizes, in turn, makes research both expensive and difficult to manage. The result is that very few autism treatment outcome studies are funded, conducted, or published. Large-scale databases that contain outcome data on real-life autism treatment hold the potential to yield answers to questions that have been difficult or impossible to address using traditional research designs. For example, if data on learning rate in ABA programs were contained in a single database, which also contained data on hundreds of other variables that might be relevant to learning outcome, research could address questions such as the optimal intensity, focus, format, and so on, of treatment for children of every conceivable age, IQ level, baseline skill level, and more. Such a database could hold promise for identifying phenotypes, or subtypes, of autism spectrum disorder (ASD) that could be helpful for predicting response to treatment, matching treatment type to child characteristics, and so on.

Skills®. CARD has developed an online treatment management platform, Skills® (www.skillsforautism.com), which includes online assessment, curriculum, and progress tracking. The Skills assessment, which has been found to have strong validity (Persicke et al., 2014), covers the eight curriculum domains described in the content section of this manual (Chapters 11–18): social, motor, language, adaptive, play, executive functions, cognition, and academic skills. In addition to the assessment being valid, the language domain of the Skills assessment has been found to be reliable (Dixon, Tarbox, Najdowski, Wilke & Granpeesheh, 2011).

When creating a Skills account for a learner and entering her birthdate, the user completes a comprehensive assessment that starts with questions about the learner's infant skills and continues up to the learner's chronological age with the goal of determining everything the learner needs to be taught in order to catch up to her typically developing, same-age peers. Each assessment question is directly linked to one or more lesson activities within any of the eight curricula of the Skills program, and each time the assessor indicates that the learner cannot perform a task, the linked lesson activities for that particular item are placed into the learner's activity library. The user is then able to choose which of the activities in this library to place into the learner's current treatment program.

The curriculum contains almost 4,000 activities, and Skills contains several tools to aid in the process of choosing which activities to prioritize for the learner. First, the lessons are all categorized by difficulty level, from 1 (easiest) to 12 (most advanced). All other things being equal, clinicians should start with lowest level lessons first. Second, all activities have a developmental age assigned to them. Generally speaking, skills that emerge earlier in typical development should be introduced before older skills, as long as they are currently relevant to the learner's life. Third, prerequisite skills are identified for all activities, so a particular activity should not be introduced before its prerequisite skills are mastered. Fourth, all the activities are categorized as one of three types: 1) building block, 2) fundamental skill, and 3) expansion skill. A building block is not a legitimate skill in and of itself; rather, it is a stepping stone toward a fundamental skill that is the real meaningful skill used in daily life. An expansion skill goes above and beyond a fundamental skill and is considered more of an enrichment activity that would be used with a child for whom one expects best outcomes. We advise clinicians to think about the profiles of their learners and choose their activities wisely. For example, when working with a child who is a fast learner, it might be unnecessary to spend time teaching building blocks. Perhaps that type of learner can go straight into learning the fundamentals and then onto expansions without every really needing building blocks. It's fine to skip building blocks because they are not the truly meaningful skill; however, it should be noted that they are important intermediate steps that can be very helpful for learners who need to learn in smaller steps. With this type of learner, the clinician might choose to start with building blocks and end at fundamental skills, ignoring expansion skills.

After choosing the activities to place in the treatment program, the clinician then teaches those skills and inputs data along the way. All authorized caregivers, health care providers, teachers, and other professionals can then track the learner's progress in Skills online. All of this information is displayed in the learner's progress charts and incorporated into her progress reports. Data on learning are automatically graphed over time. The clinician also has the ability to input data on challenging behavior, and these data are then automatically superimposed on data on learning rate in order for the clinician to observe the relationship, if any, between challenging behavior and learning rate. In addition, the clinician can input any other relevant life events that may impact challenging behavior or learning, such as medication changes, changes in school placement, illness, changes in treatment intensity, and so on. All of these variables can be viewed together or separately, so the clinician can analyze the extent to which they influence one another.

TEACHING TECHNOLOGY

Games and Applications

Hundreds, if not thousands, of teaching games and apps are currently available for children with ASD. In theory, such applications can be beneficial because they provide teaching opportunities to learners when clinicians might otherwise be unable to provide their undivided attention to the learner or when the learner is not in a direct instructional environment. In some cases, the games/apps can even be used as reinforcers for the learner during downtime. In these cases, the learner is able to continue learning even during breaks from therapist-delivered therapy.

Despite the many potential benefits of computer applications for teaching children with ASD, there are many limitations inherent in what is currently available. First, at the time of the publication of this manual, with the exception of one or two studies, none of the hundreds of currently available teaching apps have any research supporting their effectiveness. Therefore, it is presently unknown whether 99% of the currently available apps actually work.

Second, the vast majority of educational games and apps are designed by people who are not experts in treating children with ASD. Therefore, even a casual review of most apps reveals that they are not based on any principles or procedures known to be effective in teaching children with ASD. Most apps don't include even the most basic elements of effective prompting, reinforcement, and prompt-fading procedures that actually result in skill acquisition in the autism population.

A third significant limitation of teaching apps that are currently available is that the present state of technology does not yet allow most skills to be taught. Virtually all teaching apps currently require a response from the student in the form of touching a screen or clicking a mouse, so skills that require any other form of response are still a long way off from being teachable on an app. For example, expressive vocal language is difficult to teach with a computer because speech recognition technology is still primitive, although it is improving rapidly. Although it has been used successfully to teach second languages to typically developing individuals, at the time this manual goes to press, it has not yet been successfully applied to teaching children with ASD. Motion-sensing technology for teaching motor skills to children with ASD has also not yet been invented, although that is in development at several centers and will likely be available soon.

We expect that the next 5 years will bring significant advancements in the development of apps for teaching children with ASD, but we hope those advances will be accompanied by sound scientific research and that app development will be based on published research on teaching procedures that work for children with ASD. The future of autism intervention will almost certainly include an important place for technology that directly teaches learners with ASD. The first forays have already been made into this area with very mixed results, but some progress has already been made. At the moment, these types of programs should, at most, be used to supplement human-delivered ABA therapy. ABA consists of engineering the learner's teaching environment to cause learning. If a computer is made a significant part of the learner's environment (and for many learners it already is), then it follows that computers should be able to teach learners with ASD and potentially replace a significant portion of human-delivered ABA. Computerized ABA-based instruction offers many possible advantages, including increased procedural integrity, automated data collection and progress tracking, increased access to treatment, and the potential to decrease the costs of ABA treatment. To be clear, the day that research demonstrates that any portion of human-delivered ABA treatment can be replaced by computer-delivered teaching is very far off, but it seems likely that this will be the case in the future.

Robotics. At some point, it seems likely that robots will be developed that can perform at least some portion of teaching for people with and without disabilities, and there is no clear reason that children with ASD could not also benefit. Using robots to deliver instruction would essentially be the same as a child with ASD learning from an app on a tablet or computer, except that the computer can walk, talk, make facial expressions, and potentially learn from its interactions with the child. Of course, if the robot is not capable of natural social interactions, it will not be likely to be useful for teaching social skills. However, especially for children with ASD who are particularly interested in technology, robots may turn out to be an effective option for teaching nonsocial content.

COMMUNICATION APPLICATIONS

Just as people once searched for the perfect communication device, they are now on the hunt for the perfect communication application, or app. Many different communication apps are available today. Regardless of which one you choose to use with your learners, you will need to customize the vocabulary and the layout for the learner and teach him how to use it. There aren't really any communication apps that the learner can simply pick up and start using without some direct training. In fact, some learners will even need to be trained to use their index fingers properly to activate buttons correctly. Button sensitivity can be adjusted on many apps, but in an extreme case you can purchase grids that lay over the screen to physically prevent the learner from moving his finger sideways over too many buttons.

Many communication apps provide flexibility for customization by allowing you to upload your own photos, record sounds or voiceover, and so on. The advantage of using a communication app is that it provides non-vocal or limited vocal learners with a method of communication. Although the research on their effects on speech is still emerging, our clinicians anecdotally report that, in many cases, learners who use communication apps increase their vocalizations. Another advantage of communication apps is that they offer a portable solution without the requirement to print out, laminate, adhere, and keep track of (try not to misplace or lose) picture cards.

CHALLENGING BEHAVIOR MANAGEMENT

The development of technology tools for managing challenging behavior is emerging. A couple of online tools are available for conducting functional behavioral assessments (FBA) and developing behavior intervention plans (BIPs), one of which is the Skills® BIP Builder (www.skillsbipbuilder.com).

These types of tools use an indirect assessment to ask the user questions related to the function of the challenging behavior. Based on the answers to the questions and accompanying summary of the results, the user is able to identify the most plausible function. At that point, the user begins the process of building a BIP based on the hypothesized function of the challenging behavior using antecedent, replacement behavior, and consequence treatment components.

An advantage of using electronic tools for building BIPs is that, if programmed correctly, they automatically present only function and evidence-based treatment components. Moreover, by using a decision matrix based on the answers to questions about the challenging behavior, a BIP builder can be programmed to present least intrusive interventions first. This type of technology has been shown to increase the use of function-based interventions (Tarbox et al., 2013). Such tools also ensure that the clinician doesn't forget to include antecedent modifications, a replacement behavior, and consequence manipulations, while making sure the clinician also remembers all of the function and evidence-based options from which to choose. Not only does this presumably make the clinician more efficient with her time creating the BIP, but it is also a great way to give educational staff who are less familiar with writing BIPs (but whose job descriptions require it) access to tools based on best practices for writing BIPs.

OTHER CLINICAL TOOLS

Technology is useful in various capacities to assist the clinical supervisor in designing lesson activities to be carried out with learners. For example, clinicians can find 2D pictures online or via applications to use as stimuli during assessment and/or in lesson activities. Technology also offers other tools to be used during therapy, such as electronic token economies, activity schedules, and visual timers for the learner to view the passage of time when learning to "wait" or when implementing a differential reinforcement of other behavior (DRO) procedure. Pagers and special watches have been used to prompt learners (either by vibrating or beeping) to engage in appropriate behaviors, and alarms exist for teaching learners to stop bed wetting. These are just a few of the many examples of handy technology innovations meant for assisting in the delivery of autism treatment.

DATA COLLECTION

In Chapter 20, we discussed the importance of careful data collection during the course of comprehensive behavioral intervention for learners with ASD. The vast majority of data collection in behavioral intervention programs is still done with pen and paper. Paper datasheets are then stored for extended periods of time, and data from them may or may not be transferred to relatively low-tech electronic storage methods, such as Microsoft Excel files, or relatively higher-tech storage, such as networked databases. This method of data collection has served the early intensive behavioral intervention (EIBI) field well for the past several decades; however, it is outdated and unwieldy. Sometime in the near future, it seems almost certain that electronic data collection, analysis, and storage will become the norm.

Several potential benefits of electronic data collection are apparent. For example, intelligent data collection apps will allow for automated transfer of data to centralized databases, automated graphing of data for ongoing clinical analysis, and automated summary of data for reporting purposes. All of these features, if executed well, could decrease the number of person-hours required for case management and reporting, as well as make wireless, real-time clinical case management possible from anywhere in the world with an Internet connection. Just as exciting, electronic storage of data holds the promise of allowing analyses to be conducted that would have required onerous amounts of time to be allocated to data entry and analysis. For example, if 1,000 learners were receiving behavioral intervention and their data were automatically uploaded to a database that was equipped for sophisticated data mining and analytics, a vast array of clinically important questions could be addressed quantitatively. For example, What is the mean and range number of trials to acquisition for a particular skill? How do age, number of treatment hours per week, gender, treatment setting, and any other number of variables influence skill acquisition? What effects, if any, do the credentials, years of experience, number of members on a team, and a whole host of other therapist variables have on learning rate for the child? What effect, if any, do weather, region, season, or number of hours of daylight have on learning outcome? In short, if everyday autism treatment data could be analyzed from a truly "big data" standpoint, hundreds of questions could be addressed that would simply never be addressed using traditional research methodology for financial, logistical, and ethical reasons.

At the time this manual goes to press, real-time electronic data collection during behavioral intervention is still in its infancy. While apps are being marketed for this purpose, the vast majority of them fall short in a number of ways, primarily because electronic data collection has a number of inherent potential limitations.

First, therapists are still far more fluent with pencil and paper than they are with any electronic device, such that it is still almost inevitable that therapists will require more time to tap a phone or tablet than to make a brief mark on paper. As wireless devices integrate themselves into every aspect of our lives, this may change. Perhaps pens and pencils will be a thing of the past in coming decades, but a current critical concern when choosing whether to use electronic data collection is how much time it requires of the therapists. A recent study evaluating electronic data collection on handheld computers found that electronic data collection required significantly more time than pen and paper data collection and likely slowed down the pace of therapy considerably (Tarbox, Wilke, Findel-Pyles, Bergstrom & Granpeesheh, 2010).

A second potential limitation is that data collection can be limited by the interface that the application provides. In other words, one can only collect the data that the computer program allows one to collect. With pen and paper data, therapists are free to rapidly jot down notes of any sort about any topic, should the need arise. Presumably, data collection applications will be adapted to allow rapid descriptive note taking at some point, but this is a significant concern at this time.

CARD has recently developed a tablet-based software application for data collection and management called Skills LogBook™, which is designed to address the limitations described above. Skills LogBook™ runs on an iPad that each therapist uses while conducting therapy. The software allows therapists to collect acquisition and challenging behavior data and replaces a therapist's paper/pencil logbook or data sheets. Skills LogBook™ is linked directly to each individual learner's Skills account, so when therapists need to collect discrete trial training (DTT) data, they are able to select from all of the lessons that are currently in acquisition or mastered in the learner's program, as well as the particular exemplars to be taught during that session. The software automatically selects whether the lesson should be taught in mass trial, random rotation, or expanded trials (Chapter 4) based on the data that were collected the last time that lesson was taught. The supervisor has the ability to adjust mastery criteria and other details of how the software determines lesson phases. When the therapist is ready to begin conducting the lesson with the learner, the screen of the iPad resembles a standard discrete trial datasheet. At the top of the sheet is a notes section that is automatically updated with the latest notes that the supervisor entered into Skills for that particular lesson. In addition, Skills LogBook™ displays any notes regarding challenging behavior management that the supervisor has entered into the system. Each iPad is wirelessly connected to the central Skills server, so every time a lesson is conducted, the data are automatically and wirelessly updated in Skills. This gives the supervisor the ability to add notes for the therapist in real time from anywhere in the world with an Internet connection. At the time this manual goes to press, Skills LogBook™ is being used for internal purposes only, but it will be made commercially available in the near future.

CARE COORDINATION AND CASE MANAGEMENT

A new development in autism treatment is the use of technology as a means for insurance agencies to carry out care coordination and case management. Using various treatment management software programs, of which Skills is one, insurance carriers are now able to allow their case managers to log into a learner's account and view real-time progress, obtain reports, and, ultimately, make decisions about the learner's future funding. The availability of this type of technology has been useful for increasing the ability of autism treatment agencies to communicate directly with insurance carriers and for care coordination to be carried out seamlessly.

In the foreseeable future, once tens of thousands of learners' assessments and curriculum progress are saved in databases and tracked using such software programs, the face of funding for autism treatment as we know it will likely change. That is, algorithms should emerge that are capable of using individual profiles to predict a learner's potential progress within given treatment parameters. If this happens, the number of hours requested for funding should be generated directly from a computer program, eliminating the often arbitrary decision-making process of the funding agencies. If the analyses are based on valid data, then this would represent a shift toward data-based decision making on the part of funding agencies – something that is all but lacking today – while preserving the processes that enable families to challenge insurance carriers when necessary.

Such computer programs should also allow funding agencies – and potentially consumers – to view quality rankings of autism treatment agencies in terms of their level of progress with the learners they serve in relation to other agencies and even among various clinical supervisors within the same organization. This should help improve the quality of

ABA service delivery as a whole by increasing accountability within the field and eventually weeding out the less effective clinicians, as their ability to obtain funding for their services will eventually be eliminated until they receive more training and demonstrate improvement.

TRAINING

The need for global dissemination of expertise in ABA is great, and one of the largest bottlenecks is the availability of expert trainers. Web-based training is a promising method for addressing this need. Research comparing web-based training to in-person training for establishing clinical competence in ABA practitioners is still very much in its infancy, but the initial results are encouraging, both for training staff (Granpeesheh et al., 2010) and parents of children with autism (Jang et al., 2012). It seems unlikely that web-based staff training, no matter how sophisticated, will ever completely circumvent the need for human interaction in training, nor would we want it to do so. It seems likely, however, that web-based staff training will prove to increase the cost-effectiveness of disseminating staff training across longer distances and larger regions by reducing the number of hours of in-person training required and/or decreasing the number of in-person visits required by an expert trainer.

A good model for incorporating web-based training is likely to be used as a replacement for some portion of classroom didactic training. In other words, it seems likely that some or all of the time that trainees would normally spend listening to a lecture in a classroom could be replaced by self-paced web-based training as long as it is followed by in-person performance feedback and on-the-job training.

Technology-based trainings currently come in all different shapes, sizes, and modes of delivering content, including use of computer-animated videos; recorded human-delivered lecture with PowerPoint; narrated videos of procedures being carried out with learners; and interactive technology wherein trainees receive instruction and feedback while attempting to carry out procedures with a computer-animated learner.

Institute for Behavioral Training (IBT)

CARD's training materials for staff, educators, and parents are now available online in an eLearning format through the Institute for Behavioral Training (IBT; www.ibehavioraltraining.com). The format of the training is PowerPoint combined with videotaped lecture and examples of therapists demonstrating procedures with learners. These eLearning training modules are used all over the world by anyone interested in learning more about the delivery of behavioral intervention to learners with ASD.

TELEMEDICINE

The field of telemedicine is experiencing a rapid evolution in the utilization of technology to facilitate the practice of medicine across great distances. As a field, telemedicine essentially involves interacting in real time with a patient, provider, and/or caregiver via video or telephone conferencing or reviewing stored videos and patient data and includes diagnosing a problem and prescribing an intervention, as well as providing consultation to others who provide treatment. Although scientific evidence for telemedicine is still emerging, the world's leading medical institutions now have satellite hospitals, and it appears that the use of telemedicine will only continue to grow. Telemedicine is useful in the delivery of behavioral intervention to geographically remote areas in which families would otherwise go without services. Some research has shown that it can be used to train individuals to carry out specific procedures for particular behaviors. The CARD Model uses telemedicine combined with in-person training and supervision in its Remote Clinical Services model. The iPads used for Skills LogBook™ (described above) can also be used to run live videoconferencing software, so supervisors in one part of the world can watch the therapist working with the learner and give live feedback. See Chapter 28 for more details on this model.

ABA BUSINESS MANAGEMENT SOLUTIONS

In the field of ABA, most service provision agencies have been founded by clinicians providing services to individuals with ASD. However, as with any other business, many processes are required in order to effectively schedule sessions, track services rendered, submit billing, generate payroll, manage revenue, track training progress, and manage records. Technology now offers online management solutions for ABA agencies to use in conducting all of the above. While such solutions are currently in their infancy, this is an area that will likely progress quickly, resulting in streamlining the way in which ABA service agencies manage their business.

COMMUNITY OUTREACH

The basic concept behind dissemination efforts – whether in the form of web-based training, such as that contained in IBT, or writing the book you are currently reading – is to provide information that empowers families living with ASD around the world to live better lives. Recent developments in web-based social networks and social media have shown the amazing power that technology has to bring people together and share ideas, if used effectively and with noble intent. Web-based networks and video-sharing platforms have transformed commercial, social, and political life in dramatic ways to the point where political and social revolutions can be sparked by the appearance of video content that deals with the right issues at the right time. Toward this end, CARD has actively participated in a number of technology-based community outreach efforts. For example, Dr. Doreen Granpeesheh hosted a monthly web-based radio show on Autism One Radio for several years called *The ABA Piece of the Puzzle*. Each monthly show provided practical information for parents and practitioners on one specific topic within ABA. More recently, CARD founded *Autism Live*, a web show (www.autism-live.com) that is broadcast live over the web, 2 hours per day, 3 days per week. The program is hosted by Shannon Penrod (autism mom, expert, and activist) and consists of live conversations with experts from a variety of fields relevant to ASD. In addition, Autism Live contains specialty features on a wide variety of topics, ranging from cooking, to vacations with children on the spectrum, to how to have more fun in your daily life. The purpose of Autism Live is to provide genuine hope by giving information that empowers families living with ASD to live fuller lives.

SUMMARY

Technology is a powerful driving force in the future of autism treatment. While technology is currently being used in many ways to assist in the provision of services and training, the potential for future developments and their implications for the evolution of autism treatment are vast. The CARD Model values technology and is committed to leading the development of technology solutions that help achieve the mission of providing global access to top-quality treatment to as many families affected by autism as possible.

Research

Jonathan Tarbox

THE IMPORTANCE OF RESEARCH

Research plays a critical role in all areas of autism treatment. Perhaps the most important two functions of research are 1) separating what works from what doesn't and 2) providing scientific evidence that supports access to effective treatment. The first function of research, to separate effective treatments from ineffective ones, is the most obvious and fundamental role of autism treatment research. Indeed, showing what actually works is a core purpose of science in any discipline. However, autism is an area that is particularly in need of this kind of research. By some counts, upwards of 500 treatments are offered for autism, all of which have someone who is a passionate proponent. So how is a family, a school, a health insurance company, or an individual professional to choose which ones to adopt? The results of top-quality scientific research on treatment effectiveness must be the core source of information when determining which treatments to use. Human history has proven time and again that the scientific method is the only reliable way to sort out what works from what doesn't. Human judgment, intuition, feelings, beliefs, and desires have all proven to be inadequate indicators of what truly works. To err is human, and even professionals who have worked on a problem for years have been proven to make false judgments on a regular basis if those judgments are not tested carefully in an unbiased manner. This fact is not specific to autism; the history of medicine is largely a history of hunches and intuition being disproven by the scientific method. Only in recent decades have medicine and psychology begun a wholesale adoption of the ethical imperative of implementing evidence-based practices. Unfortunately, the field of education has done little to move toward evidence-based practices and continues to be more influenced by politics and budgets than by science.

The second purpose of autism treatment research, to provide information that increases access to treatment, is equally critical. For decades, funding for autism treatment was virtually non-existent. The average medical doctor, upon making an autism diagnosis, would advise the family that there was no treatment. It was only after decades of published research on the effectiveness of intervention using applied behavior analysis (ABA) that funding began to become available for treatment. And the mere publication of research was not enough. Hundreds of families had to demand that their children receive access to evidence-based treatment, and these demands had to be litigated in court before states, schools, and health insurance plans began providing funding for treatment. The outcome of these court proceedings hinged primarily on the availability of scientific evidence that demonstrates that behavioral intervention is effective and medically necessary. Had this research not been produced, it is likely that funding for autism treatment would still be unavailable today.

Importance of Single-Subject Research Methodology

Between-group, double-blind, placebo-controlled trials are considered the "gold standard" of research methodology by virtually all scientific disciplines. Research studies using these designs have many strengths, not the least of which is the fact that the studies will be taken seriously and, therefore, have a much greater impact than studies that use other designs. However, as many behavior analysts have acknowledged in the past, between-group designs also suffer from serious limitations. We will not discuss them all, as they have received thorough treatments in classic methodology textbooks (Kazdin, 2011; Hayes, Barlow, & Nelson-Gray, 1999). However, one limitation is particularly relevant to autism treatment research and, therefore, deserves special mention. All children with autism spectrum disorder (ASD) are different, and all children respond differently to treatment. Consequently, in between-group studies of treatment effectiveness, a large range in response to treatment is almost always observed. The result is that the treatment, on average, appears to produce medium effects. When group averages are considered, important differences between subgroups are masked. However, if the results for each individual are actually analyzed separately, one often sees that some individuals respond significantly more while others respond less. Those differences in response to treatment are not errors; they are a critical subject that needs to be studied in itself, and group designs mask them.

Single-subject designs are an alternative to between-group designs that do not suffer from this limitation. Indeed, the very point of single-subject designs is to identify what works for each individual participant. That is, variability among different children with ASD is not seen as a problem or an error in research. Rather, it is seen for the reality that it is: Each child is different and therefore needs customized treatment. Furthermore, single-subject designs, when done properly, can be equally experimentally valid as between-group designs (Kazdin, 2011; Hayes, Barlow, & Nelson-Gray, 1999). Unfortunately, the vast majority of the scientific community is unaware of this and still considers single-subject designs to be "pre-experimental" or "quasi-experimental." Awareness of the validity of single-subject designs is increasing, but there is still a long way to go. It should be noted that more than 90% of published research on effective autism treatment has used single-subject designs, and it would be a travesty to ignore all of that research simply because of tradition and dogma. We hope that the future brings greater awareness of single-subject designs and an acknowledgment that single-subject design is not only equal to group designs in many ways but, in fact, superior for the purposes of identifying treatment effectiveness at the level of the individual – the level at which every treatment provider works on a daily basis.

FOUNDATIONAL RESEARCH OF WHICH YOU SHOULD BE AWARE

Hundreds of studies have been published in peer-reviewed journals documenting the effectiveness of behavioral intervention for children with ASD (National Autism Center, 2009). The vast majority of these studies are small in scale and evaluate particular treatments for particular challenging behaviors or particular teaching procedures for teaching particular skills. These studies are highly useful for identifying and testing specific components of the overall early intensive behavioral intervention (EIBI) process. The content of most of Section II in this book was derived from these studies. Clearly, space does not permit even a cursory review of this vast literature. Instead, we will briefly review a small number of high-quality studies that evaluated the overall outcome of EIBI: the "greatest hits" of EIBI outcome research.

Studies

Lovaas (1987). The seminal 1987 study by O. Ivar Lovaas evaluated the outcome of the UCLA Young Autism Project and was the first controlled study to document robust global outcomes of any treatment for autism. The study compared outcomes after 2.5 years for a group of children who received 40 hours per week of EIBI to two control groups: one that received 10 hours per week of behavioral intervention and one that received approximately 10 hours per week of other interventions. The EIBI group far outperformed the two control groups on all measures, and 47% of the EIBI participants demonstrated an IQ within the average range and were succeeding in regular education without any specialized support at the end of treatment. This study clearly demonstrated that high-intensity

(40 hours per week) behavioral intervention is highly effective and, further, that low-intensity (10 hours per week) behavioral intervention is far less effective. McEachin, Smith, & Lovaas (1993) followed up with the optimal outcome participants at 13 years of age and found that eight of nine maintained their gains.

Smith, Groen, & Wynn (2000). In the only randomized controlled trial of EIBI, Smith and colleagues compared outcomes of children with autism and pervasive developmental disorder – not otherwise specific (PDD NOS) who received an average of 24.52 hours per week of behavioral intervention for 1 year with a gradual decrease in hours over the subsequent 1 to 2 years, to those of children who received only parent training for 3 to 9 months. The EIBI group outperformed the control group on tests of intelligence, visual-spatial skills, language, and academic skills, but no difference in adaptive functioning and challenging behavior was observed. The effects of this study were significantly less robust than those reported by Lovaas (1987), which makes sense, given that the participants received only 62.5% (approximately 25 hours per week, as opposed to 40) of the intervention that those in the Lovaas study received. Therefore, the study conducted by Smith and colleagues should probably be considered an evaluation of "medium-intensity" behavioral intervention.

Howard, Sparkman, Cohen, Green, & Stanislaus (2005). Howard and colleagues compared outcomes of a group of children who received intensive (i.e., 25–40 hours per week) EIBI to outcomes for two control groups, one that received high-intensity (30 hours per week) and one that received low-intensity (approximately 15 hours per week) eclectic intervention. In this study, eclectic intervention consisted of a mix of various interventions, including a small amount of discrete trial training, speech therapy, occupational therapy, TEACCH, augmentative communication, and other procedures. After 14 months of treatment, the EIBI group's mean standard scores outperformed the two control groups on cognitive, language, and adaptive standardized assessments, and progress in all domains except motor skills was statistically significant. Learning rates were also determined to be much higher for the EIBI group in comparison with the other two groups. Furthermore, the IQ scores of three participants in the 15-hour-per-week eclectic control group were lower at discharge than they were at the outset of the study. It should be noted that the eclectic treatment studied in this experiment is similar to what is commonly practiced throughout public special education, so the results of this study do not bode well for what most children with autism receive throughout the United States on a daily basis. It should also be noted that this study clearly demonstrated that EIBI is superior to eclectic treatment, even when implemented at nearly the same intensity. That is, merely providing a large number of treatment hours is not sufficient to produce treatment effects if the procedures implemented during those hours are not effective.

Sallows & Graupner (2005). Sallows and Graupner evaluated the outcome of EIBI provided at the Wisconsin Early Autism Project (WEAP). The study compared outcomes for a group that received EIBI with a high level of supervision provided by expert ABA supervisors with a group that received EIBI with a low level of supervision provided by expert ABA supervisors. The group that received less professional supervision was referred to as the "parent-directed" group because parents were trained to provide a portion of the supervision for their child's services. The therapists who delivered the therapy in both groups were professional therapists, hired and trained by WEAP. No significant difference in outcome was observed between the two groups, and both groups demonstrated very large treatment gains. Forty-eight percent of children across the two groups achieved scores in the average range on measures of cognitive, language, adaptive, social, and academic skills and were succeeding in regular education without support. In addition, the Autism Diagnostic Interview – Revised (ADI-R) was used as an outcome measure, and 8 out of 11 children labeled as "rapid learners" no longer qualified for an ASD diagnosis according to the ADI-R at the end of treatment. This study replicated the effectiveness of EIBI and suggests that some portion of professional supervision may be replaced by intensive training of parents to provide it; however, much further replication of this study would be needed before this can be concluded with any degree of certainty.

Cohen, Amerine-Dickens, & Smith (2006). Cohen and colleagues evaluated the effects of EIBI provided by a community-based service provider in central California. Participants received EIBI for 35–40 hours per week, and their outcome was compared to a similar group of children who received special education "treatment as usual," meaning the common eclectic combination of treatments that most children with ASD in the United States receive in public schools when they do not access EIBI. The children in the EIBI group far outperformed the children in the control group on IQ and adaptive behavior tests. Likewise, 6 of the 21 EIBI children were fully included in regular education placements without support and 11 more with support, while only one child in the control group was placed primarily in a regular education setting. This study is important because it provides further replication of the effects of EIBI provided by community-based service providers, not a university-based clinic.

Zachor, Ben-Itzchak, Rabinovich, & Lahat (2007). Zachor and colleagues evaluated the effects of 35 hours per week of EIBI for 1 year and compared it to outcomes of eclectic treatment for the same period of time. In addition to a variety of standardized assessment measures, the Autism Diagnostic Observation Schedule (ADOS) was used as an outcome measure. The EIBI group far outperformed the eclectic control group on language and reciprocal social interaction, and 20% of children in the EIBI group no longer qualified for an ASD diagnosis at discharge, according to the ADOS. This study is important because it included the ADOS, a gold standard diagnostic measure, at outcome and because it provided further replication of the effects of EIBI in a different region (Middle East).

Eikeseth, Smith, Jahr, & Eldevik (2007). Eikeseth and colleagues studied the effects of EIBI for slightly older children. The participants in this study were between 4 and 7 years of age at intake, whereas the children in the other studies described so far were consistently under the age of 4 years at intake. The outcome of the EIBI children was compared to that of a control group that received intensive eclectic treatment. The EIBI group outperformed the control group on tests of IQ and adaptive functioning and presented with less challenging behavior and social problems. This study is important because it shows that intensive behavioral intervention can be highly effective, even when begun slightly later. In addition, this study provides additional replication of the effects of EIBI provided on a different continent (Europe) and in a different language (Norwegian).

Remington & colleagues (2007). Remington and colleagues studied the effects of 25.6 hours per week of EIBI provided for 2 years in the United Kingdom. The effects were compared to those produced by a control group that received treatment as usual for the same duration of time. At discharge, the difference in outcome between the EIBI and control groups was deemed both clinically and statistically significant on tests of intelligence, daily living skills, language, and social behavior. Remington and colleagues also measured parent stress in an attempt to identify whether the rigorous demands of EIBI increased parent stress. Data on parent stress revealed no significant increases for the EIBI group, suggesting that EIBI did not worsen their stress.

Reviews and Meta-Analyses

Several high-quality review papers and meta-analyses have been published in recent years. Practitioners should be aware of these publications as they help summarize the "big picture" of ABA outcome research. In the most comprehensive review of autism treatment literature ever conducted, the National Standards Project, conducted by the National Autism Center (2009), reviewed and analyzed 775 autism treatment studies published in peer-reviewed journals according to strict criteria. The conclusion of the review was that a variety of ABA-based treatment strategies and components were "established" as effective treatments for autism, including comprehensive EIBI.

In a review of autism research by Dr. Sally Rogers, who is widely acknowledged as one of the world's premier autism researchers, comprehensive ABA-based intervention for children with autism was found to be "well established" (Rogers & Vismara, 2008). It is worth noting that

Dr. Rogers is not an ABA professional or researcher; rather, she is a developmental psychologist who advocates the Denver Model of autism treatment, a model oriented more to developmental than behavioral psychology. That is, Dr. Rogers has nothing to gain personally by endorsing ABA treatment and is offering her highly respected opinion from outside the discipline of ABA. Subsequent meta-analyses by Eldevik, Hastings, Hughes, Jahr, Eikeseth, & Cross (2009) and Reichow (2011) also found very strong support for the effectiveness of behavioral intervention for children with autism, and the reader is strongly encouraged to read these, as well.

Reviews by Independent Agencies and Associations

Many reviews of autism treatment research have been published by a large variety of independent bodies, and virtually all have come to the same conclusion: applied behavior analytic treatment for children with autism is well supported by scientific research. For example, in 1999, a report by the U.S. Surgeon General (U.S. Department of Health and Human Services) stated that, "Thirty years of research demonstrated the efficacy of applied behavioral methods in reducing inappropriate behavior and in increasing communication, learning, and appropriate social behavior."

Similarly, as a result of a review of autism treatment conducted by the New York State Department of Health (1999), it was reported that in all of the studies reviewed, "Groups that received the intensive behavioral intervention showed significant functional improvements compared to the control groups," and that, "Since intensive behavioral programs appear to be effective in young children with autism, it is recommended that principles of applied behavior analysis and behavioral intervention strategies be included as an important element of any intervention program."

In a thorough review of autism treatment research by the American Academy of Pediatrics (AAP), it was concluded that:

> The effectiveness of ABA-based intervention in ASDs has been well documented through five decades of research by using single subject methodology and in controlled studies of comprehensive EIBI programs in university and community settings. Children who receive early intensive behavioral treatment have been shown to make substantial, sustained gains in IQ, language, academic performance, and adaptive behavior as well as some measures of social behavior, and their outcomes have been significantly better than those of children in control groups. (*Myers & Plauché Johnson, 2007, p. 1164*)

This review is posted on the AAP website as its position statement on autism treatment.

RESEARCH AT THE CENTER FOR AUTISM AND RELATED DISORDERS

Research at the Center for Autism and Related Disorders (CARD) is guided by one primary mission: to produce information that will help people affected by ASD lead better lives. To that end, CARD has invested substantial resources in supporting research. In 2011, the Interagency Autism Coordinating Committee of the U.S. Department of Health and Human Services acknowledged CARD as the third largest non-governmental supporter of autism research in the United States. Below, we describe our primary programs of research, touching on most major topic areas relevant to the provision of ABA-based treatment for children with ASD. The vast majority of our research is devoted to treatment.

Teaching Cognitive Skills

Hundreds of studies have documented the effectiveness of ABA-based treatment for teaching relatively simple behaviors and for decreasing challenging behaviors in children with ASD. Somewhat less research has been done on procedures for establishing higher order skills. At CARD, the point of view that guides our research on teaching complex behavior is the same as that which guided our development of the CARD curriculum: if there is a skill that a child with ASD needs to learn, then it is our job to figure out how to teach it, regardless of how complex it is or how different it is from conventional skills taught in ABA therapy. If a procedure is likely to work, then it is also our job to test it rigorously via research. Therefore, one of our most active programs of research is the evaluation of ABA-based procedures for teaching skills commonly referred to as cognitive – for example, metaphorical reasoning (Persicke, Tarbox, Ranick, & St. Clair, 2012). CARD research on cognitive skills also includes acquisition research on perspective-taking skills (see Chapter 17), such as teaching children to comprehend sarcasm (Persicke, Tarbox, Ranick, & St. Clair, 2013) and teaching children to detect deception (Ranick, Persicke, Tarbox, & Kornack, 2013). In addition, we maintain an ongoing program of research on procedures for teaching executive function skills (see Chapter 18), such as working memory (Baltruschat et al., 2011a; Baltruschat et al., 2011b; Baltruschat et al., 2012) and shifting attention (Persicke et al., 2013). The general goal of research in these areas is to push the envelope in terms of the complexity and subtlety of skills that have been addressed in ABA skills acquisition research and, ultimately, to increase each learner's repertoire of skills.

Technology in Autism Treatment

As we describe in the technology chapter of this manual (Chapter 26), we believe that technological innovations will play a critical role in the future of autism treatment. Technology holds a number of potential benefits, including – at a minimum – increasing access to treatment across great distances, contributing to dissemination of knowledge of top-quality treatment, contributing to staff and parent training efforts, and simplifying data collection and analysis, as well as providing applications that directly teach learners with ASD. We view being at the forefront of technological innovation for autism treatment as a serious organizational goal. Accordingly, we maintain an active program of research focused on autism treatment technology. For example, we have studied the utility of electronic data collection methods (Tarbox, Wilke, Findel-Pyles, Bergstrom, & Granpeesheh, 2010), the validity of web-based curriculum assessments (Persicke et al., 2014), web-based training for therapists (Granpeesheh, Tarbox, Dixon, Peters, Thompson, & Kenzer, 2010), and web-based training for parents (Jang, Dixon, Tarbox, Granpeesheh, Kornack, & de Nocker, 2012). Overall, CARD research on technology aims to evaluate whether a technological innovation is useful and/or to compare it directly to more traditional, less technological options.

Challenging Behaviors

A large amount of behavioral research has already been published on the assessment and treatment of challenging behaviors; however, many idiosyncratic behaviors have been the subject of little or no previous research. CARD research on challenging behaviors generally aims to extend the scope of research to include behaviors that have not yet been researched, such as domestic pet mistreatment (Bergstrom, Tarbox, & Gutshall, 2011) and bruxism (Barnoy, Najdowski, Tarbox, Wilke, & Nollet, 2009). CARD research on challenging behaviors also focuses on developing novel non-intrusive treatments, such as new treatments for rumination (Rhine & Tarbox, 2009).

Safety Skills

As we discussed in Chapter 13, safety skills can literally make the difference between life and death for a person who has them. Unfortunately, many children with ASD do not develop critical safety skills if they are not directly taught them, and many behavioral intervention programs do not prioritize safety skills. CARD research on safety skills focuses on identifying simple but effective procedures for establishing safety skills, such as avoiding cleaning chemicals (Summers, Tarbox, Findel-Pyles, Wilke, Bergstrom, & Williams, 2011) and what to do when lost in public (Bergstrom, Najdowski, & Tarbox, 2012).

Recovery from Autism

Chapter 2 of this manual clearly defines the CARD position on recovery from autism, so we will not repeat ourselves here. It will suffice to say that some proportion of children with ASD no longer have clinically significant impairment after receiving EIBI and, therefore, are able to function successfully and in fully mainstream environments without additional support. We refer to this outcome as recovery, and we believe that a great deal more research is needed to predict which learners will achieve this outcome and to increase the percentage of learners who do. As part of our program of research on recovery, we published a retrospective analysis of clinic charts of 38 children who recovered (Granpeesheh, Tarbox, & Dixon, 2009), and the study was awarded the 2011 George Winokur Clinical Research Award by the American Academy of Clinical Psychiatrists.

Biomedical Factors

As we discuss in Chapter 24, the vast majority of leading autism researchers agree that some combination of genetic and environmental factors contribute to ASD. Hundreds of unproven theories abound, and hundreds of unproven treatments based on them are popular among parents of children with ASD. We believe that, if an unproven treatment has a reasonable medical theory behind it with at least some supporting indirect scientific evidence, and it is highly popular among parents of children with ASD, the treatment should be evaluated by sound scientific research. If unproven treatments are not evaluated, then parents are left with nothing upon which to base their decisions about which treatments to provide for their children but hunches and Internet testimonials, making parents vulnerable to ineffective treatments that may waste critical treatment time and limited financial resources. CARD conducted a study on one such treatment, hyperbaric oxygen therapy (HBOT). The study consisted of a randomized, double-blind, placebo-controlled trial that evaluated low-pressure HBOT (24% oxygen delivered at 1.3 atmospheres pressure) delivered in soft shell chambers, a format that was highly popular among parents (Granpeesheh, Tarbox, Dixon, Wilke, Allen, & Bradstreet, 2010). The effects of HBOT were evaluated across measures of all major skill and symptom areas relevant to ASD, and HBOT was found to produce no effect when compared to placebo. It is worth noting that, after the data were made public, one of the most popular autism parent conferences (Defeat

Autism Now!) barred the manufacturers of HBOT chambers from sponsoring the conference.

AUTISM RESEARCH GROUP

CARD recently founded the Autism Research Group (ARG), a nonprofit research institute dedicated to conducting research that produces meaningful differences in the lives of families living with ASD. In founding ARG, we noted that many parents of children with ASD comment that the vast majority of research on ASD that is funded by the federal government does not make a real-life difference for families living with ASD today. ARG was founded to conduct research that addresses that gap. ARG's staff is comprised of master's and doctoral-level researchers whose backgrounds are in treatment of ASD. ARG has a number of research programs, including the Parent Generated Research Initiative, that consist of research projects that are developed on the basis of parent requests. In addition to conducting research, community outreach has a large place in ARG's mission. ARG holds regular parent education seminars, free of charge and open to the public. Seminar topics vary, but they generally focus on disseminating information on evidence-based treatment for children with ASD. One such seminar was a 1-day workshop in Koreatown in Los Angeles, which targeted the Korean-speaking population of the Southern California area. The workshop consisted of presentations describing research-based treatment for ASD and was presented in English and Korean simultaneously. Dissemination to the professional community is also a priority for ARG. To this end, ARG holds regular professional development workshops, generally consisting of 1-day seminars on advanced topics in autism treatment, which also provide continuing education credit for Board Certified Behavior Analysts (BCBAs).

HOW TO STAY CONNECTED TO NEW RESEARCH

Compared to most branches of psychology, the field of ABA is characterized by a particularly close relationship between research and practice. However, even in ABA, most research is done by full-time career researchers at universities who rarely, if ever, deliver real-life services, and most service is provided by community-based practitioners who rarely, if ever, engage in research. Ethical guidelines require that BCBAs implement empirically supported procedures, and it is therefore an ethical imperative for clinicians to remain closely connected to research. Given this obligation, many have called for ways that practitioners can stay abreast of research literature, without having to take substantial time away from clinical practice. A very useful recent article (Carr & Briggs, 2010) outlines a number of recommendations for how clinicians may accomplish this, and some of those recommendations are briefly described here.

Journal Club

Holding "journal clubs" is a time-honored tradition in behavioral organizations. Journal clubs consist of regular meetings (weekly, biweekly, monthly, etc.) during which a group of professionals get together and discuss a particular journal article or book chapter. The meeting can be brief – perhaps 30 to 60 minutes – and can occur before or after work or during a lunch break while attendees eat. Typically, one member of the club acts as the leader and assigns articles that she believes would benefit the group. Alternatively, leadership of the group can rotate to a different member after each meeting, thereby giving each attendee the opportunity to influence the readings. Journal clubs are often optional, but attendance could also be written into job descriptions. Journal clubs usually work best when the atmosphere of the meetings is upbeat and casual and when the readings are relatively short, easy to consume, and directly relevant to the daily jobs of attendees. If proper procedures and guidelines are followed, attendance at journal clubs may be able to count toward BCBA continuing education units and/or BCBA supervision, but readers must check with the Behavior Analyst Certification Board (BACB) for the latest guidelines.

Journal Access

Unfortunately, most scholarly journals that publish autism treatment research have highly restricted access. Most articles are not available free of charge online, and individual articles can cost up to $30 per download, which is prohibitively expensive. However, three journals are notable exceptions: *Journal of Applied Behavior Analysis; Behavior Analysis in Practice;* and *The Analysis of Verbal Behavior.* All of these journals are peer-reviewed behavioral journals that frequently publish autism treatment research and are available in full text, free of charge, online. Typically, the most recent year or so of the journals is not available free at any given time, but a wealth of useful scientific information is available from previous years. For access to journals that do not offer free online access, a university library is almost invariably required. Most universities only offer students access to their libraries, but it is common for most schools and agencies to employ at least one person at any given time who is a current university student. Such employees can access journal articles that they can then share, for purely educational purposes, with other employees of the organization.

Continuing Education Seminars

As discussed in Chapter 22 on training and quality control, continued professional development is crucial to maintaining top-quality services, and it can also be a convenient forum for clinical staff to maintain contact with the research literature. The process for organizations to become approved providers of BACB continuing education credits is relatively straightforward, so larger organizations that employ BCBA staff who have a strong connection to the research literature are encouraged to become such providers. If an organization is not such a provider, it is highly recommended that organizations encourage clinical staff to attend continuing education opportunities, such as local and international conventions of the Association for Behavior Analysis, International, as well as other continuing education seminars, such as those offered by CARD.

HOW TO DO RESEARCH IN YOUR ORGANIZATION

There is a good reason that most practitioners don't do research and that most researchers don't do their research in the context of real-life service delivery: It's hard. Inevitably, a large number of factors work against the success of anyone trying to do research in the context of service delivery: the complexity of real-life settings, the difficulty of controlling real-life settings, the potentially conflicting priorities of fixing a clinical problem as fast as possible while also scientifically evaluating the effects of the treatment, the availability of additional staff for data collection, and the ability to ensure the fidelity of procedures and data collection, to name just a few. Despite the difficulties, it is possible to do research while also providing top-quality treatment services. Below, we will briefly describe some of the tips we have learned while developing and refining CARD's research program.

Rule #1: Make It Someone's Job to Do Research

Like any other task, if you want to get it done, research needs to be incorporated into the daily tasks of a specific individual's job description. Most service provision agencies "encourage" their clinical staff to do research. In reality, though, few agencies specifically carve out time for their staff to do research on the clock. If you simply hope that your staff will be motivated to do research in their spare or off time for the pure intellectual stimulation of it, then little, if any, research will get done. This is not because research is not interesting or because clinicians do not care about it; it is simply because research is always – and should be – less important than solving a learner's clinical problems. Therefore, when clinicians have a full clinical caseload, they will do clinical work and will rarely do research.

In our experience, there are two situations in which people reliably get research done: (1) when someone has a reduced clinical caseload and research is part of the job description or (2) when a person has to do research in order to earn a graduate degree or complete a thesis or dissertation. In the first scenario, time for research is allotted on the clock, so it need not be superseded by clinical tasks. For example, if a clinical supervisor normally supervises the cases of 10–15 children, you may consider reducing the caseload to 5–10 cases if you genuinely want research to get done. Reducing an employee's billable time clearly results in increased overhead to the organization, but meaningful research will likely contribute to your organization's clinical effectiveness and should therefore be viewed as an investment in the long-term viability of the organization. After a clinician has become a seasoned researcher, has published several publications, and is far more fluent with the research process, it may be possible that she will require less dedicated time for research and may even be able to accomplish research while also handling a full clinical caseload, but it is not reasonable to expect someone with little or no real research experience to establish a line of research while also managing a full clinical caseload. In the second scenario, since the research project is part of school, specific time is allotted to get it done. Moreover, the student experiences substantial positive consequences for getting it done (i.e., graduating) and serious negative consequences for not getting it done (i.e., not graduating).

Rule #2: Involve Someone With Research Experience

Virtually all ABA clinical procedures come from research, and the ways in which we evaluate our clinical treatments on a daily basis very much resemble the ways in which treatments are evaluated in research. This fact is a major strength of the ABA discipline, but it may also lead many to think they are cable of conducting research without the guidance of an experienced researcher. In fact, the whole process of designing and implementing research in a way that is going to be published in a peer-reviewed journal involves many individual repertoires of behavior that need to be learned, just as clinical repertoires need to be learned for someone to be a good clinician. The vast majority of research in behavioral journals is published by professional scientists whose primary activity is research, day in and day out.

To do research successfully requires the help of at least one person who has some experience and training in the research process, and merely completing a master's thesis in ABA is typically not sufficient experience. For this reason, we highly recommend that, if you are serious about establishing a line of research in your organization, hire someone who has published at least a few research articles in the past, if you do not already have such a person in your organization. If it is not possible to hire someone with research experience, a great way to start conducting research in your organization is to collaborate with an experienced researcher. Experienced researchers often need help recruiting sufficient participants for their studies, and if you have learners who may be appropriate and available to participate in those studies, your access to potential research participants can be an effective initial offering in your effort to forge a collaboration with the researcher. Most researchers would actually appreciate receiving an email from a practitioner expressing an interest in their research, and such emails often result in productive collaborations.

Rule #3: Support Conference Attendance

Establishing research capacity in a service delivery organization is about building a culture that values research. No other culture values research more than that of behavior analytic conferences. A great way to get staff interested and involved in research is to support their attendance at regional, national, and international behavior analytic conferences, particularly the annual convention of the Association for Behavior Analysis, International, and its state and regional chapter conferences.

When first establishing a line of research, it would be worthwhile to identify one or two employees who have the requisite research skills and enthusiasm and pay for them to attend one or two research conferences per year. Make sure it is possible for their clinical duties to be covered while they are gone and pay them for their time, so they are not incurring an economic hardship by attending the conference. Another incentive that can be helpful is to agree to pay for travel expenses for any employees who are presenting the results of research that they have conducted at your organization.

Rule #4: Start Small

As with any challenging enterprise, building a program of research does not happen overnight. When envisioning research, it is easy to overestimate what can reasonably be accomplished, given your current time constraints and logistical challenges. In fact, a common piece of advice to graduate students who are planning their master's theses and doctoral dissertations is, "Don't try to save the world." This warning does not mean that you shouldn't try to do something important; it merely means that your project is far more likely to get done and published if it is small and manageable. Practitioners interested in establishing research in their service provision agencies would do well to start small.

A small intervention involving only three learners that is conducted well and addresses a question of importance is enough to result in a presentation at a conference and a publication in a peer-reviewed journal. If you have three learners or students who have a similar clinical challenge and you identify a novel way to solve it, which produces new information that will be useful to clinicians, and the project is evaluated in an empirically valid manner, this may be enough to result in a publication. Projects that involve all children served at an organization, or all staff members, are far less likely to be accomplished in an experimentally sound manner. For example, if one observes that a particular prompting procedure might better be implemented in a novel way, testing it out across three learners is far more likely to be done with high integrity, inter-observer agreement data, and in a sound experimental design than if one attempts to implement it across all clients at the same time. Evaluating clinical or performance management innovations on a small scale first is also probably more sound from a clinical perspective. If the procedure you are studying is truly novel, then you don't really know if it's a good idea to do it across all learners, and it is likely therefore more responsible to try it first with a small number of learners for whom it is likely to be effective.

SUMMARY

Research evaluating autism treatment is critical because it helps to identify what actually works and because it supports access to effective treatment. Hundreds of studies of individual procedures and treatment strategies have been published documenting the effectiveness of ABA, and both meta-analyses and independent reviews substantiate the fact that ABA-based intervention is an established effective treatment for autism. To stay connected to research, you will need to support frequent contact with the research literature through efforts such as journal clubs and training seminars. To conduct research, you will need to set aside staff for it, embed it into the culture of your organization, and start with small, manageable projects.

28

Global Dissemination

Catherine Minch

The mission of the Center for Autism and Related Disorders (CARD) is to provide global access to the highest quality intervention using applied behavior analysis (ABA) to as many families living with autism spectrum disorder (ASD) as possible. CARD developed its Remote Clinical Services (RCS) model and affiliate programs to achieve this goal and to disseminate the CARD Model to families and other treatment providers across the globe. This chapter describes these two programs.

REMOTE CLINICAL SERVICES MODEL

The RCS model is used to provide services to learners and families throughout the United States and internationally who live at least 50 miles from a CARD office. RCS consists of an initial 2- to 3-day training workshop designed to assist the family in setting up an in-home ABA-based treatment program, followed by ongoing consultation with a clinical supervisor. Typically, CARD hires the therapists, although some therapists are hired by families. In all instances, a CARD clinical supervisor trains the therapists and provides ongoing supervision of the learner's program.

Initial Training Workshop

During the initial training workshop, the workshop supervisor visits the family's home and spends the first day providing instruction to the parents and therapists on the principles of ABA, skill acquisition, generalization and maintenance, behavior management techniques, and data collection. Generally, the learner is not present on the first day of training, as there is more of a didactic focus, but the learner's teacher and other members of the treatment team are invited to attend. On the second day, the learner is present, as this day is spent designing and implementing the treatment program, as well as teaching the parents and therapists how to teach skills from each lesson in the curriculum designed for the learner. The therapists and family members receive hands-on training and practice applying all concepts taught on the first day of training to the learner's specific curriculum program. Throughout this process, the RCS supervisor works directly with the learner in order to demonstrate teaching techniques and methods for managing the learner's challenging behavior. Initial workshops can be accomplished in 2 days but it is often beneficial to schedule 3 days in order to ensure that sufficient training has occurred, especially if the native language of the family is not the same as that of the RCS supervisor.

Cycle of Services

When the initial training workshop is complete, the RCS supervisor provides periodic supervision through face-to-face visits, phone conferences, video conferences, and correspondence via fax or email. Monthly supervision time can vary between 2 and 5 hours in total, which may include communicating with the family/treatment team, developing and refining the treatment program, and writing reports. These interactions afford an opportunity for the supervisor to review the current curriculum, offer suggestions about how to modify difficult lessons, advance the curriculum as needed, conduct additional training, critique therapy skills, participate in treatment team meetings and Individualized Education Program (IEP) meetings, and write reports on the learner's progress.

For an RCS program to be successful, frequent and consistent interactions between the supervisor, the treatment team, and the family are essential. Within 2 weeks of the initial visit, communication begins with a web conference call or a phone call. Between visits, regularly scheduled phone or video conferences are conducted, in addition to communication via fax or email. While email correspondence is still an acceptable means of periodic correspondence, it is imperative to have voice or face-to-face time over the Internet to remind the family and team that, despite geographical separation, the use of technology affords similar levels of support as that provided under more traditional circumstances. Because technology in some regions of the world is not as reliable, the RCS supervisor should be patient when encountering technological glitches and should also establish a backup plan for the potential failure of technology (e.g., videotaping, mailing, or uploading the videos).

The majority of face-to-face visits are held with the primary treatment team every 3 to 4 months for an average of 6 hours each day. Most families request additional time for the RCS supervisor to conduct a school observation or briefly meet school staff. For example, on any given visit, the RCS supervisor may work directly with the learner and his treatment team for a day (6 hours), plus conduct and write up a school observation for an additional 3 hours. Ideally, the RCS supervisor follows a specified cycle of services to ensure consistency and program maintenance. In general, the CARD approach is to recommend that face-to-face visits follow a 3-month delivery cycle. Specifically, after the initial workshop training, the supervisor should provide 2 months of phone, video, and email services from her local site and then visit the family in person every third month. RCS consultation hours for a 12-month period based on this standard 3-month cycle are described in Table 28.1. It should be noted that the standard RCS cycle is not always clinically appropriate. In such cases, the RCS supervisor discusses variations to the model, as needed. Providing services in countries where English is not the first language often requires a larger amount of supervision time in order to overcome language barriers. At times, it may also be necessary to hire professional translators. Naturally, the farther the RCS supervisor is located from the workshop site, the more time and financial resources must be allocated to travel.

Training Tools

The success of the workshop supervisor relies on the family's acceptance of ABA-based intervention and on their willingness and ability – as well as the ability of any other caregivers – to implement it on a daily basis. The RCS supervisor can promote successful implementation of the program through the use of varied sources of media. During the initial workshop and throughout consultation, training is conducted using a combination of both didactic and hands-on procedures. Didactic approaches include lecturing, showing the family the research that has been conducted on the effectiveness of ABA-based intervention (using the vernacular of the family and team), and presenting videos that demonstrate ABA-based techniques being performed successfully (paired with discussion of how the techniques in the video will be used with the learner and family). Hands-on procedures include modeling, role-play, rehearsal, and

TABLE 28.1 Number of Supervision Hours in the Standard 3-Month Cycle of Remote Clinical Services

	Hours
Initial in-person visit	18 hrs
Non-visit months, 8 per year	2–5 hrs
In-person visit months, 4 per year	8 hrs
Yearly total, first year	58–82 hrs
Yearly total, subsequent years	48–72 hrs

feedback. Sometimes, hands-on training begins with modeling and role-play with family members and therapists, before requiring therapists to try techniques with the learner.

Another powerful training tool involves videotaping initial workshops, follow-up visits, and therapy sessions. Such video documentation can provide families with a reliable resource to reference when needing to recall how to implement a technique. It can also be used in the future to train new team members, as prospective therapists can learn from the videos and apply the techniques via overlaps with the current team members. Furthermore, videotaped sessions provide great examples of the learner's progress over time.

The various web-based eLearning modules offered by the Institute for Behavioral Training (Chapter 26) are also critical to training parents and staff at great distances. Parents and staff at remote locations can obtain self-paced, web-based training before the RCS supervisor arrives and thereby obtain a "head start" on the training they are to receive. In addition, if a family needs to hire new therapists when the RCS supervisor is not physically present, eLearning training modules can provide a useful first step in training new staff.

Therapists

Another step in the RCS process is to identify and recruit therapists to provide the daily services to the learner. Therapists can be found by posting listings in local newspapers and at universities and colleges, specifically in the psychology, special education, and social work departments. Therapists can also be found through local religious groups, parent support groups, children's gyms, preschools, primary and secondary schools, and family friends and by word of mouth. When selecting staff, specific criteria to look for in a potential therapist include knowledge of the field (although this is not mandatory), reliability, interest in the field, ability to think quickly and problem solve, and – most importantly – demonstrated ability to play with children and establish a positive rapport. When the family's native language is not the same as that of the RCS supervisor, it is vital to attempt to hire at least some therapists who are bilingual. If this is not possible, it is important to arrange to have staff onsite who can translate, ideally staff who have some familiarity with ABA.

An additional important factor to consider during the therapist selection process is the number of therapists who will need to be trained. Every learner's program has a particular number of recommended treatment hours, so the number of therapists needed will vary. Some families prefer to train several therapists at one time and gradually weed out the less effective ones. Training more therapists than necessary can also give families a resource of potential therapists in the event a hired therapist quits. In general, each therapist should work approximately 6 to 12 hours per week with a learner. To allow for generalization across people, the total hours should be evenly distributed among the therapists, and the schedule for any one therapist should be spread out across the week as much as possible to allow for generalization across people. Generally, parents are not encouraged to be primary therapists as this may limit generalization. Parents, siblings, and other caregivers already play an important role in a learner's development, and they will be essential when generalizing skills to other environments. However, in many rural or remote locations, opportunities to recruit from outside resources simply do not exist. In such instances, parents and family members are trained to provide the treatment services.

Funding

While funding sources vary widely from state to state and, certainly, from one country to the next, remote clinical services are most often funded by one or more of three primary funding sources, including government funding (e.g., school district, department of developmental services, department of health), insurance, and private pay. With respect to health insurance coverage, different policies are offered by insurance carriers to their policyholders, and coverage varies drastically between plans and from state to state, depending on whether the state has an autism mandate and/or includes coverage for autism treatment through the Essential Health Benefits of the Affordable Care Act. When insurance isn't an option and school funding is insufficient or nonexistent – again, depending most often on local, regional, and national practices and/or laws – families may choose to pay for the services privately. All fees and services should be delineated, discussed, and agreed upon with the family prior to the RCS supervisor's first visit.

A potential variation for RCS that can decrease costs to individual families is for multiple families to share the cost of RCS supervisor visits. At the initial workshop, the costs of the first day can be shared equally by all families in attendance as long as the families and their treatment teams can benefit equally from exactly the same training. In some instances, the RCS supervisor may recommend different trainings for families if it is determined that the families have significantly different needs. When these different needs preclude the RCS supervisor from training multiple families at once, the overall travel time and travel expenses can still be split among families. Likewise, costs toward overall travel during subsequent visits can be minimized if more than one family is seen during the visit. Once an RCS supervisor is assigned and dates are confirmed, it is the responsibility of all families involved to arrange the location of the training day, the only day to be shared by the families. Although sharing costs is of considerable benefit to families, it is not always possible. For example, in the event that families are unable to agree on a location for the first day of the initial workshop, trainings will need to be conducted separately. In addition, many families may not feel comfortable with some logistical aspects of their child's treatment being affected by the needs of other families.

RCS Supervisors

The skills necessary to be an effective RCS supervisor are, for the most part, the same as those of a top-quality clinical supervisor, described in the chapters on organizational structure (Chapter 21) and clinical supervision (Chapter 19) in this manual, and additional talents contribute to the effectiveness of an RCS supervisor. For example, an RCS supervisor will achieve the most success if he is flexible, accessible to the family and treatment team, consistent with implementation, and a quick thinker. Families generally do not appreciate a rigid RCS supervisor who delivers ABA intervention in exactly the same manner in which it is delivered in his own culture or references books or colleagues in order to make treatment decisions. The RCS supervisor should be cognizant of different cultural and family practices that may require teaching approaches to be adjusted. When applying training protocols, an RCS supervisor who considers the perspectives, customs, culture, and norms of the participating family as essential variables to treatment planning is apt to be more successful. The RCS supervisor does not need to emphasize technical language and should, instead, focus on shaping the learning environment of the team and family. The goal is the successful delivery of ABA-based services regardless of the family's culture, language, and customs, and the RCS supervisor must establish rapport with the family, therapists, and learner to accomplish this.

Although the RCS supervisor provides extensive training in which the implementation of ABA may look very easy to the family, the newly trained treatment team will inevitably encounter challenges. The RCS supervisor should think of these challenges as training opportunities and focus on being positive and supportive while creating situations to promote successful demonstration of ABA techniques by the therapists. For example, rather than expecting pristine data collection and graphing, initially require that the team only provide clear and concise instructions and consequences to the learner. Newly trained staff cannot master everything all at once, so the RCS supervisor must avoid setting expectations too high; however, the RCS supervisor would do well to encourage the team to practice, practice, and practice some more! Finally, the RCS supervisor should avoid excessive focus on intensity (number of treatment hours) and urgency, as many cultures have different definitions of urgency and necessity for implementation. The more rapport the RCS supervisor can establish from the outset, the more likely the family and team will focus on acquisition of skills and aim for conducting the desired number of treatment hours.

AFFILIATE SITES

A CARD affiliate site is an agency or center that makes arrangements with CARD for staff training and program supervision needs. At least three parties are involved in the affiliate business relationship: the affiliate site, the families they are serving, and CARD. The goal of an affiliate site is to replicate the full CARD Model to the greatest extent possible in a region of the globe where it is currently not available. This is achieved by training the affiliate site's supervisors at a CARD location alongside other CARD supervisors and implementing the CARD curriculum, training, and service delivery model through an intensive consulting relationship between the affiliate site and CARD.

A new affiliate relationship begins when an agency, center, or group of parents initiates the dialog of developing an affiliation with CARD. Once the affiliate site and CARD have entered into a contract, the RCS supervisor(s) arrange the first visit. The first visit to the affiliate site involves the following: assessment of the learners, development of the learners' individual programs, training of the therapists, and parent education.

During the first visit, an RCS supervisor spends 1 to 2 days providing instruction to the affiliate site's supervisory staff and therapists on the principles of ABA, skill acquisition, generalization and maintenance, behavior management techniques, and data collection. Over several subsequent days, depending on the number of learners to be seen, the RCS supervisor spends time designing and implementing each learner's treatment program and teaching the supervisory staff, parents, and therapists how to successfully implement each learner's teaching lessons and behavior intervention plans for challenging behavior.

During subsequent months, the RCS supervisor continues to provide periodic supervision through face-to-face visits, phone conferences, and video conferences. The consultation serves as an opportunity for the RCS supervisor to review the current curriculum for each of the learners, offer suggestions about how to modify difficult lessons and advance the curriculum as needed, conduct additional staff development training, critique therapy skills and determine future visit training needs (at both the supervisor and therapist level), participate in treatment team meetings, determine parent education needs, and work with the site on staff recruitment and waitlist development.

Affiliate site visits follow a specified cycle of services to ensure consistency and program maintenance for the affiliate's current learners, ensure staff growth and development, and allow new programs to be developed for a growing clientele. In general, visits to the affiliate site occur every 1 to 3 months, depending on the needs of the site. During subsequent visits, the RCS supervisor continues to provide staff training, case supervision, and parent education, and the supervisor works with the site supervisory staff on continued staff and client recruitment. Skills® is a highly useful tool for the RCS supervisor for maintaining close contact and consultation with the affiliate site because it allows her to keep abreast of the progress of all of the affiliate site's learners from afar. A major focus of the subsequent visits is to identify staff who will be trained in lead clinical roles in which they learn to design and implement curriculum programs in order to reduce the need for visiting RCS supervisor services. The final goal of the RCS supervisor is to systematically and gradually fade consultative services according to a timetable that is determined by the affiliate site and CARD. Typically, CARD's role at an affiliate site is greatest in the first 3 to 4 years and eventually fades to a very low maintenance level. The ultimate goal of the affiliation model is to increase dissemination of best practices in autism treatment around the world, so the focus is always on establishing local excellence.

The Star Academy in South Africa is among the most successful CARD affiliate sites. Star Academy has four center-based clinics in South Africa, with two in Johannesburg, one in Pretoria, and one in Durban. In an effort to disseminate ABA treatment for children with autism beyond South Africa, Star Academy also maintains its own affiliate sites in Zimbabwe and Ghana. In addition to providing center-based ABA intervention, Star Academy clinics also provide home, school, and community-based instruction, as well as training for teachers and aides in the classroom environment. Star Academy continues to shine as an example of how high-quality ABA treatment can be disseminated to regions of the world that previously had little to no treatment available.

CULTURAL CHALLENGES

Many cultural challenges present themselves when attempting to deliver ABA-based services across a variety of different cultures, both within and outside of the United States. Specifically, dissemination barriers are observed with respect to delivery of information in the native language. Extra care has to be taken when translating ABA principles into another language, and cultural differences can affect the focus of treatment, acceptability of the diagnosis, and parental involvement.

When the first language of the supervisor and family members is not the same, a decision needs to be made about whether therapy will be delivered in the native tongue of the supervisor, if feasible, or translated into the native language of the learner. To deliver services in the learner's native language, one needs to consider the accessibility of skilled trainers who are bilingual and understand programming and behavior intervention plans in both languages. Also, when considering the translation of the program, one must determine which parts of the curriculum or services translate linguistically and culturally. For example, various possessive pronouns used in the American culture are irrelevant to everyday social interactions in the Japanese culture. In addition, most countries have very culturally specific sayings, phrases, and vocabulary, as well as differences in labels (e.g., "put this in the rubbish" versus "put this in the trash"), sentence structure, and phrases. Some also have extensive alphabets and culturally specific rules for nonvocal language.

In addition to language and general cultural considerations, the delivery of ABA-based programs in countries outside of the United States requires consideration of the applicability of the principles of reinforcement and punishment. For example, in many cultures, providing praise or tangible items as positive reinforcement is considered highly irregular. Consequently, modifications to reinforcement delivery need to be considered in order to assimilate ABA-based service delivery successfully in these cultures. Another example is the difficulty seen in the establishment of strong motivating operations (e.g., deprivation). Some parents do not want to withhold potential reinforcers (especially if maladaptive behaviors result). For this reason, it is especially critical to explain the necessity of reinforcement schedules during initial training and to achieve agreement on this issue before proceeding to any training with the learner. Differing views regarding punishment also may arise when delivering services globally. Specifically, workshop supervisors need to consider both ethical guidelines and cultural views on punishment before designing a program for learners. In many non-Western cultures, physical aversives, such as corporal punishment, are highly prevalent. Likewise, exclusionary time-out is frequently used in many cultures. Very careful consideration must be used by the RCS supervisor to tailor each intervention to the unique cultural preferences of the learner's family while simultaneously not violating the supervisor's own ethical principles.

Another barrier to treatment delivery centers on the acceptability of a comprehensive treatment program. As has been described in this book, the CARD Model of treating children with ASD focuses on creating a treatment program that addresses all areas of human functioning, including social, motor, language, adaptive, play, executive functions, cognition, and academic. Some countries, however, have a heightened focus on academics and a lack of emphasis on appropriate play skills, social skills (e.g., teaching a learner to make eye contact is seen as rude in some cultures), and adaptive skills (e.g., teaching a learner self-help skills is less important in a culture with nannies who perform those tasks for the learner). Additionally, one must consider the importance of religion and the learner's participation in religious activities when designing the learner's curriculum program.

Another barrier to treatment delivery concerns the cultural and social acceptability of the word *autism*. Often, the word *autism* is unacceptable, and there is a tendency to use the label "learning disorder." Social stigma is common for parents of children with autism and may discourage them from seeking services for their children. Thus, when they do seek services, one must determine whether to discuss treatment in terms of the diagnosis and whether alternative terms should be considered for use in practice. Additionally, many parents who experience this stigma are generally looking for a more "medical" model of treatment such that the provider "makes their child better" (as when one takes one's child to a doctor). Given this, they often prefer to go to a facility that will "fix their child" in a discrete manner. These feelings of shame can understandably be associated with limited parent involvement. Consequently, children with disabilities may not be included in family activities and are more often taken care of by nannies on a day-to-day basis. These factors need to be considered during the service delivery process, as limited parent involvement in everyday service delivery can hinder the generalization and maintenance of treatment gains.

Given the many potential cultural challenges of global dissemination, RCS supervisors should educate themselves about the specific culture in which they will be traveling and working. Treatment goals should center on the social norms of the target population and should address cultural expectations. Ultimately, RCS supervisors will be more effective if they address ethical concerns (e.g., corporal punishment) in a nonconfrontational manner. In addition, RCS supervisors should modify their technical language and be prepared to discuss procedures and principles in the family's vernacular. Finally, in order to remove the stigma associated with the diagnosis and treatment of autism, RCS supervisors should consider conducting seminars and parent workshops on autism awareness and treatment across cultures.

SUMMARY

The RCS model and affiliate programs are two methods that have facilitated the global dissemination of the CARD Model. Thousands of learners have been treated through the CARD RCS model, and multiple affiliate sites have been established across several continents. Successful implementation of the RCS model and development of affiliate sites require flexible and well-trained RCS supervisors to provide training in a culturally and linguistically appropriate manner, motivated parents and therapists who are ready to learn, and – for affiliate sites – agencies that are ready to work hard to implement the CARD Model.

A

CARD INDIRECT FUNCTIONAL ASSESSMENT (CIFA)

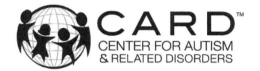

CARD Indirect Functional Assessment (CIFA)

Client name:_____   Reporter name:_____

Reporter relation to client:_____   Date:_____

Topography of behavior:_____

Directions

- Consider only the particular target behavior when completing this assessment.
- Answer every question.
- Use the following codes to answer the questions:
  - **0 = Disagree   1 = Agree   2 = Strongly Agree   n/a = Not Applicable**

	Answer
1. He/she engages in the behavior so you will tell him/her to stop.	
2. He/she engages in the behavior when alone.	
3. He/she engages in the behavior when he/she is experiencing stress.	
4. When he/she engages in this behavior, he/she appears to be saying, "I want to be the boss."	
5. He/she engages in the behavior when asked to complete a task (i.e., schoolwork, household chore, daily hygiene, etc.).	
6. He/she cries real tears when something is moved that he/she does not want moved.	
7. He/she engages in the behavior when something he/she wants is taken away (i.e., toy, game, food, etc.) or something he/she is doing is interrupted (i.e., game, TV turned off, etc.).	
8. He/she engages in the behavior so other people will pay attention to him/her.	
9. He/she engages in the behavior when he/she is bored or under-stimulated	
10. He/she engages in the behavior when worried or anxious about something.	
11. He/she engages in the behavior when people don't do what he/she asks/tells them to do.	
12. When he/she engages in this behavior, it appears he/she is saying, "I don't want to do this."	
13. He/she engages in the behavior when things are done differently (e.g., reading book in different voice, cutting food in different way, making bed with different blanket, etc.).	
14. He/she engages in the behavior when he/she is told to stop or wait for a preferred activity.	
15. He/she engages in the behavior because you are paying attention to someone else.	
16. He/she seems not to care if anyone sees him/her engage in the behavior.	
17. He/she engages in the behavior to calm himself/herself down.	

18.	He/she engages in the behavior because you are not doing what he/she wants you to do.
19.	He/she engages in this behavior when asked to do something he/she does not want to do.
20.	He/she engages in the behavior when you move objects that he/she has arranged (e.g., moved, put into a line or specific group).
21.	When he/she engages in the behavior, he/she appears to be saying, "I want that" or "Give it to me."
22.	He/she engages in the behavior when you are busy.
23.	He/she engages in the behavior when he/she is really happy or excited.
24.	He/she engages in this behavior to allow him/her to cope with being upset.
25.	He/she engages in the behavior in order to be in control of what is happening.
26.	He/she engages in the behavior to get away from work/demand situations.
27.	He/she engages in the behavior when a routine is broken.
28.	He/she engages in the behavior when he/she does not get what he/she wants.
29.	He/she looks to see if you react when he/she does the behavior.
30.	He/she engages in the behavior regardless of location or activity.
31.	He/she engages in the behavior when scared.
32.	You can prevent the behavior by allowing him/her to be in control of the situation.
33.	He/she engages in the behavior when he/she does not understand what someone is asking him/her to do.
34.	He/she engages in the behavior when something novel occurs.
35.	When you provide the toy/food/activity he/she wants, he/she stops engaging in the behavior.

The CARD Indirect Functional Assessment form. Reprinted with permission from the Center for Autism and Related Disorders.

BEHAVIOR INTERVENTION PLAN SHORT FORMAT

Name: Jimmy Smith   **Revised**: XX/XX/XXXX

Persons responsible for implementing: All therapists working with Jimmy

Operational Definition: Hitting includes all occurrences of Jimmy striking others with an open or closed fist, hard enough to make an audible sound.

Measurement System: Frequency data should be collected on hitting during all therapy sessions and converted to rate per hour. Data should be graphed at the end of each therapy session.

Antecedent Components:
- **Attention NCR.** Provide frequent positive attention to Jimmy for free, regardless of what he is doing. Give at least 10 seconds of high-quality attention every 5 minutes.
- **Teaching Attention FCT.** Prompt Jimmy to request attention from others and give lots of positive attention immediately when he requests it. Physical prompts will be used to prompt the requesting behavior. Prompt Jimmy to hand over the card at the beginning of all free play or other downtimes In addition, prompt Jimmy to hand over the card at least one time every 5 minutes, as long as he has not hit in the last 30 seconds. Add 1 minute to the interval between prompts for every day that hitting has occurred at or below one time per hour and communication has occurred at or above five times per hour.

Replacement Behavior Components:
- **Attention FCT.** The form of requesting that will be taught is handing over a communication card that says "Play with me."

Consequence Components:
- **Attention extinction for hitting.** Do not respond to hitting by providing attention in any way. If possible, act as though the behavior did not occur. If some reaction is absolutely necessary to keep yourself safe, avoid eye contact and give the minimum reaction necessary to keep people and property safe.
- **Attention reinforcement for FCT.** Every time Jimmy hands someone the attention communication card, give him a minimum of 1 minute of high-quality attention.

Appendix B. A sample short-format version of a behavioral intervention plan. This does not supplant a full, detailed plan, but rather serves as a quick reference for daily use. All staff must also read the full plan prior to working with the child. Content reprinted from the Skills® BIP Builder, with permission from the Center for Autism and Related Disorders.

C

SAMPLE CURRICULUM LESSON FROM SKILLS® (ABRIDGED FOR LENGTH), REPRINTED WITH PERMISSION FROM THE CENTER FOR AUTISM AND RELATED DISORDERS, INC.

Curriculum: Cognition
Lesson: Knowing

Purpose

The purpose of this lesson is to teach the child the concept of "knowing" and that our senses and interactions with others and our environment allow us to know things (e.g., seeing leads to knowing). The child will learn to understand the concept of "knowing" for himself / herself as well as identify what people know and how they know it. Considering what other people know is of vital importance in communicative and social interactions because it allows the speaker to judge the amount of information required by the listener in order to provide sufficient, but not excessive, background. An inability to consider others' knowledge may result in speech without context or redundant communication. Further, identification of what others know and do not know is required for other social-cognitive skills, including false beliefs and deception. This lesson aims to improve the child's identification ("Does he / she know?") and application ("If he / she doesn't know, what do I do?") of others' knowledge during communicative and social interactions.

Lesson Sections

This lesson targets the following skills:
1. Identifying What People Do and Do Not Know: 4+ yrs.
2. General Knowledge and Universally Unknown Information: Age Variable
3. Knowing About – Observation, Listening, and Reading: Age Variable
4. Knowing How – Experience, Observation, and Instruction: Age Variable
5. Applications of Knowing: 5 – 6 yrs.
6. Second-Order Knowing: Age Variable

1. Identifying What People Do and Do Not Know: 4+ yrs.

Average Age of Skills	Prerequisites
4+ yrs.: • Can explain how the child and others know something using all of the senses (i.e., one knows something because he / she can see it, hear it, etc.)	*Language Curriculum:* • Yes / No (only for *Activities* 5, 11, and 15) *Executive Functions Curriculum:* • Episodic Memory (only for *Activities* 14 – 15 if the child has difficulty recalling details about experiences)

Self Knowledge / 1st Person – Knowing by Using Senses

IEP Goal: Activities 1 – 4

- By (date), (name) will explain why he / she does / doesn't know something by referring to his / her senses, and will engage in actions to allow him / her to gain knowledge when he / she does not know, across (settings) and (people) with 100% accuracy in (# out of #) opportunities, as measured by (person responsible and data collection method).

Activity 1

SD 1a: The therapist presents an object / event and asks the child to identify the label, attributes, features, actions, etc.

R 1a: "It is (label / attribute / feature / etc.)." ⌐Metacognition⌐

SD 1b: "How do you know?"

R 1b: "Because I see / hear / smell / feel / taste it." ⌐Metacognition⌐

Examples

- SD a: The therapist cannot see Jimmy's bike because his / her view is obstructed. However, the child's view is not obstructed, so the therapist asks, "What kind of bike does Jimmy have?"
  - R a: "A batman bike."
  - SD b: "How do you know?"
  - R b: "Because I see it."
- SD a: The therapist presents orange juice to the child with pulp in it and asks, "How is it?"
  - R a: "Yucky, it has pulp in it."
  - SD b: "How do you know?"
  - R b: "Because I taste it."
- SD a: The therapist and the child are at the fair and the therapist asks, "What do you want to eat?"
  - R a: "I want to eat popcorn."
  - SD b: "How do you know there is popcorn here?"
  - R b: "Because I smell it."
- Knowledge based on seeing:
  - o The child is presented with an object / views an event / views a person and the therapist asks:
    - "What is this?"
    - "What color is it?"
    - "What's (person) doing?"
    - "What does (person) have?"
- Knowledge based on hearing:

- o The child is presented with an auditory stimulus (sight of the source of the stimulus should be obstructed):
  - ▪ The child's mom is talking loudly when the therapist asks, "Who is in the hallway?"
  - ▪ The child closes his / her eyes while the therapist claps, sneezes, breaks something, etc. Then, the therapist asks, "What am I doing?"
  - ▪ A baby is crying in the next room when the therapist asks, "What is the baby doing?"
- Knowledge based on smelling:
  - o The child is presented with an olfactory stimulus and the therapist asks (sight of the source of the stimulus should be obstructed):
    - ▪ "What is Mom cooking?"
    - ▪ Upon smelling a skunk, the therapist asks, "What animal is outside?"
- Knowledge based on touch:
  - o The child is presented with a tactile stimulus:
    - ▪ After the child touches the outside of a warm hair dryer, the therapist asks, "Was the hair dryer on recently?"
    - ▪ After the child feels the contents of a bag and identifies what is in it, the therapist asks, "What is in the bag?"
- Knowledge based on tasting:
  - o The child is presented with a gustatory stimulus:
    - ▪ After the child samples some pizza (with a blindfold on), the therapist asks, "What are you eating?"
    - ▪ The therapist and child have ice cream for a snack and the therapist asks, "What flavor do you have?"

Teaching Points

1. One way you could prompt this skill is to have a visual diagram of the five senses to which the child can refer. See the *How Do You Know?* diagram at the end of this lesson for one way you could present this.
2. When beginning to teach the concept of "knowing," you will follow the same general *Activity* progression for each of the senses / means of acquiring knowledge, beginning with the child's perspective, moving to others' perspectives, and then recalling previously acquired information. It is recommended, first, to target knowing through seeing, and then hearing, as these are most critical for social and communicative interactions. When the child is strong on these forms of knowing with the general *Activity* progression, you may then probe other means of knowing, including smelling, feeling, and tasting, as well as knowing due to experience, observation, and from being given instructions, while simultaneously moving on to the more advanced applications of knowing.

Activity 2

Setup
- The therapist sets up barriers / obstructions that prevent the child from being able to contact objects / activities using his / her senses. For example, he / she places items inside a drawer to prevent them from being seen or has people talking in another room to prevent them from being heard.

SD 2a: The therapist asks the child to identify an object / activity or an attribute or feature of the object / activity he / she cannot see / hear / smell / feel / taste (barriers / obstructions prevent contact).
R 2a: "I don't know." Metacognition
SD 2b: "Why not?"
R 2b: "Because I can't see / hear / smell / feel / taste it." Metacognition

Examples
- Setup: The therapist and the child are listening to music, and then the therapist turns down the music so the child can't hear it anymore.
  - SD a: "What song is playing?"
  - R a: "I don't know."
  - SD b: "Why not?"
  - R b: "Because I can't hear it."
- Setup: The child's friend called the child to tell him / her that he / she got a new bike today.
  - SD a: "What color is your friend's bike?"
  - R a: "I don't know."
  - SD b: "Why not?"
  - R b: "Because I can't see it."
- Setup: The therapist and the child are about to go swimming in the community pool.
  - SD a: "Is the water warm or cold?"
  - R a: "I don't know."
  - SD b: "Why not?"
  - R b: "Because I didn't feel it."
- Knowledge based on seeing:
  - The child's sight is obstructed (e.g., has eyes closed, is facing a different way, something is hidden, or items / activities are in different rooms or locations that cannot be seen). The therapist asks:
    - "What is in the box?" (the lid is on a box with no descriptors written on the outside of the box)
    - "I'm holding a penny, which hand is it in?" (both hands are closed)
    - "Do you know what color my socks are?" (socks are covered by pant leg)
    - "What is this?" (the child is blindfolded)

- "What color is it?" (while holding the object behind your back)
        - "What's Mom doing?" (Mom is in a different room)
- Knowledge based on hearing:
    - The child cannot hear:
        - The therapist is wearing headphones and asks, "What song is playing?"
        - The child sees two children outside who are playing. The therapist asks, "What are they saying?"
- Knowledge based on smelling:
    - The child cannot smell when the therapist asks:
        - "What is Dad cooking?" (cooking something that doesn't have a strong smell)
        - "Is Mom wearing perfume?"
- Knowledge based on touch:
    - The child cannot feel when asked:
        - "Is this bath warm?"
        - "Is it hot outside?"
- Knowledge based on tasting:
    - The child cannot taste when asked:
        - "What type of soda am I drinking?" (the soda is in a cup, so no labels are showing)

Teaching Points

1. Make sure the child is able to respond when you randomly rotate *Activities* 1 and 2 before moving on to the next *Activity*.
2. Ensure that there are no other stimuli present that may give away the answer. For example, if you are trying to teach knowledge based on tasting and you ask, "What type of soda am I drinking?", ensure that the child cannot see the soda can (i.e., put the soda in a glass); if you are trying to teach knowledge based on seeing and you ask, "What is your mom doing?" when the child's mother is in another room, ensure that the child cannot hear sounds that give away what his / her mother is doing.
3. To help the child learn to identify common obstructions, you could teach the child rules. For example, you could use the rule "When you are far away from an object, it looks smaller and is harder to see" or "When you are far away from something, you can't hear it" to teach the child that distance can be an obstruction to sight or hearing.

Others' Knowledge

IEP Goal: Activities 7 – 11

- By (date), (name) will identify which people know particular information and how those people know, by referring to their (third person) senses and referencing what they were told, across (settings) and (people) with 100% accuracy in (# out of #) opportunities, as measured by (person responsible and data collection method).

Activity 8

Setup
- The therapist presents an object / event (without obstructions) to a third person.

SD 8: The therapist asks a third person to identify the label, attributes, features, actions, etc. of the object / event. The third person correctly identifies the label / attribute / feature, etc. The therapist then presents the vocal stimulus, "How does (pronoun / person 1) know (information)?"

R 8: "Because (pronoun / person 1) can see / hear / smell / feel / taste it." or "Because (person 2) told (pronoun / person 1)." Social cognition

Examples
- Setup: The child's sister, Ruth, is at a baseball game with the child and the therapist. Ruth can see the scoreboard.
  - SD: The therapist asks Ruth what the score of the game is. Ruth says, "Two to zero." The therapist asks the child, "How does Ruth know the score?"
  - R: "Because she can see the scoreboard."
- Setup: The child's sister, Ruth, tastes onions in the casserole that Mom made.
  - SD: The therapist asks Ruth if she knows if there are onions in the casserole. Ruth says, "Yes." The therapist asks the child, "How does Ruth know there are onions in the casserole?"
  - R: "She can taste them."
- The examples of knowledge based on seeing / hearing / smelling / touch / tasting listed in the *Examples* for *Activity* 1 also apply to this *Activity*, except the questions should be directed toward a third person.

Teaching Points
1. *Teaching Point* 1 for *Activity* 1 also applies to this *Activity*.
2. For "knowledge based on being told," if the child's response is to say that someone knows something because he / she was told, make sure to ask the child whether the person knows immediately after the child sees the person being told.
3. Have the child put his / her body under the same conditions (same position to visual / auditory / olfactory stimulus) that the third person is experiencing so that the child is able to identify how the person knows information.

Activity 9

Setup

- The therapist sets up barriers / obstructions that prevent a third person from being able to contact objects / activities using his / her senses. For example, he / she places items inside a drawer to prevent them from being seen or has people talking in another room to prevent them from being heard.

SD 9:   The therapist asks a third person to identify an object / activity or an attribute or feature of the object / activity he / she cannot see / hear / smell / feel / taste (barriers / obstructions prevent contact). The third person says, "I don't know." The therapist then presents to the child the vocal stimulus, "Why doesn't (<u>pronoun / third person</u>) know?"

R 9:   "Because (<u>pronoun / third person</u>) can't see / hear / smell / feel / taste it." or "Because (<u>person / nobody</u>) didn't tell / told (<u>pronoun / third person</u>)." Social cognition

Examples

- Setup: The child's sister, Ruth, does not know that their mother put onions in the casserole.
  - SD: The therapist asks Ruth if she knows that there are onions in the casserole. Ruth says, "I don't know." The therapist asks the child, "Why doesn't Ruth know?"
  - R: "Because she hasn't tasted / didn't see Mom put onions in the casserole yet."
- Setup: The child's sister, Ruth, is at a baseball game with the child and the therapist. Ruth cannot see the scoreboard because a pole is in the way.
  - SD: The therapist asks Ruth what the score of the game is. Ruth says, "I don't know." The therapist asks the child, "Why doesn't Ruth know?"
  - R: "Because there is a pole in the way, so she can't see the score."
- The examples of knowledge based on seeing / hearing / smelling / touch / tasting listed in the *Examples* for *Activity 2* also apply to this *Activity*, except the questions should be directed toward a third person.

Teaching Points

1. *Teaching Point 3* for *Activity 2* also applies to this *Activity*.
2. *Teaching Points 2 – 3* for *Activity 8* also apply to this *Activity*.

CARD LANGUAGE CURRICULUM

I. Level One
- a. Echoics
    - i. Establishing New Sounds in Children With Limited Echoics: 0 – 12 mos.
    - ii. Echoic Sounds: 0 – 12 mos.
    - iii. Echoic Blends: 0 – 12 mos.
    - iv. Echoic Chains: 0 – 12+ mos.
    - v. Echoic Words: 0 – 6 yrs.
    - vi. Echoic Phrases and Sentences: 1 – 8 yrs.
- b. Basic Mands
    - i. Mands for Cessation: 0 – 2 yrs.
    - ii. Mands for People: 1 – 3 yrs.
    - iii. Mands for Objects: 1 – 3 yrs.
    - iv. Mands for Actions: 1 – 3 yrs.
- c. Objects
    - i. Matching: 1 – 2 yrs.
    - ii. Receptive: 1 – 2 yrs.
    - iii. Sorting: 2 – 3 yrs.
    - iv. Mands: 1 – 3 yrs.
    - v. Tacts: 1 – 3 yrs.
    - vi. Tacts With the Conjunction "And": 4 – 5 yrs.
- d. Following Instructions
    - i. One-Step Instructions: 0 – 2 yrs.
    - ii. Two-Step Instructions: 1 – 3 yrs.
    - iii. Three-Step Instructions: 3+ yrs.
    - iv. Complex Instructions of Four+ Steps: Age Variable

II. Level Two
- a. Choices
    - i. Child's Desires: Age Variable
    - ii. Factual Choices: Age Variable
    - iii. Receptive Either / Or: 3+ yrs.
    - iv. Others' Desires: 3 – 5 yrs.
- b. People
    - i. Mands: 1 – 3 yrs.
    - ii. Matching: Age Variable
    - iii. Receptive: 1 – 2 yrs.
    - iv. Tacts: 1 – 3 yrs.
    - v. Identifying People by Possessions or Actions: Age Variable
- c. Body Parts
    - i. Receptive: 1 – 6 yrs.
    - ii. Matching: 1 – 2+ yrs.
    - iii. Mands: 2+ yrs.
    - iv. Tacts: 2 – 7 yrs.

    d. Yes / No
       i. Mands: 0 – 2 yrs.
       ii. Responding to Yes / No: 1 – 2 yrs.
       iii. Tacts and Intraverbals: 2 – 3 yrs.
    e. Sound Discrimination
       i. Receptive: Age Variable
       ii. Intraverbals: 1 – 2 yrs.
       iii. Mands: 2 – 3 yrs.
       iv. Tacts: Age Variable
    f. Locations
       i. Matching: Age Variable
       ii. Receptive: Age Variable
       iii. Mands: 2 – 3 yrs.
       iv. Tacts: 2 – 3 yrs.
       v. Intraverbals: 3 – 7 yrs.
    g. SD Rotations
       i. Responding to Randomly Rotated SDs: Age Variable
    h. Actions
       i. Present Tense Matching: Age Variable
       ii. Present Tense Receptive: Age Variable – 3 yrs.
       iii. Present Tense Mands: 1 – 3 yrs.
       iv. Present Tense Tacts: 2 – 4 yrs.
       v. Present Tense Extended Descriptions of Actions: Age Variable
       vi. Past Tense Tacts: 3 – 8 yrs.
       vii. Future Tense Tacts and Intraverbals: 3+ yrs.
       viii. Intraverbals – Actions of People and Animals: Age Variable
       ix. Noun-Verb Agreement: 6 – 8 yrs.
    i. Gestures
       i. Mands: 0 – 2 yrs.
       ii. Receptive: 1 – 5+ yrs.
       iii. Tacts and Intraverbals: 5+ yrs.
III. Level Three
    a. I Have / I See
       i. I Have: 2 – 3 yrs.
       ii. I See: 2 – 3 yrs.
       iii. I Have / I See Using the Conjunction "And": 4 – 5 yrs.
    b. Functions
       i. Manual Expression: 1 – 2+ yrs.
       ii. Receptive: 2 – 3 yrs.
       iii. Mands: 2 – 6 yrs.
       iv. Fill-In Intraverbals: 2 – 7 yrs.
       v. Intraverbals: 2 – 7 yrs.
    c. Manding for Information
       i. "What" and "Where" Questions: 2 – 3 yrs.
       ii. "Why," "How," "Who," and "When" Questions: 3 – 4 yrs.
       iii. Asking Questions With Inverted Auxiliary Verbs: Age Variable
       iv. Persisting in Getting Questions Answered: Age Variable
       v. "Which" Questions: Age Variable
       vi. Asking for Definitions of Words / Phrases and Using New Words: 4 – 6 yrs.
       vii. Asking Complex Questions: Age Variable

    d. Categories
- i. Matching / Sorting: Age Variable
- ii. Receptive: 3 – 7 yrs.
- iii. Mands: 4 – 5 yrs.
- iv. Intraverbals: 4 – 6 yrs.

    e. Gender
- i. Matching: Age Variable
- ii. Receptive: 1 – 2 yrs.
- iii. Mands: 2 – 3 yrs.
- iv. Making People: Age Variable
- v. Tacts: 2 – 3 yrs.
- vi. Intraverbals: 2 – 3+ yrs.

    f. Prepositions
- i. Matching: Age Variable
- ii. Receptive: 2 – 8 yrs.
- iii. Mands: 2 – 7 yrs.
- iv. Tacts: 2 – 7 yrs.

IV. Level Four

    a. Features
- i. Matching: Age Variable
- ii. Receptive: 2 – 3 yrs.
- iii. Part / Whole: Age Variable
- iv. Tacts: Age Variable
- v. Intraverbals: Age Variable

    b. What Goes With
- i. Matching: Age Variable
- ii. Receptive: Age Variable
- iii. Intraverbals: Age Variable

    c. Attributes
- i. Matching: Age Variable
- ii. Sorting: 2 – 7 yrs.
- iii. Receptive: 2 – 7 yrs.
- iv. Mands: 2 – 7 yrs.
- v. Tacts: 2 – 7 yrs.
- vi. Intraverbals: 3 – 7 yrs.
- vii. Comparatives – Receptive: 4 – 5 yrs.
- viii. Comparatives – Mands: 4 – 5 yrs.
- ix. Comparatives – Tacts: 4 – 5 yrs.
- x. Comparatives – Intraverbals: Age Variable
- xi. Superlatives – Receptive: 4 – 5 yrs.
- xii. Superlatives – Mands: Age Variable
- xiii. Superlatives – Tacts: 4 – 5 yrs.
- xiv. Superlatives – Intraverbals: Age Variable
- xv. Classifying by Attributes: 6 – 7 yrs.

    d. Opposites
- i. Matching: Age Variable
- ii. Receptive: Age Variable
- iii. Tacts: Age Variable
- iv. Intraverbals: 3 – 4 yrs.

e. Pronouns
  i. Demonstrative Pronouns: Age Variable
  ii. Possessive Pronouns / Nouns: 2 – 3+ yrs.
  iii. Possessive Pronouns / Nouns With Nouns: 2 – 4 yrs.
  iv. Personal Pronouns: 2 – 3 yrs.
  v. Objective Pronouns: 2 – 3+ yrs.
  vi. Reflexive Pronouns: Age Variable
  vii. Double Pronouns: 3 – 4 yrs.
  viii. Indefinite Pronouns: Age Variable
f. Describe
  i. Manding by Description: Age Variable
  ii. Identifying by Description: 4 – 7 yrs.
  iii. Intraverbals – Describing: 4+ yrs.
  iv. Sorting by Description: Age Variable
g. Plurals
  i. Matching: Age Variable
  ii. Receptive: Age Variable
  iii. Mands: 2 – 5 yrs.
  iv. Tacts: 2 – 5 yrs.
h. Language Fluency
  i. Combining Accuracy With Speed: Age Variable
  ii. Using Language Concepts With Peers / Others: Age Variable

V. Level Five
a. Negation
  i. Don't: 2 – 3+ yrs.
  ii. Not: Age Variable – 4 yrs.
  iii. Can't: 2 – 3+ yrs.
  iv. Won't: Age Variable
  v. Doesn't: Age Variable
  vi. Didn't: Age Variable
  vii. Couldn't: Age Variable
  viii. Shouldn't: Age Variable
  ix. Wouldn't: Age Variable
  x. Except: 4 – 6 yrs.
b. Wh- Discrimination
  i. Matching: Age Variable
  ii. Receptive: Age Variable
  iii. Tacts: 2 – 5 yrs
  iv. Intraverbals: 3 – 7 yrs.
c. Statement-Statement
  i. Statement-Positive Statement: Age Variable
  ii. Statement-Negative Statement: Age Variable
d. I Don't Know
  i. Tacts: Age Variable
  ii. Intraverbals: Age Variable

  e. Sequences – First, Then, Last
    i. Receptive: 3+ yrs.
    ii. Following Instructions: Age Variable
    iii. Mands: Age Variable
    iv. Following Instructions With Recall: Age Variable
    v. Sequencing Pictures and Use of Procedural Discourse: 5 – 6 yrs.
    vi. Giving Instructions and Use of Procedural Discourse: 6 – 8 yrs.
  f. Sequences – Before / After
    i. Picture Sequences: Age Variable
    ii. Following Instructions: Age Variable – 5 yrs.
    iii. Choices: Age Variable
    iv. Following Instructions With Immediate Recall: Age Variable

VI. Level Six
  a. Adverbs
    i. Mands: 2 – 5 yrs.
    ii. Receptive: Age Variable
    iii. Tacts: 2 – 8 yrs.
    iv. Intraverbals: Age Variable
    v. Comparative Adverbs – Tacts and Intraverbals: Age Variable
    vi. Superlative Adverbs – Tacts and Intraverbals: Age Variable
  b. Same / Different
    i. Matching: Age Variable
    ii. Receptive: 4 – 5 yrs.
    iii. Mands: Age Variable
    iv. Tacts: 4 – 6 yrs.
    v. Intraverbals: 4 – 7 yrs.
  c. Sequencing
    i. Part-to-Whole Picture Sequences: Age Variable
    ii. Daily Activity Sequences: 4 – 5 yrs.
    iii. Life Cycle Picture Sequences: Age Variable
    iv. Attribute Sequences: 4 – 5 yrs.
    v. Story Sequences: Age Variable

VII. Level Seven
  a. Tell a Story
    i. Contributing to Telling a Story: Age Variable
    ii. Independently Telling a Story: Age Variable
  b. Statement-Question
    i. Responding to Statements With Questions: 5+ yrs.
  c. Barrier Games
    i. Giving Specific Instructions: Age Variable
  d. Relationships
    i. Matching / Sorting: Age Variable
    ii. Receptive: Age Variable
    iii. Tacts: Age Variable
    iv. Intraverbals: Age Variable

VIII. Level Eight
  a. Ask and Tell
    i. Tell: 2 – 3 yrs.
    ii. Ask: Age Variable

E

CARD PLAY CURRICULUM

I. LEVEL ONE

a. Interactive Play
- **i.** Early Social Games.
  1. Imitation: 1–3 yrs.
  2. Receptive: 1–2 yrs.
  3. Initiating Play: 1–3 yrs.
- **ii.** Peer Play.
  1. Imitative Play: 1–2 yrs.
  2. Parallel Play: 2–3 yrs.
  3. Associative Play: 2–7 yrs.
  4. Joining and Initiating Play: 3–5+ yrs.
  5. Cooperative Play: 3–6 yrs.

b. Independent Play
- **i.** Sensorimotor and Manipulative Play.
  1. Non-vocal Imitation: 1–2+ yrs.
  2. Independent Play: 1–3 yrs.
  3. Initiating Play: 2–3 yrs.

II. LEVEL TWO

a. Interactive Play
- **i.** Treasure Hunt.
  1. Object Permanence: 0–12 mos.
  2. Visual and Vocal Cues: 1–2 yrs.
  3. Vocal Cues: 1–5 yrs.
  4. Map: 3–4 yrs.
  5. Textual Cues: Age Variable.
- **ii.** Music and Movement.
  1. Dancing: 1–3 yrs.
  2. Singing: 1–5 yrs.
  3. Initiating Play: 2–3 yrs.

        4. Motions That Go With Songs: 2–3 yrs.

        5. Singing With Motions: Age Variable.

        6. Playing Instruments: Age Variable.

    iii. Read-to-Me Books and Nursery Rhymes.

        1. Receptive: 1–3 yrs.

        2. Reciting Nursery Rhymes: Age Variable–8 yrs.

        3. Initiating Play: 2–3 yrs.

        4. Answering Questions: 2–5 yrs.

b. Independent Play

  i. Task Completion Play.

      1. Non-vocal Imitation: 1–2+ yrs.

      2. Independent Play: 1–5 yrs.

      3. Initiating Play: 2–3 yrs.

c. Pretend Play

  i. Functional Pretend Play.

      1. Imitation: 1–2+ yrs.

      2. Initiating Play: 1–4 yrs.

      3. Conversation: 2–7 yrs.

III. LEVEL THREE

a. Pretend Play

  i. Symbolic Play.

      1. Imitation: 1–2+ yrs.

      2. Initiating Play: 1–4 yrs.

      3. Conversation: 2–7 yrs.

b. Constructive Play

  i. Block Constructions.

      1. Matching: Age Variable.

      2. Structure Identification: Age Variable.

      3. Imitation: 1–6 yrs.

      4. Initiating Play: 2–3 yrs.

      5. Creative Building: 3–4 yrs.

  ii. Clay Constructions.

      1. Matching: Age Variable.

      2. Structure Identification: Age Variable.

      3. Creating Constructions: 3+ yrs.

      4. Initiating Play: 3+ yrs.

      5. Conversation: 3–5 yrs.

  iii. Sand and Water Constructions.

      1. Matching: Age Variable.

      2. Structure Identification: Age Variable.

      3. Creating Constructions: 3+ yrs.

      4. Initiating Play: 3+ yrs.

      5. Conversation: 3–5 yrs.

IV. LEVEL FOUR

a. Interactive Play
  i. Locomotor Play.
     1. Playing Games: 4–12 yrs.
     2. Initiating Play: 4–12 yrs.
     3. Conversation: 4–12 yrs.
b. Independent Play
  i. Play Stations.
     1. Sustaining Play: 3–4 yrs.
c. Constructive Play
  i. Arts and Crafts.
     1. Matching: Age Variable.
     2. Structure Identification: Age Variable.
     3. Creating Constructions: 3–7 yrs.
     4. Initiating Play: 3+ yrs.
     5. Conversation: 3–5 yrs.
  ii. Structure Building.
     1. Matching: Age Variable.
     2. Structure Identification: Age Variable.
     3. Creating Constructions: 3–4 yrs.
     4. Initiating Play: 3–4 yrs.
     5. Conversation: 3–5 yrs.

V. LEVEL FIVE

a. Pretend Play
  i. Role-Taking and Sociodramatic Play.
     1. Imitation of Roles: 3–5 yrs.
     2. Initiating Play: 3–6 yrs.
     3. Sociodramatic Play: 4–7 yrs.
  ii. Imaginary Play.
     1. Imitation: 4–5 yrs.
     2. Initiating Play: 4–5 yrs.
     3. Conversation: 4–7 yrs.

VI. LEVEL SIX

a. Interactive Play
  i. Card and Board Games.
     1. Playing Games: 3–7 yrs.
     2. Initiating Play: 3+ yrs.
     3. Conversation: 3–7 yrs.

VII. LEVEL EIGHT

a. Electronic Play
  i. Audio and Video Play.
   1. Initiating Play: 2–3 yrs.
   2. Equipment Identification: 2–4 yrs.
   3. Operating the System: 2–4 yrs.
   4. Equipment Functions: 2–6 yrs.
   5. Conversation: 2–7 yrs.
  ii. Computer Play.
   1. Initiating Play: 3+ yrs.
   2. Equipment Identification: 3+ yrs.
   3. Operating the System: 3–7 yrs.
   4. Equipment Functions: 3+ yrs.
   5. Conversation: 3–7 yrs.
  iii. Video Games.
   1. Initiating Play: 3+ yrs.
   2. Equipment Identification: 3+ yrs.
   3. Operating the System: 3+ yrs.
   4. Equipment Functions: 3+ yrs.
   5. Conversation: 3–7 yrs.

CARD ADAPTIVE CURRICULUM

I. LEVEL ONE

a. Personal
  i. Feeding.
    1. Self-feeding Finger Foods: 0–12+ mos.
    2. Introducing New Foods: 0–12 mos.
    3. Drinking From a Cup: 0–2 yrs.
    4. Introducing New Beverages: Age Variable.
    5. Using a Straw: 1–2 yrs.
    6. Using a Spoon: 1–7 yrs.
    7. Using a Fork: 1–7 yrs.
    8. Using a Napkin: 2–7 yrs.
    9. Using a Knife: 4–7 yrs.

II. LEVEL TWO

a. Personal
  i. Undressing.
    1. Socks: 1–2 yrs.
    2. Shoes: 1–3 yrs.
    3. Front-opening Clothing: 2–4 yrs.
    4. Pull-down Clothing: 2–6 yrs.
    5. Getting Undressed: 3–6 yrs.
    6. Pull-over Clothing: 4–5 yrs.
    7. Gloves: Age Variable.
  ii. Unfastening.
    1. Unzipping: 1–5 yrs.
    2. Untying Bows: 2–3 yrs.
    3. Unbuttoning: 2–6 yrs.
    4. Unsnapping: 3–5 yrs.
    5. Unbuckling: Age Variable.

       6. Unlacing: Age Variable.

       7. Untying Knots: Age Variable.

b. Domestic

   i. Tidying.

       1. Putting Items Away After Use: 1–6 yrs.

       2. Closing Cabinets/Drawers: Age Variable.

       3. Turning the Lights Off: Age Variable.

c. Safety

   i. Safety Awareness.

       1. Following Safety Instructions: Age Variable.

       2. Following Safety Rules: 3–7 yrs.

       3. Identifying Safe/Dangerous: 3–6 yrs.

       4. Identifying Relationship-Appropriate Safety Behavior: 5–7 yrs.

       5. Identifying Safety Signs: 5–7 yrs.

III. LEVEL THREE

a. Personal

   i. Dressing.

       1. Front-opening Clothing: 2–7 yrs.

       2. Pull-up Clothing: 2–7 yrs.

       3. Socks: 3–4 yrs.

       4. Pull-over Clothing: 3–7 yrs.

       5. Shoes: 4–6 yrs.

       6. Gloves: Age Variable.

       7. Getting Dressed: 4–7 yrs.

       8. Coordinating Clothing: Age Variable.

       9. Selecting Clothing: Age Variable.

       10. Dressing for Weather: 5–7 yrs.

   ii. Toileting.

       1. Routine Training: 2–5 yrs.

       2. Bladder Training: 2–5 yrs.

       3. Bowel Training: 2–5 yrs.

       4. Indication Training: 2–5 yrs.

       5. Independent Toileting: 2–5+ yrs.

       6. Nocturnal Toileting: 4–8 yrs.

   iii. Preventing the Spread of Germs.

       1. Washing and Drying Hands: 2–3+ yrs.

       2. Blowing Nose: 2–6 yrs.

       3. Covering Mouth: 5–6 yrs.

       4. Avoiding Individuals With Contagious Illnesses: 8–9 yrs.

  iv. Teeth Care.
     1. Brushing Teeth: 3–7 yrs.
     2. Using Mouthwash: 6+ yrs.
     3. Flossing: Age Variable.
  v. Fastening.
     1. Fastening Zippers: 3–7 yrs.
     2. Fastening Buttons: 3–6 yrs.
     3. Fastening Snaps: 3–6 yrs.
     4. Lacing: Age Variable–5 yrs.
     5. Buckling: 4–5 yrs.
     6. Tying Shoes: 5–6 yrs.
     7. Tying a Knot: 6+ yrs.

IV. LEVEL FOUR

a. Personal
  i. Adaptive Fluency.
     1. Combining Accuracy With Speed: Age Variable.
b. Domestic
  i. Snacks and Meals.
     1. Obtaining a Snack: Age Variable.
     2. Obtaining a Drink: 3–4+ yrs.
     3. Assisting With Meal Preparation: 5–6 yrs.
     4. Using Appliances: 7–10 yrs.
     5. Independent Meal Preparation: Age Variable.
     6. Preparing School Lunch: Age Variable.
  ii. Clothing Care.
     1. Placing Dirty Clothing in Hamper: Age Variable.
     2. Sorting Clothing: Age Variable.
     3. Putting Away Folded/Hung Clothing: 4–5+ yrs.
     4. Removing Clothing From the Dryer: Age Variable.
     5. Folding/Hanging Clothing: 5+ yrs.
     6. Putting It All Together: 7–10 yrs.

V. LEVEL FIVE

a. Personal
  i. Hair Care.
     1. Brushing/Combing Hair: 5–6 yrs.
     2. Styling Hair: Age Variable.
     3. Using a Hair Dryer: 7+ yrs.

VI. LEVEL SIX

a. Personal
   i. Bathing.
      1. Using the Faucet: 3–7 yrs.
      2. Washing and Drying Face: 3–4+ yrs.
      3. Drying Hair and Body: 4–6 yrs.
      4. Washing Hair: 7+ yrs.
      5. Bathing/Showering: 7+ yrs.
b. Domestic
   i. Setting and Clearing the Table.
      1. Clearing the Table: 1–10 yrs.
      2. Wiping the Table: Age Variable.
      3. Setting the Table: 4–8 yrs.

VII. LEVEL SEVEN

a. Domestic
   i. Making a Bed.
      1. Making a Bed: 6–7 yrs.
b. Community
   i. Shopping.
      1. Placing Items in a Cart: Age Variable.
      2. Using a Cart: Age Variable.
      3. Manding for Information/Assistance: 5+ yrs.
      4. Making Small Purchases: Age Variable.
   ii. Restaurant Readiness.
      1. Disposing of Unwanted Foods: 5+ yrs.
      2. Ordering From the Menu: 8+ yrs.
      3. Buffet Lines: Age Variable.

VIII. LEVEL EIGHT

a. Safety
   i. Safety Equipment.
      1. Putting on Safety Equipment: 6–7 yrs.
      2. Removing Safety Equipment: 6–7 yrs.
      3. Putting It All Together: 6–7 yrs.

IX. LEVEL TEN

a. Personal
   i. Health Care.
      1. Applying Lotion: Age Variable.

    2. Caring for Minor Cuts: 7+ yrs.
    3. Following Special Diets: 7+ yrs.
    4. Taking Medicine: 7+ yrs.
b. Community
  i. Telephone Skills.
    1. Answering the Phone: 3–8 yrs.
    2. Summoning Others to the Phone: 5–8 yrs.
    3. Taking a Message: 5–7 yrs.
    4. Making Phone Calls: 6–8 yrs.
    5. Finding a Phone Number: Age Variable.

X. LEVEL ELEVEN

a. Personal
  i. Nail Care.
    1. Filing Nails: Age Variable.
    2. Cleaning Nails: 6–7 yrs.
    3. Clipping Nails: Age Variable.
b. Domestic
  i. Cleaning.
    1. Taking the Trash Out: Age Variable.
    2. Cleaning up Spills/Broken Items: 5+ yrs.
    3. Dusting the Furniture: Age Variable.
  ii. Gardening.
    1. Watering the Plants: 5+ yrs.
    2. Raking the Leaves: 8–11 yrs.

XI. LEVEL TWELVE

a. Domestic
  i. Pet Care
    1. Feeding the Pet: 1–6 yrs.
    2. Letting the Pet Out: Age Variable.
    3. Brushing the Pet: 5–6 yrs.
    4. Walking the Dog: Age Variable.
    5. Bathing the Dog: Age Variable.
    6. Picking up Feces: Age Variable.

G

CARD MOTOR CURRICULUM

I. LEVEL ONE

a. Gross Motor
  i. Rolling Over.
   1. Rolling From Stomach to Back: 0–12 mos.
   2. Rolling From Back to Stomach: 0–12 mos.
  ii. Sitting.
   1. Sitting Unsupported: 0–12 mos.
   2. Rising to a Sitting Position: 0–12 mos.
   3. Rotating Trunk/Pivoting Buttocks While Sitting: 0–12 mos.
  iii. Creeping/Crawling.
   1. Creeping: 0–12 mos.
   2. Crawling: 0–12 mos.
  iv. Standing.
   1. Standing Up: 0–2 yrs.
   2. Standing on One Foot: 1–6 yrs.
  v. Walking.
   1. Walking Forward: 0–2 yrs.
   2. Walking Sideways: 1–2 yrs.
   3. Walking Backward: 1–3 yrs.
   4. Walking Forward Heel-to-Toe: 3–5 yrs.
   5. Walking Backward Toe-to-Heel: 5–7 yrs.
b. Fine Motor
  i. Hand Skills.
   1. Reaching: 0–12 mos.
   2. Grasping and Releasing: 0–2 yrs.
   3. Pulling: 0–12+ mos.
   4. Squeezing: 0–12+ mos.
   5. Twisting: 0–5 yrs.
  ii. Finger Skills.
   1. Pointing: 0–12 mos.
   2. Pincer Grasp: 0–12+ mos.

   3. Object Manipulation: 0–6 yrs.
   4. Turning the Pages of a Book: 1–5 yrs.
   5. Stringing Beads: 2–3 yrs.
c. Oral Motor
  i. Oral Motor.
   1. Mouth Movements: 1–3 yrs.
   2. Tongue Movements: 1–7 yrs.
   3. Velar Movements: 2–4 yrs.

II. LEVEL TWO

a. Visual Motor
  i. Ocular Motility.
   1. Fixation: 0–12+ yrs.
   2. Pursuits: 0–12+ mos.
   3. Saccades: Age Variable.
   4. Scanning: Age Variable.
  ii. Binocular Vision Skills.
   1. Convergence: 1–2 yrs.
   2. Stereopsis: 1–4 yrs.
b. Gross Motor
  i. Stairs and Climbing.
   1. Creeping/Crawling Upstairs: 1–2 yrs.
   2. Creeping/Crawling Downstairs Backward: 1–2 yrs.
   3. Climbing on/off Household Objects: 1–3 yrs.
   4. Walking Upstairs: 1–4 yrs.
   5. Climbing on/off Playground Equipment: 1–7 yrs.
   6. Walking Downstairs: 2–4 yrs.
  ii. Rolling/Throwing/Dribbling.
   1. Rolling a Ball: 1–2+ yrs.
   2. Throwing a Ball: 2–7 yrs.
   3. Throwing a Bounced Ball: Age Variable.
   4. Dribbling a Ball: Age Variable.
  iii. Running
   1. Running, Turning, and Stopping: 2–6 yrs.
   2. Galloping: 4–7 yrs.
   3. Skipping: 4–6 yrs.
  iv. Balance Beam.
   1. Standing on a Balance Beam: 1–3 yrs.
   2. Walking Sideways on a Balance Beam: Age Variable–6 yrs.
   3. Walking Forward on a Balance Beam: 1–6 yrs.
   4. Walking Backward on a Balance Beam: Age Variable–7 yrs.

     v. Riding Foot-Propelled Vehicles.
        1. Riding a Small Car: Age Variable.
        2. Riding a Scooter: Age Variable.
        3. Riding a Skateboard: Age Variable.
    vi. Catching.
        1. Catching a Rolled Ball: Age Variable.
        2. Catching a Thrown Ball: 3–7 yrs.
        3. Catching a Bounced Ball: 3–6+ yrs.
    vii. Jumping.
        1. Bending the Knees: Age Variable.
        2. Jumping Independently: 2–3 yrs.
        3. Jumping Forward/Over Objects: 2–5 yrs.
        4. Jumping Backward: 4–7 yrs.
        5. Jumping Rope: 5–7 yrs.
c. Fine Motor
  i. Coloring.
      1. Using a Crayon: 1–5 yrs.
      2. Using Multiple Colors: Age Variable.
      3. Coloring Inside the Lines: 5–6 yrs.
      4. Using Realistic Colors: Age Variable.

III. LEVEL THREE

a. Visual Motor
  i. Visual Perception.
      1. Visual Form Perception: 2–5 yrs.
      2. Visual Spatial/Orientation Relations: 3–6+ yrs.
      3. Visual Form Constancy: 3+ yrs.
      4. Visual Figure-Ground Discrimination: 4–5 yrs.
      5. Visual Closure: 4+ yrs.
b. Gross Motor
  i. Kicking.
      1. Kicking: 2–5 yrs.
      2. Kicking a Ball: 2–7 yrs.
  ii. Hopping.
      1. Hopping on Preferred Foot: 2–6 yrs.
      2. Hopping on Other Foot: 2–6 yrs.
  iii. Riding a Tricycle/Bicycle.
      1. Riding a Tricycle: 3–4 yrs.
      2. Riding a Bicycle: Age Variable–7 yrs.
c. Fine Motor
  i. Prehandwriting.

   1. Holding a Piece of Paper in Place: 1–2 yrs.
   2. Scribbling: 1–3 yrs.
   3. Imitating Strokes: 2–3 yrs.
   4. Using a Tripod Grasp: 3–5 yrs.
   ii. Cutting With Scissors.
      1. Scissor Manipulation: 2–3 yrs.
      2. Cutting: 2–7 yrs.
d. Motor Fluency
   i. Motor Fluency.
      1. Combining Accuracy With Speed: Age Variable.

IV. LEVEL FOUR

a. Fine Motor
   i. Drawing.
      1. Drawing Shapes/Simple Symbols: 3–7 yrs.
      2. Drawing Complex Forms: 4–7 yrs.
      3. Drawing With Tools: 6+ yrs.

V. LEVEL FIVE

a. Gross Motor
   i. Swinging a Bat/Racquet/Paddle.
      1. Hitting a Ball With a Bat: Age Variable.
      2. Hitting a Ball With a Racquet or Paddle: Age Variable.

VI. LEVEL SIX

a. Gross Motor
   i. Physical Education Readiness.
      1. Stretching the Major Muscle Groups: Age Variable.
      2. Warm-up Exercises: Age Variable.
      3. Obstacle Course: 6–7 yrs.

H

CARD ACADEMIC CURRICULUM

I. LEVEL THREE

a. Math
  i. Quantitative Concepts.
   1. Requests: 1–7 yrs.
   2. Receptive: 2–7 yrs.
   3. Naming: Age Variable.
   4. Representing: 2–7 yrs.

II. LEVEL FOUR

a. Language Arts
  i. Colors.
   1. Matching/Sorting: 2–3 yrs.
   2. Receptive: 3–5 yrs.
   3. Naming: 3–6 yrs.
   4. Requests: Age Variable.
   5. Colors of Objects: Age Variable.
   6. Mixing Colors: Age Variable.
  ii. Letters.
   1. Reciting the Alphabet: Age Variable–5 yrs.
   2. Matching: 3–4+ yrs.
   3. Receptive: 3–5 yrs.
   4. Naming: 4–6 yrs.
   5. Same/Different: 5–7 yrs.
   6. Sequencing – Before/After: Age Variable–7 yrs.
   7. Uppercase vs. Lowercase Letters: 5–6 yrs.
   8. Writing the Alphabet: 5–6 yrs.
  iii. Community Helpers.
   1. Matching: Age Variable.
   2. Receptive: Age Variable.

3. Naming: Age Variable.
4. Functions of Community Helpers: 5–7 yrs.
5. Locations of Community Helpers: Age Variable.
6. Features of Community Helpers: Age Variable.
7. Making Inferences: Age Variable.

b. Math
  i. Counting and Quantities.
    1. Rote Counting: 2–7 yrs.
    2. One-to-One Correspondence: Age Variable.
    3. Rational Counting and Cardinal Numbers: 3–6 yrs.
    4. Requests: Age Variable.
    5. Representing Groups: 4–6 yrs.
    6. Matching Numerals to Groups: 4–6 yrs.
  ii. Shapes.
    1. Matching/Sorting: 2–3 yrs.
    2. Receptive: 3–8 yrs.
    3. Naming: 4–7 yrs.
    4. Requests: Age Variable.
    5. Same/Different: 5–6 yrs.
    6. Shapes of Objects: 5–6 yrs.
    7. Creating Shapes and Objects out of Shapes: Age Variable.
    8. Describing Shapes: 5–8 yrs.
    9. Comparing Shapes: 5–7 yrs.
    10. Classifying Shapes: 7–8 yrs.
  iii. Numbers.
    1. Matching: 3–4 yrs.
    2. Receptive: 4–7 yrs.
    3. Naming: 4–8 yrs.

III. LEVEL FIVE

a. Language Arts
  i. Handwriting and Penmanship.
    1. Writing Uppercase Letters: 4–6 yrs.
    2. Writing Lowercase Letters: Age Variable–6 yrs.
    3. Writing Numbers: Age Variable–8 yrs.
    4. Copying Words and Sentences: 4–5+ yrs.
    5. Erasing: 6–7 yrs.
  ii. Listening Comprehension – Retelling Stories.
    1. Filling in a Story: 3–4 yrs.
    2. Retelling the Entire Story: 4–7 yrs.
  iii. Phonics – Single Letter-Sound Correspondence.
    1. Receptive: Age Variable.
    2. Naming: 5–6 yrs.

b. Math
  i. Patterning.
   1. Copying Patterns: 4–5 yrs.
   2. Identifying and Describing Patterns: 5–6 yrs.
   3. Extending Patterns: 5–6 yrs.
   4. Creating Patterns: 5–6 yrs.
   5. Transferring Patterns: 5–6 yrs.
   6. Problem Solving – "What's Missing?/What's Wrong?" 5–7 yrs.
  ii. Quantitative Comparisons.
   1. Comparing Groups – Receptive: 4–6 yrs.
   2. Comparing Groups – Naming: 4–6 yrs.
   3. Comparing Groups – Estimation: 5–6 yrs.
   4. Comparing Numerals: 6–8 yrs.

IV. LEVEL SIX

a. Language Arts
  i. Phonemic Awareness – Minimal Pairs.
   1. Same/Different: 4–6 yrs.
   2. Detecting Word Changes: Age Variable.
   3. Receptive: Age Variable.
   4. Yes/No: Age Variable.
   5. Imitation: Age Variable.
  ii. Phonological Awareness – Words and Syllables.
   1. Word Segmentation: 5–6 yrs.
   2. Onset and Rime Blending: 5–6 yrs.
   3. Syllable Blending: 5–6 yrs.
   4. Syllable Segmentation: 5–6 yrs.
   5. Syllable Deletion: 6–7 yrs.
   6. Syllable Addition: Age Variable.
  iii. Phonological Awareness – Rhyming.
   1. Rhyme Recognition: 5–6 yrs.
   2. Rhyme Production: 5–6 yrs.
  iv. Sight-Words.
   1. Matching: 5–6 yrs.
   2. Receptive: 5–8 yrs.
   3. Naming: 5–8 yrs.
  v. Decoding.
   1. Blending Single Sounds Into Words: 5–6 yrs.
   2. Word Families: 5–7 yrs.
   3. Consonant Blends and Digraphs: 6–7 yrs.
  vi. Phonemic Awareness – Phoneme Isolation.
   1. Phoneme Isolation – Initial Sounds: 5–7 yrs.

2. Phoneme Isolation – Final Sounds: 5–7 yrs.
3. Phoneme Isolation – Position and Order of Sounds: 5–6 yrs.
4. Phoneme Isolation – Medial Sounds: 6–7 yrs.

vii. Phonemic Awareness – Phoneme Blending and Segmentation.
1. Phoneme Blending: 5–7 yrs.
2. Phoneme Segmentation: 5–6 yrs.

V. LEVEL SEVEN

a. Language Arts
  i. Phonemic Awareness – Phoneme Matching.
    1. Phoneme Matching – Initial Sounds: 5–6 yrs.
    2. Phoneme Matching – Final Sounds: 5–6 yrs.
  ii. Phonemic Awareness – Phoneme Manipulation.
    1. Phoneme Deletion: 5–6 yrs.
    2. Phoneme Addition: 5–6 yrs.
    3. Phoneme Substitution: 5–6 yrs.
  iii. Print Concepts.
    1. Reading and Organization of Printed Materials: 4–6 yrs.
    2. Parts of a Book: 5–7 yrs.
b. Math
  i. Calendar.
    1. Reciting – Days and Months: 5–6 yrs.
    2. Textual Days of the Week – Receptive and Naming: Age Variable.
    3. Textual Months of the Year – Receptive and Naming: Age Variable.
    4. Using a Calendar: 5–6+ yrs.
    5. Seasons: 6–7 yrs.
    6. Calendar Units – Identifying and Naming Without a Calendar: Age Variable–8 yrs.
  ii. Ordinal Numbers.
    1. Receptive – Positions: 5–6 yrs.
    2. Naming – Positions: 5–6 yrs.
    3. Reading Ordinal Numbers: 6–7 yrs.
    4. Problem Solving and Reasoning: Age Variable.
  iii. Addition.
    1. Joining Groups: 4–6 yrs.
    2. Addition Problems Using Concrete Objects: 5–6 yrs.
    3. Addition Problems Using Pictures: 5–6 yrs.
    4. Decomposition of Numbers: 5–6 yrs.
  iv. Time of Day and Daily Activities.
    1. Time of Day: 3–5 yrs.
    2. Time to the Hour: 5–6 yrs.
    3. Relating Time to Daily Activities – Before/After: 6–7 yrs.

VI. LEVEL EIGHT

a. Language Arts
  i. Listening Comprehension – Answering and Asking Questions.
    1. Answering Questions – Story Elements: 4–6 yrs.
    2. Answering Questions – Connecting Life Experiences: 5+ yrs.
    3. Group Reading: 5+ yrs.
    4. Answering Questions – Identifying Reasons That Support Key Points in Texts: 5+ yrs.
    5. Answering Questions – Fantasy Versus Realistic Text: 5+ yrs.
    6. Asking Questions: 5+ yrs.
  ii. Phonics – Initial Consonants.
    1. Matching: 6–7 yrs.
    2. Receptive: 6–7 yrs.
    3. Naming: 6–7 yrs.
  iii. Phonics – Final Consonants.
    1. Matching: 6–7 yrs.
    2. Receptive: 6–7 yrs.
    3. Naming: 6–7 yrs.
b. Math
  i. Sequencing Numerals and Ordering Groups.
    1. Sequencing Numerals: 5–8 yrs.
    2. Ordering Groups: 5–6 yrs.
    3. Before/After: 5–7 yrs.
    4. Writing Numerals in Sequence: 5–7 yrs.
  ii. Charts and Graphs.
    1. Concrete Graphs: 6–7 yrs.
    2. Picture Graphs: 6–7 yrs.
    3. Tally Tables: 6–7 yrs.
    4. Bar Graphs: 6–7 yrs.
  iii. Skip Counting.
    1. Counting by 10s, 5s, and 2s: 5–6 yrs.
    2. Problem Solving – Number Patterns: 6–8 yrs.

VII. LEVEL NINE

a. Language Arts
  i. Phonics – Short Vowels.
    1. Matching: 6–7 yrs.
    2. Receptive: 6–7 yrs.
    3. Naming: 6–7 yrs.
  ii. Grammar and Writing Mechanics.
    1. Capitalization: 5–6 yrs.
    2. Punctuation: 5–6 yrs.

      iii. Spelling.
          1. Personal Data: 5–6 yrs.
          2. Consonant-Vowel-Consonant Words: 5–6 yrs.
      iv. Phonics – Consonant Blends and Digraphs.
          1. Letter-Sound Correspondence: Receptive: Age Variable.
          2. Letter-Sound Correspondence: Naming: 6–7 yrs.
          3. Matching to Pictures – Initial Consonant Blends and Digraphs: 6–7 yrs.
          4. Receptive – Initial Consonant Blends and Digraphs: 6–7 yrs.
          5. Matching to Pictures – Final Consonant Blends and Digraphs: Age Variable.
          6. Receptive – Final Consonant Blends and Digraphs: Age Variable.
b. Math
      i. Money.
          1. Matching/Sorting Coins: 5–6 yrs.
          2. Receptive Coins/Dollar Bill: 5–7 yrs.
          3. Naming Coins/Dollar Bill: 5–7 yrs.
          4. Monetary Value – Single Coin/Dollar Bill: 5–7 yrs.
          5. Monetary Symbols and Decimal Notation, Counting and Totaling Value of Coins of Single Denomination: 5–8 yrs.
          6. Monetary Value – Equivalent Forms: 5–7 yrs.
          7. Counting and Totaling Value of Coins of Mixed Denominations: 6–8 yrs.
      ii. Telling Time.
          1. Features on a Clock Face: 5+ yrs.
          2. Telling and Writing Time: 6–7 yrs.
          3. Time and Schedules: 6–7 yrs.
          4. Comparing Duration of Activities: 6–7 yrs.
          5. Equivalent Units of Time: 7–8 yrs.
          6. a.m./p.m.: 7–8 yrs.
          7. Elapsed Time: 7–8 yrs.
      iii. Subtraction
          1. Taking Apart Groups: 5–6 yrs.
          2. Subtraction Problems Using Concrete Objects: 5–6 yrs.
          3. Subtraction Problems Using Pictures: 5–6 yrs.

VIII. LEVEL TEN

a. Language Arts
      i. Listening Comprehension – Story Prediction.
          1. Making Predictions Using Books With Repetitive Story Patterns: 5–6 yrs.

2. Making Predictions Using Picture Clues and Listening to Text: 5–6 yrs.
3. Making Predictions Using Picture Clues and Confirming Predictions by Listening to Text: 5–6 yrs.

ii. Reading Comprehension.
 1. Single Words – Matching: 5–6 yrs.
 2. Connected Text – Accuracy: 5–7 yrs.
 3. Connected Text – Matching: 5–7 yrs.
 4. Following Instructions: 6–7 yrs.
 5. Connected Text – Answering Questions: 6–7 yrs.

iii. Independent Writing.
 1. Sentence Frames: 5–6 yrs.
 2. Guided Writing: 5–6 yrs.

CARD SOCIAL CURRICULUM

I. LEVEL ONE

a. Non-vocal Social Behavior
  i. Eye Contact.
    1. Gaining Eye Contact Through Social Games: 0–12 mos.
    2. Responding to Requests for Eye Contact: 0–12+ mos.
  ii. Non-vocal Imitation.
    1. Imitation of Actions With Objects: 0–2 yrs.
    2. Gross Motor Imitation: 1–4 yrs.
    3. Fine Motor Imitation: 2–3 yrs.
    4. Multiple-Step Imitation: Age Variable.
b. Social Rules
  i. Compliance.
    1. In Child's Home: 0–5 yrs.
    2. In the Community: 0–5 yrs.
c. Social Interaction
  i. Joint Attention.
    1. Responding to Joint Attention Bids: 0–3 yrs.
    2. Initiating Joint Attention Bids: 0–3 yrs.
    3. Interactive Joint Attention: 1–3 yrs.

II. LEVEL TWO

a. Social Interaction
  i. Gaining Attention.
    1. Gaining Attention – Basic Behavior: 0–3 yrs.
    2. Basic Persistence and Alternative Strategy: Age Variable.
    3. Contextual Recognition: Age Variable.
    4. Gaining Attention – Considering Context: Age Variable.
  ii. Assertiveness
    1. Being Assertive – Basic Skills: 1–3 yrs.
    2. Following Rules for Being Assertive – Getting What I Want: 3+ yrs.

    3. Following Rules for Being Assertive – Disagreement: 4+ yrs.
    4. Following Rules for Being Assertive – Refusal Skills: 5+ yrs.
  iii. Social Referencing
    1. Engaging With Novel Objects: 0–1 yr.
    2. Changing Behavior in Response to Emotional Expression: 0–1 yr.

III. LEVEL THREE

a. Social Interaction
  i. Sharing and Turn-Taking.
    1. Turn-Taking: 3–5 yrs.
    2. Responding to Direct Requests to Share: 3–5 yrs.
    3. Making Requests of Others to Share: 3–5 yrs.
    4. Making Offers of Sharing and Turn-Taking: 4–5+ yrs.
b. Social Language
  i. Personal Information.
    1. Answering Personal Information Questions: 1–7 yrs.
  ii. Greetings and Salutations.
    1. Responding to Greetings and Salutations – Basic Behavior: 1–2 yrs.
    2. Initiating Greetings and Salutations – Basic Behavior: 2–3 yrs.
  iii. Prosody.
    1. Volume, Pitch, and Speed: 1–8 yrs.
    2. Statement Versus Question Intonation: 2–8 yrs.
    3. Emotional Prosody: Age Variable.
    4. Intonation and Inflection to Change Meaning: Age Variable–7+ yrs.
c. Social Context
  i. Basic Social Cues.
    1. Recognizing and Responding to Environmental Cues: Age Variable.
    2. Recognizing and Responding to Overt Behavioral Cues: 3–6 yrs.
d. Self-Esteem
  i. Positive Self-Statements.
    1. Making Positive Statements: 3+ yrs.
    2. Identifying Strengths and Weaknesses: Age Variable.
    3. Social Impression Management: 5–6 yrs.

IV. LEVEL FOUR

a. Social Rules
  i. Following Rules.
    1. Rules Specifying the Behavior and Preferred Consequence: 3+ yrs.

    2. Rules Specifying the Behavior and Non-preferred Consequence: 3+ yrs.

    3. Rules Specifying the Antecedent and Behavior: 3+ yrs.

    4. Rules Specifying the Antecedent, Behavior, and Consequence: 3+ yrs.

    5. Following Established Rules: 5+ yrs.

  ii. Say-Do Correspondence.

    1. Connection Between "Saying" and "Doing": 3–8 yrs.

    2. Correspondence Training: 3+ yrs.

  iii. Politeness and Manners.

    1. Following Rules of Politeness and Manners: 3–8 yrs.

    2. Identifying Polite and Impolite Behavior: 4–7 yrs.

b. Social Language

  i. General Knowledge.

    1. General Knowledge: Age Variable.

    2. Popular Culture: Age Variable.

c. Group-Related Behavior

  i. Responding in Unison.

    1. Responding to Questions and Instructions in Unison: Age Variable.

    2. Songs in Unison: Age Variable.

d. Absurdities

  i. What's Wrong?

    1. What's Wrong With This? Age Variable.

V. LEVEL FIVE

a. Social Interaction

  i. Compliments.

    1. Responding to Compliments – Following a Direction: 3 yrs.

    2. Recognizing and Responding to Compliments: 3–5+ yrs.

    3. Giving Compliments: 3+ yrs.

  ii. Introductions.

    1. Responding to Introductions: 3–4 yrs.

    2. Introducing Self to Others: Age Variable–3+ yrs.

    3. Introducing Others: 5+ yrs.

b. Social Language

  i. Initiating Conversation.

    1. Gaining the Listener's Attention: 4–7 yrs.

    2. Introducing a Topic: 5+ yrs.

  ii. Ending Conversation.

    1. Responding to Others' Attempts to End Conversation: Age Variable.

    2. Ending Conversation: 5–7 yrs.

c. Social Context
    i. Learning Through Observation.
        1. What's Missing?: Age Variable.
        2. Observing Actions: 3–6 yrs.
        3. Observing Speech: 3–4 yrs.

VI. LEVEL SIX

a. Non-vocal Social Behavior
    i. Body Language and Facial Expressions.
        1. Basic Body Language and Facial Expressions: 5+ yrs.
        2. Body Language and Facial Expressions – Adding Context: 5+ yrs.
        3. Recognizing Behavior in Self and What It Means to Others: 5+ yrs.
        4. Rules for Body Language and Facial Expressions: Age Variable.
b. Social Language
    i. Repairing Conversation.
        1. Responding to Requests for Clarification: 4–7 yrs.
        2. Asking for Clarification: 4–7 yrs.
        3. Clarifying Spontaneously: 7+ yrs.
        4. Preventing Conversation Breakdown During a Disruption: 7+ yrs.

VII. LEVEL SEVEN

a. Social Rules
    i. Community Rules.
        1. Following Vocal Community Rules: 5+ yrs.
        2. Identifying Community Signs: 6–7 yrs.
        3. Following Community Signs: 7+ yrs.
b. Social Language
    i. Listening to Conversation.
        1. Active Listening: 5+ yrs.
        2. Topic Identification: Age Variable.
c. Social Interaction
    i. Personality Attributes.
        1. Identifying Personal Characteristics: 4 yrs.
d. Social Context
    i. Complex Social Cues.
        1. Recognizing and Responding to Body Language, Facial Expression, and Tone of Voice: 5+ yrs.
        2. Recognizing Whether Behaviors Match and Identifying the Intended Message: 5+ yrs.
        3. Following Rules for Responding to Complex Social Cues: Age Variable.

VIII. LEVEL EIGHT

a. Non-vocal Social Behavior
  i. Gestures to Regulate Social Interaction.
    1. Responding to Gestures in a Social Setting: 5+ yrs.
    2. Using Gestures in a Social Setting: 5+ yrs.
b. Social Interaction
  i. Apologizing.
    1. Following Instructions to Give and Accept Apologies: Age Variable.
    2. Giving Apologies: 5+ yrs.
    3. Accepting Apologies: Age Variable.
  ii. Compromise, Collaboration, and Negotiation.
    1. Making Concessions: Age Variable.
    2. Compromising and Negotiating: 4–7 yrs.
    3. Offering Help: 5+ yrs.
c. Self-Esteem
  i. Dealing With Conflict.
    1. Identifying Basic Conflict: 3–5 yrs.
    2. Responding to Conflict – Rule Following: 3–5+ yrs.
    3. Identifying Complex Conflict – Perspective Taking: Age Variable.
d. Absurdities
  i. Figures of Speech.
    1. Identifying Meaning and Responding to Figures of Speech: 6+ yrs.
    2. Using Figures of Speech: 6+ yrs.

IX. LEVEL NINE

a. Social Language
  i. Physical Context of Conversation.
    1. Identifying the Physical Context: Age Variable.
    2. Identifying Volume and Gestures: Age Variable.
    3. Demonstrating Appropriate Speaking for Physical Context: 5+ yrs.
    4. Selecting Appropriate Conversation Opportunities in Physical Context: Age Variable.
    5. Demonstrating Appropriate Spatial Proximity for Physical Context: 6–9 yrs.
  ii. Conversational Audience.
    1. Audience Identification: 5–7 yrs.
    2. Speaking Appropriately to the Audience: 5–7+ yrs.
  iii. Transitioning Topics of Conversation.
    1. Identifying Transition in Conversation Topics: Age Variable.

2. Responding to Others' Attempts to Transition Topics: Age Variable.
3. Transitioning Topics: 5–7+ yrs.
   iv. Maintaining Conversation.
1. Using Boundary Markers: 5+ yrs.
2. Turn-Taking: 5+ yrs.
3. Topic Maintenance: 5–7+ yrs.
b. Group-Related Behavior
   i. Group Discussions.
1. Child as Participant: 5–8 yrs.
2. Child as Discussion Leader: 6–8 yrs.

X. LEVEL TEN

a. Social Interaction
   i. Levels of Friendship and Relationships.
1. Developing and Maintaining Friendships: 5+ yrs.
2. Identifying Levels of Friendship and Relationships: 5–7 yrs.
3. Relationship-Appropriate Behavior: 5–6 yrs.
b. Self-Esteem
   i. Winning and Losing.
1. Demonstrating Good Sportsmanship: 5–7 yrs.
c. Absurdities
   i. Humor and Jokes.
1. Identifying and Explaining Humor and Why We Engage in Humorous Behavior: Age Variable.
2. Facial Expression and Non-vocal Cues That Indicate Humor: Age Variable.
3. Learning to Respond to Humor – Recognizing Humor: Age Variable.
4. Learning to Respond to Humor – Determining Intent: Age Variable.
5. Following Rules for Responding to Humor: Age Variable.
6. Engaging in Humorous Behavior: Age Variable.
7. Following Rules for Engaging in Humorous Behavior: Age Variable.

XI. LEVEL ELEVEN

a. Social Interaction
   i. Regulating Others.
1. Reminding: 5+ yrs.
2. Delineating Personal Claims: 5+ yrs.

      3. Delaying or Hurrying Actions of Self or Others: 5+ yrs.

      4. Persuading: 5+ yrs.

   ii. Borrowing and Lending.

      1. Identifying Personal Property From Another's Property: 5+ yrs.

      2. Lending: 5+ yrs.

      3. Asking to Borrow/Use: 7+ yrs.

      4. Returning Borrowed Items: 7+ yrs.

b. Social Language

   i. Joining Conversation.

      1. Responding to Others' Attempts to Join a Conversation: Age Variable.

      2. Joining Conversation: 5+ yrs.

   ii. Conversation: Putting It All Together

      1. Engaging in Conversation: 5+ yrs.

XII. LEVEL TWELVE

a. Self-Esteem

   i. Constructive Criticism.

      1. Responding to Constructive Criticism: Age Variable.

      2. Identifying Constructive Versus Destructive Criticism: Age Variable.

      3. Responding to Destructive Criticism: Age Variable–5+ yrs.

      4. Giving Constructive Criticism: Age Variable.

J

CARD COGNITION CURRICULUM

I. LEVEL TWO

a. Desires
  - **i.** Expressing Own Desires: 1–3 yrs.
  - **ii.** Responding to Others' Requests for Desired Items: 1–2 yrs.
  - **iii.** Inferring Others' Desires: 1–2+ yrs.
  - **iv.** Finding Out Others' Desires: Age Variable.
  - **v.** Wishes and Hopes: Age Variable.
  - **vi.** Changing One's Mind: Age Variable.
  - **vii.** Disguised Mands: 4–7 yrs.

II. LEVEL FOUR

a. Emotions
  - **i.** Matching: Age Variable.
  - **ii.** Receptive: Age Variable.
  - **iii.** Naming Emotions: 3–7 yrs.
  - **iv.** Desire-Based Emotions: 3–5 yrs.
  - **v.** Emotional Prediction and Effect: 3+ yrs.
  - **vi.** Causal Identification of Emotions: 3+ yrs.
  - **vii.** Identifying Emotions Based on Desires and Preferences: 3–8 yrs.
  - **viii.** Predicting Emotions Based on Desires and Preferences: 3–8 yrs.
  - **ix.** Predicting Emotions Based on Beliefs: 4–6 yrs.
  - **x.** Considering Emotions in Social Behavior Management: Age Variable.

III. LEVEL SIX

a. Senses
  - **i.** Sight: Age Variable.
  - **ii.** Touch: 2–5 yrs.

    iii. Taste: Age Variable.
    iv. Hear: Age Variable.
    v. Smell: Age Variable.
    vi. Seeing Versus Hearing: Age Variable.
    vii. Sensory-Based Mands: Age Variable.
b. Physical States
    i. Matching: Age Variable.
    ii. Receptive Identification of Physical States in Others: Age Variable.
    iii. Naming Physical States of Others: 3–4 yrs.
    iv. Receptive Identification of Physical States of Self: Age Variable.
    v. Naming Physical States of Self: Age Variable.
    vi. Physical State Prediction and Effect in Self: 3–5 yrs.
    vii. Causal Identification of Physical States of Self: 3–5 yrs.
    viii. Requesting With Expression of Physical States: Age Variable.
    ix. Physical State Prediction and Effect in Others: 3–5 yrs.
    x. Causal Identification of Physical States of Others: 3–5 yrs.

IV. LEVEL SEVEN

a. Thinking
    i. Thinking as Suggestion for Action: 3–5 yrs.
    ii. Thinking When Uncertain: 3–5 yrs.
    iii. Thinking About…: 3–5+ yrs.
    iv. Inferring Others' Thoughts Based on Non-vocal Cues: Age Variable.
    v. Thinking as Opinion/Judgment: 4–7 yrs.
    vi. Inferring Others' Thoughts Based on Preferences: Age Variable.
    vii. Relationship Between Thinking, Feeling, Saying, and Doing: Age Variable.
    viii. Thinking About Consequences Before Doing: Age Variable.

V. LEVEL EIGHT

a. Sensory Perspective Taking
    i. Visual Perspective Taking: 3–4+ yrs.
    ii. Tactile Perspective Taking: Age Variable.
    iii. Gustatory Perspective Taking: Age Variable.
    iv. Olfactory Perspective Taking: Age Variable.
    v. Auditory Perspective Taking: Age Variable.
    vi. Visual Versus Auditory Perspective Taking: Age Variable.

b. Cause and Effect
    i. Identifying and Predicting Effect: 3–4+ yrs.
    ii. Identifying Cause: 3–4 yrs.
    iii. Predicting Comparatively: Age Variable.
    iv. Identifying and Predicting Cause and Effect – Increasing Spontaneity: Age Variable.
    v. Multiple Possible Effects/Causes: Age Variable.
    vi. Inferences: Age Variable.

VI. LEVEL NINE

a. Preferences
    i. Identifying Own Preferences: 3–4+ yrs.
    ii. Identifying Others' Preferences: Age Variable.
    iii. Inferring Preferences: 3–4+ yrs.
    iv. Application of Preferences to Social Behavior: Age Variable.
    v. Inferring and Predicting Behavior Based on Preferences: Age Variable.
b. Knowing
    i. Identifying What People Do and Do Not Know: 4+ yrs.
    ii. General Knowledge and Universally Unknown Information: Age Variable.
    iii. Knowing About – Observation, Listening, and Reading: Age Variable.
    iv. Knowing How – Experience, Observation, and Instruction: Age Variable.
    v. Applications of Knowing: 5–6 yrs.
    vi. Second-Order Knowing: Age Variable.

VII. LEVEL TEN

a. Beliefs
    i. Identifying Beliefs and False Beliefs: 4–5 yrs.
    ii. Predicting Beliefs and False Beliefs: 4–5 yrs.
    iii. Predicting Belief-Based Actions/Identifying Beliefs Leading to Action: 4–5 yrs.
    iv. Second-Order Beliefs: 6+ yrs.
    v. Third-Order Beliefs: Age Variable.
b. Deception
    i. Playing Tricks for Amusement: 4+ yrs.
    ii. Identifying Deception in Others: 4+ yrs.
    iii. Advanced Deception (Lies, Secrets, Bluffs, White Lies, and Advanced Tricks): Age Variable–5+ yrs.

VIII. LEVEL ELEVEN

a. Detecting Sarcasm

    i. Understanding and Responding to Sarcasm: Age Variable.

IX. LEVEL TWELVE

a. Intentions

    i. Inferring Intentions of Previous Actions: 3–4+ yrs.

    ii. Inferring Intentions of Current, Incomplete Actions: 3–4 yrs.

    iii. Responding to Intentional/Unintentional Actions: 5–6 yrs.

K

CARD EXECUTIVE FUNCTIONS CURRICULUM

I. LEVEL ONE

a. Attention
   i. Stimulus Orienting.
      1. Non-social Orienting: 0–12 mos.
      2. Social Orienting: 0–12 mos.
b. Inhibition
   i. Waiting.
      1. Basic Waiting: 1–3 yrs.
      2. Waiting Rules: 3–6 yrs.
      3. Delay of Gratification: 4+ yrs.
c. Planning
   i. Activity Schedules and To-Do Lists.
      1. Learning First Schedule With Mastered Activities: 2+ yrs.
      2. Learning New Schedules: 2+ yrs.
      3. Learning an Unknown Activity: Age Variable.
      4. Choosing Own Reinforcers: 2+ yrs.
      5. Sequencing Own Schedule: Age Variable.
      6. Using a To-Do List: Age Variable.
d. Problem Solving
   i. Simple Problem Solving.
      1. Using Mands to Solve Simple Problems: 1–3 yrs.

II. LEVEL TWO

a. Attention
   i. Disengagement.
      1. Visual Disengagement: 0–12 mos.
      2. Auditory Disengagement: Age Variable.
      3. Vocal/Thought Disengagement: Age Variable.
      4. Combinations of Visual, Auditory, and/or Vocal/Thought Disengagement: Age Variable.

b. Inhibition
  i. Non-vocal Inhibition.
    1. Inhibition of Prepotent Non-vocal Behavior: 1–4+ yrs.
    2. Inhibition of Socially Inappropriate Behavior: 3+ yrs.
    3. Inhibition During Games: 4–7 yrs.
    4. Inhibition During Paper and Pencil Tasks: 5–8 yrs.
c. Planning
  i. Organizing Materials.
    1. Toys: 1–6 yrs.
    2. Storage Areas at School: Age Variable.
    3. Locations of Household Items and Personal Belongings: Age Variable.
    4. Bookshelf: Age Variable.
    5. Clothing: 5–10 yrs.
    6. Bathroom: Age Variable.
    7. Carrying Items: Age Variable.
    8. Backpack/Bag: Age Variable.
    9. Suitcase: Age Variable.
    10. Organizing Papers: 5–8 yrs.
    11. Desk: 5+ yrs.
    12. Creating Organizational Schemes: Age Variable.

III. LEVEL THREE

a. Attention
  i. Shifting Attention.
    1. Shifting Between Non-social/Social Stimuli: Age Variable.
    2. Shifting Between Tasks and Task Components: Age Variable.
    3. Shifting Attention in the Social Setting: Age Variable.
  ii. Sustained Attention.
    1. Sustaining Attention to Stimuli: Age Variable..
    2. Task Persistence: 4–7 yrs.
b. Flexibility
  i. Non-social Flexibility.
    1. Recognizing and Reporting on Rule Changes: 3+ yrs.
    2. Inhibition of Previous Response and Demonstration of New Response: 4+ yrs.
    3. Spontaneous Generation of New Responses: Age Variable.
  ii. Social Flexibility.
    1. Recognizing and Reporting on Social Changes: Age Variable.
    2. Going Along With Social Changes: Age Variable.
    3. Generating Alternative Social Strategies: Age Variable.

c. Memory
   i. Auditory Memory.
      1. Identity Matching: Age Variable.
      2. Echoics: 2–8 yrs.
      3. Arbitrary Matching: Age Variable.
      4. Receptive: 3–8 yrs.
      5. Impure Tacts: Age Variable.
   ii. Visual Memory.
      1. Identity Matching: Age Variable.
      2. Arbitrary Matching: Age Variable.
      3. Non-vocal Imitation: 3–7 yrs.
      4. Impure Tacts: Age Variable – 5+ yrs.
      5. Environmental Visual Memory: Age Variable.

IV. LEVEL FOUR

a. Inhibition
   i. Vocal Inhibition.
      1. Inhibition of Prepotent Vocal Behavior: 3+ yrs.
      2. Inhibition of Socially Inappropriate Behavior: 3+ yrs.
b. Memory
   i. Spatial Memory.
      1. Receptive: 1–2 yrs.
      2. Identity Matching: Age Variable.
      3. Non-vocal Imitation: 2–8 yrs.
      4. Impure Tacts: Age Variable.
      5. Environmental Spatial Memory: Age Variable.

V. LEVEL FIVE

a. Flexibility
   i. Language Flexibility.
      1. Manding in More Than One Way: 1–3 yrs.
      2. Questions: 2–3 yrs.
      3. Synonyms: 4+ yrs.
b. Metacognition
   i. Self-Management.
      1. Identifying the Target Behavior: Age Variable.
      2. Self-Monitoring: Age Variable.
      3. Self-Evaluation: Age Variable.
      4. Self-Reinforcement: Age Variable.
      5. Creating Self-Management Contingencies: Age Variable.

c. Planning
    i. Adaptive Planning.
        1. Simple Academic Planning: 3–5+ yrs.
        2. Goal Setting: 5–7+ yrs.
        3. Action Plan: 5–14 yrs.
        4. Task Initiation: Age Variable.
        5. Monitoring/Evaluating Progress: Age Variable.
        6. Putting It All Together: Age Variable.
    ii. Academic Planning.
        1. Simple Academic Planning: Age Variable.
        2. Goal Setting: 5–7+ yrs.
        3. Action Plan: 5–14 yrs.
        4. Task Initiation: Age Variable.
        5. Checking Work: 5+ yrs.
        6. Monitoring/Evaluating Progress: Age Variable.
        7. Putting It All Together: Age Variable.

VI. LEVEL SIX

a. Attention
    i. Divided Attention.
        1. Simultaneous Stimuli from Different Sensory Modalities: Age Variable.
        2. Simultaneous Stimuli from a Single Sensory Modality: Age Variable.
        3. Simultaneous Stimuli Related to Functional Skills: Age Variable.
b. Flexibility
    i. Shades of Gray.
        1. Establishment of a Concept-Based Continuum: 3+ yrs.
        2. Establishment of a Rule-Based Continuum: 4+ yrs.
c. Memory
    i. Working Memory.
        1. Backward Span – Mixed Operants: 3–7 yrs.
        2. Impure Tacts: Age Variable.
        3. Intraverbals: Age Variable.
        4. Environmental Working Memory: Age Variable.
    ii. Episodic Memory.
        1. Current Events: Age Variable.
        2. Immediate Recall: 3–5 yrs.
        3. Recalling Past Events – Same Day: Age Variable–5 yrs.
        4. Recalling Past Events – Yesterday and Beyond: Age Variable–7 yrs.
d. Metacognition
    i. Emotional Self-Control.

1. Simple Emotional Self-Control: 3+ yrs.
2. Advanced Emotional Self-Control: 6–8 yrs.

VII. LEVEL SEVEN

a. Attention
  i. Determining Saliency.
    1. Visual Saliency: Age Variable.
    2. Auditory Saliency: Age Variable.
    3. Social Saliency: Age Variable.
    4. Textual Saliency: Age Variable.

VIII. LEVEL NINE

a. Problem Solving
  i. Non-social Problem Solving.
    1. Identifying the Problem: 3–5 yrs.
    2. Responding to Presented Solutions: Age Variable.
    3. Selecting and Evaluating Effectiveness of a Solution: Age Variable.
    4. Persisting When Solutions Fail: Age Variable.
    5. Solving Problems Independently: 6+ yrs.
    6. Preventing Future Problems: 6+ yrs.
    7. Paper/Pencil Problem Solving: Age Variable.

IX. LEVEL TEN

a. Metacognition
  i. Self-Awareness.
    1. Identifying Presence and Degree of Behavior in Self: Age Variable.
    2. Identifying Strengths and Weaknesses: Age Variable.
    3. Identifying Liked and Disliked Activities: Age Variable.
    4. Identifying Liked and Disliked Qualities of Self: Age Variable.
    5. Describing Self: Age Variable.
b. Problem Solving
  i. Social Problem Solving.
    1. Identifying Basic Social Problems: 3–5 yrs.
    2. Responding to Social Problems – Rule Following: 3–5 yrs.
    3. Identifying Complex Social Problems – Perspective Taking: Age Variable.

4. Responding to Presented Solutions: Age Variable.
5. Selecting and Evaluating Effectiveness of a Solution: Age Variable.
6. Persisting When Solutions Fail: Age Variable.
7. Solving Problems Independently: 6+ yrs.

X. LEVEL ELEVEN

a. Metacognition
  i. Metamemory.
    1. Using Strategies to Remember Things: Age Variable.
b. Planning
  i. Social Planning.
    1. Simple Social Planning: 3–5 yrs.
    2. Goal Setting: 5–7+ yrs.
    3. Action Plan: 5–14 yrs.
    4. Task Initiation: Age Variable.
    5. Monitoring/Evaluating Progress: Age Variable.
    6. Putting It All Together: Age Variable.

XI. LEVEL TWELVE

a. Attention
  i. Summarizing.
    1. Summarizing Spoken Information: Age Variable.
    2. Summarizing Stories: 6–7 yrs.
    3. Summarizing Written Information: Age Variable.
  ii. Paraphrasing.
    1. Paraphrasing Spoken Information: 7–8 yrs.
    2. Paraphrasing Written Information: Age Variable.
b. Planning
  i. Using a Weekly Homework Sheet.
    1. Using the Teacher's Homework Sheet: 6–8 yrs.
    2. Filling in a Blank Homework Sheet: 7–8 yrs.
  ii. Using a Planner.
    1. Navigating a Planner: Age Variable.
    2. Storing Information Into a Planner: Age Variable.
    3. Checking a Planner and Remaining on Schedule: Age Variable.

References

Adams, L. (1998). Oral-motor and motor-speech characteristics of children with autism. *Focus on Autism and Other Developmental Disabilities, 13,* 108–112.

Allen, K. D., & Cowan, R. J. (2008). Naturalistic teaching. In J. K. Luiselli, D. C. Russo, W. P. Christian, & S. M. Wilczynski (Eds.), *Effective practices for children with autism: Educational and behavior support interventions that work* (pp. 213–226). New York, NY: Oxford University Press, Inc.

American Psychiatric Association. (2013). *Diagnostic and statistical manual of mental disorders* (5th ed.). Washington, DC: American Psychiatric Association.

American Psychological Association. (2010). *Ethical principles of psychologists and code of conduct.* Retrieved August 28, 2013, from, www.apa.org/ethics/code/principles.pdf. Accessed 04.08.14.

Azrin, N. F., & Foxx, R. M. (1974). *Toilet training in less than a day.* New York, NY: Pocket Books.

Baer, D. M., Wolf, M. M., & Risley, T. R. (1968). Some current dimensions of applied behavior analysis. *Journal of Applied Behavior Analysis, 1,* 91–97.

Bailey, J., & Burch, M. (2013). *Ethics for behavior analysts: A practical guide to the Behavior Analyst Certification Board guidelines for responsible conduct.* New York, NY: Routledge.

Baltruschat, L., Hasselhorn, M., Tarbox, J., Dixon, D. R., Najdowski, A. C., Mullins, R. D., et al. (2011a). Addressing working memory in children with autism through behavioral intervention. *Research in Autism Spectrum Disorders, 5,* 267–276.

Baltruschat, L., Hasselhorn, M., Tarbox, J., Dixon, D. R., Najdowski, A. C., Mullins, R. D., et al. (2011b). Further analysis of the effects of positive reinforcement on working memory in children with autism. *Research in Autism Spectrum Disorders, 5,* 855–863.

Baltruschat, L., Hasselhorn, M., Tarbox, J., Dixon, D. R., Najdowski, A. C., Mullins, R. D., et al. (2012). The effects of multiple exemplar training on a working memory task involving sequential responding in children with autism. *The Psychological Record, 62,* 549–562.

Barnoy, E. L., Najdowski, A. C., Tarbox, J., Wilke, A. E., & Nollet, M. D. (2009). Replication of a multicomponent intervention for diurnal bruxism in a young child with autism. *Journal of Applied Behavior Analysis, 42,* 845–848.

Baron-Cohen, S., Leslie, A., & Frith, U. (1985). Does the autistic child have a theory of mind? *Cognition, 21,* 37–46.

Bayley, N. (1993). *Bayley scales of infant development* (2nd ed.). San Antonio, TX: Psychological Corp.

Behavior Analyst Certification Board. (2012). *BACB guidelines for responsible conduct for behavior analysts.* Retrieved August 28, 2013, from, www.bacb.com/Downloadfiles/BACBguidelines/BACB_Conduct_Guidelines.pdf. Accessed 04.08.14.

Bergstrom, R., Najdowski, A. C., & Tarbox, J. (2012). Teaching children with autism to seek help when lost in public. *Journal of Applied Behavior Analysis, 45,* 191–195.

Bergstrom, R., Najdowski, A. C., & Tarbox, J. (in press). A systematic replication of teaching children with autism to respond appropriately to lures from strangers. *Journal of Applied Behavior Analysis.*

Binder, C. (1996). Behavioral fluency: Evolution of a new paradigm. *The Behavior Analyst, 19,* 163–197.

Bowers, L., Huisingh, R., & LoGiudice, C. (2005). *Test of problem solving 3 – Elementary.* East Moline, IL: LinguiSystems.

Carr, J. E., & Briggs, A. M. (2010). Strategies for making regular contact with the scholarly literature. *Behavior Analysis in Practice, 3,* 13–18.

Charlop-Christy, M. H., Carpenter, M., Le, L., LeBlanc, L. A., & Kellet, K. (2002). Using the picture exchange communication system (PECS) with children with autism: Assessment of PECS acquisition, speech, social-communicative behavior, and problem behavior. *Journal of Applied Behavior Analysis, 35*(3), 213–231.

Cohen, H., Amerine-Dickens, M., & Smith, T. (2006). Early intensive behavioral treatment: Replication of the UCLA model in a community setting. *Developmental and Behavioral Pediatrics, 2,* 145–157.

Cooper, J. O., Heron, T. E., & Heward, W. L. (2007). *Applied behavior analysis* (2nd ed.). Upper Saddle River, N.J.: Pearson Prentice Hall.

Delprato, D. J. (2001). Comparisons of discrete-trial and normalized behavioral language intervention for young children with autism. *Journal of Autism and Developmental Disorders, 31,* 315–325.

Dewey, D., Cantell, M., & Crawford, S. G. (2007). Motor and gestural performance in children with autism spectrum disorders, developmental coordination disorder, and/or attention deficit hyperactivity disorder. *Journal of the International Neuropsychological Society, 13,* 246–256.

Dixon, D. R., Tarbox, J., Najdowski, A. C., Wilke, A. E., & Granpeesheh, D. (2011). A comprehensive evaluation of language for early behavioral intervention programs: The reliability of the SKILLS language index. *Research in Autism Spectrum Disorders, 5,* 506–511.

Dyck, M. J., Piek, J. P., Hay, D. A., & Hallmayer, J. F. (2007). The relationship between symptoms and abilities in autism. *Journal of Developmental and Physical Disabilities, 19,* 251–261.

Eikeseth, S., Smith, T., Jahr, E., & Eldevik, S. (2007). Outcome for children with autism who began intensive behavioral treatment between ages 4 and 7: A comparison controlled study. *Behavior Modification, 31,* 264–278.

Eldevik, S., Hastings, R. P., Hughes, J. C., Jahr, E., Eikeseth, S., & Cross, S. (2009). Meta-analysis of early intensive behavioral intervention for children with autism. *Journal of Clinical Child and Adolescent Psychology, 38,* 439–450.

Fein, D., Barton, M., Eigsti, I. M., Kelley, E., Naigles, L., Schultz, R. T., et al. (2013). Optimal outcome in individuals with a history of autism. *Journal of Child Psychology and Psychiatry, 54*(2), 195–205.

Fisher, W., Piazza, C. C., Bowman, L. G., Hagopian, L. P., Owens, J. C., & Slevin, I. (1992). A comparison of two approaches for identifying reinforcers for persons with severe and profound disabilities. *Journal of Applied Behavior Analysis, 25,* 491–498.

Foxx, R. M. (1996). Translating the covenant: The behavior analyst as ambassador and translator. *The Behavior Analyst, 19,* 147–162.

Frost, L., & Bondy, A. (2002). *The picture exchange communication system training manual* (2nd ed.). Newark, DE: Pyramid Educational Consultants.

Gioia, G. A., Espy, K. A., & Isquith, P. K. (2003). *Behavior rating inventory of executive function-preschool version (BRIEF-P).* Odessa, FL: Psychological Assessment Resources.

Gotham, K., Risi, S., Pickles, A., & Lord, C. (2007). The autism diagnostic observation schedule: Revised algorithms for improved diagnostic validity. *Journal of Autism and Developmental Disorders, 37*(4), 613–627.

Gould, E., Tarbox, J., O'Hora, D., Noone, S., & Bergstrom, R. (2011). Teaching children with autism a basic component skill of perspective-taking. *Behavioral Interventions, 26,* 50–66.

Granpeesheh, D., Tarbox, J., & Dixon, D. (2009). Applied behavior analytic interventions for children with autism: A description and review of treatment research. *Annals of Clinical Psychiatry, 21,* 162–173.

Granpeesheh, D., Tarbox, J., Dixon, D. R., Carr, E., & Herbert, M. (2009). Retrospective analysis of clinical records in 38 cases of recovery from autism. *Annals of Clinical Psychiatry, 21*(4), 195–204.

Granpeesheh, D., Tarbox, J., Dixon, D. R., Peters, C. A., Thompson, K., & Kenzer, A. (2010). Evaluation of an eLearning tool for training behavioral therapists in academic knowledge of applied behavior analysis. *Research in Autism Spectrum Disorders, 4*(1), 11–17.

Granpeesheh, D., Tarbox, J., Dixon, D., Wilke, A. E., Allen, A., & Bradstreet, J. J. (2010). Randomized trial of hyperbaric oxygen therapy for children with autism. *Research in Autism Spectrum Disorders, 4,* 268–275.

Granpeesheh, D., Tarbox, J., & Persicke, A. (2014). Prevention and recovery. In J. Tarbox, D. Dixon, P. Sturmey, & J. Matson (Eds.), *Early intervention for autism spectrum disorders: Research, policy, and practice.* New York, NY: Springer.

Greer, R. D., Stolfi, L., & Pistoljevic, N. (2007). Emergence of naming in preschoolers: A comparison of multiple and single exemplar instruction. *European Journal of Behavior Analysis, 8,* 109–131.

Gresham, F. M., & Elliott, S. N. (2008). *Social skills improvement system (SSIS) rating scales.* Minneapolis, MN: NCS Pearson.

Harris, R. (2012). *The reality slap: Finding peace and fulfillment when life hurts.* Oakland, CA: New Harbinger Publications.

Hastings, R. P., & Johnson, E. (2001). Stress in UK families conducting intensive home-based behavioral intervention for their young child with autism. *Journal of Autism and Developmental Disorders, 31,* 327–336.

Hayes, S. C., Barlow, D. H., & Nelson-Gray, R. O. (1999). *The scientist practitioner: Research and accountability in the age of managed care.* New York, NY: Allyn and Bacon.

Hayes, S. C., Barnes-Holmes, D., & Roche, B. (Eds.) (2001). *Relational frame theory: A post-Skinnerian account of human language and cognition.* New York, NY: Springer.

Howard, J. S., Sparkman, C. R., Cohen, H. G., Green, G., & Stanislaw, H. (2005). A comparison of intensive behavior analytic and eclectic treatments for young children with autism. *Research in Developmental Disabilities, 26*(4), 359–383.

Jang, J., Dixon, D. R., Tarbox, J., Granpeesheh, D., Kornack, J., & de Nocker, Y. (2012). Randomized trial of an eLearning program for training family members of children with autism in the principles and procedures of applied behavior analysis. *Research in Autism Spectrum Disorders, 6,* 852–856.

Kazdin, A. E. (2011). *Single-case research designs: Methods for clinical and applied settings.* New York, NY: Oxford University Press.

Kenzer, A. L., & Bishop, M. R. (2011). Evaluating preference for familiar and novel stimuli across a large group of children with autism. *Research in Autism Spectrum Disorders, 5,* 819–825.

Korkman, M., Kirk, U., & Kemp, S. (2007). *NEPSY* (NEPSY-II) (2nd ed.). San Antonio, TX: Harcourt Assessment.

Krantz, P. J., & McClannahan, L. E. (2014). Picture activity schedules. In J. Tarbox, D. Dixon, P. Sturmey, & J. Matson (Eds.), *Handbook of early intervention for autism spectrum disorders: Research, policy, and practice.* New York, NY: Springer.

Kubina, R. M., Jr., & Wolfe, P. (2005). Potential applications of behavioral fluency for students with autism. *Exceptionality, 13,* 35–44.

Kubina, R. M., & Yurich, K. K. L. (2012). *The precision teaching book.* Lemont, PA: Greatness Achieved.

Kurtz, L. A. (2006). *Visual perception problems in children with AD/HD, autism, and other learning disabilities: A guide for parents and professionals.* Philadelphia, PA: Jessica Kingsley Publishers.

Le Couteur, A., Rutter, M., Lord, C., Rios, P., Robertson, S., Holdgrafer, M., et al. (1989). Autism diagnostic interview: A standardized investigator-based instrument. *Journal of Autism and Developmental Disorders, 19*(3), 363–387.

Lord, C., Rutter, M., DiLavore, P., & Risi, S. (1999). *Autism diagnostic observation schedule manual.* Los Angeles, CA: Western Psychological Services.

Lord, C., Rutter, M., Goode, S., Heemsbergen, J., Jordan, H., Mawhood, L., et al. (1989). Autism diagnostic observation schedule: A standardized observation of communicative and social behavior. *Journal of Autism and Developmental Disorders, 19*(2), 185–212.

Lord, C., Rutter, M., & Le Couteur, A. (1994). Autism diagnostic interview-revised: A revised version of a diagnostic interview for caregivers of individuals with possible pervasive developmental disorders. *Journal of Autism and Developmental Disorders, 24*(5), 659–685.

Lovaas, I. O. (1987). Behavioral treatment and normal educational and intellectual functioning in young autistic children. *Journal of Consulting and Clinical Psychology, 55*, 3–9.

Lovaas, O. I., Koegel, R., Simmons, J. Q., & Long, J. S. (1973). Some generalization and follow-up measures on autistic children in behavior therapy. *Journal of Applied Behavior Analysis, 6*, 131–166.

Martin, D. J., Garske, J. P., & Davis, M. K. (2000). Relation of the therapeutic alliance with outcome and other variables: A meta-analytic review. *Journal of Consulting and Clinical Psychology, 68*, 438–450.

Matson, J. L. (1995). *Diagnostic assessment for the severely handicapped-II.* Baton Rouge, LA: Disability Consultants.

Matson, J. L. (Ed.). (2012). *Functional assessment for challenging behaviors.* New York, NY: Springer.

Matson, J. L., Belva, B. C., Hattier, M. A., & Matson, M. L. (2012). Scaling methods to measure psychopathology in persons with intellectual disabilities. *Research in Developmental Disorders, 33*(2), 549–562.

Matson, J. L., Boisjoli, J., & Wilkins, J. (2007). *The baby and infant screen for children with autism traits (BISCUIT).* Baton Rouge, LA: Disability Consultants, LLC.

Matson, J. L., & Nebel-Schwalm, M. (2007). Assessing challenging behaviors in children with autism spectrum disorders: A review. *Research in Developmental Disabilities, 28*, 567–579.

Matson, J. L., & Vollmer, T. (1995). *Questions about behavioral function (QABF).* Baton Rouge, LA: Scientific.

Mayes, S. D., & Calhoun, S. L. (2006). Frequency of reading, math, and writing disabilities in children with clinical disorders. *Learning and Individual Differences, 16*, 145–157.

McEachin, J. J., Smith, T., & Ivar Lovaas, O. (1993). Long-term outcome for children with autism who received early intensive behavioral treatment. *American Journal of Mental Retardation, 97*, 359–372.

Montes, G., & Halterman, J. S. (2006). Characteristics of school-age children with autism. *Developmental and Behavioral Pediatrics, 27*, 379–385.

Mullen, E. M. (1995). *Mullen scales of early learning.* Circle Pines, MN: American Guidance Services, Inc.

Myers, S. M., & Plauché Johnson, C. (2007). Management of children with autism spectrum disorders. *Pediatrics, 120*, 1162–1182.

Najdowski, A. C., Chilingaryan, V., Bergstrom, R., Granpeesheh, D., Balasanyan, S., Aguilar, B., et al. (2009). Comparison of data collection methods in a behavioral intervention program for children with pervasive developmental disorders: A replication. *Journal of Applied Behavior Analysis, 42*, 827–832.

Najdowski, A. C., & Gould, E. R. (2014). Behavioral family intervention. In J. K. Luiselli (Ed.), *Children and youth with autism spectrum disorder (ASD): Recent advances and innovations in assessment, education, and intervention.* New York, NY: Oxford University Press.

Najdowski, A. C., Gould, E. R., Lanagan, T. M., & Bishop, M. R. (2014). Designing curriculum programs for children with autism. In J. Tarbox, D. Dixon, P. Sturmey, & J. L. Matson (Eds.), *Handbook of early intervention and autism spectrum disorders: Research, practice, and policy.* New York, NY: Springer.

National Autism Center. (2009). *National standards report: The national standards project – Addressing the need for evidence-based practice guidelines for autism spectrum disorders.* Randolph, MA: National Autism Center.

New York State Department of Health, Early Intervention Program. (1999). *Clinical practice guideline: Report of the recommendations: Autism / Pervasive developmental disorders: Assessment and intervention for young children (Age 0–3 years).*

Newcomer, P. L., & Hammill, D. D. (2008). *Test of language development-primary* (TOLD-P:4) (4th ed.). Austin, TX: Pro-Ed.

Ozonoff, S., Young, G. S., Goldring, S., Greiss-Hess, L., Herrera, A. M., Steele, J., et al. (2008). Gross motor development, movement abnormalities, and early identification of autism. *Journal of Autism and Developmental Disorders, 38,* 644–656.

Pace, G. M., Ivancic, M. T., Edwards, G. L., Iwata, B. A., & Page, T. J. (1985). Assessment of stimulus preference and reinforcer value with profoundly retarded individuals. *Journal of Applied Behavior Analysis, 18,* 249–255.

Persicke, A., Bishop, M. R., Coffman, C. M., Najdowski, A. C., Tarbox, J., Chi, K., et al. (2014). Evaluation of the concurrent validity of a skills assessment for autism treatment. *Research in Autism Spectrum Disorders, 8,* 281–285.

Persicke, A., St. Clair, M., Tarbox, J., Najdowski, A., Ranick, J., Yu, Y., et al. (2013). Teaching children with autism to attend to socially relevant stimuli. *Research in Autism Spectrum Disorders, 7,* 1551–1557.

Persicke, A., Tarbox, J., Ranick, J., & St. Clair, M. (2012). Establishing metaphorical reasoning in children with autism. *Research in Autism Spectrum Disorders, 6,* 913–920.

Persicke, A., Tarbox, J., Ranick, J., & St. Clair, M. (2013). Teaching children with autism to detect and respond to sarcasm. *Research in Autism Spectrum Disorders, 7,* 193–198.

Phelps-Terasaki, D., & Phelps-Gunn, T. (2007). *Test of pragmatic language* (TOPL-2) (2nd ed.). Austin, TX: Pro-Ed.

Ranick, J., Persicke, A., Tarbox, J., & Kornack, J. A. (2013). Teaching children with autism to detect and respond to deceptive statements. *Research in Autism Spectrum Disorders, 7,* 503–508.

Reichow, B. (2011). Overview of meta-analyses on early intensive behavioral intervention for children with autism spectrum disorders. *Journal of Autism and Developmental Disorders, 42,* 512–520.

Remington, B., Hastings, R. P., Kovshoff, H., Espinosa, F. E., Jahr, E., Brown, T., et al. (2007). Early intensive behavioral intervention: Outcomes for children with autism and their parents after two years. *American Journal on Mental Retardation, 112,* 418–438.

Rhine, D., & Tarbox, J. (2009). Chewing gum as a treatment for rumination in a child with autism. *Journal of Applied Behavior Analysis, 42,* 381–385.

Rogers, S. J., & Vismara, L. A. (2008). Evidence-based comprehensive treatments for early autism. *Journal of Clinical Child and Adolescent Psychology, 37,* 8–38.

Roid, G. H., & Miller, L. J. (1997). *Leiter international performance scale-revised.* Wood Dale, IL: Stoelting Co.

Roid, G. H., & Sampers, J. L. (2004). *Merrill-Palmer – Revised scales of development.* Wood Dale, IL: Stoelting.

Ross, D. E., & Greer, R. D. (2003). Generalized imitation and the mand: Inducing first instances of speech in young children with autism. *Research in Developmental Disabilities, 24,* 58–74.

Sallows, G. O., & Graupner, T. D. (2005). Intensive behavioral treatment for children with autism: Four-year outcome and predictors. *American Journal on Mental Retardation, 110,* 417–438.

Sautter, R. A., & LeBlanc, L. A. (2006). Empirical applications of Skinner's analysis of verbal behavior with humans. *The Analysis of Verbal Behavior, 22,* 35–48.

Semel, E., Wiig, E. H., & Secord, W. A. (2003). *Clinical evaluation of language fundamentals* (CELF-4) (4th ed.). Toronto, Ontario, Canada: The Psychological Corporation/A Harcourt Assessment Company.

Shafer, E. (1994). A review of interventions to teach a manding repertoire. *The Analysis of Verbal Behavior, 12,* 53–66.

Simonoff, E., Pickles, A., Charman, T., Chandler, S., Loucas, T., & Baird, G. (2008). Psychiatric disorders in children with autism spectrum disorders: Prevalence, comorbidity, and associated factors in a population-derived sample. *Journal of the American Academy of Child and Adolescent Psychiatry, 47*, 921–929.

Skinner, B. F. (1957). *Verbal behavior*. Acton, MA: Copley Publishing Group.

Skinner, B. F. (1974). *About behaviorism*. New York, NY: Vintage Books.

Smith, T., Groen, A. D., & Wynn, J. W. (2000). Randomized trial of intensive early intervention for children with pervasive developmental disorder. *American Journal on Mental Retardation, 105*, 269–285.

Sparrow, S. S., Cicchetti, D. V., & Balla, D. A. (2005). *Vineland adaptive behavior scales (Vineland-II)*. Livonia, MN: Pearson Assessments.

Stokes, T. F., & Baer, D. M. (1977). An implicit technology of generalization. *Journal of Applied Behavior Analysis, 10*, 349–367.

Summers, J., Tarbox, J., Findel-Pyles, R. S., Wilke, A., Bergstrom, R., & Williams, W. L. (2011). Teaching two household safety skills to children with autism. *Research in Autism Spectrum Disorders, 5*, 629–632.

Tarbox, J., Dixon, D. R., Sturmey, P., & Matson, J. L. (Eds.). (2014). *Handbook of early intervention for autism spectrum disorders: Research, practice, and policy*. New York, NY: Springer.

Tarbox, J., Najdowski, A. C., Bergstrom, R., Wilke, A., Bishop, M., Kenzer, A., et al. (2013). Randomized evaluation of a web-based tool for designing function-based behavioral intervention plans. *Research in Autism Spectrum Disorders, 7*, 1509–1517.

Tarbox, J., Persicke, A., & Kenzer, A. (2013). Home-based services. In D. D. Reed, F. D. DiGennaro Reed, & J. K. Luiselli (Eds.), *Handbook of crisis intervention for individuals with developmental disabilities*. New York, NY: Springer.

Tarbox, J., Wilke, A. E., Findel-Pyles, R. S., Bergstrom, R. M., & Granpeesheh, D. (2010). A comparison of electronic to traditional pen-and-paper data collection in discrete trial training for children with autism. *Research in Autism Spectrum Disorders, 4*(1), 65–75.

Tarbox, J., Zuckerman, C. K., Bishop, M. R., Olive, M. L., & O'Hora, D. P. (2011). Rule-governed behavior: Teaching a preliminary repertoire of rule-following to children with autism. *The Analysis of Verbal Behavior, 27*, 125–139.

Tsiouri, I., & Greer, R. D. (2003). Inducing vocal verbal behavior in children with severe language delays through rapid motor imitation responding. *Journal of Behavioral Education, 12*(3), 185–206.

U.S. Department of Health and Human Services. (1999). *Mental health: A report of the surgeon general*. Rockville, MD: U.S. Department of Health and Human Services, Substance Abuse and Mental Health Services Administration, Center for Mental Health Services, National Institutes of Health, National Institute of Mental Health.

Wechsler, D. (2002a). *The Wechsler preschool and primary scale of intelligence* (WPPSI-III) (3rd ed.). San Antonio, TX: The Psychological Corporation.

Wechsler, D. (2002b). *Wechsler individual achievement test* (WIAT-II) (2nd ed.). San Antonio, TX: Psychological Corp.

Wechsler, D. (2003). *Wechsler intelligence scale for children* (WISC-IV) (4th ed.). San Antonio, TX: Harcourt Assessment.

White, S. H. (2000). Conceptual foundations of IQ testing. *Psychology, Public Policy, and Law, 6*(1), 33–43.

Woodcock, R. W., McGrew, K. S., & Mather, N. (2001). *Woodcock-Johnson III*. Rolling Meadows, IL: Riverside Publishing.

Zachor, D. A., Ben-Itzchak, E. L., Rabinovich, A. L., & Lahat, E. (2007). Change in autism core symptoms with intervention. *Research in Autism Spectrum Disorders, 1*, 304–317.

Zimmerman, I. L., Steiner, V. G., & Pond, R. E. (2002). *Preschool language scale* (4th ed.). San Antonio, TX: Harcourt Assessment.

Glossary

Abolishing Operation: An antecedent event or condition that temporarily decreases the value of a reinforcer and decreases the likelihood of behaviors that have been reinforced by that reinforcer in the past. For example, satiation of something desirable, such as food, decreases the effectiveness of receiving food as a reinforcer and decreases the likelihood of behaviors that have resulted in food in the past: for example, someone is not likely to ask for food when she is full. See also **motivating operation** and **establishing operation.**

Abolishing Operation (EO): See **motivating operation.**

Antecedent: Anything that occurs or is present immediately before a behavior.

Antecedent Manipulations: Modifying environmental conditions prior to the occurrence of a behavior in order to make that behavior more or less likely to occur. Common antecedent manipulations include noncontingent reinforcement, prompting, response effort, motivating operations, behavioral momentum, demand fading, and discriminative stimuli.

Applied Behavior Analysis (ABA): A scientific discipline that applies behavior analytic principles of learning and motivation to solving problems of social significance. Autism treatment is the application for which ABA is most well known.

Attention: Behavior that results in gaining positive or negative attention from others. See also **functions of behavior, attention, automatic reinforcement, escape,** and **tangible.**

Automatic Reinforcement: Behavior that is reinforcing in and of itself. That is, the behavior feels good; e.g., scratching an insect bite. See also **functions of behavior, attention, escape,** and **tangible.**

Aversive: The technical definition is a stimulus that is undesirable and functions as punishment if it is delivered as a consequence of behavior and functions as negative reinforcement if it is removed as a consequence of behavior. In everyday usage in the lay community, the word *aversive* usually refers to harsh punishment procedures that cause pain or discomfort, but that is not the technical meaning of the term.

Backward Chaining: Backward chaining involves teaching the terminal behavior in the chain first until independent, then adding the second-to-last behavior, and so on. See also **chaining procedures, forward chaining,** and **total task.**

Baseline: The period during which a behavior is measured before an intervention is implemented. The effects of an intervention are then compared against the baseline level of the behavior.

Behavior: Anything a person says or does. Same definition as response. Overt behaviors are observable by others, for example, saying "car" aloud. Covert behaviors are not observable by people other than the one who is engaging in it, for example, saying "car" silently "in one's head," as in thinking about the word *car.*

Behavior Chain: A sequence of component behaviors that comprise a more complex task or activity. For example, tooth brushing requires multiple component behaviors such as removing the toothpaste cap, squeezing the toothpaste onto the toothbrush, turning on the water, etc. Each behavior in the chain serves as a discriminative stimulus for the next behavior and a conditioned reinforcer for the previous behavior.

Behavior Intervention Plan (BIP): A document describing the treatment procedures to be used for decreasing a challenging behavior and replacing it with a more adaptive replacement behavior. BIPs are based on the results of Functional Behavioral Assessments. A BIP typically includes an operational definition of the challenging behavior and replacement behavior, how both behaviors will be measured, measurable goals for both behaviors, a hypothesis as to the function of the challenging behavior, and a clear description of the intervention strategies, who is to implement them, and in what settings.

Behavioral Skills Training (BST): A package intervention for teaching skills. BST typically includes the following components: instructions, modeling, role-play and rehearsal, feedback, and can be supplemented with *in situ* training if necessary.

Chaining Procedures: Procedures used to teach behavior chains. See also **backward chaining, forward chaining,** and **total task.**

Conditioned Reinforcer: A previously neutral stimulus that was conditioned to be a reinforcer through pairing with an established reinforcer. For example, vocal praise that has been paired with a primary reinforcer (such as food) may become a conditioned reinforcer, so now praise will function as a reinforcer when previously it did not.

Consequence: Any event that occurs directly after the behavior. As opposed to the negative connotation that the word *consequence* has in everyday usage, in technical terms, consequence has neither a positive nor a negative connotation.

Consequence Manipulations: Modifying environmental conditions after the occurrence of a behavior in order to produce an increase or decrease in the future occurrence of the behavior. Consequence manipulations generally consist of reinforcement or extinction.

Contingency or Contingent: Dependent upon. Reinforcers are delivered contingent upon behavior, meaning that they are delivered as a consequence for the behavior, according to the schedule specified in the treatment program.

Continuous Reinforcement: Every occurrence of a behavior results in reinforcement. See also **schedules of reinforcement** and **intermittent reinforcement.**

Demand Fading: An antecedent modification in which the amount of work or task demands is reduced initially to make the task easier for the learner to complete, followed by systematic increases of demands until the learner is able to follow through with the original task/activity/response. If demands are non-preferred, then demand fading works by making the learner less motivated to escape the work because a lower amount of work is less non-preferred than a larger amount of work.

Differential Reinforcement: A procedure wherein reinforcement is delivered in some circumstances and not others. Generally speaking, behaviors that are more desirable are reinforced to a greater degree than behaviors that are less desirable. For example, once the child has learned to request what she wants using full sentences, the therapist will use differential reinforcement by no longer giving the learner what she wants when she asks using single-word requests. This should result in an increase in full-sentence requests and a decrease in single-word requests.

Differential Reinforcement of Alternative Behavior (DRA): A differential reinforcement procedure in which an alternative, more appropriate behavior is reinforced instead of the undesirable behavior. This procedure is commonly used to decrease challenging behavior by giving the learner reinforcement when she engages in an alternative behavior (asking for attention) instead of the challenging behavior (tantrums for attention).

Differential Reinforcement of High Rates of Behavior (DRH): A differential reinforcement procedure in which reinforcement is delivered only when a desirable behavior has occurred above a particular rate. For example, a learner is given reinforcement if he makes five or more social initiations during a 10-minute play period.

Differential Reinforcement of Incompatible Behavior (DRI): A form of DRA wherein the alternative behavior is physically incompatible with the undesirable behavior. For example, petting a dog softly is incompatible with hitting it.

Differential Reinforcement of Low Rates of Behavior (DRL): A differential reinforcement procedure in which reinforcement is delivered only if a behavior occurs at or below a particular rate. DRL is generally used for behaviors that are not completely undesirable but merely occur at too high a rate. For example, a child who attempts to comment on every single thing the teacher says during class might be given reinforcement if he makes one comment or fewer during every 5-minute period.

Differential Reinforcement of Other Behavior (DRO): A time-based differential reinforcement procedure in which reinforcement is delivered when the undesirable behavior has not occurred for a specified period of time. DRO does not help establish a specific replacement behavior.

Discrete Trial Training (DTT): A structured one-to-one teaching procedure involving the presentation of a clear (discrete) instruction, an opportunity for the learner to respond, and then a clear consequence for the learner response, depending on whether it is correct or incorrect – generally positive reinforcement for correct responses and error correction for incorrect responses.

Discrimination Training: The process by which a particular behavior is reinforced only in the presence of a specific antecedent stimulus and not reinforced in the presence of other antecedent stimuli. As a result, the behavior becomes more likely when that specific stimulus is presented because that stimulus comes to have stimulus control over the behavior. That stimulus is then referred to as the discriminative stimulus or SD.

Discriminative Stimulus (S^D): The discriminative stimulus (S^D) signals that reinforcement for a particular response is available because that stimulus was present when the behavior was reinforced in the past (see discrimination training above). An S^D can be any environmental stimulus (or combination of stimuli), including a vocal instruction, question or statement given by another person or the presentation or removal of a particular item/activity/action/person, etc. Instructions during acquisition phases of ABA therapy are commonly referred to as S^Ds, but this usage is generally incorrect because those instructions have not become S^Ds yet, as that is the purpose of the acquisition phase of treatment.

Distractor: A stimulus other than the target stimulus, presented during discrimination training. For example, during receptive discrimination, the therapist might place a fork, knife, and spoon on the table and ask the learner to point to the fork. In this trial, the knife and spoon are distractor stimuli. Distractors may be known (mastered) or unknown (not yet mastered).

Duration: Amount of time that passes while the behavior is occurring. For example, a child may engage in a tantrum that lasts 30 minutes.

Echoic: A verbal operant that consists of repeating what is heard. For example, saying "car" after hearing someone say "car."

Error Correction: Procedures used during teaching programs after an incorrect response is made as a means to correct errors prior to the presentation of subsequent learning opportunities or trials. Error correction procedures generally consist of a prompt that will help the learner respond correctly.

Escape: Behavior that results in the escape, avoidance, or lessening of non-preferred demands or tasks. See also **functions of behavior, attention, automatic reinforcement,** and **tangible.**

Establishing Operation: An antecedent event or condition that temporarily increases the value of a reinforcer and evokes behaviors that have been reinforced by that reinforcer in the past. For example, deprivation of something desirable, such as attention, increases the effectiveness of receiving attention as a reinforcer and momentarily evokes behaviors that have resulted in attention in the past. See also **motivating operation** and **abolishing operation.**

Establishing Operation (EO): See **motivating operation.**

Exemplar: An example of a skill or concept that you are trying to teach. For example, one picture of a dog is an exemplar of dogs, five pictures of different dogs are multiple exemplars of dogs.

Extinction: The process by which a previously reinforced behavior no longer receives reinforcement and therefore decreases. For example, if a child tantrums to get candy and his parents no longer give him candy when he has a tantrum, they are implementing extinction and tantrums will decrease.

Extinction Burst: A temporary increase in the rate or intensity of a behavior when that behavior is placed on extinction.

Fading: Gradually changing the physical properties of a stimulus. Stimuli may be faded in (as in the case of gradually adding distracters to a field) or faded out (as in the gradual removal of a prompt). See also: prompt Fading.

FBA (Functional Behavioral Assessment): An assessment conducted to determine the ongoing source of reinforcement for a challenging behavior. The source of reinforcement is referred to as the function of the behavior. FBAs typically include operational definitions of the behavior of interest, indirect functional assessments (interviews and record review), direct assessments (observation), and experimental functional analyses, as needed.

FCT (Functional Communication Training): A form of DRA in which communication is taught as a replacement behavior for a challenging behavior. The learner is taught to request the functional reinforcer, rather than engaging in the challenging behavior to get it. The challenging behavior is placed on extinction, if possible. FCT is generally considered the gold standard first-line treatment for challenging behavior.

Feedback: A consequence for a behavior that describes the desirable aspects and/or undesirable aspects of the behavior. Feedback is the most widely effective procedure for training and managing staff and parent performance.

Field: The set of stimuli the therapist presents during discrimination training. A single item presented alone at the beginning of discrimination training is referred to as a "field of one." Three items presented simultaneously are referred to as a "field of three."

Fluency: Responding with both speed and accuracy. Although little research has evaluated it, it is generally agreed upon that learners who are fluent in a particular skill will be able to execute that skill more readily when they need to use it in the course of their daily lives.

Forward Chaining: Forward chaining involves teaching each component behavior of the chain starting from the first behavior in the chain. The first behavior is taught until independent, then the second behavior is added to the first, and so on until the entire behavior chain is successfully performed. See also **chaining procedures, backward chaining,** and **total task.**

Frequency: Number of occurrences of a behavior.

Functions of Behavior: The source of reinforcement for the behavior; what the learner gets out of the behavior; what the learner is trying to get when he engages in the behavior. Research has shown that most challenging behaviors displayed by people with developmental disabilities have one or more of the following four functions: a) **automatic reinforcement,** b) **attention,** c) **escape,** and/or d) **tangible.**

Generalization: A spreading of the effects of treatment to other stimuli or behaviors than those directly targeted during treatment. Generalization applies to both adaptive behavior and challenging behavior. Generalization consists of **stimulus generalization** and **response generalization.**

Gestural Prompt: Pointing or gesturing to the correct stimulus, resulting in a correct response. See also **prompt, model prompt, physical prompt, proximity prompt,** and **within-stimulus or intra-stimulus prompt.**

High-Probability Request Sequence/Behavioral Momentum: The presentation of multiple high-probability responses that do not evoke challenging behavior immediately prior to the presentation of a low-probability response that usually evokes challenging behavior.

Impure Intraverbal: An impure intraverbal response occurs in response to a word or phrase with the addition of other stimuli or prompts. For example, the child's response to the instruction, "Tell me a farm animal," is impure if there are also pictures of farm animals presented because it is partially also a tact (in response to the non-verbal stimulus of a picture). It is also impure if the child repeats part of what was said in the instruction, making it partially an echoic. Teaching intraverbals typically progresses from impure to pure. See also **intraverbal** and **pure intraverbal.**

Impure Mand: A mand that depends on additional sources of support, other than a motivating operation. In other words, a request that is made in the presence of additional stimuli or prompts. For example, saying, "I want a cookie," is an impure mand if the child says it when he sees cookies or if the therapist has first asked, "What do you want?" See also **mand** and **pure mand.**

Impure Tact: An impure tact occurs in the presence of prompts. For example, the therapist points to a tree, and the child says, "I see a tree." A comment that is produced in response to the comments of others is also impure, as it is partially an intraverbal. In addition, a tact that occurs as a result of an establishing operation (EO), such as saying "cookie" in the presence of a cookie, is impure, as it is partially a mand. See also **tact** and **pure tact.**

In Situ: Training that occurs in the actual environment where the behavior or skill needs to be used. For example, teaching a child to cross the street at a real street intersection.

In Vivo **Training:** Training occurring in the natural environment.

Individualized Education Program (IEP): A legal special education document developed by educational professionals outlining the student's unique needs, along with specific goals and how these goals will be achieved over the course of the school year.

Intermittent Reinforcement: Only some occurrences of a behavior result in reinforcement. See also **schedules of reinforcement** and **continuous reinforcement.**

Interval Recording: A data collection procedure involving the division of observation time into equal shorter intervals and calculating the percentage of intervals in which behavior was observed. See also **partial interval, whole interval,** and **momentary time sampling.**

Intraverbal: A verbal behavior where the antecedent stimulus is verbal and the response is verbal but the antecedent and response do not match. Examples of intraverbal behavior include fill-ins, such as saying "star" upon hearing "Twinkle twinkle little…" or answering the question, "How are you?" Intraverbal behavior may be divided into **impure intraverbals** and **pure intraverbals.**

Latency: Duration of time between the presentation of an instruction or discriminative stimulus and the initiation of the response.

Leading Questions: A prompt in the form of questions used to help guide the learner to a correct response without directly telling the learner the correct response.

Least-to-most: Prompting hierarchies that begin with no prompts and then are faded in contingent on incorrect responding. These procedures are often used during maintenance or with experienced learners. See also **prompt hierarchy** and **most-to-least.**

Maintenance: The persistence of the effects of an intervention over time after the intervention has been discontinued.

Mand: A verbal behavior that is under the antecedent control of a motivating operation and which describes its own reinforcer. In lay terms, a mand is a request for a reinforcer, including food, objects, people, attention, actions, locations, cessation, and so on. Mands may be divided into **impure mands** and **pure mands.**

Mass Trial: Repeated, consecutive trials of the same instruction and response. For example, if the label "shirt" is to be introduced in mass trial, the therapist will deliver the instruction "give me shirt" for a several consecutive trials.

Mastered: Accurate responding (typically above either 80% or 90%) that is stable (typically across 2 days and two different therapists).

Model Prompt: Demonstrating the behavior that is expected of the child. For example, when introducing the instruction "jump," the therapist also jumps. Model prompts can be physical or vocal: for example, saying a word or part of a word that you want the child to say or jumping when you want the child to jump. See also **prompt, gestural prompt, physical prompt, proximity prompt,** and **within stimulus or intra-stimulus prompt.**

Momentary Time Sampling: Each interval during a recording period is scored as a plus only if the behavior occurs at the moment the interval elapses.

Most-to-least: Prompting hierarchies that begin with the largest prompts and then are faded out contingent on correct responding. These procedures are typically used when teaching new responses and/or when working with early learners. See also **prompt hierarchy** and **least-to-most.**

Motivating Operation: An antecedent event or condition that temporarily changes the value of a reinforcer and changes the momentary probability of behaviors that have been reinforced by that reinforcer in the past. Motivating operations consist of **establishing operations** and **abolishing operations.**

Natural Consequence: A consequence for behavior that occurs naturally in the environment from engaging in that behavior. For example, the natural consequence of making a sandwich is getting to eat the sandwich.

Natural Environment Training (NET): Teaching a skill in the context in which that skill will normally be used in the course of everyday life. NET teaching opportunities are learner-initiated, include prompts as needed, and deliver functionally related reinforcers whenever possible.

Negative Reinforcement: The removal of a stimulus after the behavior occurs, resulting in a higher probability of the behavior occurring in the future: for example, a child asks for non-preferred music to be turned off, and the parent turns it off. See also **reinforcement** and **positive reinforcement.**

Noncontingent Reinforcement (NCR): An antecedent procedure for decreasing the rate of a behavior in which a reinforcer (generally the functional reinforcer for a challenging behavior) is delivered according to a time-based schedule, rather than contingent on the challenging behavior or any other behavior. In other words, reinforcement is given for free.

Novel Tasks or Exemplars: Tasks or exemplars that have never been directly taught.

Operant: Behavior that is influenced by its consequences. Most human behavior is operant behavior. Operant behavior does not include reflexes, which are not affected by their consequences (e.g., blinking when air is blown into your eye).

Partial Interval: Each interval during the recording period is scored as a plus if the behavior occurred at all during that interval and scored as a minus if it did not occur at all during that interval.

Physical Prompt: Using physical guidance to help the learner correctly engage in the target response. For example, when teaching receptive identification of body parts, the instructor will present the instruction "touch head," followed by a hand-over-hand physical prompt guiding the learner's hand to touch her head. See also **prompt, gestural prompt, model prompt, proximity prompt,** and **within-stimulus or intra-stimulus prompt.**

Positive Reinforcement: The addition of a stimulus after the behavior occurs, resulting in a higher probability of the behavior occurring in the future: for example, giving a child a teddy bear when she asks for it. See also **reinforcement** and **negative reinforcement.**

Preference Assessment: A procedure used to determine a child's preferred items that might function as reinforcers. For example, before beginning a teaching session, the therapist presents three or more likely preferred items and asks the learner to choose the preferred item for which she would like to work. The item that the learner chooses is then used as the reinforcer for correct responding for the next 5 minutes.

Probe: A brief test without prompting or reinforcement. Probes are usually used to determine which items or skills a child already has mastered before teaching them (e.g., during baseline) or after multiple exemplar training in order to assess for generalization of the newly trained skill to untrained items.

Prompt: An additional stimulus that evokes a correct response. By definition, prompts are additional help or assistance, which must be faded after they are used (see **prompt fading** below). See also **gestural prompt, model prompt, physical prompt, proximity prompt,** and **within-stimulus or intra-stimulus prompt.**

Prompt Dependent: When a learner continues to depend on prompting in order to respond correctly due to a failure in the prompt fading process. See also **prompt hierarchy** and **least-to-most.**

Prompt Fading: Gradually fading out prompts across learning opportunities, with the goal of eventually removing prompts altogether. Since prompts are, by definition, an unwanted source of stimulus control, prompts must eventually be faded out.

Prompt Hierarchy: Referring to the order in which prompts will be delivered dependent on previous responding. See also **least-to-most** and **most-to-least.**

Proximity Prompt: Positioning the correct stimulus closer to the learner. See also **prompt, gestural prompt, model prompt, physical prompt,** and **within-stimulus or intra-stimulus prompt.**

Punishment: Any consequence that results in a decrease in the future probability of a behavior.

Pure Intraverbal: A pure intraverbal response occurs in response to a word or phrase without the presence of other non-vocal or echoic prompts. No part of the word or phrase to which the learner is responding is repeated in the response; otherwise, the response would be partially echoic. Independent participation in conversation is an example of pure intraverbal behavior. See also **intraverbal** and **impure intraverbal.**

Pure Mand: A pure mand is a mand that is evoked purely by a motivating operation without the presence of additional stimuli or prompts. In other words, it is a request that a learner makes independently, purely because she wants something. For example, a learner has not seen his mom in a while (motivating operation is deprivation of mom's attention), she is not physically present (maybe in the other room), and he requests to see her. For a mand to be pure, it cannot depend on the learner being able to sense (see, hear, smell, taste, or feel) the reinforcer at the time of the request, and it cannot be in response to someone asking the learner, "What do you want?" Pure mands are important because they show that the child can independently communicate what she wants and that she does not rely on reminders or prompts from others. See also **mand** and **impure mand.**

Pure Tact: A pure tact occurs spontaneously in response to a non-verbal stimulus without prompting. For example, a child sees an airplane flying across the sky and says, "Airplane." Additionally, in order to be considered a pure tact, there must be no establishing operation present, and the comment must not be produced in response to the comment of another person. See also **tact** and **impure tact.**

Random Rotation: A procedure used during discrimination training in which the target is interspersed randomly with other targets. For example, the target "shoe" could be randomly rotated with "fish," "brush," and "swing" wherein the therapist will ask, "What is it?" in the presence of each stimulus in a random order. One could also randomly rotate across vocal instructions. For example, the target "clap hands" could be randomly rotated with "stand up," "sit down," and "jump."

Rate: Frequency per unit time of observation (e.g., 10 times per minute) calculated by dividing the frequency by the total observation time.

Receptive: Nonvocal responding to instructions: for example, touching a picture of a shoe when told to "touch shoe."

Redirection: Attempting to direct the learner to engage in a different, more appropriate behavior using prompting strategies.

Reinforcement: The process by which the consequence of a behavior increases or maintains the future probability of that behavior. For example, if the child appropriately requests hugs and receives hugs, the child is likely to continue to appropriately request hugs in future. See also **negative reinforcement** and **positive reinforcement.**

Repertoire: The learner's current skill set: for example, what she is capable of doing based on what behaviors have been acquired in the past.

Replacement Behavior: Adaptive behaviors that serve the same function as challenging behaviors: for example, asking for a break instead of having a tantrum to get a break.

Response: A single occurrence of a behavior.

Response Blocking: An intervention strategy used to prevent a response from occurring by physically intervening at the initiation of the response so that the full response cannot be completed.

Response Effort: The amount of effort required by the learner to engage in a behavior.

Response Generalization: The effects of intervention on one behavior produce the same effect on a different behavior. For example, reinforcing plural use of some words results in plural use of other, untrained words. Or placing aggression on extinction results in a reduction in property destruction. See also **generalization** and **stimulus generalization.**

Role-Play: Acting out specific responses as practice using contrived scenarios that resemble real-life situations.

Rule-Governed Behavior: Behavior under control of verbal antecedent stimuli, or rule statements. For example, when a rule is stated, "If the phone rings, answer it," the learner will engage in the behavior described in the rule without requiring direct training.

Schedules of Reinforcement: The schedule with which reinforcement will be provided. See also **continuous reinforcement** and **intermittent reinforcement.**

Shaping: Teaching through differential reinforcement of successive approximations of the response until the entire response is learned. For example, you would teach the learner to say "mama" by first reinforcing the "mm" sound until independent, then differentially reinforcing "ma," and finally, "mama." See also **schedules of reinforcement and continuous reinforcement.**

Spontaneous: Behaviors that occur under naturally occurring contingencies without prompting or contrivance.

Stereotypy: Behaviors that occur the same way repeatedly.

Stimulus: Any environmental event to which a person can respond. Overt stimuli are stimuli in the outside environment to which others can also respond, such as objects, sounds, the behavior of others, and so on. Covert stimuli are stimuli to which others cannot respond, including internal physiological states, such as a toothache, and covert products of one's own covert behavior, as in cases of remembering, imagining, and visualizing. For example, one can respond today to the remembered sight of something that occurred yesterday. Plural: stimuli.

Stimulus Generalization: Can occur across people, settings, or stimuli. For example, a learner begins to say "hi" to family members when they enter the room, although the learner has only been explicitly trained to greet the therapist (generalization across people). A learner begins to indicate when he wishes to use the toilet at pre-school, although he has only been explicitly taught to do so at home (generalization across settings). A learner begins to identify numbers on mailboxes while out on a walk, although he has only been explicitly taught to identify numbers on flashcards (generalization across stimuli). See also **generalization** and **response generalization.**

Tact: A verbal behavior under the antecedent control of a non-verbal stimulus. In lay terms, tacts include comments, names, and labels. For example, a child sees a plane and says, "Plane"; a child hears a dog and says, "I hear a dog barking." Tacts may be divided into **impure tacts** and **pure tacts.**

Tangible: Behavior that results in gaining access to preferred items or activities. See also **functions of behavior, attention, automatic reinforcement,** and **escape.**

Task Analysis (TA): Dividing a larger task into its component step-by-step responses to create manageable teaching steps. TAs are used during chaining procedures.

Token Economy: The use of tangible items (tokens) delivered as conditioned reinforcers to reinforce desirable behavior. Tokens can later be exchanged for a back-up reinforcer (an item or activity already established to be reinforcing for the child). For example, the therapist may present the child with a button after every correct response during a lesson. When the child has earned five buttons, she can exchange them for a preferred reinforcer, such as 5 minutes of a video or jumping on the trampoline. Money is a commonly used token for typically developing adults in daily life.

Topography: The physical form of the behavior, that is, what the behavior looks or sounds like.

Total Task: Each component behavior is taught during each presentation. See also **chaining procedures, backward chaining,** and **forward chaining.**

Verbal Operant: A functional unit of language, defined by the sources of antecedent control and reinforcers. *Echoics, mands, tacts,* and *intraverbals* are examples of verbal operants. See the individual definitions of the verbal operants listed in this glossary.

Whole Interval: Each interval during a recording period is scored as a plus if the behavior occurred for that entire interval and scored as a minus if the behavior did not occur for the entire interval.

Within-stimulus or Intra-stimulus prompt: Modifying the stimulus in a way that prompts the learner to respond correctly: for example, making the target stimulus a larger size than distractor stimuli. See also **prompt, gestural prompt, model prompt, physical prompt,** and **proximity prompt.**

Index

Note: Page numbers followed by *ge* indicate glossary, *f* indicate figures and *t* indicate tables.

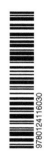